VisualDx: Essential Adult Dermatology

SENIOR EDITORS:

Noah Craft, MD, PhD, DTM&H
Assistant Professor of Dermatology
Divisions of Dermatology and Adult Infectious Diseases
Harbor-UCLA Medical Center
Los Angeles Biomedical Research Institute
David Geffen School of Medicine at UCLA
Torrance, California

Lindy P. Fox, MD
Assistant Professor of Clinical Dermatology
Director, Hospital Consultation Service
Department of Dermatology
University of California, San Francisco
San Francisco, California

ASSOCIATE EDITORS:

Lowell A. Goldsmith, MD, MPH
Professor of Dermatology
Department of Dermatology
University of North Carolina-Chapel Hill
Chapel Hill, North Carolina

Art Papier, MD
Associate Professor of Dermatology and Medical Informatics
Department of Dermatology
University of Rochester School of Medicine and Dentistry
Rochester, New York

ASSISTANT EDITORS:

Ron Birnbaum, MD
Resident in Dermatology
Harbor-UCLA Medical Center
Torrance, California

Priya M. Rajendran, MD
Resident in Dermatology
University of California, San Francisco
San Francisco, California

Mary Gail Mercurio, MD
Associate Professor of Dermatology
Department of Dermatology
University of Rochester School of Medicine and Dentistry
Rochester, New York

Michael Rosenblum, MD, PhD
Resident In Dermatology
University of California, San Francisco
San Francisco, California

Daniel Miller, MD
Resident in Dermatology
University of California, San Francisco
San Francisco, California

Emma Taylor, MD
Resident in Dermatology
David Geffen School of Medicine at UCLA
Los Angeles, California

Paul Camille Tumeh, MD
Resident in Dermatology
Harbor-UCLA Medical Center
Torrance, California

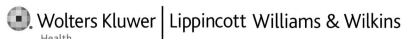

Wolters Kluwer | Lippincott Williams & Wilkins
Health

Philadelphia • Baltimore • New York • London
Buenos Aires • Hong Kong • Sydney • Tokyo

Acquisitions Editor: Sonya Seigafuse
Product Manager: Kerry Barrett
Vendor Manager: Alicia Jackson
Senior Manufacturing Manager: Ben Rivera
Marketing Manager: Kim Schonberger
Design Coordinator: Teresa Mallon
Production Service: SPi Technologies

© 2010 by LIPPINCOTT WILLIAMS & WILKINS, a WOLTERS KLUWER business
530 Walnut Street
Philadelphia, PA 19106 USA
LWW.com

Printed in China.

Library of Congress Cataloging-in-Publication Data
  VisualDx : Essential adult dermatology / senior editors, Noah Craft, Lindy P. Fox ; associate editors, Lowell A. Goldsmith, Art Papier ; assistant editors, Ron Birnbaum ... [et al.].
       p. ; cm.
  Includes bibliographical references and index.
  ISBN 978-1-60831-805-6 (alk. paper)
  1. Dermatology—Textbooks. 2. Dermatology—Atlases. I. Craft, Noah. II. Fox, Lindy P. III. Title: Essential adult dermatology.
  [DNLM: 1. Skin Diseases—diagnosis. 2. Skin Diseases—therapy. 3. Adult. 4. Skin Manifestations. WR 140 V834 2010]
  RL71.V57   2010
  616.5—dc22
                                                                                                    2009052719

Care has been taken to confirm the accuracy of the information presented and to describe generally accepted practices. However, the authors, editors, and publisher are not responsible for errors or omissions or for any consequences from application of the information in this book and make no warranty, expressed or implied, with respect to the currency, completeness, or accuracy of the contents of the publication. Application of the information in a particular situation remains the professional responsibility of the practitioner.

The authors, editors, and publisher have exerted every effort to ensure that drug selection and dosage set forth in this text are in accordance with current recommendations and practice at the time of publication. However, in view of ongoing research, changes in government regulations, and the constant flow of information relating to drug therapy and drug reactions, the reader is urged to check the package insert for each drug for any change in indications and dosage and for added warnings and precautions. This is particularly important when the recommended agent is a new or infrequently employed drug.

Some drugs and medical devices presented in the publication have Food and Drug Administration (FDA) clearance for limited use in restricted research settings. It is the responsibility of the health care provider to ascertain the FDA status of each drug or device planned for use in their clinical practice.

To purchase additional copies of this book, call our customer service department at (800) 638-3030 or fax orders to (301) 223-2320. International customers should call (301) 223-2300.

Visit Lippincott Williams & Wilkins on the Internet: at LWW.com. Lippincott Williams & Wilkins customer service representatives are available from 8:30 am to 6 pm, EST.

10 9 8 7 6 5 4 3 2 1

Dedication

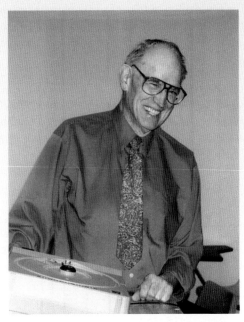

Victor D. Newcomer, MD (1916–2002)

Victor Newcomer was a legendary dermatologist and a resident of California for more than 50 years. He was Clinical Professor of Medicine/Dermatology at the University of California, Los Angeles, for more than 40 years. He was an esteemed and beloved educator and a mentor to physicians and students throughout the city and state. He was strongly dedicated to his patients, to patient advocacy, and to issues surrounding patients' rights.

Dr. Newcomer was renowned for being a superb teacher and role model for generations of dermatologists. He was so beloved by his students that, in 1988, they established the Victor D. Newcomer, MD Award for Excellence in Teaching. Among his other honors was the Golden Apple Award, an annual award given to the most outstanding teacher in the UCLA medical school. Additionally, he received Excellence in Teaching recognition from the Virginia and the California Medical Association; the Thomas L. Stern Award for Excellence in Clinical Teaching from Santa Monica Hospital; the J.N. Taub International Memorial Award for Psoriasis Research; the Clark W. Finnerud Award from the Dermatology Foundation; and the Everett C. Fox, MD Memorial Lectureship. And he is one of a select few Masters in Dermatology, awarded by the American Academy of Dermatology.

Dr. Newcomer had a long and distinguished career and served as a member of prestigious boards, committees, foundations, associations, societies, academies, and task forces. In addition, he published more than 152 articles and book chapters. Passionate about medical photography, throughout his career he used his collection of 40,000 clinical images to train residents and medical students. Many of his excellent images are in this book.

Dr. Newcomer was a dedicated physician, a tireless and enthusiastic teacher, and a patient's best advocate. He was a true healer, a rigorous scholar, a stoic comedian, and a student's dream. When a medical student or a resident or a junior faculty member or a colleague or the chair of dermatology asked Dr. Newcomer for his thoughts about a patient, they were not asking for a differential diagnosis; they were asking for THE diagnosis. His collection of slides of patients over a long and productive career in dermatology cataloged over half of a century in Los Angeles. He began his career at a time when clinical diagnosis was still a fine art. Though in person he was a humble giant, through his work, he became an institution. Over 50 years, he personally taught an enormous percentage of practicing dermatologists in Los Angeles, using this slide collection that has since been digitized and archived. It is only through the efforts of rigorous clinician-scientists like Dr. Newcomer that we can define the range of dermatologic disease presentations accurately and improve the ability of doctors to recognize variations of disease severity and quality.

Aside from dermatology, he was dedicated to conservation, preservation of water sources, wildlife, and plants. His contributions to his patients and students and to the field of medicine were immeasurable and speak volumes as to the quality of human being he was. Quality of excellence was the standard in all that he did.

Humor was a close ally. Some favorite sayings were, "Always clean the manure and chicken droppings from under your fingernails before seeing patients," "A good remedy smells bad, is brightly colored, and stains people's clothes," "That's tinea corporis every day of the week, spreading across the skin like a Santa Monica brush fire," and "Hello, I'm Dr. Newcomer, rhymes with cucumber."

"Nothing is so contagious as enthusiasm…[it] is the genius of sincerity, and truth accomplishes no victories without it."—Edward G. Bulwer-Lytton

Noah Craft, MD, PhD, DTM&H
Worked as a medical student and dermatology resident
with Victor Newcomer from 1998 to 2002

Table of Contents

Preface

VisualDx: Essential Adult Dermatology is a foundation textbook for diagnosing and managing common and serious adult skin diseases. The authors of this text are practicing dermatologists who have seen and cared for thousands of adults with common, rare, and very unusual skin diseases at the Harbor-UCLA Medical Center and the University of California, Los Angeles; the University of California, San Francisco; the University of Rochester; and the University of North Carolina. In addition to knowledge that can be referenced, it is the combined experience of the editors that brings special value to this book for practicing clinicians. It should be particularly useful to those who see adults with skin disease either very frequently or infrequently, those who see patients with severe and challenging skin diseases, and those who consult for hospitalized patients with skin problems. The chapters emphasize important details that are not often discussed in other texts, including the approach to the patient and office-based diagnostic and biopsy procedures. The book also dedicates an entire chapter to summarizing the details of dermatologic therapy. Special diagnostic issues that may be present in the skin of heavily pigmented patients or immunosuppressed patients are also clearly addressed. This is a modern textbook that is in touch with newer ways of learning and using information.

VisualDx: Essential Adult Dermatology is a complete diagnostic system with an additional online decision support resource. Over 800 images in the book are reinforced by thousands of additional online images and extensive references for each condition, differentiating this textbook from other traditional textbooks with online images and text. In addition to functionality that allows searching for a differential diagnosis and therapeutic information by diagnosis, the VisualDx decision support system—a powerful point-of-care clinical tool—also allows its users to search by problem, lesion features, symptoms, and other pertinent patient findings. This book is complementary to *VisualDx: Essential Pediatric Dermatology* and its online decision support resource that emphasizes skin disease in children and adolescents.

As educators and clinicians, we aim to be at the forefront of developments combining the best features of all media for education and patient care. Lippincott Publishing is an enthusiastic partner with us in these endeavors.

Lindy P. Fox, MD
Noah Craft, MD, PhD, DTMH
Art Papier, MD
Lowell A. Goldsmith, MD, MPH

Acknowledgments

Many of the photographs in this book are part of a collection of dermatology conditions taken by Dr. Victor D. Newcomer during his outstanding career as a clinician and educator that have been contributed to Logical Images. Other photographs are from institutions that have donated clinician photographs to Logical Images, which include the slide collections of the Departments of Dermatology at New York University and the School of Medicine and Dentistry of the University of Rochester and their editors and authors. Additional photographs were contributed from the collections of Charles Crutchfield III, MD; Nancy Esterly, MD; Art Papier, MD; Stephen Estes, MD; Robert Chalmers, MD; Steven Oberlender, MD, PhD; Lowell A. Goldsmith, MD, MPH; Karen Wiss, MD; Robert Baran, MD; Noah Craft, MD, PhD; Mary Gail Mercurio, MD; David Elpern, MD; Lawrence Parish, MD; David C. Foster, MD, MPH; Lynette J. Margesson, MD; Sook-Bin Woo, MS, DMD, MMSc; Carl M. Allen, DDS, MSD; Tor Shwayder, MD; Frances J. Storrs, MD; Benjamin Fisher, MD; Shahbaz A. Janjua, MD; Karen McKoy, MD; Elaine Siegfried, MD; William Bonnez, MD; Robert T. Brodell, MD; Ncoza Dlova, MD; Kenneth Greer, MD; Robert Kalb, MD; Mark Malek, MD, MPH; Ricardo Mandojana, MD; Larry Millikan, MD; Christopher J. Rapuano, MD; and William Van Stoecker, MD.

Illustrations of morphologic lesion types were created by Glen Hintz, MS, Professor of Medical Illustration at Rochester Institute of Technology.

All the authors and editors are grateful for the meticulous care that Frances Reed gave to the preparation and redaction of this text and the precision and professional skill with which Stephanie Piro prepared the large number of clinical photographs for this text. Sonya Seigafuse, Kim Schonberger, and Kerry Barrett at Lippincott Williams & Wilkins helped make this complex project a reality.

Introduction to the VisualDx: Essential Dermatology Series

Welcome to the *VisualDx: Essential Dermatology* series. The goal of this series is to assist you in making the diagnosis and planning for the treatment of the most common skin disorders you will encounter in your daily clinical practice.

With *VisualDx: Essential Adult Dermatology*, you have two stand-alone and complementary products:

1. Book: The book contains an approach to adult patients, techniques of diagnosis and laboratory testing, a special approach leading you to the correct diagnosis and differential diagnosis, and typically four color figures showing the clinical variation of the condition. The book is designed for quick use while the patient is still in your office.

   Each disease, or set of related diseases, has special sections of text on the diagnostic criteria, skin characteristics, best laboratory tests, differential diagnosis, special characteristics of the condition in immunocompromised patients and those with darker skin color, and treatments.

2. Online: The Web-based decision support system combines the power of a comprehensive medical image collection with expert-reviewed clinical information. Features include:

   - Illustrative lesion icons for easy dermatologic diagnosis search. Also search by body location, signs, symptoms, past medical history, medications, and more.
   - The ability to build a patient-relevant differential. Build a patient-relevant visual differential diagnosis based on observable symptoms you see in your patient.
   - Clickable printouts for sharing information with your patients or coworkers.
   - Thousands of medical images that represent variations of disease presentations, with zoom capability for quick side-by-side comparison to your patient.

We certainly hope that this product will be useful to you and the patients you care for.

Please look for other titles in the *VisualDx: Essential Dermatology* series.

Introduction to VisualDx: Essential Adult Dermatology Online

To see the chapter, go to www.essentialdermatology.com/ adult and register using the code found in the front of this book.

VisualDx is a diagnostic clinical decision support system that integrates search, imagery, and text in an easy-to-use Web browser–based system. VisualDx allows you to simultaneously "look up" information by multiple parameters rather than by a single index term, as found in print-based resources. It is important to know that VisualDx online does not work by a simple search of this textbook or a search of text in an online database. Our authors and editors have reviewed the medical literature and created a search technology that allows you, the user, to search by patient findings. Through organization by patient characteristics such as symptoms, signs, visual clues, laboratory, etc., you will receive highly relevant information results. This distinction is important: when using a search engine such as Google or Yahoo, one is searching millions of pages of text; in decision support systems such as VisualDx, you do not experience the randomness of millions of pages of search and results, and you are searching purposefully designed medical relationships derived from the medical literature. The search results are more accurate, easier to read, and more comprehensive from the point of view of clinical differential diagnosis. And the process takes much less time than it took to read this paragraph! Investigate this distinction, and prove it for yourself. Start by registering your VisualDx online account by visiting www.essentialdermatology.com/adult as instructed on the inside cover of this book. Then complete the following scenarios:

Scenario 1:
1. Open an Internet search engine or a medical electronic resource.
2. Type the following search terms into the search box: adult, toxic, pustules, and widespread.
3. View the results.

Scenario 2:
1. Log in to VisualDx and follow the choice/path for building a differential diagnosis.

2. Enter age, characteristics of a widespread location/ distribution, (Fig. 1) and lesion morphology of pustule (Fig. 2).

3. View the results.

Compare the results of the information display optimized for medical diagnosis (Fig. 3) with those from a generic search engine or medical reference system organized by diagnosis, and you will immediately recognize the difference between search engines that search text and a clinical decision support system designed to search structured relationships between findings and diagnoses.

In addition to a structured search of medical findings-to-diagnosis relationships, the VisualDx interface is optimized to display images prominently. The information task our engineers are addressing is best summarized by the question, "What am I looking at?" To address this universal information need for the health care professional, we have

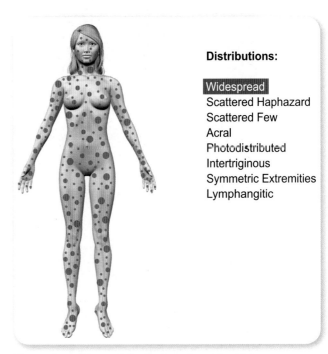

Distributions:

Widespread
Scattered Haphazard
Scattered Few
Acral
Photodistributed
Intertriginous
Symmetric Extremities
Lymphangitic

Figure 1 A Widespread distribution selected for Adult.

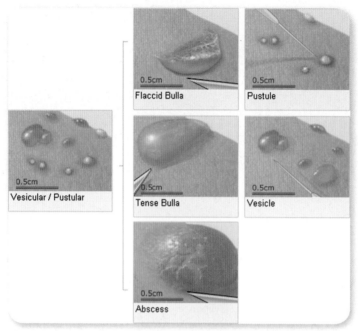

Figure 2 Vesicular/Pustular lesion morphology and its subtypes, including Pustule.

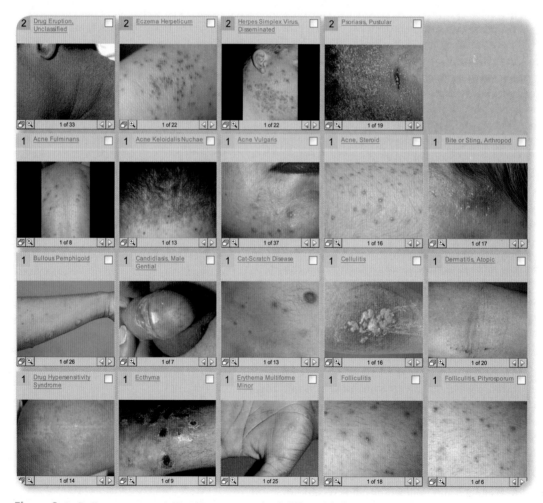

Figure 3 As findings are entered, VisualDx returns a visual differential diagnosis organized by the diagnoses with most matched findings.

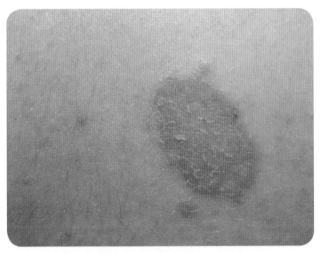

Figure 4 Classic plaque in pityriasis rosea. In light skin, a "classic" oval erythematous, scaly herald plaque.

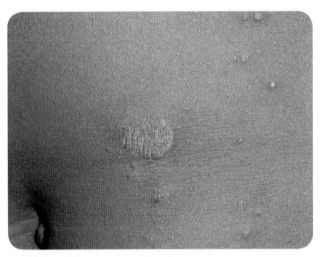

Figure 5 In dark skin, small papules are common as well as the more typical scaly plaques in pityriasis rosea.

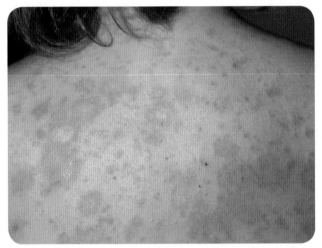

Figure 6 Pityriasis rosea. In light skin, classic morphology with thin, scaly, salmon-colored plaques; however, this patient does not have a "Christmas tree" pattern to the lesions, which is often cited as a clue to this diagnosis.

designed the VisualDx interface around pictures, diagrams, and graphics. This allows the search by findings to result in a visual differential diagnosis. The near-limitless ability to electronically access pictures means that our authors can go beyond displaying the "classic" examples of disease. Online VisualDx presents the typical *and* the common—and even very unusual—variants (Figs. 4–6). The computer interface has a unique "stacking" of each diagnosis thumbnail that is dependent on the entered morphology search term; the picture variants re-sort within the stacks to match the morphology you search. This means that in addition to the differential diagnosis created by your patient factors, VisualDx will also display extra relevant image examples. Moreover, while this textbook is typically limited to four images per disease, VisualDx has thousands of pictures. The images are organized by your search entry and displayed in uniform color and standard size.

Be sure to register for your free subscription to VisualDx online at www.essentialdermatology.com/adult, and start accessing VisualDx to:

- Develop a differential diagnosis using the data from the actual patients being examined. This process fulfills practice-based learning goals and allows more comprehensive and relevant differential diagnoses as you work.
- If you have an exam room computer, log in and bookmark VisualDx so that you can quickly search for images to use for patient education and reassurance. There is nothing like a picture to reassure a patient that a rash is common and there is no need to worry.
- Use the LearnDerm link for interactive training in dermatology exam, morphology, and disease variation.
- Review many more diagnoses and pictures.

CHAPTER 1

Approach to the Dermatology Patient

History

Is the approach to the dermatology patient any different than the approach to a patient with a general medical problem such as hypertension, chest pain, or a cough? Indeed. For starters, because most problems on the skin are visible, dermatology patients, and often those around them, are acutely aware of the problem at hand. Many times, patients seek dermatologic advice because a family member or casual observer suggested they "get it checked out." Having a skin problem can be very distressing and stigmatizing. In today's world, the role of the physician or caregiver is rapidly changing. Especially in dermatology, many patients have already tried to self-diagnose and self-treat using advice they have gathered from friends, family, and the Internet. Some have even ordered prescription medications over the Internet. Thus, many patients have a different type of anxiety about the problem than they might when they are going to have a breast or a prostate examination.

Compared to the typical patient-doctor interaction, the approach to a specific dermatologic problem can be focused early during the visit. Patients will usually offer their own opinions about when and how a skin condition began, what caused it, what helped it, what did not help it, and what the condition means for the patient and his or her family. However, a preliminary objective assessment of the problem can help incorporate the subjective thoughts of the patient into the course of information gathering. One effective method to develop rapport during initial data gathering is to examine patients while they are voicing their concerns. For example, saying to the patient "Show me while you are explaining what you think caused your skin problem" can be helpful. With dermatologic issues, it is useful to examine the patient in the first few minutes of the visit to get a sense of what types of primary lesions (if any) are involved. Naturally, the initial examination can be tailored depending on whether the visit is intended for prevention, diagnosis, or ongoing treatment of the skin problem at hand.

Once the physician determines the nature of the skin problem by a physical examination, a more focused and detailed history can be obtained. After building the differential diagnosis based on the primary lesion morphologies and anatomic distribution, the physician can gather information to support or refute the various diagnoses. Occam's razor has a two-sided blade. In the perfect diagnostic world, all the skin lesions of an individual and their history would mesh congruently. However, this is not always the case; the skin lesions may have nothing to do with other signs or symptoms, or individuals may have two different skin diseases simultaneously. Diagnosis of skin diseases is a learned skill that is always improved with practice and feedback from the reality of each patient.

The dermatologic history includes time of onset, duration of the problem, and a history of prior episodes. Associated symptoms, aggravating or relieving factors, and previous therapies tried may be helpful information as well. A thorough review of systems can be useful if the skin condition could be associated with other systemic problems (e.g., pyoderma gangrenosum in a patient with ulcerative colitis and gastrointestinal complaints). Review of medications is important (including topical, over-the-counter, and herbal medications). Alterations to medication regimens may be relevant when a cutaneous reaction is suspected. Certain skin conditions are associated with underlying medical diseases (e.g., acanthosis nigricans and diabetes), have a genetic component (e.g., neurofibromatosis), or are associated with or exacerbated by social habits or exposures. Review of the past medical history, the social history, and the family history, therefore, may be relevant depending on the problem being addressed. Obtaining a history may be especially challenging when the patient's native language is not the one the physician can speak, the patient communicates with sign language, or ethnic or religious reasons prevent full frankness of discussion. Social and occupational histories, a focused family history, and a noncutaneous medical history establish the full and rich substrate for the physician-patient relationship. This approach remains an essential part of exemplary patient care, as many dermatologic diseases are influenced by environmental, genetic, and occupational factors.

After the initial screening examination is completed and a thorough history obtained, a more detailed physical examination can be performed. Thoroughness establishes the physician as the consummate professional and expert. Looking in the mouth and between the toes, careful parting of the hair to examine the scalp, and inspection of all of the nails may not have been performed by previous examiners. The patient will be positively impressed by the assiduous search for disease and etiology. Talking with the patient and explaining what you are observing makes the patient a part of the process and ultimately enlists him or her in the diagnostic, prevention, or treatment plans. Explaining the need for photographs, with the reassurance of confidentiality, is also logically done at this stage.

In patients where the diagnosis is already confirmed and the problem is not contagious, clinicians can reassure the patients by touching the skin. This is especially important in skin diseases such as psoriasis, where the patient may feel disfigured. If the skin lesions are not contagious (as with many skin problems), *do not wear gloves* while touching the patient.

The process of gathering and integrating information from the history and physical examination directly influences what additional information a physician decides to gather; however, physicians do face challenges that may impair their ability to effectively do so. *Cognitive bias* describes the phenomenon whereby physicians see what they think they should be seeing rather than being a critical observer of what actually exists on the patient being examined. Examples of this bias include being misled by a false "clue" from the history, a recent patient, another physician's previous diagnosis, or an article that was read just before seeing the patient. In addition, due to the evolving nature of skin lesions and the diseases associated with them, a diagnosis may not be possible at the time of the initial visit; this unsettling fact must be communicated to the patient with compassion and knowledge.

Biopsies and Laboratory Testing

Biopsies and laboratory tests are most useful when purposely performed to establish an important diagnosis. In many parts of the world, these tests may cost the patients, their insurers, or their governments more than the physicians' visits. Significant judgment goes into the decision to do tests, especially when genetic testing is contemplated. Classical psoriasis with multiple plaques covering 10% of the body or classical acanthosis nigricans in an obese adolescent or adult is not an indication for a biopsy. If a diagnosis is made clinically, it may be worthwhile to explain why no tests are needed to make the diagnosis. Likewise, the physician should discuss with the patient why a biopsy or any laboratory test will be performed. Whenever considering any laboratory test, the clinician should have a solid understanding of the limitations of the test about to be ordered and an idea of what diagnoses are under consideration *before* the test is ordered.

The approach to the biopsy is an important concept and interlocks with the discussion about when to refer a patient to a dermatologist. Not all patients or settings permit a skin biopsy; furthermore, in certain situations, pathology or dermatology services may not be available at all. Thus, after building a differential diagnosis, carefully evaluate the potential serious diagnoses and the risks and benefits of performing a biopsy. Weigh this against the risks of empirically treating the patient without a biopsy, the likelihood that a patient will be able to follow up, and the accessibility of a dermatology consultation should one be necessary.

Before performing a biopsy, a clinician should have a reasonable differential diagnosis in mind, as most biopsy results require clinicopathologic correlation. If a clinician has no idea what the diagnosis could be, a biopsy is unlikely to yield useful information. In these cases, it may be prudent to refer the patient to a dermatologist for evaluation before performing a biopsy. However, in cases where a clinician is trying to decide between three and four possible diagnoses or, at the very least, is trying to confirm a single diagnosis, a biopsy would be indicated. Destruction of a skin lesion such as a seborrheic keratosis or an actinic keratosis should be performed only when there is certainty in the diagnosis. Many malpractice suits have come from destruction of a lesion that has turned out to be a malignancy.

Deciding which type of biopsy to perform is important. Shave biopsies, punch biopsies, and excisional biopsies can be used in various circumstances. Shave biopsies are preferred for diseases that primarily involve the epidermis or superficial dermis (most inflammatory diseases such as eczema and psoriasis and nonmelanoma skin cancers), while punch biopsies are preferred for lesions where the suspected infiltrate is deeper (sarcoidosis, erythema nodosum, dermal neoplasm, etc.). An excisional biopsy is preferred for subcutaneous nodules. When biopsying annular lesions (e.g., erythema annulare centrifugum or porokeratosis), the leading edge of the lesion is usually preferable to biopsy.

Evaluation of pigmented lesions is challenging. It is important to remember that no matter what technique is used, if a melanoma is diagnosed, additional surgery will be required. Thus, a biopsy performed by the primary care provider can save the patient many weeks or months of waiting for an appointment. In some settings, this fact alone can justify performing a biopsy with the best technique available. General rules of thumb follow. When suspicion for melanoma is high, excisional biopsy is the preferred technique. When evaluating a pigmented lesion and suspicion for melanoma is present but very low (e.g., a clinically apparent seborrheic keratosis), a shave biopsy can be used to remove the lesion with optimized cosmetic results. If the biopsy results are not as expected, a larger excisional biopsy can be performed at follow-up to evaluate the full extent of the melanoma. Performing a small punch biopsy of a much larger pigmented lesion is not recommended, as it can mistakenly capture a benign component of a malignant process (i.e., a melanoma arising in a nevus or associated with a seborrheic keratosis). Know the qualifications of the pathologist interpreting the skin biopsy. Dermatopathology is a recognized subspecialty because of the complexity and variations in inflammatory skin diseases; general pathologists are competent to diagnose neoplastic lesions. Pigmented premalignant lesions are often sources of alternative interpretations, even among experts in the histopathology of these lesions.

In many kinds of lesions, rebiopsy of a different portion of the lesion, biopsy of another lesion, or rebiopsy as a lesion evolves is necessary for a diagnosis. The complexity of biopsy interpretation should not dissuade a physician from performing a biopsy; it is equally important to note that there are circumstances in which the patient should not be left with the unrealistic expectation that the biopsy will answer everything.

Referral

Referral to a dermatologist is indicated for widespread blistering, pustules, or erosions; total body skin pain with erythroderma (total body erythema); or widespread purpura or eschars. In immunocompromised patients, these criteria are even more important. If the primary clinician feels incapable of proper evaluation in an expedient time frame, patients with suspicious pigmented skin lesions should be referred to a dermatologist on an urgent, but not emergent, basis.

Communication

Communication of biopsy and laboratory test results is important for continued patient rapport. This can be performed over the phone, but additional communication by letter or e-mail is useful, even if the patient is to be seen again. This completes the communication loop and is appreciated by the patient.

The diagnosis, prognosis, and available treatment options are what the patient carries away from the visit. In today's world, patients will certainly go home and read about their diagnosis and treatment on the Internet. Providing patients with handouts and/or specific links to trusted Internet sites, such as www.skinsight.com, can be a useful way to engage patients in the understanding of the disease and the available treatment options. Topical medicines, especially corticosteroids, are often confusing to patients. Comparing the strengths of various topical corticosteroids to the strengths of a bicycle, a Honda, a Mercedes, and—when occlusion is used—a supercharged Mercedes can be helpful, as patients remember this therapeutic ladder more easily than chemical names. Although many patients like certainty of diagnosis and treatment, this is not always possible. Confession about the uncertainty of a diagnosis is acceptable as long as a clear plan to pursue a more certain diagnosis or treatment regimen is conveyed to the patient at the same time. In all cases, reassuring a patient that his or her problem is not cancer and not contagious (when appropriate) can relieve much of the potential anxiety while he or she awaits laboratory results.

Disclosing bad news to patients is always a difficult part of the practice of medicine. Strategies for disclosing bad news to patients include this ABCDE mnemonic: **A**dvance preparation, **B**uild a therapeutic relationship and environment, **C**ommunicate well, **D**eal with the reactions of the patient and family, and **E**ncourage and validate emotions.[1] Additional potentially helpful strategies are described below:

- Avoid disclosing extremely bad news over the telephone.
- For possibly very upsetting information, suggest to the patient that he or she may want to bring a family member or friend for support.
- Touch the affected patient with obvious care.
- Show a caring and compassionate sense of connection with the patient.
- Pace the discussion to the emotional state of the patient.
- Avoid jargon.
- Ensure that patients do not blame themselves or others for the problem.
- Write out the name of the illness for the patient, or present him or her with a handout or link to a trusted Internet site.
- Confirm effective transmission of information by asking the patient to use his or her own words to explain what you discussed.
- Address the implications that could affect the patient's future.
- Acknowledge the patient's emotions, and be prepared for tears and the need for time.
- Avoid being aloof or detached.
- Give patients time to integrate the information and formulate additional questions.
- Be able to recommend community-based resources, where appropriate.
- Arrange a follow-up plan and an appointment for continued conversation.

Abuse

Physical and sexual abuse can occur at any age and must be considered in disorders affecting the genitals and when the physical signs suggest an external etiology of the lesions. Some key points for addressing potential abuse are described as follows:

- If there is any suspicion of sexual or physical abuse, report it to the appropriate local social services agency.
- A full physical examination looking for signs of abuse should be performed on all patients in whom sexual or physical abuse is suspected.
- In patients with symptoms suggestive of a sexually transmissible infection (STI), test for other common STIs before initiating any treatment that may interfere with their diagnosis.
- If unsure whether to report, discuss the case with local adult or elder abuse consultants.

Hospitalized Patients

The hospitalized patient presents a unique dermatologic scenario. Despite a growing movement to establish hospitalist dermatology practices,[2] dermatologists are available for inpatient consultations less and less.[3] Therefore, this responsibility may rest on the shoulders of the admitting clinicians. It is not uncommon for patients to develop skin problems while in the hospital that could be clues to underlying systemic medical problems or reactions to other pharmacologic interventions. Often, the skin holds the key to serious medical diagnoses (e.g., splinter hemorrhages and subacute bacterial endocarditis or skin pain and impending toxic epidermal necrolysis).

When a hospitalized patient has cutaneous manifestations of underlying systemic diseases or a drug eruption is suspected, a biopsy should be performed expediently. Because skin biopsies are performed at the bedside, it is best to have all the materials needed for a biopsy ready ahead of time. Expedited processing of the specimen should be requested when possible. If an infection is suspected, an additional skin biopsy specimen should be sent to the microbiology laboratory for bacterial, fungal, mycobacterial, and viral cultures.

International Travel

When patients who have recently traveled to international destinations or who have emigrated from other countries present with an acute skin complaint, diseases endemic to the country of origin or places the patient visited should be considered. Many infectious diseases have specific geographic distributions that will determine the possibilities of diagnosis. For example, fever and an eschar after returning from Botswana suggest African tick bite fever, while a nonhealing ulcer on the cheek that started 3 weeks after returning from the jungles of Costa Rica suggests leishmaniasis. If one is unfamiliar with the potential parasites and infections, decision support tools and Internet resources are available. Additionally, the dermatologic clinician can play an important role in pretravel counseling about sun protection and insect avoidance (including the use of DEET and bed nets to prevent malaria, leishmaniasis, etc.).

Summary

In general, because skin problems can be manifestations of so many different disease processes, the approach to patients with dermatology issues should be an iterative process that results in a focused, yet thorough, history and examination. Appreciation of special circumstances surrounding your patient is essential (i.e., institutionalized patients, hospitalized patients, prisoners, immigrants, or travelers). After examining and questioning your patient, it is critical to form a differential diagnosis based on lesion morphology and distribution before deciding on which laboratory test or biopsy to perform. Finally, communicating to your patient your diagnosis (or working plan to arrive at a diagnosis) and treatment plan must be done while paying careful attention to the patient's cultural and social background, assuring understanding before the patient leaves the room.

References

1. VandeKieft GK. Breaking bad news. *Am Fam Physician.* 2001;64(12):1975–1978.
2. Fox LP, Cotliar J, Hughey L, et al. *J Am Acad Dermatol.* 2009;61(1):153–154.
3. Helms AE, Helms SE, Brodell RT. Hospital consultations: Time to address an unmet need? *J Am Acad Dermatol.* 2009;60(2):308–311.

CHAPTER 2

Examination of the Skin

Examining the Skin

The Patient

It is best to first interact with the patient and then quickly acknowledge and identify the patient's support team. We prefer to have patients identify their relationship with others in the room because complications may ensue when you assume who the spouse, parents, grandparents, and other friends or family members are.

The patient should completely undress for a comprehensive skin examination. When patients ask the physician to examine a particular lesion or area of involved skin, the physician often focuses only on the patient's complaint without looking elsewhere. Looking at an isolated lesion without examining the patient completely, however, may lead to a misdiagnosis or nondiagnosis of potentially serious lesions. Encourage your patient to completely disrobe and wear a gown, explaining how other clues or problems might be hidden on skin covered by clothing.

Once the patient is prepared for the examination, it is more acceptable and less invasive to start with the fingers and nails. After establishing comfort and observing for nail-related findings, the examiner can work his or her way to the rest of the body, verbalizing where he or she is going in advance and what is being seen. Verbalizing your findings allows for patient input, reassurance, and confidence in the clinical interaction and distracts the patient from potential fear.

When performing a skin examination, the entire skin surface should be examined, including the scalp, oral cavity, genitals, and nails. Gloves are worn for examination of the genitals, intraoral palpation, and palpation of potentially infectious lesions that are moist, hemorrhagic, or crusted. Gloves are not necessary for examination elsewhere unless there is a concern about infection. In fact, wearing gloves for the complete examination may cause the patient to feel embarrassed or self-conscious. Further, in patients with common, easily diagnosed, and noninfectious conditions such as psoriasis, touching the patient's psoriatic plaques can make him or her feel normal and comfortable. This can

be reassuring to the patient as well as to family members, illustrating that he or she is not contagious.

Lighting

Good lighting, either artificial or natural, is essential for a good skin examination. Fixed or standing lighting frees both hands for examination and manipulation of lesions. Oblique illumination (side lighting) of a slightly elevated papule confirms its raised character by the shadow it casts. This should be done in a dimly lit or dark room (Fig. 2-1). Intense light (e.g., the head of an ophthalmologic penlight) is used to transilluminate cystic lesions and reveal the homogeneity of the structure. Focused, intense light should not be used for the complete examination because it can wash out important details.

Wood Light

The Wood lamp (black light) produces long-wave ultraviolet rays (365 nm peak UVA range) with relatively low energy. No special precautions are required for its routine use, except that

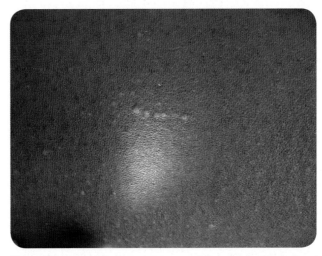

Figure 2-1 Side lighting. Faint degrees of elevation can be detected by side lighting, as seen in this side lighting of the tiny linear papules of lichen nitidus.

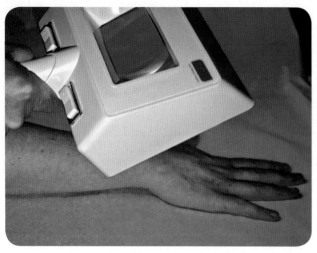

Figure 2-2 Wood lamp. Small degrees of decreased or increased pigmentation can be seen with the Wood lamp after visual adaptation to the dark.

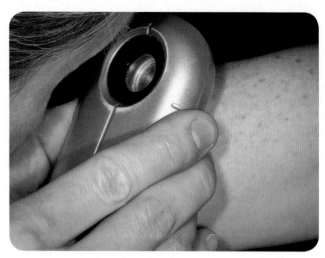

Figure 2-3 Episcope. Especially pigmented and vascular lesions can be examined in more detail by the use of bright optics and polarization.

the room should be as dark as possible (Fig. 2-2). Melanin absorbs strongly at 365 nm, so that minor losses of melanin are accentuated. Hypopigmented areas are paler than normal skin, and depigmented areas are stark or milk white under Wood light. The Wood lamp is especially useful in the diagnosis of vitiligo or in seeing the hypopigmentation of tinea versicolor in early stages. Certain conditions have characteristic fluorescent patterns (Table 2-1). The Wood lamp is also useful for checking urine specimens for uroporphyrins (pink fluorescence), which are characteristic of porphyria cutanea tarda. Multiple exogenous substances, including markers, lint, dyes, and lipstick, can fluoresce on the skin.

Magnification

Magnifying lenses (5× to 10×) should be strong enough to allow the physician to easily observe lesions. Lenses are especially useful for detecting altered skin markings and contours in tumors, especially melanoma. Lenses are also used to observe nail-fold telangiectasia in connective tissue diseases and to detect the subtle surface changes (Wickham striae) in lichen planus. When mineral oil or immersion oil is placed on the skin, the stratum corneum becomes more transparent, revealing deeper structures in more detail. This technique

allows easier visualization of telangiectases, Wickham striae, and similar findings. Episcopes or dermatoscopes allow the examination of skin lesions under magnification with excellent illumination and permit resolution of fine detail and size (Fig. 2-3). They are especially useful for viewing complex pigmented lesions and melanomas.

Compression

Observing the changes in a skin lesion with compression (diascopy) is often useful in the diagnosis of skin diseases. Compression may be performed with a magnifying glass, microscope slide, or clear plastic plate. These instruments are all considered *diascopes*. Blue to red lesions that blanch when compressed are vascular lesions, and their gradual refilling is observed by seeing the red color return. Purpuric lesions do not blanch completely with pressure; raised, purpuric, non-blanchable lesions indicate cutaneous small vessel vasculitis. Compression of brown to yellow-brown papules may reveal the apple-jelly nodules of granulomatous diseases (e.g., sarcoidosis, tuberculosis).

Palpation of Skin Lesions

Palpation reveals the lesion's depth, extension, texture, firmness, and fixation to underlying structures of skin. Light pressure can reveal a thrill in a vascular lesion, implying an arteriovenous malformation. Lateral compression of dermatofibromas causes them to become depressed and to indent the overlying skin (Fitzpatrick sign). Firm stroking of apparently normal skin can induce histamine release, redness, and edema; this phenomenon, known as dermographism, is accentuated in urticaria (Fig. 2-4). Stroking of individual papules leading to local erythema and edema (and, rarely, vesiculation) is diagnostic of urticaria pigmentosa. This phenomenon is named Darier sign (Fig. 2-5). Stroking the skin of atopic patients produces a white line without a red phase

TABLE 2-1 Fluorescent Characteristics of Certain Conditions	
Characteristics	**Conditions**
Yellow-green fluorescence of hair	*Microsporum canis*
Yellow-green fluorescence of skin	*Pseudomonas* infection
Pink fluorescence of urine	Uroporphyrins of porphyria cutanea tarda
Coral fluorescence of toes, axillae, groin	Erythrasma infection

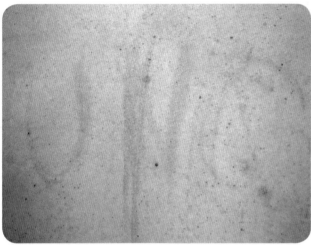

Figure 2-4 Dermographism. Histamine release is accentuated in patients with reactive vasculature in hypersensitivity reactions.

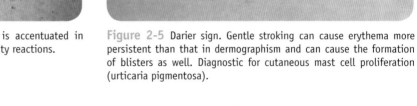

Figure 2-5 Darier sign. Gentle stroking can cause erythema more persistent than that in dermographism and can cause the formation of blisters as well. Diagnostic for cutaneous mast cell proliferation (urticaria pigmentosa).

(white dermographism). In nevus anemicus, firm rubbing makes the surrounding normal skin bright red but does not induce erythema in the hypopigmented skin. In blistering diseases, rubbing apparently normal skin may induce new blisters; this occurs in patients with pemphigus vulgaris and toxic epidermal necrolysis (Nikolsky sign). Extension of an intact blister by application of pressure to the lesion (Asboe-Hansen sign) indicates an intraepidermal blister.

Special Diagnostic Procedures

Organism Detection and Presumptive Identification

Organism identification is essential for the rational treatment of skin infections and infestations. Procedures important for dermatology are outlined in this section; standard infectious disease and microbiology texts should be consulted for further details. Superficial crusts, exudates, and topical medications should be swabbed with alcohol to remove saprophytes and secondary contaminating bacteria.

Potassium Hydroxide (KOH) Preparation for Fungus

1. With an alcohol swab, cleanse the skin of any ointment.
2. With the edge of a microscope slide or scalpel, vigorously scrape the skin onto a second microscope slide. The best areas for scraping are the following:
   - Inner surface of a blister roof or the blister base
   - Moist, macerated areas, such as between toes, at the edge of the lesion, away from potential secondary infections that may interfere with fungal growth
   - Rim or leading edge of lesions
   - Under a nail or under a paronychial fold
   - Base of a plucked hair
3. Place a drop of 10% to 20% KOH on the scale-covered slide and apply a coverslip.

4. Warm gently. Avoid actual boiling, as this causes the KOH to crystallize (Fig. 2-6).
5. Examine with a microscope by scanning at 10× and then confirming hyphae with the 40× objective at low illumination. This is achieved by setting a low level of light. Close the condenser diaphragm iris all the way to enhance the contrast (Fig. 2-7).

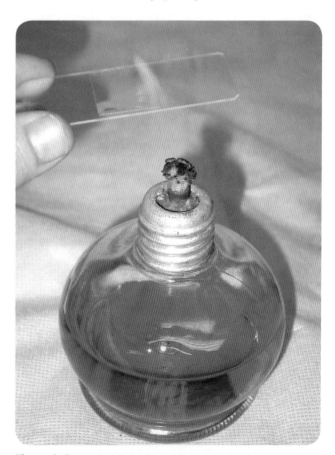

Figure 2-6 Gentle heating of a small amount of scale with KOH over an alcohol lamp is the key for a useful fungal preparation.

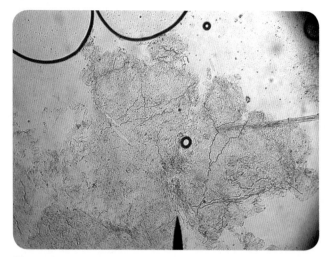

Figure 2-7 Identification of hyphal elements with a 10× objective and low illumination allows hyphae to show up as dark objects against the background. Using a 40× objective confirms the diagnosis.

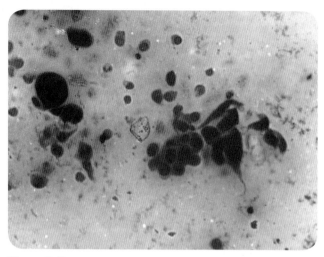

Figure 2-8 Multinucleated cells or giant nuclei characterize herpes simplex or herpes zoster infections of the skin.

Small amounts of scrapings on a slide frequently yield the best results because the coverslip rests on the slide, producing the best optical properties. KOH hydrolyzes the epidermal proteins but not the fungal elements. The cell envelopes of the stratum corneum remain and should not be confused with fungi.

Tzanck Smear for Giant Cells

A Tzanck smear is very important for the rapid diagnosis of patients with vesicles and does not require special techniques such as PCR or fluorescent microscopy. The demonstration of multinucleated giant cells indicates that the causative agent is either herpes simplex virus or varicella-zoster virus. The procedure is as follows:

1. Select a fresh umbilicated vesicle.
2. Unroof the vesicle with a scalpel blade.
3. Gently scrape the base of the vesicle with the scalpel, and smear scrapings onto a microscope slide.
4. Fix with 95% alcohol.

5. Stain with Wright or Giemsa stain, using the technique that is used for routine white cell differential counts.
6. Examine under the microscope using the 10× or 40× objective. A positive preparation demonstrates very large multinucleated giant cells with a high nuclear-cytoplasmic ratio. Examination with the oil immersion objective is often required in equivocal cases (Fig. 2-8).

Examination for Lice

Nits (eggs of lice) on pubic, axillary, scalp, or other hairs may be directly examined with the microscope. Organisms or empty, highly refractile egg cases are easily observed with the 10× objective (Fig. 2-9). Adult lice can be seen with the naked eye and are dramatic under the lower objective (Fig. 2-10).

Examination for Scabies

Scabetic mites may be removed from burrows with a scalpel after applying 10% KOH or mineral oil to the suspected

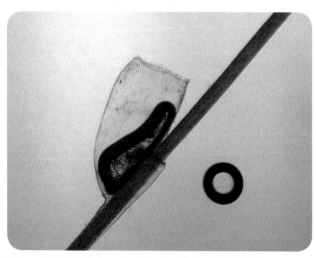

Figure 2-9 Hair with a louse egg case (nit). 10× objective.

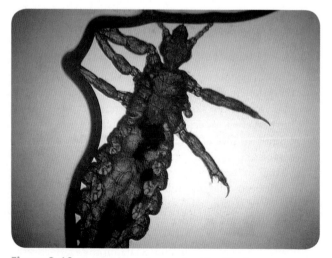

Figure 2-10 An adult louse from scalp. 10× objective.

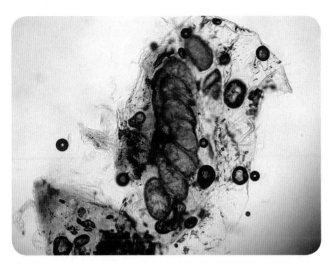

Figure 2-11 Scraping from a burrow with an adult *Sarcoptes* mite, in lower-left corner, and a string of eggs containing organisms.

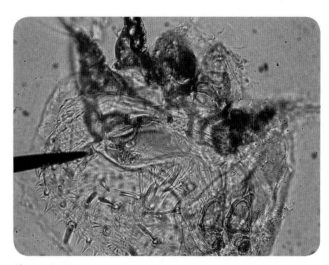

Figure 2-12 Close-up of an adult *Sarcoptes* mite, the cause of scabies.

burrow. The oil optically clears the stratum corneum, enhancing visualization of the mite. Application of a tetracycline solution (500 mg tetracycline in 20 mL glycerin and 80 mL absolute ethanol), followed 1 min later by shining a Wood lamp on the skin, accentuates the burrow. Burrows fluoresce a brilliant green, allowing easy removal of a suspected organism. Alternatively, a small drop of ink placed on the opening of the burrow that is then rapidly wiped away with a tissue may also reveal tracks (**Figs. 2-11–2-13**).

Gram Stain for Bacteria and *Candida*

1. Air-dry the slide.
2. Cover with 1% crystal violet for 15 s. Wash with water.
3. Cover with Gram iodine for 15 s. Wash with water.
4. Decolorize for 15 s with acetone alcohol. Wash with water.
5. Cover with 2.5% safranin for 15 s. Wash with water and air-dry.
6. Examine with 10×, 40×, and oil immersion lenses.

Special Techniques Usually Not Performed in the Primary Care Office

Patch Testing

Patch testing is done to determine delayed hypersensitivity to exogenous substances. The materials are specially prepared or may be available in the form of kits (e.g., T.R.U.E. TEST [Allerderm, Phoenix, AZ]). The patches are applied for 48 h under occlusion and then examined for a delayed hypersensitivity that may vary from mild edema to actual vesiculation (**Fig. 2-14**). False-negative tests are frequent, and many positives (e.g., to nickel) may not be clinically relevant to the condition at hand.

Culture Techniques

Sabouraud medium is useful for the isolation of most fungi. It is commercially available, stored cool, and then incubated with specimens at room temperature. Sabouraud medium with cycloheximide (actidione) and chloramphenicol

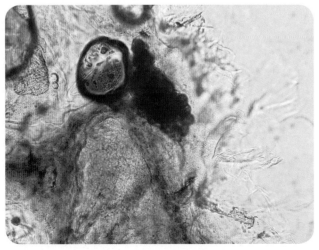

Figure 2-13 Clump of scabies feces. The presence of this alone is diagnostic of scabies.

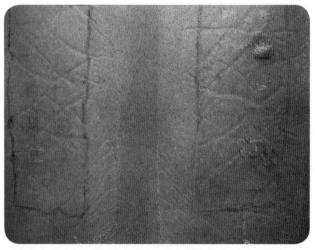

Figure 2-14 Vesicular patch test reaction. Patch test material is often applied on a small disc under occlusion.

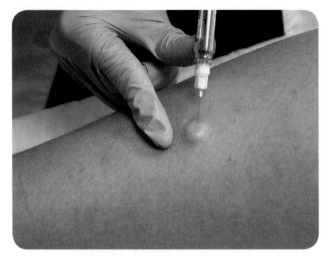

Figure 2-15 Biopsy. Intradermal injection of a local anesthetic using a 30-gauge needle.

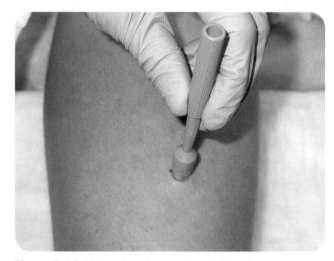

Figure 2-16 Biopsy. Firm pressure is applied to the cutaneous surface while rotating the punch biopsy instrument between the thumb and the forefinger.

suppresses bacteria and saprophytic fungi. It is very important to avoid the use of this medium if *Cryptococcus* is suspected because cycloheximide suppresses the growth of *Cryptococcus*.

India Ink Stain for *Cryptococcus*

A smear of an exudate is mixed with one small drop of commercial India ink, and a coverslip is applied. If the preparation is too dark, water may be added to dilute the ink. The large, translucent capsules of *Cryptococcus*, with a small central nucleus that may contain a nucleolus, can be seen. The buds have a narrow base; blastomycosis and other fungi have a broad base.

Acid-Fast Stain

In suspected lepromatous leprosy and orificial tuberculosis, direct stains may be positive. In other forms of cutaneous leprosy and cutaneous tuberculosis, the chance of a positive smear is so small that a direct smear is not indicated. *Nocardia* in mycetomas will also stain with the acid-fast stain.

Punch Biopsy

The punch biopsy is a common biopsy used by dermatologists. When properly performed, the procedure can be done rapidly with a very low incidence of adverse events or significant scarring.

1. Prepare a punch biopsy tray: Include alcohol pads, local anesthetic, gloves, punch instrument, forceps, scissors, gauze, needle driver, and suture.
2. Prepare the patient: Explain the procedure to the patient step by step in a gentle, reassuring manner. Ideally, the patient should be reclining or supine during the procedure to avoid an accident if he or she loses consciousness.
3. Anesthetize the patient: Topical anesthetics, such as topical lidocaine or EMLA, under occlusion may be used to reduce the discomfort caused by needle sticks, but they

are not usually necessary. If using a topical anesthetic, once the cutaneous surface is appropriately anesthetized, wipe the area clean with an alcohol pad and use a syringe with a 30-gauge needle to inject a local anesthetic into the deep dermis (Fig. 2-15).
4. Punch biopsy: Apply gentle lateral traction around the area of skin to be biopsied. The punch biopsy is then performed by applying slight downward pressure on the skin while rotating the punch instrument clockwise and counterclockwise (Fig. 2-16). One will feel a gentle pop as the instrument penetrates the dermis into the subcutaneous tissue.
5. Remove the biopsy tissue: Gently grasp the sample with forceps, lift until resistance is felt, and cut the tissue free at the subcutaneous level.
6. Close the defect with one to three simple interrupted sutures (Fig. 2-17): Choose the appropriate suture based on the patient's age, anatomic site, and size of the biopsy.

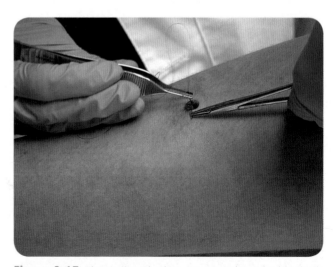

Figure 2-17 Biopsy. Wound edges are approximated with simple interrupted sutures.

In general, nonabsorbable (nylon or polypropylene) 4-0 suture is appropriate for superficial suturing of lesions on the trunk and extremities, and 5-0 suture is preferred for the face and genitalia.

7. Dress the wound: Apply a thin layer of white petrolatum or antibiotic ointment, cover the area with a nonadherent pad (e.g., Telfa [Kendall, Mansfield, MA]), and secure the pad with adhesive tape.

8. Provide the patient with written postoperative instructions explaining proper wound care, activity restrictions, and a number to call in case an adverse event occurs.

9. Remove sutures: The patient should return in 5 to 7 days for the removal of facial sutures and 10 to 14 days for the removal of sutures on the torso and extremities.

Shave Biopsy

The shave biopsy is another common biopsy technique used by dermatologists. When properly performed, the procedure can be done rapidly with a very low incidence of adverse events or significant scarring. Shave biopsy is most commonly performed when ruling out skin cancer in an exophytic lesion.

1. Prepare a shave biopsy tray: Include alcohol pads, local anesthetic, gloves, flexible or rigid scalpel, forceps, gauze, an agent for hemostasis (20% aluminum chloride solution), and bandage.

2. Prepare the patient: Explain the procedure to the patient step by step in a gentle, reassuring manner. Ideally, the patient should be reclining or supine during the procedure to avoid an accident if he or she loses consciousness.

3. Anesthetize the patient: Topical anesthetics, such as topical lidocaine or EMLA, under occlusion may be used to reduce the discomfort caused by needle sticks, but they are not usually necessary. If using a topical anesthetic, once the cutaneous surface is appropriately anesthetized, wipe the area clean with an alcohol pad and use a syringe with a 30-gauge needle to inject local anesthetic into the deep dermis (Fig. 2-15).

4. Shave biopsy: Apply gentle lateral traction around the area of skin to be biopsied. The shave biopsy is then performed using the scalpel to gently cut through the base of the lesion using a side-to-side sawing motion. If needed, use the back of a cotton swab to cut against when the final attachment of the tissue is reached. Alternatively, forceps can be used to grab the specimen.

5. Remove the biopsy tissue.

6. Using a cotton swab, apply aluminum chloride solution to the area as an agent of hemostasis. Vigorous rubbing can help stop bleeding more quickly. This technique should not be used near the eyes. If bleeding is persistent, continued pressure or electrocautery may be required to achieve hemostasis.

7. Dress the wound: Apply a thin layer of white petrolatum or antibiotic ointment, cover with a nonadherent pad (e.g., Telfa), and secure the pad with adhesive tape.

8. Provide the patient with written postoperative instructions explaining proper wound care, activity restrictions, and a number to call in case an adverse event occurs.

CHAPTER 3

Morphology and Distribution

Learning to describe skin findings is the fundamental and essential skill of dermatologic diagnosis. Learn to describe what you see with the words defined in this chapter and online at www.essentialdermatology.com. In this chapter, there are precise definitions of the key morphologic terms with illustrative case examples. Online, there are additional images, an interactive self-assessment, and further training in configurations, distributions, and a lesson in variants of disease presentation. Master these definitions in this chapter and online.

Morphology

The ability to use the standard morphologic descriptive terminology of dermatology has been the key to developing accurate skin-based differential diagnoses for over a century. The characterization of visual skin findings requires both careful observation and the use of universally accepted terminology. Once you know these terms, you will be able to use the differential diagnosis index in Chapter 4 and use the online differential diagnosis engine of VisualDx more effectively. In this section, as in VisualDx, the primary morphologic terms are grouped into logical categories. For example, vesicles, bullae, and pustules are grouped because these are terms that represent fluid-filled lesions. The grouping is purposeful. As you examine the patient, ask yourself questions such as, Are these lesions raised? Are these lesions solid or fluid filled? Do these lesions blanch, or are they nonblanching as in the purpuras? The categories match the skin exam method. In addition to the main categories, further describe papules and plaques by checking for surface change such as scale or crust. Visit www.essentialdermatology.com for access to the LearnDerm interactive tutorial. The tutorial includes more images, image descriptions, and an interactive self-study test with virtual examination tools.

Group	Lesion Type	Definition
FLAT	Macule	A flat, generally less than 0.5 cm area of skin or mucous membranes with different color from surrounding tissue. Macules may have nonpalpable, fine scale (Fig. 3-1).
	Patch*	A flat, generally greater than 0.5 cm area of skin or mucous membranes with different color from surrounding tissue. Patches may have nonpalpable, fine scale. *When used to describe an early clinical stage of cutaneous T-cell lymphoma (mycosis fungoides), the term patch may include fine textural change such as "cigarette paper" thinning, poikilodermatous atrophy, or slickness secondary to follicular loss (Fig. 3-2).
RAISED AND SMOOTH	Papule	A discrete, solid, elevated body usually less than 0.5 cm in diameter. Papules are further classified by shape, size, color, and surface change (Fig. 3-3).
	Plaque	A discrete, solid, elevated body usually broader than it is thick, measuring more than 0.5 cm in diameter. Plaques may be further classified by shape, size, color, and surface change (Fig. 3-4).
	Nodule	A dermal or subcutaneous firm, well-defined lesion usually greater than 0.5 cm in diameter (Fig. 3-5).
	Cyst	A closed cavity or sac containing fluid or semisolid material. A cyst may have an epithelial, endothelial, or membranous lining (Fig. 3-6).
SURFACE CHANGE	Crust	A hardened layer that results when serum, blood, or purulent exudate dries on the skin surface. Crusts may be thin or thick and can have varying color. Crusts are yellow-brown when formed from dried serum, green or yellow-green when formed from purulent exudate, or red-black when formed by blood (Fig. 3-7).
	Scale	Excess stratum corneum accumulated in flakes or plates. Scale usually has a white or gray color (Fig. 3-8).

(Continued)

Group	Lesion Type	Definition
FLUID-FILLED	Abscess	A localized accumulation of pus in the dermis or subcutaneous tissue. Frequently red, warm, and tender (Fig. 3-9).
	Bulla	A fluid-filled blister greater than 0.5 cm in diameter. Fluid can be clear, serous, hemorrhagic, or pus filled (Fig. 3-10).
	Pustule	A circumscribed elevation that contains pus. Pustules are usually less than 0.5 cm in diameter (Fig. 3-11).
	Vesicle	Fluid-filled cavity or elevation less than 0.5 cm in diameter. Fluid may be clear, serous, hemorrhagic, or pus filled (Fig. 3-12).
RED BLANCHABLE	Erythema	Localized, blanchable redness of the skin or mucous membranes (Fig. 3-13).
	Erythroderma	Generalized, blanchable redness of the skin that may be associated with desquamation (Fig.3-14).
	Telangiectasia	Visible, persistent dilation of small, superficial cutaneous blood vessels. Telangiectasias will blanch (Fig. 3-15).

(Continued)

(Continued)		
Group	**Lesion Type**	**Definition**
PURPURIC 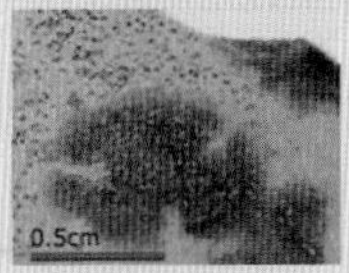	Ecchymosis 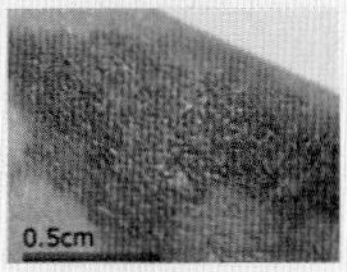	Extravasation of blood into the skin or mucous membranes. Area of flat color change may progress over time from blue-black to brown-yellow or green (Fig. 3-16).
	Petechiae 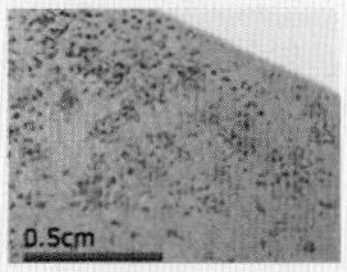	Tiny 1–2 mm, initially purpuric, nonblanchable macules resulting from tiny hemorrhages (Fig. 3-17).
	Palpable Purpura 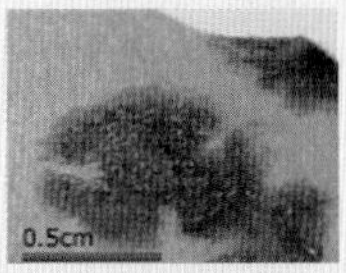	Raised and palpable, nonblanchable, red or violaceous discoloration of skin or mucous membranes due to vascular inflammation in the skin and extravasation of red blood cells (Fig. 3-18).
SUNKEN 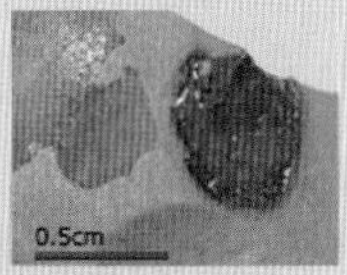	Atrophy 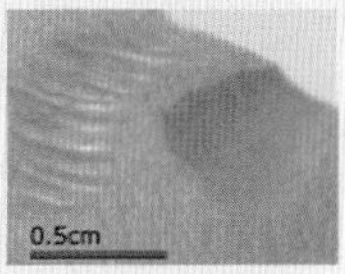	A thinning of tissue defined by its location, such as epidermal atrophy, dermal atrophy, or subcutaneous atrophy (Fig. 3-19).
	Erosion 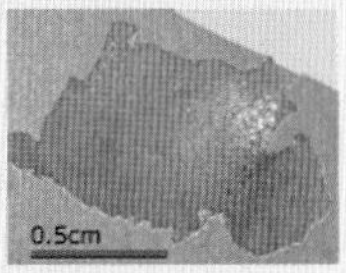	A localized loss of the epidermal or mucosal epithelium (Fig. 3-20).
	Ulcer 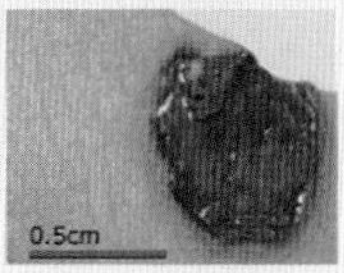	A circumscribed loss of the epidermis and at least upper dermis. Ulcers are further classified by their depth, border/shape, edge, and tissue at its base (Fig. 3-21).
GANGRENE	Gangrene 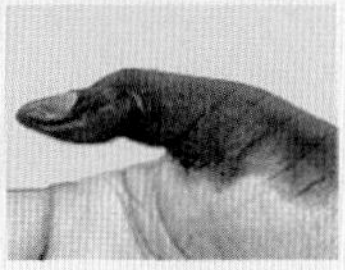	Necrotic, usually black, tissue due to obstruction, diminution, or loss of blood supply. Gangrene may be wet or dry (Fig. 3-22).
ESCHAR	Eschar 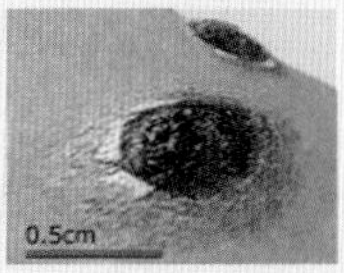	An adherent thick, dry, black crust (Fig. 3-23).

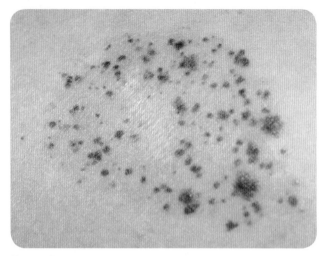

Figure 3-1 Speckled lentiginous nevus (nevus spilus) is macular lesions with a faint brown background and multiple darker macules of varying sizes.

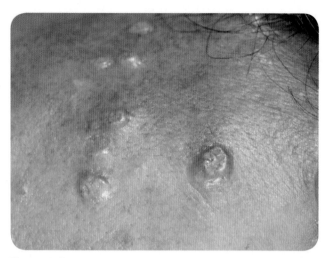

Figure 3-3 Molluscum contagiosum with multiple papules, many of which have central umbilications.

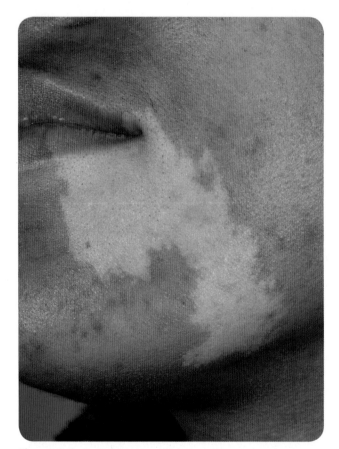

Figure 3-2 Hypopigmented macule of vitiligo with sharp borders between depigmented and uninvolved skin. Small pigmented macules may persist in the depigmented macule.

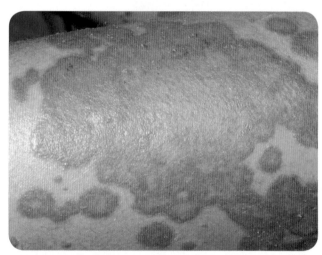

Figure 3-4 Psoriasis with papules of various sizes and then large raised plaques that arise from confluent papules.

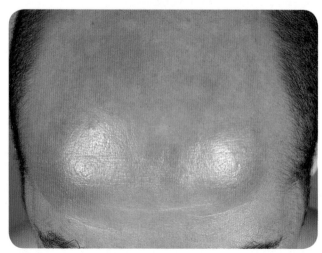

Figure 3-5 Nodules of T-cell lymphoma have a surface component and a deeper component.

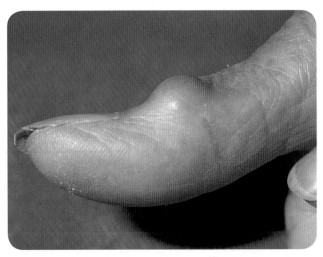

Figure 3-6 Myxoid cysts (mucoid cysts) contain mucinous fluid and are deep lesions in the dermis that most frequently arise from the distal joint of a finger.

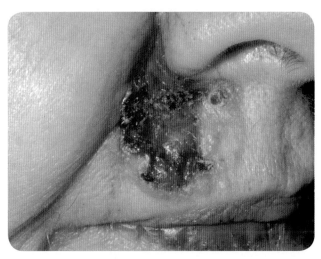

Figure 3-7 Irregular crust on an eroded basal cell carcinoma.

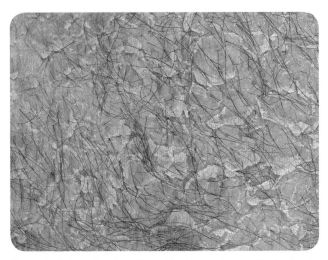

Figure 3-8 Irregular plate-like scales characterize lamellar ichthyosis.

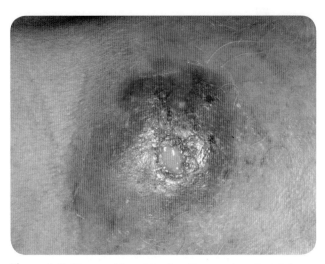

Figure 3-9 Abscess with peripheral erythema and purulent drainage.

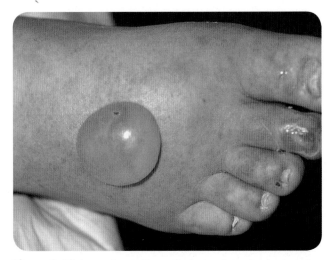

Figure 3-10 Large clear bulla on the foot or lower leg is characteristic of diabetic bullae. They are typically not infected.

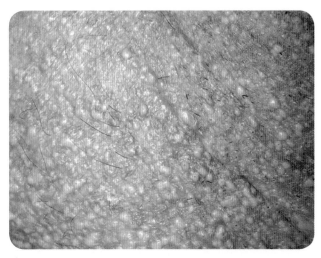

Figure 3-11 Multiple pustules characterize acute generalized exanthematous pustulosis, which is usually caused by a drug eruption.

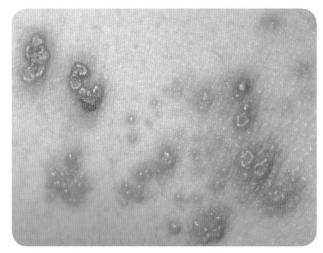

Figure 3-12 Multiple vesicles due to the varicella-zoster virus. Many of the vesicles are grouped and some are umbilicated. Herpes simplex causes similar lesions.

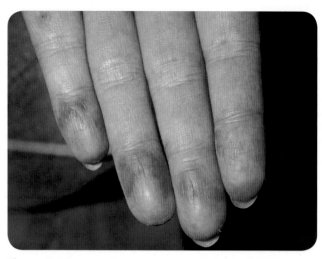

Figure 3-13 Erythema may be the only presenting feature of lupus erythematosus.

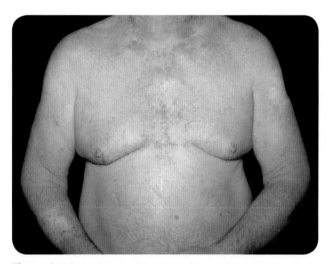

Figure 3-14 Persistent erythroderma due to enalapril maleate.

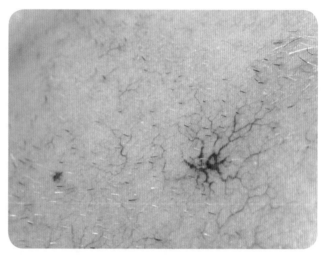

Figure 3-15 One or more telangiectasias are common in sun-exposed skin above the waist.

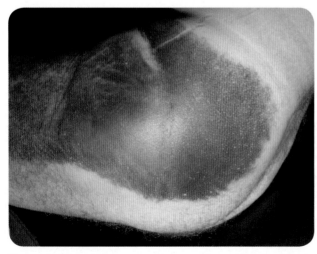

Figure 3-16 Ecchymoses secondary to a bike accident in a healthy adult.

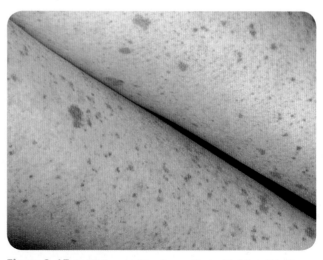

Figure 3-17 Multiple petechiae in a patient with idiopathic thrombocytopenic purpura.

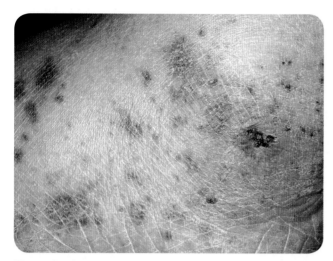

Figure 3-18 Palpable purpura in leukocytoclastic vasculitis is characteristically on the lower extremities.

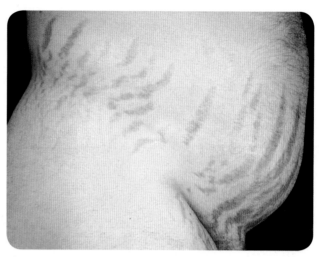

Figure 3-19 Striae caused by steroid atrophy in a male after high-dose oral cortisone to treat pemphigus vulgaris.

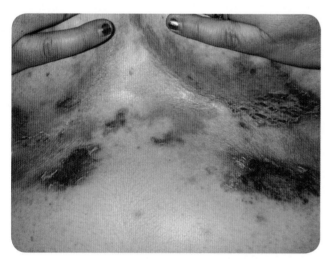

Figure 3-20 Inframammary erosions are characteristic of benign familial pemphigus.

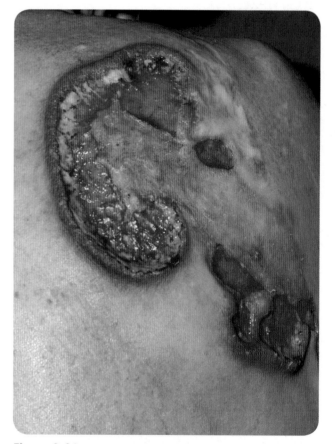

Figure 3-21 Raised, undermined border in an ulcerated lesion is characteristic of pyoderma gangrenosum.

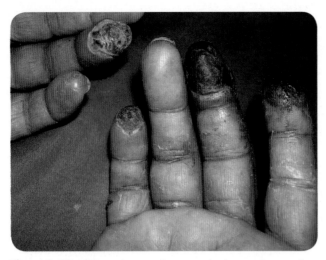

Figure 3-22 Different degrees of gangrene in the vascular complications of Buerger disease.

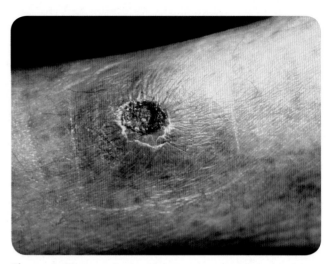

Figure 3-23 Hemorrhagic adherent crust associated with rickettsialpox.

Distributions

Skin lesions can occur at a discrete body location or form a distribution pattern by involving multiple body surfaces. Distribution refers to the pattern in which multiple lesions are arranged. Both location and distribution can be powerful clues in the process of developing a differential diagnosis. Learn the most important distributions in this section and visit www.essentialdermatology.com for additional definitions and an interactive self-study quiz.

Distribution	Definition
Acral 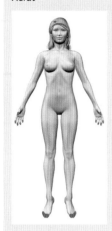	An acral pattern of skin lesions involves the distal aspects of the head (ears and nose) and the extremities (hands, fingers, feet, and toes).
Dermatomal 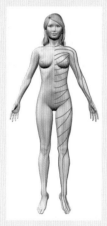	Dermatomal distribution includes an area of skin following the sensory skin innervation of a particular nerve root. Dermatomal distributions do not cross the midline of the body.
Intertriginous 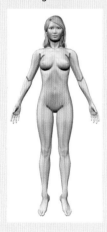	Intertriginous distribution involves skin creases and folds. An intertriginous pattern includes involvement of the axillae, crural fold, gluteal crease, and possibly the inframammary fold.

(Continued)

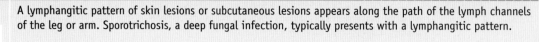

(Continued)	
Distribution	**Definition**
Lymphangitic 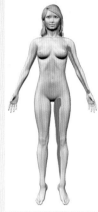	A lymphangitic pattern of skin lesions or subcutaneous lesions appears along the path of the lymph channels of the leg or arm. Sporotrichosis, a deep fungal infection, typically presents with a lymphangitic pattern.
Photodistributed 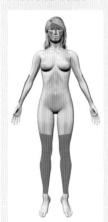	A photodistributed pattern follows the sun-exposed skin. Typical areas of involvement are the forehead, chest, upper back, upper ears, nose, cheeks, upper lip, neck, forearms, and dorsum of the hands.
Scattered 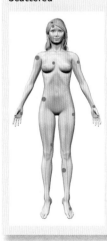	Skin lesions occurring across many body locations can appear to be distributed randomly or haphazardly. A severe case of poison ivy dermatitis could appear widely scattered.

(Continued)

(Continued)	
Distribution	Definition
Symmetric	Skin lesions that are found symmetrically on the extremities can be indicative of diagnoses of many etiologies, including infectious, metabolic, genetic, and inflammatory causes.
Widespread	A widespread distribution involves the entire—or almost the entire—body.

CHAPTER 4

Essential Adult Skin Diseases

This chapter contains 195 diseases and disorders organized according to their common presentations. These clinical presentations are divided by morphology and are in the order as shown in Morphology Indexes 4-1 and 4-2 for multiple lesions; Morphology Index 4-3 for lesions that are often present as solitary or few growths; and Morphology Index 4-4 for lesions on the scalp, nails, the genital region, or in the mouth. One major challenge of clinical diagnosis is disease variability. These lists are guides for those using this text book alone. The complexity and number of disorders in adults should encourage the user to refer to the VisualDx online diagnostic resource that accompanies this book. Using the online system is a powerful way to assist with building a differential diagnosis. Start by going to www.essentialdermatology.com to activate your free 1-year subscription. Further instructions and your activation product code are detailed on the inside front cover of this book.

Alphabetical Index 4-5 contains all of the discrete diseases in an alphabetical list with the appropriate page number for the disorder.

Because the timing of disease presentation is usually critical to developing a differential diagnosis, we have listed disorders that are often of acute onset (i.e., hours to a few days) in italics.

MORPHOLOGY INDEX 4-1 Multiple Lesions or Rash in the Well Adult

(Continued)

MORPHOLOGY INDEX 4-1 *(Continued)*

MORPHOLOGY INDEX 4-2 Multiple Lesions or Rash in the Febrile, Ill, or Toxic-Appearing Adult

MORPHOLOGY INDEX 4-3 Single Lesion or Growth

Lumps and Bumps

MORPHOLOGY INDEX 4-4 Special Locations

Scalp

Nails

Perineum

Mouth

ALPHABETICAL INDEX 4-5 Alphabetical List of All Adult Essential Skin Disease

ALPHABETICAL INDEX 4-5   *(Continued)*

Dermatographism

Diagnosis Synopsis

Dermatographism is the most common form of physical urticaria and manifests as an exaggerated wheal and flare reaction of the skin induced by pressure. In dermatographism, inadvertent stroking or rubbing of the skin will result in corresponding linear wheals. The wheals usually persist for 15 to 30 min. It is usually asymptomatic, but some forms are associated with pruritus. The exact cause of dermatographism is unknown. An increased incidence has been reported during pregnancy, in individuals with Behçet disease, thyroid disorders, infections, and atopic dermatitis. It affects approximately 2% to 5% of the population and is more common in young adults.

Look For

Linear wheals or geometric shapes are suggestive of external provocation such as stroking or rubbing the skin (Figs. 4-1–4-4). The extent of the white inner portion and the extent of the wheal are more than the normal triple response of Lewis (wheal and flare reaction).

Dermatographism may occur on any body surface, but the scalp and genitalia are less frequently involved.

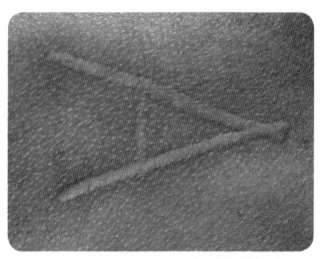

Figure 4-1 Dermatographism is an exaggerated response to pressure.

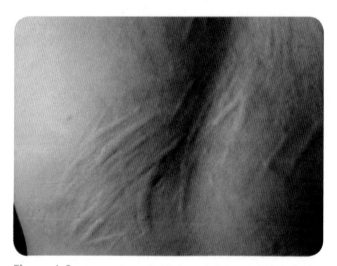

Figure 4-2 Pressure from clothing or sitting can bring out dermatographism.

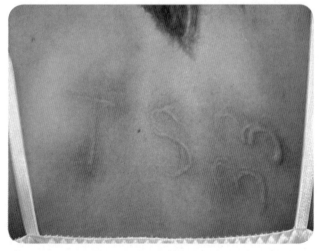

Figure 4-3 Central edema and peripheral erythema characterize dermatographism.

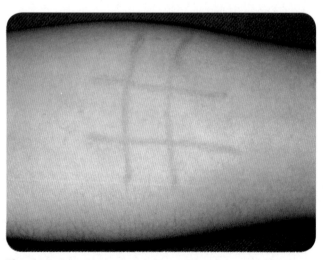

Figure 4-4 Resolving dermatographism, with erythema and most edema gone.

Diagnostic Pearls

- Folds from clothing may produce complex patterns.
- Dermatographism may occur concomitantly with other physical urticarias such as cold or pressure-induced urticaria. Pressure urticaria may be delayed and is usually painful, while dermatographism develops over minutes and is asymptomatic or pruritic. Most patients with active urticaria also manifest dermatographism.

 ## Differential Diagnosis and Pitfalls

- Early contact dermatitis may present with linear urticarial lesions.
- Urticaria pigmentosa
- Lesions from strongyloides (cutaneous larva migrans) may resemble rapidly moving urticarial wheals.
- The early stages of bullous pemphigoid may manifest with urticarial plaques.
- Systemic mastocytosis
- Urticaria
- Angioedema

 ## Best Tests

- Reproduce lesions by firm, slow pressure with the dull end of a pen cap or a ballpoint pen tip (retracted). Test yourself at the same time for comparison.

Management Pearls

- If treatment is desired by the patient, be sure to warn him/her about the sedating effects of certain antihistamines.

Therapy

Most cases can be managed with an H1 antihistamine. Using a second/third-generation antihistamine is recommended because they cause less sedation and have a longer half-life. H1 and H2 antihistamines may be combined in severe cases.

First-Generation Antihistamines
- Diphenhydramine hydrochloride (25, 50 mg tablets or capsules): 25 to 50 mg nightly or every 6 h, as needed
- Hydroxyzine (10, 25 mg tablets): 12.5 to 25 mg, every 6 h, as needed

Second-Generation Antihistamines
H1 Blockers
- Cetirizine 10 mg daily or twice daily
- Loratadine 10 mg daily or twice daily
- Fexofenadine 120 to 180 mg daily

H2 Blockers
- Cimetidine 400 mg two to three times daily
- Ranitidine 150 mg twice daily

Psoralen plus UVA (PUVA) has been reported to help several symptomatic patients by decreasing pruritus.

Suggested Readings

James WD, Berger TG, Elston DM. Erythema and urticaria. In: James WD, Berger TG, Elston DM, Odom RB, eds. *Andrews' Diseases of the Skin: Clinical Dermatology.* 10th Ed. Philadelphia, PA: Saunders Elsevier; 2006:153.

Wong RC, Fairley JA, Ellis CN. Dermographism: A review. *J Am Acad Dermatol.* 1984 Oct;11(4 Pt 1):643–652.

Diagnosis Synopsis

Drug-induced photosensitivity can be divided into two kinds of reactions: phototoxic and photoallergic.

Drug-induced phototoxicity results in a rash similar to sunburn. The rash is thought to result from systemic drug (circulating in superficial dermal blood vessels) absorbing ultraviolet light (UVL) and releasing free radicals and reactive oxygen species, which damage or "burn" the skin in only those areas exposed to the UV source. All drugs that cause such a reaction absorb UV and/or visible radiation. The effects are dependent on both the dose of the drug and the amount of UVL that the person is exposed to.

In general, patients with a phototoxic drug eruption complain of burning.

Three types of clinical reactions can occur:

- Immediate/Mild—Immediate onset of erythema occurring approximately 30 min after UVL exposure. This reaction is associated with burning and pruritus but minimal edema. It usually lasts for 1 to 2 days after stopping UVL exposure.
- Immediate/Wheals—Immediate onset of transient wheals associated with burning. This reaction can occur with room light (non-UVL) and resolves rapidly after light exposure is stopped.
- Delayed/Severe—Onset is 8 to 24 h after UVL exposure. This reaction is associated with dark erythema, edema, and hyperpigmentation. Blistering may occur with severe reactions. It usually lasts 2 to 4 days after UVL exposure is stopped, but in some instances, it may persist for months.

Phototoxic drug reactions are predictable and dose related in the sense that all patients exposed to enough drugs and enough UV exposure will develop phototoxicity. Some of the more common offenders include the following: antiarrhythmics (amiodarone and quinidine), antifungals (voriconazole), diuretics (furosemide and thiazides), NSAIDs (nabumetone, naproxen, and piroxicam), phenothiazines (chlorpromazine, and prochlorperazine), psoralens (5-methoxypsoralen and 8-methoxypsoralen), quinolones (ciprofloxacin, lomefloxacin, nalidixic acid, and sparfloxacin), tetracyclines (doxycycline, and demeclocycline), St. John's wort, topical tar.

Drug-induced photoallergic reactions are allergic reactions due to UVL-induced alteration of a drug. They are dose independent and do not occur in all patients. Patients typically complain of itching rather than burning, and symptoms tend to be chronic. Common offenders include the following: sunscreens (oxybenzone), fragrances (musk ambrette and sandalwood oil), topical antimicrobial agents (chlorhexidine, fenticlor, and hexachlorophene), NSAIDs (diclofenac, ketoprofen, and piroxicam), phenothiazines (chlorpromazine and promethazine), antiarrhythmics (quinidine), antifungals (griseofulvin), antimalarials (quinine), quinolones (enoxacin, lomefloxacin), and sulfonamides.

◉ Look For

Phototoxic drug reaction: In sun-exposed areas, a bright red, confluent rash, sometimes accompanied by edema, weeping, blistering, and later desquamation. Patients may complain of a burning or stinging sensation with onset of the rash.

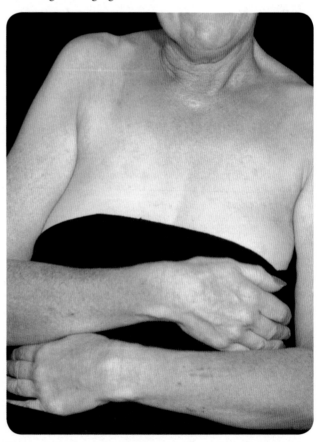

Figure 4-6 Upper chest photosensitivity reaction to meprobamate.

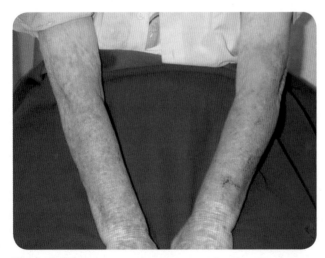

Figure 4-5 Extensor arms are very common locations for photosensitivity reactions.

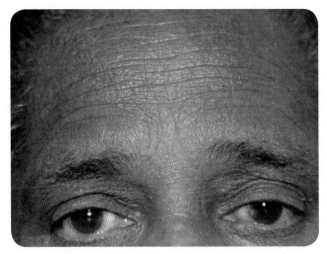

Figure 4-7 Chronic photosensitivity reaction to glyburide.

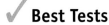

Erythema most prominent at the forehead, superior cheeks, lips, the "V" of the chest, extensor arms, and dorsum of the hands (Figs. 4-5–4-7). There are often sharp cutoffs where clothing and other barriers have blocked UV rays (Fig. 4-8).

Photoallergic reaction: Lesions are dermatitic (papular with or without pinpoint vesicles and/or scale) or lichen planus-like (flat topped and hyperpigmented). Lesions begin in photo-exposed areas but may generalize to include photo-protected areas.

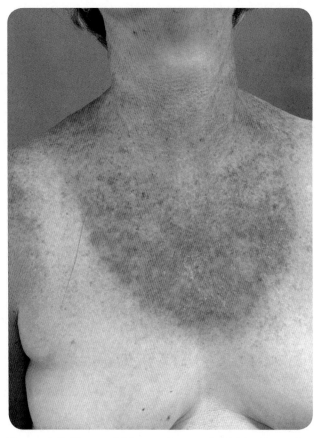

Figure 4-8 Photosensitivity reaction to griseofulvin. Upper chest involvement is common.

Diagnostic Pearls

- Skin under the nose, chin, and other areas protected from direct exposure to the sun may be rash-free. Drug-induced photosensitivity is often related to acute, intense sun exposure.

Differential Diagnosis and Pitfalls

- Sunburn
- Systemic lupus erythematosus
- Dermatomyositis
- Porphyria cutanea tarda
- Pseudoporphyria
- Airborne contact dermatitis
- Autoimmune blistering disease (in severe reactions)
- Phytophotodermatitis
- Widespread dermatitis
- Lichen planus (if lichenoid papules are present)

Best Tests

- This is typically a clinical diagnosis but can be confirmed by biopsy.

- Take a careful medication history in any patient presenting with a photodistributed rash. Although glass greater than 0.6 cm thick filters UVB, UVA is generally not filtered by standard glass. Because most phototoxic drug reactions occur in the UVA spectrum, a careful history of light exposure through window glass should be taken.
- Phototesting can be performed to confirm the diagnosis. A positive phototest will show a decreased minimal erythema dose to UVA.
- Additional testing, such as urinary porphyrin levels and screening for autoantibodies, is occasionally done to rule out other photosensitive dermatoses.

Management Pearls

- To prevent sunburn, impress upon patients to avoid sun exposure at midday (10:00 AM to 3:00 PM), use barrier protectants (tightly woven clothes and hats), and apply sunscreen that includes both UVA and UVB ("broad-spectrum") coverage and is at least SPF (sun protection factor) 30.
- Eliminate the medication from the patient's regimen if at all possible. If this cannot be done, counsel the patient about sun protection and sun avoidance.

Therapy

Treatment is supportive and involves decreasing the dose of or eliminating altogether the use of the drug and limiting exposure to UV sources. The patient should use combined UVB/UVA sunscreens (with titanium dioxide or with the UVA blocker Parsol 1789).

Phototoxic

Cool compresses will provide some symptomatic relief. Cool milk or Burow solution soaks are an alternative.

Nonsteroidal anti-inflammatory agents (NSAIDs) may help decrease the degree of erythema and will help with the discomfort. NSAIDs should not be used if they have been used by the patient prior to the onset of the rash, as this class of agents is known to be a photosensitizer.

For severe reactions, early administration of prednisone (40 to 60 mg per day for only a few days with no taper) may also help reduce the inflammation.

In very rare instances, patients may develop severe second-degree sunburns necessitating an aggressive skin care regimen, electrolyte management, and fluid replacement.

Photoallergic

Although removal of the offending medication often provides relief, the reaction may take several months, rarely years, to resolve.

Topical corticosteroids can be used for symptomatic relief. Patients whose photosensitivity persists for months or years require a dermatologic evaluation and may benefit from psoralen plus UVA (PUVA), hydroxychloroquine, or azathioprine.

Suggested Readings

Allen JE. Drug-induced photosensitivity. *Clin Pharm.* 1993 Aug;12(8): 580–587.

Gould JW, Mercurio MG, Elmets CA. Cutaneous photosensitivity diseases induced by exogenous agents. *J Am Acad Dermatol.* 1995 Oct;33(4): 551–573; quiz 574–576.

Kaidbey KH, Mitchell FN. Photosensitizing potential of certain nonsteroidal anti-inflammatory agents. *Arch Dermatol.* 1989 Jun;125(6):783–786.

Moore DE. Drug-induced cutaneous photosensitivity: Incidence, mechanism, prevention and management. *Drug Saf.* 2002;25(5):345–372.

Nedorost ST, Dijkstra JW, Handel DW. Drug-induced photosensitivity reaction. *Arch Dermatol.* 1989 Mar;125(3):433–434.

Erythema Multiforme Minor

Diagnosis Synopsis

Erythema multiforme (EM) is an acute, self-limited inflammatory skin reaction characterized by the sudden onset of erythematous papules in an acral distribution. The lesions of EM are classically described as targetoid. In contrast to Stevens-Johnson syndrome (SJS) and toxic epidermal necrolysis (TEN), EM is most often precipitated by viral or other infectious pathogens, not medications. It is now recognized that EM does not progress to TEN. Two subtypes exist: EM major and EM minor. Key differences between the EM subtypes include mucosal involvement and systemic symptoms such as fever, arthralgias, and asthenias seen in the major subtype. Both subtypes can occur at any age, in both sexes, and in any ethnicity but are seen most commonly in young adults following herpes simplex virus (HSV) infection.

While the etiology remains unclear, genetically susceptible individuals with certain HLA subtypes (HLA-DRw53, HLA-DQw3, and HLA-Aw33) may trigger aberrant cellular and humoral responses after exposure to infection. The majority of EM cutaneous eruptions are believed to be in response to HSV-1 or HSV-2 infections. Other known precipitating pathogens include varicella, parapoxvirus, adenovirus, coxsackievirus, HIV, hepatitis, *Mycoplasma pneumonia*, *Salmonella*, and *Histoplasma capsulatum*.

The progression of the cutaneous eruption of EM is usually complete within 72 h. It remains fixed for up to 2 weeks and resolves without sequelae. While the face and upper extremities are the most commonly affected sites, EM can appear on the palms, neck, trunk, and, less commonly, on the legs. Pruritus is a commonly associated feature.

The following points should be kept in mind when a diagnosis of EM is being considered:

- Herpes labialis may precede, develop concomitantly, or manifest after the onset of EM. In almost half of all cases, herpes labialis precedes EM.
- Although a strong association exists with HSV and EM, a direct immunofluorescence test or viral culture for HSV will be negative in EM lesions.
- Classical target lesions are well-defined circular lesions that are less than 3 cm in diameter, have three distinct color zones, and a central zone that has a bulla or crust.
- Atypical target lesions are palpable, poorly defined, circular lesions that have two distinct color zones.
- EM minor can demonstrate classical target lesions, atypical target lesions, or both concomitantly.
- EM, SJS, and TEN can clinically resemble each other. Clinical differences include the following: EM has characteristic target lesions and occurs on the extremities more often than trunk. In over 90% of cases, the precipitating factor is a viral infection, not medications. Lesions are often papular, and the Nikolsky sign is negative.
- EM is not considered within the same disease spectrum as SJS/TEN and confers no risk in progressing to TEN.

Immunocompromised Patient Considerations

HIV infection is a known cause of EM minor.

Look For

Classical target lesions are well-defined, circular, erythematous macules or papules that are less than 3 cm in diameter, have three distinct color zones, and a central zone that has a bulla or crust (Figs. 4-9–4-12).

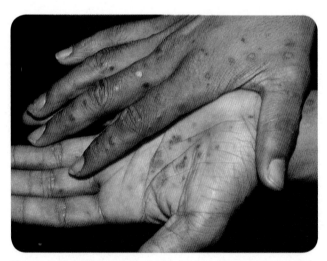

Figure 4-9 Multiple papules on the dorsum and volar surfaces of the hands and small erosions on the dorsum in EM minor.

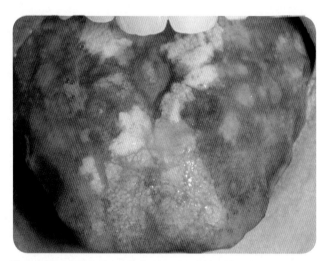

Figure 4-10 EM minor of the tongue with red erosions and white hyperkeratosis.

35

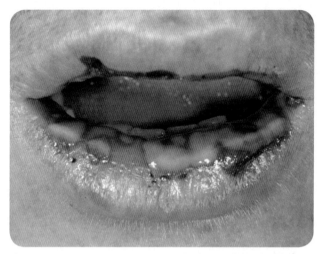

Figure 4-11 Lip ulcerations sparing the vermillion border in EM minor.

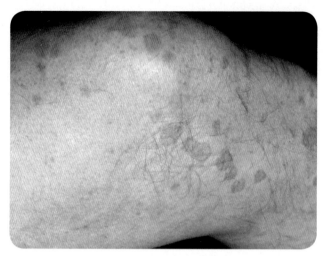

Figure 4-12 EM minor in a patient with HIV; there are suggestions of target lesions within some of the red plaques.

Atypical target lesions are poorly defined, circular, erythematous papules that have two distinct color zones.

Diagnostic Pearls

- Recurrent EM eruptions can occur and are more likely if the inciting cause is an HSV infection.
- Postinflammatory hyper- or hypopigmentation are unlikely but may occur.

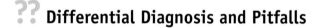

?? Differential Diagnosis and Pitfalls

- SJS/TEN—Histological features may not differentiate EM from SJS/TEN. Clinically, however, look for irregularly shaped, dusky red macular- or patch-like lesions on the trunk, face, and palms/soles. A positive Nikolsky sign can be found; mucosal involvement, including the eyes, lips, mouth, and genitalia. Look for hemorrhagic crust, bullae, and denudation in these areas. Systemic symptoms are commonly present but not invariable. Lesions are more pronounced on the trunk than on the extremities. Precipitating factors are usually medications.
- Urticaria—New lesions appear daily; lesions are transient and last less than 24 h, associated with the edema of lips, face, hands, and feet. No evidence of epidermal damage in the center of urticarial lesions. Subcutaneous epinephrine injections will clear urticarial lesions but not EM lesions.
- Generalized fixed drug eruption—Look for erythematous plaques that develop on the lips, face, distal extremities, and genitalia 1 to 2 weeks after medication ingestions. Oral mucosa can be involved. Histology will differentiate fixed drug eruption from EM.
- Erythema annulare centrifugum (EAC)—Erythematous, annular patches and plaques that are idiopathic in nature;

can last from days to months, no systemic symptoms, lesions commonly appear on hips and thighs. Biopsy will differentiate EAC and EM.
- Lichen planus—Very pruritic, sometimes associated with hepatitis C. Biopsy will differentiate EM from lichen planus.
- Subacute cutaneous lupus erythematosus (SCLE)—Check ANA, will be positive in majority of lupus patients. SCLE is characterized by annular plaques with raised borders and central clearing or papulosquamous lesions that are restricted to sun-exposed skin.
- Secondary syphilis—Scattered scaling papules and plaques; check RPR, check for the history of primary chancre and systemic symptoms.
- Leukocytoclastic vasculitis (LCV)—Palpable purpura is the most common finding, consisting of nonblanching 1 to 3 mm, violaceous, round papules, characteristically involving the lower extremities. Biopsy will differentiate fixed LCV from EM.
- Arthropod bites—Haphazard distribution of erythematous papules.
- Id reaction
- Viral exanthem
- If the patient has systemic symptoms or oral mucosal involvement, consider EM major.

✓ Best Tests

- EM minor is largely a clinical diagnosis, based on history and the classic appearance and location of skin lesions.
- Skin biopsy for histological examination and direct immunofluorescence may help to rule out other bullous disease.
- If grouped vesicles are present, culture them for HSV and/or perform HSV PCR.

▲▲ Management Pearls

- Discontinue any possible causative drug.
- Treat any secondarily infected lesions with the appropriate topical or systemic antibiotic.
- Consider a dermatology consultation.

Immunocompromised Patient Considerations

In recurrence, treating the underlying cause early in the course with systemic anti-herpetic agents is a reasonable approach.

Therapy

Treat any identifiable underlying condition. The following treatment strategy will be focused on EM minor.

Because EM minor is typically self-limited, it only requires symptomatic relief. NSAIDs can be used for the relief of minor discomfort. Cool compresses may be soothing. Oral antihistamines may be prescribed in cases in which pruritus is a factor, as can mild-to-mid-potency topical steroid preparations.

Antihistamines

- Diphenhydramine hydrochloride (25, 50 mg tablets or capsules): 25 to 50 mg nightly or every 6 h, as needed
- Hydroxyzine (10, 25 mg tablets): 12.5 to 25 mg every 6 h, as needed
- Cetirizine hydrochloride (5, 10 mg tablets): 5 to 10 mg per day
- Loratadine (10 mg tablet): 10 mg once daily

Mid-potency topical corticosteroids (Classes 3 and 4)

- Triamcinolone cream or ointment—apply twice daily (15, 30, 60, 120, 240 g)
- Mometasone cream or ointment—apply twice daily (15, 45 g)
- Fluocinolone ointment or cream—apply twice daily (15, 30, 60 g)

Mild-potency topical corticosteroids (Class 6 or 7)

- Desonide cream or lotion—apply twice daily (15, 30, 60 g)
- Hydrocortisone cream 2.5%—apply twice daily (1, 2 oz)

Recurrent EM minor (more than six attacks per year) may respond to long-term acyclovir (400 mg p.o. twice daily) or valacyclovir (500 mg p.o. daily).

See HSV therapy sections for primary or recurrent HSV infections.

Azathioprine (100 to 150 mg p.o. daily) has been reported to be useful in several cases, as has dapsone (100 to 150 mg daily) and thalidomide (25 to 200 mg p.o. daily).

Systemic corticosteroids are not recommended in mild cases due to HSV because they may actually lead to continuing EM eruptions.

Suggested Readings

Auquier-Dunant A, Mockenhaupt M, Naldi L, et al.; SCAR Study Group. Severe cutaneous adverse reactions. Correlations between clinical patterns and causes of erythema multiforme majus, Stevens-Johnson syndrome, and toxic epidermal necrolysis: Results of an international prospective study. *Arch Dermatol*. 2002 Aug;138(8):1019–1024.

Bastuji-Garin S, Rzany B, Stern RS, et al. Clinical classification of cases of toxic epidermal necrolysis, Stevens-Johnson syndrome, and erythema multiforme. *Arch Dermatol*. 1993 Jan;129(1):92–96.

Gober MD, Laing JM, Burnett JW, et al. The Herpes simplex virus gene Pol expressed in herpes-associated erythema multiforme lesions upregulates/activates SP1 and inflammatory cytokines. *Dermatology*. 2007;215(2):97–106.

Grosber M, Alexandre M, Poszepczynska-Guigné E, et al. Recurrent erythema multiforme in association with recurrent Mycoplasma pneumoniae infections. *J Am Acad Dermatol*. 2007 May;56(5 Suppl.):S118–S119.

Marzano AV, Frezzolini A, Caproni M, et al. Immunohistochemical expression of apoptotic markers in drug-induced erythema multiforme, Stevens-Johnson syndrome and toxic epidermal necrolysis. *Int J Immunopathol Pharmacol*. 2007 Jul–Sep;20(3):557–566.

Olut AI, Erkek E, Ozunlu H, et al. Erythema multiforme associated with acute hepatitis B virus infection. *Clin Exp Dermatol*. 2006 Jan;31(1):137–138.

Weston WL. Herpes-associated erythema multiforme. *J Invest Dermatol*. 2005 Jun;124(6):xv–xvi.

Williams PM, Conklin RJ. Erythema multiforme: A review and contrast from Stevens-Johnson syndrome/toxic epidermal necrolysis. *Dent Clin North Am*. 2005 Jan;49(1):67–76, viii.

▪▪ Diagnosis Synopsis

Primary human immunodeficiency virus (HIV) infection (PHI) syndrome, also called acute retroviral syndrome, is an acute flu-like illness that develops anywhere from 1 to 6 weeks following an exposure to HIV. PHI is believed to occur in 40% to 80% of newly infected individuals. Symptoms are variable: fever, headache, lymphadenopathy, nausea, diarrhea, rash, and pharyngitis are usually present. Other symptoms include vomiting, arthralgias, and photophobia.

The cutaneous eruption is characteristically a morbilliform exanthem resembling a simple drug or viral exanthem. The palms and soles are usually spared, and lymphadenopathy is usually present. It may last for a few days to several weeks, with most cases resolving within 4 to 5 days. The eruption is self-limited.

PHI occurs prior to the development of sufficient HIV antibodies for an individual to test positive on enzyme-linked immunosorbent assay (ELISA) or western blot. These antibodies can take 2 to 4 months to develop. PHI is also important to recognize from a public health perspective. Patients with PHI are ten times more likely to transmit HIV as compared to the chronic phase of HIV infection. Patients with PHI are most likely to present to primary care physicians, emergency rooms, urgent care and walk-in centers, or general medicine clinics. Approximately 90% of cases are not diagnosed at the primary encounter.

◉ Look For

A transient, blanching morbilliform eruption, primarily involves the trunk (Fig. 4-13). Lymphadenopathy is usually prominent. Oral and penile ulcers in males are findings that have also been associated with PHI.

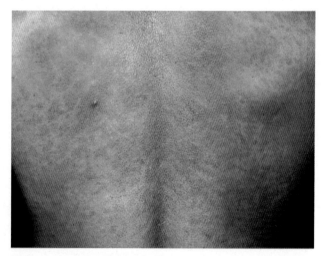

Figure 4-13 Fine, discrete, confluent papules on the upper back.

●● Diagnostic Pearls

- Diagnosis is based on clinical suspicion in those at risk, such as the sexually promiscuous, intravenous drug users, and men who have sex with men.
- Consider the diagnosis of PHI in any individual with flu-like symptoms and risk factors for HIV. Specifically, fever for greater that 7 days, morbilliform eruption, lymphadenopathy, elevated liver enzymes, and reversal of the CD4:CD8 ratio warrant HIV viral load testing, even if clear risk factors for HIV are not elicited by history.

?? Differential Diagnosis and Pitfalls

- Clinically similar to mononucleosis
- Consider any viral-induced exanthem
- Influenza
- Viral hepatitis
- Measles
- Rubella
- Exanthematous drug eruption if there is a history of preceding medication use
- Cytomegalovirus infection
- Secondary syphilis
- Toxoplasmosis
- Brucellosis
- Malaria

✓ Best Tests

- In the acute stage of infection, viral RNA can be detected by polymerase chain reaction methods prior to the formation of antibodies. An HIV viral load and CD4+ T-cell count should be performed at initial presentation.
- The diagnosis of primary HIV infection should be confirmed with ELISA in the weeks that follow. Furthermore, western blot analysis should be used as a confirmatory test on all ELISAs yielding a positive result.
- Skin biopsy is nonspecific and will usually not help to make the diagnosis.

▲▲ Management Pearls

- Sequential HIV antibody tests are recommended when clinical suspicion is high.
- Immediate partner notification is essential in any patient with PHI. Have Department of Health notify partners and recommend or obtain HIV testing.

Therapy

When and if therapy is to be instituted is controversial. Points in favor of treatment include decreasing or preventing the seeding of central nervous system (CNS), decreasing HIV transmission, and preserving HIV-directed cytotoxic T lymphocyte. Points against treatment include toxicity, increased risk of resistance, cost of treatment, and the possibility of treating a potential long-term nonprogressor. Consultation with infectious disease specialists may be warranted.

Suggested Readings

Dybul M, Fauci AS, Bartlett JG, et al.; Panel on Clinical Practices for the Treatment of HIV. Guidelines for using antiretroviral agents among HIV-infected adults and adolescents. Recommendations of the Panel on Clinical Practices for Treatment of HIV. *MMWR Recomm Rep*. 2002 May;51(RR-7):1–55.

Graziosi C, Soudeyns H, Rizzardi GP, et al. Immunopathogenesis of HIV infection. *AIDS Res Hum Retroviruses*. 1998 Jun;14 (Suppl. 2):S135–S142.

Huang ST, Lee HC, Liu KH, et al. Acute human immunodeficiency virus infection. *J Microbiol Immunol Infect*. 2005 Feb;38(1):65–68.

Kahn JO, Walker BD. Acute human immunodeficiency virus type 1 infection. *N Engl J Med*. 1998 Jul;339(1):33–39.

Macneal RJ, Dinulos JG. Acute retroviral syndrome. *Dermatol Clin*. 2006 Oct;24(4):431–438, v.

Pilcher CD, Eron JJ, Galvin S, et al. Acute HIV revisited: New opportunities for treatment and prevention. *J Clin Invest*. 2004 Apr;113(7):937–945.

Soogoor M, Daar ES. Primary HIV-1 infection: Diagnosis, pathogenesis, and treatment. *Curr Infect Dis Rep*. 2005 Mar;7(2):147–153.

Sterling TR, Chaisson RE. General clinical manifestations of human immunodeficiency virus (inlcuding the acute retroviral syndrome and oral, cutaneous, renal, ocular, and cardiac diseases). In: Mandell GL, Bennett JE, Dolin R, eds. *Principles and Practice of Infectious Diseases*. 6th Ed. Philadelphia, PA: Elsevier; 2005:1546–1566.

Zetola NM, Pilcher CD. Diagnosis and management of acute HIV infection. *Infect Dis Clin North Am*. 2007 Mar;21(1):19–48, vii.

Livedo Reticularis

■■ Diagnosis Synopsis

Livedo reticularis is a vascular reaction pattern characterized by a reticular (netlike) discoloration on the extremities and trunk. It is caused by decreased blood flow to the skin or impaired outflow in the dermal venous plexus and stagnation of the blood within these vessels. The darker, discolored areas represent the accumulation of deoxygenated blood. Etiologic categories include vasospasm, vessel wall dysfunction (e.g., vasculitis), and vascular flow compromise as in coagulopathies. Livedo reticularis is exacerbated by cold temperatures. It may be physiologic (cutis marmorata), a primary disease (as in idiopathic cases), or associated with other conditions such as collagen vascular diseases. Livedo reticularis is frequently seen in patients with Raynaud disease.

Localized forms may be associated with vasculitis. In severe cases, the extremities are cold and ulcers may form. Sneddon syndrome is extensive diffuse livedo reticularis in a typical racemose, or broken, pattern with cerebrovascular disease (from transient ischemic attacks to frank cerebrovascular accidents); hypertension and antiphospholipid antibodies are often present. Livedo reticularis is also seen in patients with poor vascular flow (e.g., peripheral vascular disease and cardiac failure). There is strong literature evidence for currently used drugs—amantadine, quinidine, and catecholamines—as triggers. Drugs used in the past to treat syphilis—bismuth and arsphenamine—also caused livedo reticularis.

Immunocompromised Patient Considerations

In the immunosuppressed patient, angioinvasive infections should be considered. These may include aspergillosis and other deep fungal infections, strongyloidiasis, and mycobacterial infections.

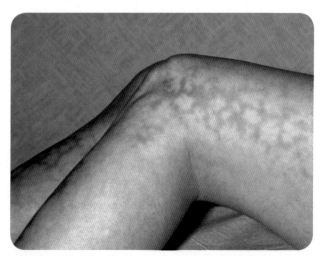

Figure 4-14 Netlike vascular pattern of livedo reticularis.

Look For

Reticular violet to bluish patches on the extremities (Figs. 4-14–4-17).

Dark Skin Considerations

Livedo reticularis was more prevalent in a Latin American subgroup versus whites/Europeans in a study of patients with antiphospholipid syndrome.

●● Diagnostic Pearls

- Elevating the extremity may lessen the color change by increasing venous outflow. The physiologic form of livedo reticularis responds to rewarming.

?? Differential Diagnosis and Pitfalls

Look for associated diseases and/or triggers:

- Collagen vascular diseases or vasculitides (polyarteritis nodosa, systemic lupus erythematosus, rheumatoid arthritis, and dermatomyositis)

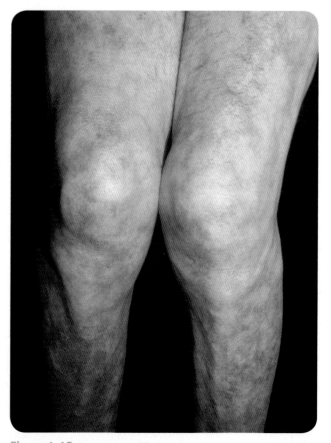

Figure 4-15 Extensive netlike vascular pattern of livedo reticularis.

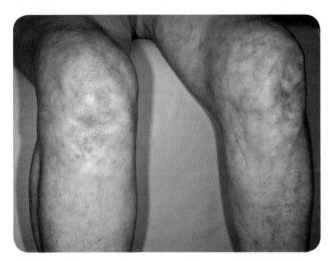

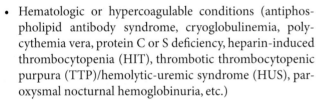

Figure 4-16 Netlike skin, vascular pattern with whitish hypopigmentation of the skin.

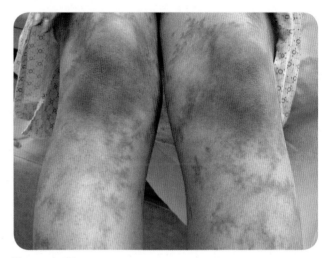

Figure 4-17 Livedo reticularis may be fixed and purpuric, as is this case due to vasculitis.

- Hematologic or hypercoagulable conditions (antiphospholipid antibody syndrome, cryoglobulinemia, polycythemia vera, protein C or S deficiency, heparin-induced thrombocytopenia (HIT), thrombotic thrombocytopenic purpura (TTP)/hemolytic-uremic syndrome (HUS), paroxysmal nocturnal hemoglobinuria, etc.)
- Livedoid vasculopathy
- Embolic phenomena (cholesterol, fat, and septic emboli)
- Deposition diseases (calciphylaxis and oxalosis)
- Medications (amantadine, warfarin, interferon, minocycline, gemcitabine, quinidine, etc.)
- Infections (hepatitis C, *Mycoplasma*, endocarditis, meningococcemia, syphilis, *Rickettsia, M. leprae* [Lucio phenomenon], etc.)
- Neoplasms (renal cell carcinoma, pheochromocytoma, and some hematologic malignancies)
- Neurologic disorders (multiple sclerosis, Parkinson disease, reflex sympathic dystrophy, and Sneddon syndrome)
- Endocrine/metabolic conditions (hypercalcemia, hypothyroidism, and carcinoid)
- Miscellaneous (chronic pancreatitis, heart failure, and Degos disease)
- Pernio is cold-induced distal blisters or ulcers associated with cold and high humidity.
- Erythema ab igne is a form of fixed reticulate dyspigmentation in skin with chronic repeated heat exposure.
- Reticular erythematous mucinosis is a form of cutaneous mucinosis affecting the upper chest with prominent redness.

✓ Best Tests

- Skin biopsy for microscopy and direct immunofluorescence may be helpful if vasculitis is suspected.
- A workup for underlying disease is often indicated:
- CBC with differential

- Serum electrolytes including renal function (blood urea nitrogen [BUN]/Cr)
- Coagulation profile
- Serum lipid profile
- Cryoglobulins
- Cold agglutinins
- Hypercoagulable workup including antiphospholipid antibodies, protein C and S levels, antithrombin III, factor V Leiden mutation, and homocysteine
- Paraproteins
- Antinuclear antibodies, rheumatoid factor, ANCA

▲▲ Management Pearls

- In cases of physiologic livedo reticularis, minimize cold exposure and encourage the use of warm clothing. Gently rewarm the affected area(s).
- Depending on the underlying cause of the livedo reticularis, varying consultations may be needed from clinicians in such specialties as hematology/oncology, rheumatology, infectious diseases, neurology, etc.

Therapy

The cutaneous manifestations of livedo reticularis itself are difficult to treat and do not require any treatment per se. The identification and treatment of the underlying etiology is most important. Be sure to withdraw any medication that may be offending, if possible.

Patients diagnosed with Sneddon syndrome should receive antithrombotic treatment, such as aspirin.

Pentoxifylline (400 mg twice daily) in livedoid vasculopathy.

(Continued)

Psoralen plus UVA (PUVA) has been reported to help two patients with ulcers and recalcitrant livedo reticularis/ livedoid vasculopathy.

Patients with cholesterol emboli as a cause of their disease may benefit from treatment with a statin.

Suggested Readings

Baker C, Kelly R. Other vascular disorders. In: Bolognia J, Jorizzo JL, Rapini RP, eds. *Dermatology*. 2nd Ed. St. Louis, MO: Mosby; 2008:1615–1618.

Blume JE, Miller CC. Livedo reticularis with retiform purpura associated with gefitinib (Iressa). *Int J Dermatol*. 2007 Dec;46(12):1307–1308.

Fleischer AB, Resnick SD. Livedo reticularis. *Dermatol Clin*. 1990 Apr;8(2):347–354.

García-Carrasco M, Galarza C, Gómez-Ponce M, et al. Antiphospholipid syndrome in Latin American patients: clinical and immunologic characteristics and comparison with European patients. *Lupus*. 2007;16(5): 366–373.

Gibbs MB, English JC, Zirwas MJ. Livedo reticularis: an update. *J Am Acad Dermatol*. 2005 Jun;52(6):1009–1019.

Hayes BB, Cook-Norris RH, Miller JL, et al. Amantadine-induced livedo reticularis: a report of two cases. *J Drugs Dermatol*. 2006 Mar;5(3): 288–289.

Marion DF, Terrien CM. Photosensitive livedo reticularis. *Arch Dermatol*. 1973 Jul;108(1):100–101.

Toubi E, Shoenfeld Y. Livedo reticularis as a criterion for antiphospholipid syndrome. *Clin Rev Allergy Immunol*. 2007 Apr;32(2):138–144.

Lupus Erythematosus, Discoid

Diagnosis Synopsis

Discoid lupus erythematosus (DLE) is a scarring photosensitive autoimmune disease and the most common form of chronic cutaneous lupus erythematosus. It has a characteristic clinical appearance consisting of red, scaly plaques with resulting pigmentary changes; the plaques are frequently found on the face and scalp. DLE most commonly afflicts women in the third and fourth decades of life, though it may occur at any age. Black and Latino patients are at increased risk. Only 5% to 10% of patients demonstrate systemic involvement or will go on to develop systemic lupus erythematosus (SLE). Squamous cell carcinoma may develop in chronic DLE scars, especially in sun-exposed areas.

Look For

Raised or scar-like, atrophic, red plaques. The plaques are often covered with adherent scales and will heal so as to leave atrophy, scarring, and depigmentation in the center of the lesion with a peripheral rim of hyperpigmentation (Fig 4-18). In the most common localized form of the disease, only areas above the neck such as the scalp, bridge of the nose, cheeks (Fig. 4-19), lower lip, and ears (Fig. 4-20) are affected by the lesions. The generalized form of the disease affects the torso and upper extremities as well as areas above the neck. Scarring alopecia may be seen (Fig. 4-21). Mucosal lesions and nail involvement may also be seen.

Variants include hyperkeratotic DLE and palmoplantar DLE.

Dark Skin Considerations

Raised or scar-like, dull, edematous, red plaques, especially on the sun-exposed areas of the face and arms. The plaques are often covered with adherent scales and will heal to leave atrophy, telangiectasia, follicular keratotic plugs, depigmentation in the center of the lesion, and hyperpigmentation at the periphery, especially in blacks. The black patient can also present with scaly, hyperkeratotic, inflammatory lesions that are often mistaken for seborrheic dermatitis or eczema. The DLE lesions of people of color classically have a well-demarcated, deep violaceous border surrounding an atrophic hypopigmented plaque.

Diagnostic Pearls

- Only 5% to 10% of patients with DLE will progress to SLE. However, discoid rash is one of the 11 diagnostic criteria for SLE, and 20% of patients with SLE will manifest discoid lesions.
- There may be a positive family history of lupus or connective tissue disease.
- It is unusual to see DLE below the neck if there is no disease above the neck. Patients with disease above and below the neck are said to have generalized DLE and may be at increased risk of developing SLE.
- Peeling back scale in lesions of DLE may reveal follicle-based keratotic spikes. This is known as "the carpet tack sign."

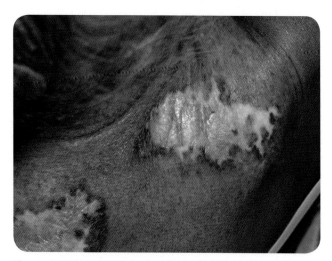

Figure 4-18 Atrophic hypopigmented plaques of discoid lupus often have a rim of hyperpigmented papules.

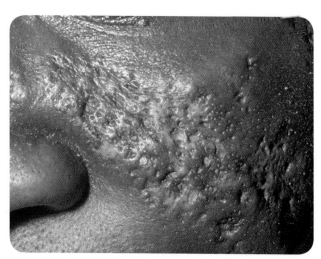

Figure 4-19 Multiple sites of cribriform (ice-pick) scarring are characteristic of discoid lupus.

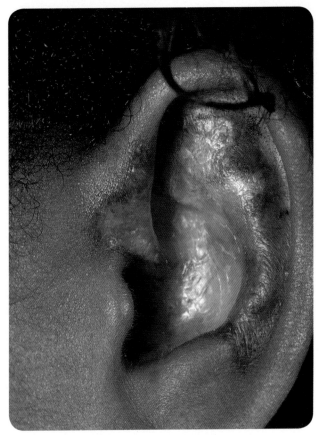

Figure 4-20 Discoid lupus frequently involves the ear, including the concha.

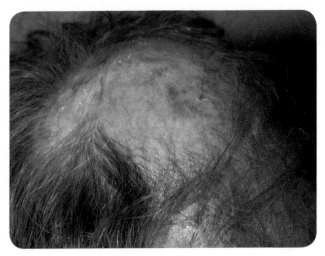

Figure 4-21 Discoid lupus frequently involves the scalp with scarring alopecia.

- Granuloma annulare
- Granuloma faciale
- Dermatomyositis
- Psoriasis
- Syphilis
- Porphyria
- Squamous cell carcinoma
- Sarcoidosis

✓ Best Tests

- Skin biopsy. In addition to typical findings on H&E stained sections, direct immunofluorescence on biopsy specimens may show a "lupus band."
- Autoantibody studies (ANA, anti-Ro [SSA] and anti-La [SSB]) may be helpful, especially in cases where systemic signs and symptoms are present.
- Other routine laboratory tests that may demonstrate findings in the case of systemic involvement include CBC with differential, erythrocyte sedimentation rate (ESR), chemistry panel, and urinalysis.

▲▲ Management Pearls

- Avoid sunlight exposure. Sunscreens with both UVB and UVA blockers (avobenzone with octocrylene, titanium dioxide, and zinc oxide) are recommended. Excessive heat, excessive cold, and trauma to the affected regions have been shown to worsen the condition. Smoking worsens cutaneous lupus.
- The alopecia is considered to be scarring, and patients should be advised that there is little chance of hair regrowth.
- Camouflage cosmetics may be employed.
- Patients with systemic involvement may require referral to a rheumatologist and/or a nephrologist.

Dark Skin Considerations

Other forms of scarring alopecia, especially the follicular degeneration syndrome in blacks, should be considered.

?? Differential Diagnosis and Pitfalls

- *Trichophyton tonsurans* (tinea capitis) infections of the scalp can be very inflammatory and should be ruled out.
- Acute early lesions may resemble polymorphous light eruptions.
- DLE lesions have been associated with chronic granulomatous disease. In familial cases, check for complement deficiency.
- Other forms of scarring alopecia, such as the follicular degeneration syndrome.
- Lichen planus
- Lichen planopilaris
- Burn scar
- Chronic radiation dermatitis
- Subacute cutaneous lupus erythematosus
- Rosacea

Therapy

High-potency topical steroids, flurandrenolide impregnated tape, and/or intralesional corticosteroids (triamcinolone 3 to 10 mg/cc infiltrated into the dermal plaque). Patient use of topical steroids should be monitored closely due to the risk of atrophy. Special care should be taken with facial skin.

High-potency topical corticosteroids should be limited to the hypertrophic lesions.

High-potency topical corticosteroids (classes 1 and 2)

- Clobetasol cream or ointment—apply twice daily
- Fluocinonide cream or ointment—apply twice daily
- Desoximetasone cream or ointment—apply twice daily
- Halcinonide cream or ointment—apply twice daily
- Amcinonide ointment—apply twice daily

Topical immunosuppressive agents: tacrolimus 0.1% ointment or pimecrolimus 1% cream do not cause atrophy, but may be less helpful in very hyperkeratotic lesions.

Systemic therapies targeting the prevention of progression require knowledge of the drugs and specific monitoring.

Antimalarials (hydroxychloroquine 200 mg twice daily alone or in combination with quinacrine 100 mg per day) can be employed for cases not adequately treated with topical or local agents.

Systemic retinoids—acitretin 25 to 50 mg p.o. daily, or isotretinoin 40 to 80 mg p.o. daily for 4 months should be considered as second-line therapy.

Dapsone (100 to 200 mg p.o. daily), methotrexate, mycophenolate mofetil, and other immunosuppressives have also been used. Oral gold has also been reported to be helpful.

Recent studies have shown thalidomide (50 to 100 mg p.o. daily) to be an effective therapy, but it should be reserved for severe cases that are unresponsive to other measures. Caution is advised due to the potential teratogenic and neurologic side effects.

Suggested Readings

Costner ML, Sontheimer RD. Lupus erythematosus. In: Fitzpatrick TB, Wolff K, eds. *Fitzpatrick's Dermatology in General Medicine*. 7th Ed. New York, NY: McGraw-Hill; 2008:1515–1535.

Hordinsky M. Cicatricial alopecia: Discoid lupus erythematosus. *Dermatol Ther*. 2008 Jul–Aug;21(4):245–248.

Jessop S, Whitelaw D, Jordaan F. Drugs for discoid lupus erythematosus. *Cochrane Database Syst Rev*. 2001;(1):CD002954.

Kluger N, Bessis D, Guillot B. Chronic cutaneous lupus flare induced by systemic 5-fluorouracil. *J Dermatolog Treat*. 2006;17(1):51–53.

Koga M, Kubota Y, Kiryu H, et al. A case of discoid lupus erythematosus of the eyelid. *J Dermatol*. 2006 May;33(5):368–371.

Kyriakis KP, Kontochristopoulos GJ, Panteleos DN. Experience with low-dose thalidomide therapy in chronic discoid lupus erythematosus. *Int J Dermatol*. 2000 Mar;39(3):218–222.

Lee LA. Lupus erythematosus. In: Bolognia J, Jorizzo JL, Rapini RP, eds. *Dermatology*. 2nd Ed. St. Louis, MO: Mosby; 2008:561–573.

Lo JS, Berg RE, Tomecki KJ. Treatment of discoid lupus erythematosus. *Int J Dermatol*. 1989 Oct;28(8):497–507.

Rothfield N, Sontheimer RD, Bernstein M. Lupus erythematosus: Systemic and cutaneous manifestations. *Clin Dermatol*. 2006 Sep–Oct;24(5): 348–362.

Sugano M, Shintani Y, Kobayashi K, et al. Successful treatment with topical tacrolimus in four cases of discoid lupus erythematosus. *J Dermatol*. 2006 Dec;33(12):887–891.

Wollina U, Hansel G. The use of topical calcineurin inhibitors in lupus erythematosus: an overview. *J Eur Acad Dermatol Venereol*. 2008 Jan;22(1):1–6.

Wozniacka A, Salamon M, Lesiak A, et al. The dynamism of cutaneous lupus erythematosus: Mild discoid lupus erythematosus evolving into SLE with SCLE and treatment-resistant lupus panniculitis. *Clin Rheumatol*. 2007 Jul;26(7):1176–1179.

■■ Diagnosis Synopsis

Cutaneous lesions of lupus erythematous can be classified into specific and nonspecific types. Within the group of specific lesions, there are three main subtypes based on chronicity, association with systemic lupus erythematosus (SLE), and location/depth of inflammatory infiltrate. They are as follows:

- Acute cutaneous lupus erythematosus (ACLE)
  - Transient cutaneous findings typified by malar erythema without scarring
  - Strongly associated with systemic findings
  - Inflammatory infiltrate seen in the superficial dermis on biopsy
- Subacute cutaneous lupus erythematosus (SCLE)
  - Photosensitive cutaneous eruption lasting longer than ACLE but without scarring
  - 10% to 15% of patients go on to have systemic findings
  - Inflammatory infiltrate seen in the upper dermis on biopsy
- Chronic cutaneous lupus erythematosus
  - Also known as discoid lupus erythematosus

- Chronic discoid lesions with permanent disfiguring scars
- 5% to 10% of patients go on to develop systemic findings
- Significant inflammatory infiltrate seen in superficial and deep dermis as well as prominent involvement of the adnexa on biopsy

SCLE is characterized by annular plaques with raised borders and central clearing or papulosquamous lesions that are restricted to sun-exposed skin. The sides of the face, the lower neck, and the extensor surfaces of the arms are the most commonly affected sites. Although scarring is not a characteristic finding, dyspigmentation is common sequelae.

While the etiology remains poorly understood, there is a strong association with anti-Ro antibodies and SCLE. It is hypothesized that a complex interplay between genetic proclivity and environmental influences leads to a perpetuated autoimmune response. In addition, specific HLA types (HLA-B8, DR3, DRw52, DQ1) have been shown to be associated with lupus erythematosus. Risk factors for developing cutaneous lesions include sex (3:1 female-to-male ratio, especially during child-bearing years) and ethnicity, with blacks demonstrating a higher incidence when compared to whites.

Of note, certain drugs such as hydrochlorothiazide, terbinafine, and other antihypertensives, such as calcium channel blockers and ACE inhibitors, and nonsteroidal anti-inflammatory drugs have been reported to trigger SCLE. These drug-induced SCLE lesions run an unpredictable course, and they may not clear after discontinuing the offending drug.

As previously mentioned, about 10% to 15% of patients with SCLE will go on to develop SLE. In addition, anti-Ro antibodies are also seen in Sjögren syndrome, and some patients can have both SCLE and Sjögren syndrome.

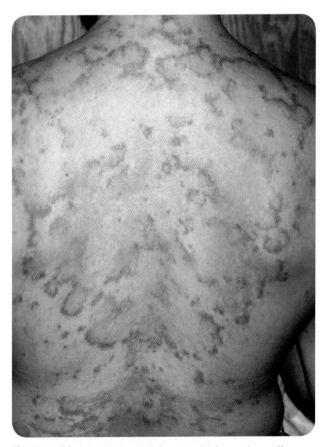

Figure 4-22 Subacute lupus. A few or multiple annular, scaling papules on the sun-exposed portions of the back.

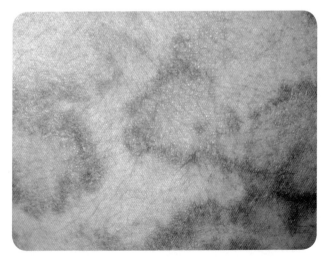

Figure 4-23 Annular, erythematous lesion of subacute lupus.

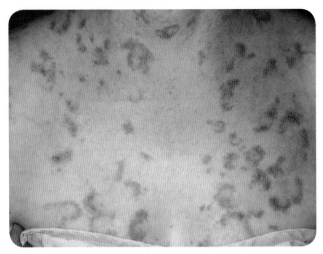

Figure 4-24 Multiple arcuate lesions of subacute lupus.

Look For

Lesions are nonscarring and nonindurated (secondary to inflammatory infiltrate being confined to superficial dermis) (Figs. 4-22–4-25). They are generally of two types:

- Annular type—Photodistributed annular or polycyclic plaques with a raised, erythematous border and central clearing.
- Papulosquamous type—Photodistributed erythematous scaly papules and plaques that may look eczematous in nature.

Diagnostic Pearls

- SCLE is more common in sun-exposed areas of the neck, shoulders, upper extremities, and trunk, whereas ACLE is more frequent on the cheeks.

Differential Diagnosis and Pitfalls

Annular Variant

- Granuloma annulare—Mainly in children and young adults, biopsy will help differentiate granuloma annulare and SCLE; facial lesions are extremely rare.
- Tinea corporis—Usually has scale at the leading edge. Check KOH.
- Erythema marginatum—Seen more commonly in children; cutaneous feature of acute rheumatic fever.
- Polymorphic light eruption—Most lesions resolve within several days.
- Erythema multiforme—Characteristic targetoid lesions; tends to involve the palms.
- Annular psoriasis—Biopsy will assist in differentiating psoriasis from SCLE.

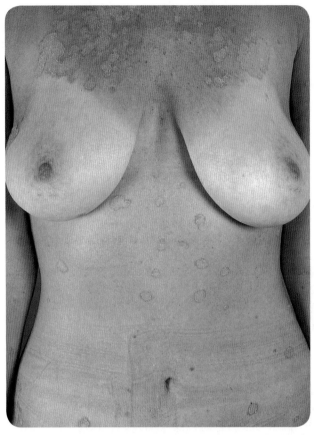

Figure 4-25 Lupus lesions are not present where the skin was covered by a bathing suit and had little sun exposure.

- Annular urticaria—Wheals that are characteristically pruritic.

Papulosquamous Variant

- Erythema annulare centrifugum (EAC)—Mostly seen on hips and thighs in patients in their 50s; biopsy can help differentiate EAC from SCLE. Usually has scale trailing the leading edge.
- Sarcoidosis—More infiltrative plaques.
- Lichen planus—Pruritic, scaly papules that involve wrists, forearms, genitalia, and presacral area; biopsy will assist in differentiating lichen planus from SCLE.
- Syphilis—Check RPR.

Best Tests

- Most patients demonstrate positive titers of antinuclear antibodies as well as anti-Ro (SS-A) and, to a lesser extent, anti-La (SS-B) cytoplasmic antibodies. Antibodies to double-stranded DNA (anti-dsDNA) are more commonly found in SLE.

- Lesional skin biopsies are positive (60% of the time) for basement membrane zone–bound immunoglobulin using direct immunofluorescence techniques.
- Be sure to take a thorough medication exposure history. Patients with SCLE merit a full evaluation to exclude systemic disease, including a CBC, urinalysis, electrolytes, blood urea nitrogen (BUN) and creatinine, erythrocyte sedimentation rate (ESR), complement levels, and, often, a chest X-ray and ECG.

▲▲▲ Management Pearls

- Withdraw any potential inciting medication.
- There is extreme sensitivity to ultraviolet light, UVB more than UVA. Opaque sunscreens may be necessary.
- Systemic manifestations, such as renal and central nervous system diseases, are present in 10% to 15% of patients, and patients must be followed with these potential complications in mind. Consultations with rheumatology, nephrology, neurology, and/or dermatology are recommended.

Therapy

The main goals of treatment are to improve the patient's appearance and to prevent additional lesions from developing. Sunscreens, sun-protective clothing, and sun avoidance are essential components of therapy. Topical corticosteroids and antimalarials are first-line therapy.

High-to-mid-potency topical corticosteroids may be used on truncal and extremity skin.

High-potency topical corticosteroids (class 2)

- Fluocinonide cream or ointment—apply twice daily (15, 30, 60, 120 g)
- Desoximetasone cream or ointment—apply twice daily (15, 60, 120 g)
- Halcinonide cream or ointment—apply twice daily (15, 60, 240 g)
- Amcinonide ointment—apply twice daily (15, 30, 60 g)

Mid-potency topical corticosteroids (classes 3 and 4)
The main goals of treatment are to improve the patient's appearance and to prevent additional lesions from developing. Sunscreens, sun-protective clothing, and sun avoidance are essential components of therapy. Topical corticosteroids and antimalarials are first-line therapy.

Mid-potency topical corticosteroids (classes 3 and 4)

- Triamcinolone cream or ointment—apply twice daily (15, 30, 60, 120, 240 g)
- Mometasone cream or ointment—apply twice daily (15, 45 g)
- Fluocinolone ointment or cream—apply twice daily (15, 30, 60 g)

Use milder-potency topical steroids on thinner skin and classes 6 and 7 steroids on the face and intertriginous areas (desonide cream, lotion, or ointment twice daily).

Antimalarials
Hydroxychloroquine 200 to 400 mg p.o. daily or chloroquine 250 to 500 mg p.o. daily.
Note: before starting these agents, liver and renal function tests should be obtained. Ophthalmologic baseline examination should be performed at or near the time these agents are started. Patients on antimalarials should be seen for ophthalmologic testing every 6 to 12 months.

Topical retinoids (tretinoin and tazarotene), dapsone (100 to 200 mg p.o. daily), oral retinoids (acitretin 25 to 50 mg p.o. daily or isotretinoin 40 to 60 mg p.o. daily), gold (auranofin 6 mg p.o. daily), thalidomide (100 to 300 mg p.o. daily), and other immunomodulating drugs such as methotrexate, azathioprine, and mycophenolate mofetil are also used. Systemic corticosteroids may be quite effective but are not considered first-line therapy due to the side effects of long-term use.

Suggested Readings

Abdel-Aziz K, Goodfield M. Evaluation of the cutaneous lupus activity and severity score in the assessment of lupus erythematosus skin disease. *Br J Dermatol*. 2008 Jan;158(1):181–182.

Bano S, Bombardieri S, Doria A, et al. Lupus erythematosus and the skin. *Clin Exp Rheumatol*. 2006 Jan–Feb;24(1 Suppl. 40):S26–S35.

Bleumink GS, ter Borg EJ, Ramselaar CG, et al. Etanercept-induced subacute cutaneous lupus erythematosus. *Rheumatology (Oxford)*. 2001 Nov;40(11):1317–1319.

Callen JP. Update on the management of cutaneous lupus erythematosus. *Br J Dermatol*. 2004 Oct;151(4):731–736.

Chaudhry SI, Murphy LA, White IR. Subacute cutaneous lupus erythematosus: A paraneoplastic dermatosis?. *Clin Exp Dermatol*. 2005 Nov;30(6):655–658.

Clayton TH, Ogden S, Goodfield MD. Treatment of refractory subacute cutaneous lupus erythematosus with efalizumab. *J Am Acad Dermatol*. 2006 May;54(5):892–895.

Costner ML, Sontheimer RD. Lupus erythematosus. In: Fitzpatrick TB, Wolff K, eds. *Fitzpatrick's Dermatology in General Medicine*. 7th Ed. New York, NY: McGraw-Hill; 2008:1515–1535.

Hivnor CM, Hudkins ML, Bonner B. Terbinafine-induced subacute cutaneous lupus erythematosus. *Cutis*. 2008 Feb;81(2):156–157.

Kuhn A, Sontheimer RD. Cutaneous lupus erythematosus: Molecular and cellular basis of clinical findings. *Curr Dir Autoimmun*. 2008;10:119–140.

Lee HJ, Sinha AA. Cutaneous lupus erythematosus: Understanding of clinical features, genetic basis, and pathobiology of disease guides therapeutic strategies. *Autoimmunity*. 2006 Sep;39(6):433–444.

Neri R, Mosca M, Bernacchi E, et al. A case of SLE with acute, subacute and chronic cutaneous lesions successfully treated with Dapsone. *Lupus*. 1999;8(3):240–243.

Parodi A, Rivara G, Guarrera M. Possible naproxen-induced relapse of subacute cutaneous lupus erythematosus. *JAMA*. 1992 Jul;268(1):51–52.

Pelle MT. Issues and advances in the management and pathogenesis of cutaneous lupus erythematosus. *Adv Dermatol*. 2006;22:55–65.

Sontheimer RD. Subacute cutaneous lupus erythematosus: A decade's perspective. *Med Clin North Am*. 1989 Sep;73(5):1073–1090.

Wenzel J, Brähler S, Bauer R, et al. Efficacy and safety of methotrexate in recalcitrant cutaneous lupus erythematosus: Results of a retrospective study in 43 patients. *Br J Dermatol*. 2005 Jul;153(1):157–162.

Lyme Disease

Diagnosis Synopsis

Lyme disease is an immune-mediated inflammatory disease resulting from infection with the spirochete *Borrelia burgdorferi sensu lato*, composed of three distinct genospecies: *Borrelia burgdorferi sensu stricto*, *Borrelia garinii*, and *Borrelia afzelii*.

In the United States, Lyme disease is primarily seen in New England, the Midwest states, and the west coast. It is also endemic to most of Europe. The ticks that transmit Lyme disease are of the genus *Ixodes*. Mice and deer are the major animal reservoirs. Transmission occurs most commonly in the spring and summer months.

Lyme disease is subdivided clinically into three phases:

1. Early localized disease
2. Early disseminated disease
3. Chronic disease

Early Localized

Early localized disease presents a few days to a month after a tick bite. The characteristic lesion of Lyme disease, erythema migrans, develops at the site of the tick bite in approximately 60% to 90% of those diagnosed. If left untreated, the disease disseminates to lymph nodes and hematogenously. In Europe, early lesions sometimes present as *Borrelia* lymphocytomas.

Early Disseminated

Multiple smaller skin lesions can represent hematogenous spread or, in rare cases, multiple independent primary tick bites. Burning and itching can occur at the site of the tick bite and in erythema migrans lesions. Initial infection is typically associated with flu-like symptoms, headache, arthralgias, and neck pain. Early neurologic symptoms can include facial nerve paralysis (Bell palsy). Atrioventricular block can develop and persist from several days to a few weeks. Lyme disease–associated arthritis usually develops from a few months to 2 years after initial infection.

Chronic

Acrodermatitis chronicum atrophicans is a manifestation of chronic Lyme disease in Europe. Untreated cases can also lead to chronic arthritis, encephalopathy, and neuropathy.

Look For

Early Localized

A red macule or edematous plaque initially develops at the site of the tick bite. The lesion expands centrifugally, eventually forming a characteristic targetoid, or "bull's-eye," lesion (Figs. 4-26–4-29). Lymphocytomas can present as bluish-red nodules or plaques on the ear lobe, nipples, or scrotum.

Early Disseminated

Multiple erythematous, blanching patches, and minimally elevated targetoid plaques can be present in a scattered distribution.

Chronic

Acrodermatitis chronica atrophicans typically presents with chronic blue-red plaques on the acral extremities, with associated edema and "doughy" texture of the involved skin. Later, involved skin becomes atrophic and shiny. Occasionally, these areas are indurated and can be associated with peripheral neuropathy and local lymphadenopathy.

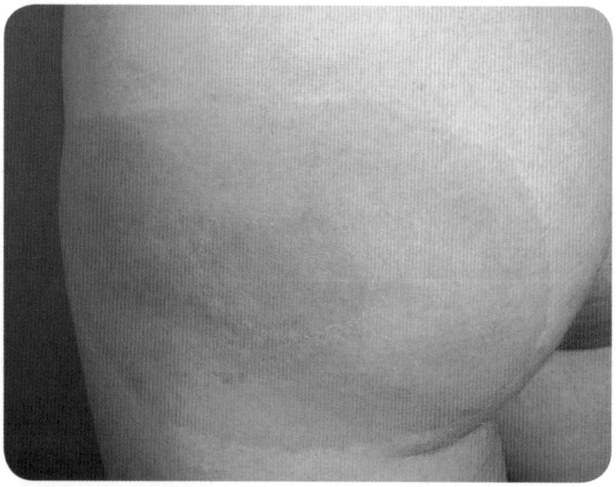

Figure 4-26 Large annular lesion with central bull's-eye.

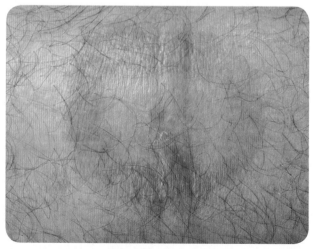
Figure 4-27 Bull's-eye rim of erythema with a central rim of clearing.

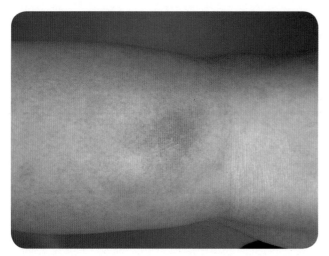

Figure 4-28 Lyme disease with a cellulitis-like plaque and central raised papules.

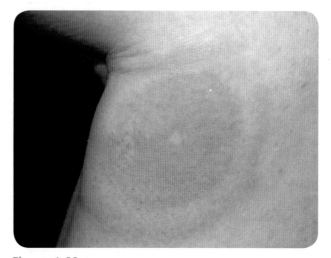

Figure 4-29 Annular zones of erythema and clearing in Lyme disease.

Diagnostic Pearls

- The characteristic lesion is an expanding targetoid, erythematous patch.
- The transmission of Lyme borreliosis takes 24 to 48 h of tick attachment and feeding. Therefore, a brief tick exposure (<24 h) should not be sufficient to contract Lyme disease.

Differential Diagnosis and Pitfalls

Early

- Erythema annulare centrifugum has a fine collarette of scaling inside the border of the lesion (trailing scale).
- Southern tick–associated rash illness clinically presents with erythema migrans but is transmitted by the tick *Amblyomma americanum*, possibly caused by *Borrelia lonestari*.
- Arthropod bite develops rapidly after bite.
- Fixed drug reactions tend to be pigmented and do not expand.
- Tinea corporis—Associated lesions have overlying scale.
- Contact dermatitis develops vesicles or bullae within lesion.
- Erysipelas/cellulitis has a more rapid onset with homogenous erythema as it expands from the site of initial infection.

Early Disseminated

Multiple Lesions

- Erythema multiforme lesions tend to have a dusky center; are symmetrically distributed favoring the dorsal hands, face, and forearms; and are usually with associated herpes infection.
- Secondary syphilis can have a characteristic "rust" color and overlying scale.
- Pityriasis rosea presents with a herald patch and lesions in characteristic "fir tree" distribution over the trunk with overlying fine scale.
- Urticarial lesions are edematous, pruritic, and typically resolve within 24 h.

Lymphocytoma

- Nodular scabies are more common in the groin and extremely pruritic.
- Arthropod bite develops rapidly after bite.
- Arthropod bite granuloma can be firm and typically does not expand.
- Malignancy (e.g., breast cancer) presents with firm papules and nodules.
- Granuloma faciale.
- Sarcoidosis lesions are characteristically violaceous.

Late

- Circulatory insufficiency.
- Dermatomyositis has a characteristic heliotrope rash; Gottron papules over dorsal distal inter-phalangeal (DIP), proximal inter-phalangeal (PIP), metacarpophalangeal (MCP) joints; and a "shawl sign."
- Lupus presents with photosensitivity, malar rash, and systemic symptoms of myalgias, arthralgias, and other organ involvement.

✓ Best Tests

- The diagnosis of Lyme disease is based on a high clinical index of suspicion in an endemic area, with the detection of *Borrelia* spirochete from tissues (either lesional or blood). Current serologic tests can be unreliable, however, especially when the pretest likelihood is low.

- The FDA currently recommends a two-step testing regimen for suspected cases:
  1. ELISA for either total or IgM or IgG antibodies. If there is a negative or equivocal result, complete step 2.
  2. Perform a western blot (immunoblot) as a second-line test.
- Tests can be falsely negative if taken too early in infection (window period of seroconversion) and should be repeated between 2 to 4 weeks after the initial tick bite if clinical suspicion remains high.
- Biopsy is not specific but can aid in diagnosis.

▲▲ Management Pearls

- Patients with neurologic or cardiac involvement or those with arthritis that fail oral therapy should be treated with parenteral antibiotics.

Therapy

Infectious Diseases Society of America Guidelines:

Prophylaxis*
Within 72 h of tick bite, doxycycline, 200 mg in a single dose.

Prophylaxis is indicated only when *all* of the following conditions are met:

- *The attached tick is identified as an *Ixodes scapularis* tick that has been attached for approximately 36 h (determined by the degree of engorgement of the tick with blood or certainty of the time of exposure).
- Post-exposure prophylaxis is started within 72 h of tick removal.
- The local rate of infection with *B. burgdorferi* is at least 20%.
- Doxycycline is not contraindicated.

Observation is recommended if these criteria are not met.

Treatment
Early Localized Disease
Preferred oral regimens for adults and children aged older than 8 years:

- Doxycycline 100 mg p.o. every 12 h for 14 to 21 days
- Preferred oral regimen for pregnant women and children aged younger than 8 years:
- Amoxicillin 500 mg p.o. every 8 h for 14 to 21 days

Alternative Regimens

- Cefuroxime axetil 500 mg p.o. every 12 h for 14 to 21 days
- Azithromycin 500 mg daily for 7 to 10 days
- Clarithromycin 500 mg twice daily for 14 to 21 days
- Erythromycin 500 mg 4 times daily for 14 to 21 days

Mild Early Disseminated Disease or Chronic Disease
Preferred oral regimen for adults and children aged older than 8 years:

- Doxycycline 100 mg p.o. every 12 h for 14 to 28 days

Preferred oral regimen for pregnant women and children aged younger than 8 years: Amoxicillin 500 mg p.o. every 8 h for 14 to 28 days

Alternative Regimen

- Cefuroxime axetil 500 mg p.o. every 12 h for 14 to 28 days

Severe Early Disseminated Disease or Chronic Disease
Preferred parenteral regimen:

- Ceftriaxone 2 g IV daily for 14 to 38 days (duration dependent upon the severity of infection)

Alternative Parenteral Regimens

- Cefotaxime 2 g IV every 8 h for 14 to 28 days (duration dependent upon the severity of infection)
- Penicillin G 18 to 24 MU IV daily, in divided doses every 4 h for 14 to 28 days (duration dependent upon the severity of infection)

Suggested Readings

Belongia EA, Reed KD, Mitchell PD, et al. Clinical and epidemiological features of early Lyme disease and human granulocytic ehrlichiosis in Wisconsin. *Clin Infect Dis*. 1999 Dec;29(6):1472–1477.

Bratton RL, Whiteside JW, Hovan MJ, et al. Diagnosis and treatment of Lyme disease. *Mayo Clin Proc*. 2008 May;83(5):566–571.

Cameron D, Gaito A, Harris N, et al.; ILADS Working Group. Evidence-based guidelines for the management of Lyme disease. *Expert Rev Anti Infect Ther*. 2004;2(1 Suppl.):S1–S13.

Centers for Disease Control and Prevention (CDC). Lyme disease—United States, 2003–2005. *MMWR Morb Mortal Wkly Rep*. 2007 Jun;56(23): 573–576.

Centers for Disease Control and Prevention (CDC). Recommendations for test performance and interpretation from the Second National Conference on Serologic Diagnosis of Lyme Disease. *MMWR Morb Mortal Wkly Rep*. 1995 Aug;44(31):590–591.

España A. Figurate erythemas. In: Bolognia J, Jorizzo JL, Rapini RP, eds. *Dermatology*. 2nd Ed. St. Louis, MO: Mosby/Elsevier; 2008:282–284.

Medical Letter. Treatment of Lyme disease. *Med Lett Drugs Ther.* 2005 May;47(1209):41–43.

Steere AC, McHugh G, Damle N, et al. Prospective study of serologic tests for Lyme disease. *Clin Infect Dis.* 2008 Jul;47(2):188–195.

Steere AC. Lyme disease. *N Engl J Med.* 2001 Jul;345(2):115–125.

Tibbles CD, Edlow JA. Does this patient have erythema migrans? *JAMA.* 2007 Jun;297(23):2617–2627.

Wharton M, Chorba TL, Vogt RL, et al. Case definitions for public health surveillance. *MMWR Recomm Rep.* 1990 Oct;39(RR-13):1–43.

Wormser GP, Dattwyler RJ, Shapiro ED, et al. The clinical assessment, treatment, and prevention of Lyme disease, human granulocytic anaplasmosis, and babesiosis: Clinical practice guidelines by the Infectious Diseases Society of America. *Clin Infect Dis.* 2006 Nov;43(9):1089–1134.

Phytophotodermatitis

Diagnosis Synopsis

Phytophotodermatitis is a cutaneous phototoxic eruption caused by the interaction of furocoumarins found in some common plants with solar UVA radiation. Approximately 24 h after plant contact with subsequent exposure to sunlight, a burning erythema develops. Limes, other citrus fruits, celery, wild parsnip, figs, meadow grass, certain weeds, and oil of bergamot are frequently causative. Common scenarios include squeezing limes outdoors, gardening and agricultural work, and hiking in areas of causative plants. There is no predilection for any age or ethnicity or either sex, although phytophotodermatitis may be more noticeable in fair skin types. The condition is benign and self-limited, and treatment is supportive.

The term "Berloque dermatitis" refers to phytophotodermatitis from the natural oil of bergamot in perfumes. This eruption is typically seen on the face and neck of women applying aerosolized fragrances. This has become rare since the introduction of artificial oil of bergamot.

Look For

Bizarre linear or haphazard erythema and edema with or without vesiculation occur in areas of exposure to both the sensitizing compound and light (Figs. 4-30–4-33). Handprints and other geographic shapes may correspond to physical contact with objects carrying furocoumarins. This presentation may cause confusion with physical abuse, especially when appearing in children. Blisters usually occur a day or so after the erythema, followed by hyperpigmentation, which typically appears 1 to 2 weeks later and may persist for weeks, months, or, rarely, years.

Dark Skin Considerations

Blistering disease is rare in blacks, and the reaction is usually limited to mild erythema followed by the usual hyperpigmentation observed in all races, which may persist for months.

Diagnostic Pearls

- Take a careful history, including occupation and hobbies.
- Linearity and stroke-like lesions are characteristic of phytophotodermatitis.
- Bartenders, agricultural workers, and grocers are particularly prone to lesions on the hands, from limes and celery in particular.

Differential Diagnosis and Pitfalls

- Phototoxic reaction due to another cause (e.g., medication)
- Immunobullous disease

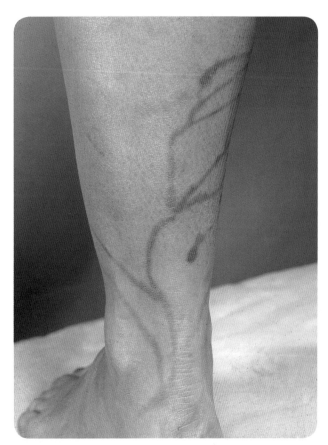

Figure 4-30 Lime juice coupled with sunlight produced this example of phytophotodermatitis.

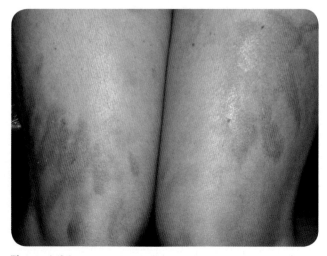

Figure 4-31 Phytophotodermatitis due to lime.

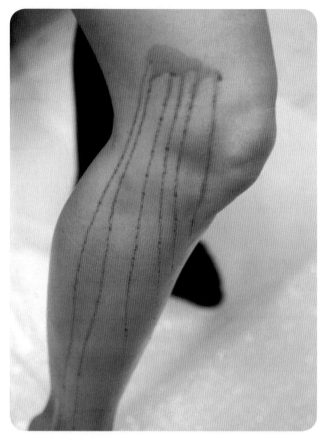

Figure 4-32 Phytophotodermatitis due to lemon. Notice lines that represent areas where lemon juice dripped down the leg.

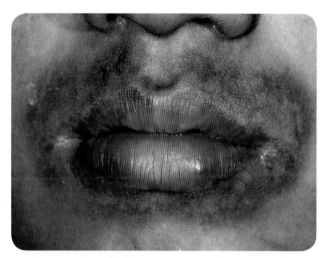

Figure 4-33 Hyperpigmentation from sucking limes and then going out in the sun.

▲▲ Management Pearls

- Reassure patients of the self-limited nature of the condition, but warn them that the postinflammatory hyperpigmentation may persist for some time.
- The prevention of future eruptions should be one of the primary goals of management. Patients should be educated as to common plants causing eruptions. Those with future exposures to known agents should promptly wash affected skin with soap and water.

Therapy

Eliminate the source of furocoumarin exposure, and encourage the use of sunscreens and sun-protective clothing.

Treat discomfort with cool soaks and compresses. An oral antihistamine may be prescribed if needed for pruritus:

- Diphenhydramine hydrochloride (25, 50 mg tablets or capsules): 25 to 50 mg nightly or every 6 h as needed
- Hydroxyzine (10, 25 mg tablets): 12.5 to 25 mg, every 6 h as needed
- Cetirizine hydrochloride (5, 10 mg tablets): 5 to 10 mg per day
- Loratadine (10 mg tablets): 10 mg once daily

A short course of oral corticosteroids (i.e., prednisone 1 mg/kg daily tapered over 1 to 2 weeks) may be necessary in severe cases. Indomethacin (200 mg p.o. two to four times daily for 5 to 7 days) may be given for skin discomfort and

(Continued)

- Erythema multiforme (early stage)
- Fixed drug reaction (late stage and if limited to one to three lesions)
- Contact dermatitis
- Heat or chemical burn
- Physical abuse—handprint or drip patterns are sometimes seen
- Sunburn
- Porphyria cutanea tarda
- Cnidaria (jellyfish) stings or other marine envenomation
- Factitial dermatitis

✔ Best Tests

- This is a clinical diagnosis based on careful history and physical examination.
- The following tests may be performed to rule out other diagnoses:
  - Serum, urine, or stool porphyrin levels (porphyria cutanea tarda)
  - Photopatch testing (photoallergic reaction)
  - Skin biopsy (numerous others)

may offer some protection against UVA-induced epidermal apoptosis.

Topical corticosteroids in conjunction with a combined UVA/UVB sunscreen to the site will help with fading the postinflammatory hyperpigmentation (classes 6 and 7 for face and classes 2 to 4 for trunk and arms).

High-potency topical corticosteroids (class 2)

- Fluocinonide cream, ointment—apply twice daily (15, 30, 60, 120 g)
- Desoximetasone cream, ointment—apply twice daily (15, 60, 120 g)
- Halcinonide cream, ointment—apply twice daily (15, 60, 240 g)
- Amcinonide ointment—apply twice daily (15, 30, 60 g)

Mid-potency topical corticosteroids (classes 3 and 4)

- Triamcinolone cream, ointment—apply twice daily (15, 30, 60, 120, 240 g)

- Mometasone cream, ointment—apply twice daily (15, 45 g)
- Fluocinolone ointment, cream—apply twice daily (15, 30, 60 g)

Mild-potency topical corticosteroids (class 6 or 7)

- Desonide cream, lotion—apply twice daily (15, 30, and 60 g)
- Hydrocortisone cream 2.5%—apply twice daily (1, 2 oz)

Suggested Readings

Bowers AG. Phytophotodermatitis. *Am J Contact Dermat.* 1999 Jun;10(2):89–93.

Egan CL, Sterling G. Phytophotodermatitis: a visit to Margaritaville. *Cutis.* 1993 Jan;51(1):41–42.

Hipkin CR. Phytophotodermatitis, a botanical view. *Lancet.* 1991 Oct;338(8771):892–893.

McGovern TW. Dermatoses due to plants. In: Bolognia J, Jorizzo JL, Rapini RP, eds. *Dermatology.* 2nd Ed. St. Louis, MO: Mosby; 2008:249–252.

Weber IC, Davis CP, Greeson DM. Phytophotodermatitis: The other "lime" disease. *J Emerg Med.* 1999 Mar–Apr;17(2):235–237.

Polymorphous Light Eruption

Diagnosis Synopsis

Polymorphous light eruption (PMLE), or polymorphic light eruption, is a common acquired cutaneous disorder that is characterized by a pathological response to ultraviolet radiation. Erythematous papules, vesicles, and plaques (hence the name "polymorphous") develop minutes to hours after exposure to sunlight or a tanning bed. The lesions are often pruritic, non-scarring, and are always restricted to sun-exposed areas. Systemic symptoms such as fever, malaise, headache, myalgias, and arthralgias are usually absent. While lesions can last up to several weeks, most resolve within several days' time.

PMLE is most commonly seen in fair-skinned women aged 20 to 30, but it can occur in either sex, all ages, and all ethnicities. Attacks most commonly occur during the spring and early summer months and disappear during the winter. While the etiology is not well-defined, investigations support a type IV delayed-type hypersensitivity reaction.

Although the condition frequently recurs, the tendency toward the development of PMLE and the severity of the eruption diminishes with repeated sunlight exposure. This key concept in the management of PMLE is termed "hardening." As the summer proceeds, it has been observed that the incidence of new eruptions decreases. Prophylactic phototherapy supports this concept of hardening or tolerance.

Of note, despite the variability of presentations, individual patients tend to experience the same clinical manifestations with each episode.

Look For

As the name suggests, there are a variety of morphologic types. The most common are the papular and papulovesicular forms. These are erythematous, small papules and vesicles distributed in sun-exposed areas (Figs. 4-34–4-37). Variants include an eczematous-like form as well as a vesiculobullous form. Some lesions may be difficult to distinguish from erythema multiforme.

Dark Skin Considerations

Grouped 1 to 2 mm papules are often seen in darkly pigmented skin.

Diagnostic Pearls

- Ten percent of the population has this reaction, often with the first episode of sun exposure each season (especially in those from a northern climate who visit a sunny vacation spot). The distribution of lesions is more useful in suggesting this diagnosis than the morphology.
- PMLE may occasionally occur in the winter as the result of the reflection of UV rays off of snow (more common in those who participate in winter sports).
- As a distinction from the ordinary sunburn eruption, people sensitive to longer wavelengths (UVA) can erupt when light goes through window glass (e.g., a bus or car window).

Differential Diagnosis and Pitfalls

- Systemic lupus erythematosus—Check for circulating ANA and other associated lupus antibodies, direct immunofluorescence will be positive, skin lesions can be located on sun-exposed and sun-protected areas (in contrast to PMLE, which is primarily in sun-exposed sites).

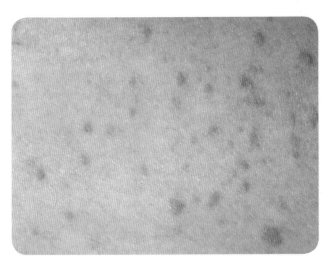

Figure 4-34 Multiple monomorphous papules is one morphology of PMLE.

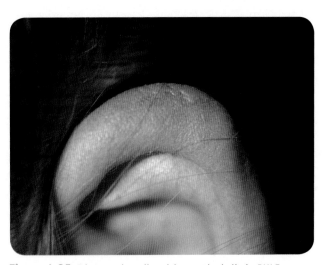

Figure 4-35 Edema and small vesicles on the helix in PMLE.

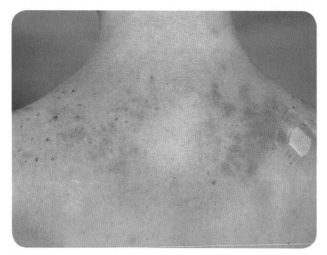

Figure 4-36 PMLE on the sun-exposed area of the upper back.

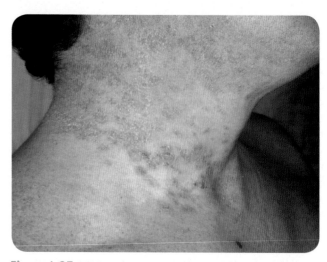

Figure 4-37 PMLE on the sun-exposed area of the neck, stopping at the collar line of the shirt.

- Sunburn
- Solar urticaria—Shorter time course with urticarial lesions lasting 1 to 2 h.
- Erythema multiforme—Characteristic target lesions, systemic symptoms are prominent (in contrast to PMLE, where fever, malaise, nausea, and headache are rare).
- Hydroa vacciniforme
- Transient acantholytic dermatosis (Grover disease)—Peak incidence in winter months; lesions are frequently crusted over, and there is more trunk involvement than extremities and face.
- Porphyria cutanea tarda—Will have abnormal porphyrin profile (elevated urine uroporphyrin and stool isocoproporphyrin).
- Erythropoietic protoporphyria—Lesions are very painful, and there is an elevated red blood cell protoporphyrin concentration.
- Photoallergic drug reaction—Investigate for drug history; not seasonally associated and does not improve over time.
- Phototoxic drug reaction
- Airborne contact dermatitis

✓ Best Tests

- Skin biopsy is suggestive of the diagnosis but is not always necessary.
- Laboratory investigations may be done to rule out other diagnoses. Obtaining ANA, SS-A, and SS-B titers and urine, stool, and serum porphyrin levels will rule out lupus erythematosus and porphyria. In addition, a direct

immunofluorescence will be positive in lupus and negative in PMLE.
- Note, however, that previous studies have shown that up to 19% of patients with PMLE can be ANA positive. A recent long-term follow-up study of patients with PMLE demonstrated that although ANA positive, these patients did not have clinical, histopathological, or laboratory abnormalities suggestive of lupus erythematosus. An ANA alone may not be sufficient in differentiating PMLE from lupus. Skin biopsy may not definitively distinguish PMLE for lupus erythematosus.
- Phototesting with UVA, UVB, and visible light sources may be helpful. Photopatch testing can rule out photoallergic or airborne contact dermatitis.

▲▲ Management Pearls

- Prevention is often the best treatment. Instruct patients to limit their sunlight exposure, especially in the early morning and late afternoon hours. The use of tanning beds should be stopped. Patients should also be encouraged to wear protective clothing and use a sunscreen that blocks both UVA and UVB rays, as UVB blocking alone may exacerbate the rash.
- Sunscreens that have high sun protection factor have not demonstrated efficacy in protecting against UVA-induced PMLE. A recent randomized, placebo-controlled trial demonstrated that the addition of a potent antioxidant (such as vitamin E) to a broad-spectrum sunscreen may be much more effective than the sunscreen alone.
- Refer severe and/or recalcitrant cases to a dermatologist.

Therapy

Preventative measures as above should be instituted.

Phototherapy

Prophylactic phototherapy two to three times/week for an average of 5 weeks in early spring with the following:

- Psoralen plus UVA (PUVA) 0.5 to 0.6 mg/kg of 8-methoxypsoralen 1 h prior to UVA exposure
- Narrow-band (311 nm) UVB phototherapy can be efficacious

In both forms of phototherapy, oral prednisone (1 mg/kg) can be administered for the first week of treatment to minimize erythema and photoexacerbation.

Corticosteroids

- Topical corticosteroids may provide some symptomatic relief (classes 6 and 7 for face and classes 2 to 4 for trunk and arms).

High-potency topical corticosteroids (class 2)

- Fluocinonide cream or ointment—apply twice daily (15, 30, 60, 120 g)
- Desoximetasone cream or ointment—apply twice daily (15, 60, 120 g)
- Halcinonide cream or ointment—apply twice daily (15, 60, 240 g)
- Amcinonide ointment—apply twice daily (15, 30, 60 g)

Mid-potency topical corticosteroids (classes 3 and 4)

- Triamcinolone cream or ointment—apply twice daily (15, 30, 60, 120, 240 g)
- Mometasone cream or ointment—apply twice daily (15, 45 g)
- Fluocinolone ointment or cream—apply twice daily (15, 30, 60 g)

Mild-potency topical corticosteroids (class 6 or 7)

- Desonide cream or lotion—apply twice daily (15, 30, 60 g)
- Hydrocortisone cream 2.5%—apply twice daily (1, 2 oz)

Antihistamines are helpful for pruritus.

Systemic corticosteroids may be needed to suppress severe, generalized eruptions:

- Prednisone 0.5 to 2 mg/kg p.o. daily divided twice daily, taper over 1 to 2 weeks.

Antimalarials

A course of antimalarials may also be helpful in the treatment and prevention of severe cases:

- Hydroxychloroquine 200 mg p.o. twice daily for 2 to 3 months in early springtime.

Vitamins

- Beta-carotene 30 to 300 mg p.o. daily
- Nicotinamide 1 g p.o. three times daily

Immunomodulators

- Thalidomide 50 to 200 mg p.o. nightly

Suggested Readings

Dummer R, Ivanova K, Scheidegger EP, et al. Clinical and therapeutic aspects of polymorphous light eruption. *Dermatology*. 2003;207(1):93–95.

Fesq H, Ring J, Abeck D. Management of polymorphous light eruption: Clinical course, pathogenesis, diagnosis and intervention. *Am J Clin Dermatol*. 2003;4(6):399–406.

Hawk JLM, Ferguson J. Abnormal responses to ultraviolet radiation: Idiopathic, probably immunologic, and photo-exacerbated. In: Fitzpatrick TB, Wolff K, eds. *Fitzpatrick's Dermatology in General Medicine*. 7th Ed. New York, NY: McGraw-Hill; 2008:816–818.

Hönigsmann H. Polymorphous light eruption. *Photodermatol Photoimmunol Photomed*. 2008 Jun;24(3):155–161.

Ling TC, Gibbs NK, Rhodes LE. Treatment of polymorphic light eruption. *Photodermatol Photoimmunol Photomed*. 2003 Oct;19(5):217–227.

Naleway AL, Greenlee RT, Melski JW. Characteristics of diagnosed polymorphous light eruption. *Photodermatol Photoimmunol Photomed*. 2006 Aug;22(4):205–207.

Norris PG, Hawk JL. Polymorphic light eruption. *Photodermatol Photoimmunol Photomed*. 1990 Oct;7(5):186–191.

Tutrone WD, Spann CT, Scheinfeld N, et al. Polymorphic light eruption. *Dermatol Ther*. 2003;16(1):28–39.

Tzaneva S, Volc-Platzer B, Kittler H, et al. Antinuclear antibodies in patients with polymorphic light eruption: A long-term follow-up study. *Br J Dermatol*. 2008 May;158(5):1050–1054.

Pruritic Urticarial Papules and Plaques of Pregnancy

■■ Diagnosis Synopsis

Pruritic urticarial papules and plaques of pregnancy (PUPPP) is the most common specific eruption of pregnancy. The etiology is unknown, but it may be related to skin distension. It is a benign condition that almost always begins in the third trimester of a first pregnancy and resolves around the time of delivery. The lesions are associated with striae gravidarum (striae distensae). Pruritus can be severe, leading to sleep disturbance. PUPPP is associated with a higher frequency of multiple gestations. It is important to note that there is no association with adverse fetal or maternal outcomes. Recurrence with subsequent pregnancies is uncommon.

◉ Look For

Erythematous papules and plaques occur over the course of a few days (Figs. 4-38–4-41). They begin on the abdomen in areas of striae gravidarum and spread to involve the buttocks and proximal thighs. (They are seen less often on the arms and distal legs.) The immediate periumbilical area is spared. A few vesicles may be noted, as may the rare targetoid lesion or annular wheal. The face, palms, and soles are spared.

●● Diagnostic Pearls

- Lesions are very itchy and are usually very small (1 to 2 mm) initially.
- The finding of frank bullae should suggest the rarer disorder pemphigoid gestationis.

?? Differential Diagnosis and Pitfalls

- Impetigo herpetiformis has distinct vesicles.
- Prurigo gestationis

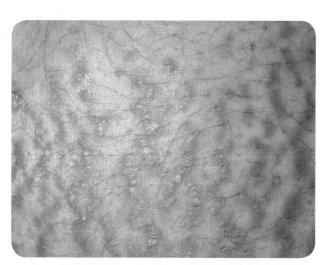

Figure 4-38 PUPPP lesions typically present in striae.

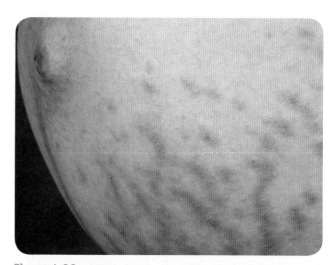

Figure 4-39 PUPPP lesions are typically uniform in size.

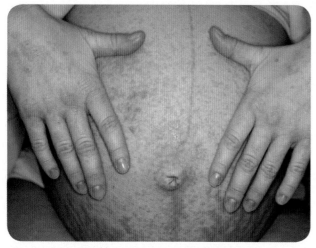

Figure 4-40 PUPPP lesions of the abdomen and hands.

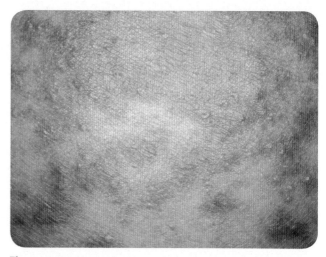

Figure 4-41 PUPPP papules can coalesce into plaques.

- Pemphigoid (herpes) gestationis is an autoimmune blistering disease that occurs in pregnancy wherein the lesions have definite vesicles and bullae.
- Urticaria
- Cholestasis
- Erythema multiforme
- Drug eruption
- Insect bites
- Contact dermatitis
- Seabather's eruption
- Scabies

✓ Best Tests

- PUPPP is an ill-defined entity because of its variable clinical presentation and lack of specific laboratory abnormalities.
- Skin biopsy for direct immunofluorescence is not specific but helps to eliminate pemphigoid gestationis and impetigo herpetiformis.
- Serum may also be submitted for indirect immunofluorescence to rule out pemphigoid gestationis.

▲▲▲ Management Pearls

- Patients should be provided with continual reassurance that the itching rapidly clears after delivery and that there is no evidence that the eruption is associated with any fetal distress or poor fetal outcome.

Therapy

Treatment is symptomatic.

The itching is intense and responds poorly to topical steroids.

Cool soaks and bland emollients often provide some symptomatic relief.

When the itching is severe, consider the use of a first-generation antihistamine such as diphenhydramine 25 to 50 mg every 6 h or a long-acting antihistamine once daily such as cetirizine, levocetirizine, loratadine, or fexofenadine (under obstetrical guidance).

Rarely, severe cases of PUPPP warrant systemic corticosteroids. Consult with an obstetrician first if considering this treatment.

Suggested Readings

Aronson IK, Bond S, Fiedler VC, et al. Pruritic urticarial papules and plaques of pregnancy: Clinical and immunopathologic observations in 57 patients. *J Am Acad Dermatol.* 1998 Dec;39(6):933–939.

Brzoza Z, Kasperska-Zajac A, Oleś E, et al. Pruritic urticarial papules and plaques of pregnancy. *J Midwifery Womens Health.* 2007 Jan–Feb;52(1):44–48.

Kroumpouzos G, Cohen LM. Specific dermatoses of pregnancy: An evidence-based systematic review. *Am J Obstet Gynecol.* 2003 Apr;188(4): 1083–1092.

Matz H, Orion E, Wolf R. Pruritic urticarial papules and plaques of pregnancy: Polymorphic eruption of pregnancy (PUPPP). *Clin Dermatol.* 2006 Mar–Apr;24(2):105–108.

Ohel I, Levy A, Silberstein T, et al. Pregnancy outcome of patients with pruritic urticarial papules and plaques of pregnancy. *J Matern Fetal Neonatal Med.* 2006 May;19(5):305–308.

Diagnosis Synopsis

Raynaud phenomenon is a vascular disorder characterized by intermittent arteriolar vasospasm of the digits and occurs in two settings: primary and secondary Raynaud phenomenon. Primary Raynaud phenomenon is also called Raynaud disease or Raynaud syndrome. It is characterized by the occurrence of vasospasm without ischemic injury or underlying associated disease. This variant is most commonly encountered in otherwise healthy adolescent girls and young women. Individuals suffer from digital pallor, cyanosis, and sharply bordered redness, and the disease is often associated with numbness of the fingers. Vasoconstriction is most often triggered by cold exposure and stress. Patients with primary Raynaud phenomenon have a younger age of onset, normal nailfold capillaries, and negative or low titers of autoantibodies. Primary Raynaud phenomenon usually involves all fingers in a symmetric distribution, and pain is usually absent to minimal. Smoking is contraindicated in these patients, as it may worsen the condition.

Secondary Raynaud phenomenon is characterized by an underlying disease where vasospasm can result in ischemic injury. It is commonly seen in patients with collagen vascular disorders, particularly systemic sclerosis, and in approximately 20% of lupus patients. Additional associations include rheumatoid arthritis, pulmonary hypertension, frostbite, hematologic malignancies, polyvinyl chloride exposure, cryoglobulinemia, reflex sympathetic dystrophy, repeated trauma/vibration, arteriovenous fistulae, intra-arterial drug administration, thoracic outlet syndrome, thromboangiitis obliterans, and Takayasu arteritis.

Look For

Affected digits commonly demonstrate at least two color changes—white (pallor) (Figs. 4-42–4-44), blue (cyanosis), and/or red (hyperemia)—and usually, but not always, in that order.

Ulcers and necrosis may form due to ischemia in secondary Raynaud phenomenon (Fig. 4-45).

Dark Skin Considerations

Cyanosis is challenging to observe in darkly pigmented skin, but pallor is usually obvious in the earliest stages of presentation.

Diagnostic Pearls

- Primary Raynaud: symmetrical, absent to minimal pain, normal nailfold capillaries, negative or low titers of autoantibodies, absence of ulcers and necrosis.
- Secondary Raynaud: asymmetrical, significant pain with ulcers and necrosis, high levels of autoantibodies, dilated nailfold capillaries.
- If you see digital ulcers and necrosis secondary to ischemia, aggressively pursue an underlying cause. Primary Raynaud phenomenon is not associated with these irreversible findings.

Differential Diagnosis and Pitfalls

- Carefully evaluate for cervical ribs and other causes of thoracic outlet syndromes.
- Carpal tunnel syndrome
- Reflex sympathetic dystrophy
- Paroxysmal hemoglobinuria
- Deep vein thrombosis (Paget-von Schrötter syndrome)
- Cryoglobulinemia

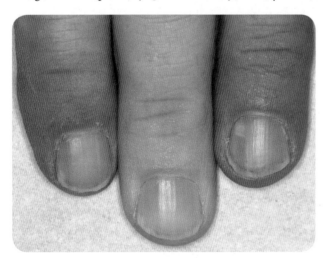

Figure 4-42 White finger of Raynaud syndrome with two fingers slightly redder than normal.

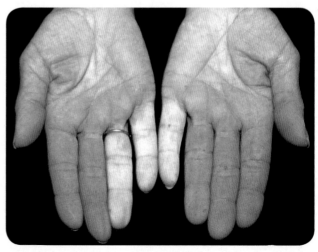

Figure 4-43 Dramatic blanching of fingers on both hands in Raynaud phenomenon.

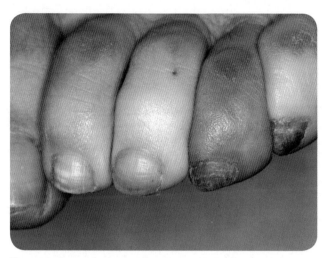

Figure 4-44 White constriction of four of five toenails.

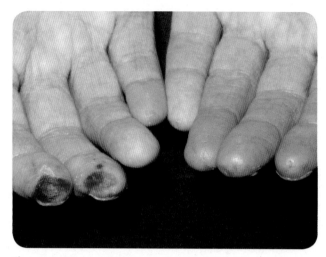

Figure 4-45 Raynaud phenomenon secondary to bleomycin.

- Waldenstrom macroglobulinemia, multiple myeloma, and other hematology malignancies
- Various hypercoagulable disorders, including antithrombin deficiency, antiphospholipid antibody syndrome, protein C or S deficiency, etc.
- Drug effects such as ergots, vinblastine, methysergide, beta blockers, caffeine, nicotine, oral contraceptives, and bleomycin
- Toxicity from arsenic, polyvinylchloride (PVC), cocaine, cyanide, or lead
- Livedo reticularis
- Acrocyanosis
- Atherosclerosis
- Thromboangiitis obliterans
- Vasculitis
- Erythromelalgia

✓ Best Tests

- Take a thorough medication history. Nailfold capillaroscopy in the appropriate setting may be beneficial.
- Obtain basic hematologic studies, such as a CBC, chemistry panel, and a coagulation profile.
- If an autoimmune connective tissue disease is suspected:
  - ANA titers
  - Anti-dsDNA, anti-Scl-70 (anti-topoisomerase I), anti-centromere, anti-Ro, anti-La, anti-RNP, and rheumatoid factor antibodies
  - ESR
  - Cryoglobulins

▲▲ Management Pearls

- Avoidance of exposure to cold temperatures and smoking cessation (if applicable) is essential.

- In cases of Raynaud phenomenon, maximize treatment of the underlying disorder. Eliminate any environmental, occupational, or drug exposures.
- Patients with Raynaud phenomenon may require consultation with a rheumatologist, hematologist, or vascular surgeon.

Therapy

Treatment regimens can be divided based on the severity of digital ischemia and whether the patient has primary or secondary Raynaud phenomenon.

Primary Raynaud Phenomenon
Lifestyle modification

- Smoking cessation, minimizing exposure to cold environments, avoidance of caffeine, discontinuing medications that cause vasoconstriction

Nitric oxide derivatives

- Topical 1% nitroglycerin
- Topical L-arginine (useful in patients with baseline low blood pressure)

Calcium channel blockers (dihydropyridine class)

- Nifedipine 10 to 30 mg three times daily
- Felodipine 2.5 to 10 mg daily
- Diltiazem, sustained release 120 to 300 mg daily
- Verapamil 40 to 120 mg three times daily

Phosphodiesterase inhibitors

- Sildenafil 50 mg twice daily

(Continued)

Vasodilators

- L-arginine 2 to 8 g daily

ACE inhibitors

- Losartan 50 mg daily

Selective serotonin reuptake inhibitors

- Fluoxetine 20 mg daily for 6 weeks

Miscellaneous (useful in patients with baseline low blood pressure)

- Vitamin E 500 U daily
- Aspirin 81 mg daily
- Slo-niacin 250 mg daily
- Pentoxifylline 400 mg three times daily
- Griseofulvin 500 mg daily

Secondary Raynaud Phenomenon
Treat the underlying disease. Treatment regimens can be further divided into etiology.

Non-Rheumatological Causes
Vascular occlusive diseases

- Smoking cessation
- Statin therapy
- Pentoxifylline 400 mg three times daily

Anatomical diseases

- Surgical evaluation

Drug-induced diseases

- Discontinuation of medication

Rheumatological Causes
Systemic Sclerosis

Lifestyle modification

- Smoking cessation, minimizing exposure to cold environments, avoidance of caffeine, discontinuation of medications that cause vasoconstriction

Nitric oxide derivatives

- Topical 1% nitroglycerin
- Topical L-arginine (useful in patients with baseline low blood pressure)
- Statins
- Atorvastatin 40 mg daily

Calcium channel blockers

- Nifedipine 10 to 30 mg three times daily
- Felodipine 2.5 to 10 mg daily
- Diltiazem, sustained release 120 to 300 mg daily
- Verapamil 40 to 120 mg three times daily

Phosphodiesterase inhibitors

- Sildenafil 50 mg twice daily

Miscellaneous (useful in patients with baseline low blood pressure)

- Vitamin E 500 U daily
- Aspirin 81 mg daily
- Slo-niacin 250 mg daily
- Pentoxifylline 400 mg three times daily
- Griseofulvin 500 mg daily

Vasculitis

- Azathioprine
- Cyclophosphamide
- Plasmapheresis

Hypercoagulable States

- Aspirin 325 mg daily
- Warfarin (low dose)
- Plaquenil

Suggested Readings

Bakst R, Merola JF, Franks AG, et al. Raynaud's phenomenon: Pathogenesis and management. *J Am Acad Dermatol.* 2008 Oct;59(4):633–653.

Boin F, Wigley FM. Understanding, assessing and treating Raynaud's phenomenon. *Curr Opin Rheumatol.* 2005 Nov;17(6):752–760.

Bowling JC, Dowd PM. Raynaud's disease. *Lancet.* 2003 Jun;361(9374): 2078–2080.

Comparison of sustained-release nifedipine and temperature biofeedback for treatment of primary Raynaud phenomenon. Results from a randomized clinical trial with 1-year follow-up. *Arch Intern Med.* 2000 Apr;160(8):1101–1108.

Cooke JP, Marshall JM. Mechanisms of Raynaud's disease. *Vasc Med.* 2005 Nov;10(4):293–307.

Pope J. Raynaud's phenomenon (primary). *Clin Evid.* 2005 Jun;13: 1546–1554.

Raynaud's disease. Cold hands, slowed blood flow. *Mayo Clin Health Lett.* 2007 May;25(5):7.

Thompson AE, Pope JE. Calcium channel blockers for primary Raynaud's phenomenon: A meta-analysis. *Rheumatology (Oxford).* 2005 Feb;44(2): 145–150.

Vinjar B, Stewart M. Oral vasodilators for primary Raynaud's phenomenon. *Cochrane Database Syst Rev.* 2008 Apr;(2):CD006687.

Diagnosis Synopsis

Sunburn (solar erythema) is the skin's reaction to excessive ultraviolet light exposure. It presents as reddening and tenderness of the skin that typically appears 30 min to 8 h after exposure and peaks between 12 and 24 h after exposure. UVB radiation is much more potent than UVA at inducing erythema; the 300 nm wavelength within the UVB range is the most erythemogenic. Severe sunburn can evolve into edema, blistering, and desquamation, the latter of which occurs 4 to 7 days after the exposure as the erythema is fading. Extreme reactions may include systemic symptoms such as chills and malaise and may necessitate hospitalization and management similar to that for thermal burns. Sunburn incidence is increased in areas that are closer to the equator and higher in altitude. Sunburn occurs more frequently in fairer-skinned individuals and in younger age groups. Darker skin types are more resistant to photodamage due to increased epidermal melanin content and different melanosome dispersion patterns. Skin phototypes (Fitzpatrick classification) are classified on the basis of susceptibility to sunburn and ability to tan:

Skin Phototype:

1. Always burns, never tans
2. Frequently burns, rarely tans
3. Infrequently burns, usually tans
4. Low susceptibility to sunburn, light brown skin color
5. Very low susceptibility to sunburn, brown skin color
6. Extremely low susceptibility to sunburn, dark brown skin color

Although sunburn is self-limiting, there is morbidity and mortality associated with long-term sun exposure in the form of a heightened risk of skin cancer.

Look For

Immediate erythema within 4 h following exposure followed by deep redness, vesiculation, and bullae formation in severe cases (Figs. 4-46–4-49). There is often warmth, tenderness, and edema. Erythema may persist for days to weeks following the acute burn.

Solar erythema is limited to sun-exposed areas of the body; therefore, sharp lines of demarcation may be present at sites where clothing or other barriers have shielded UV rays. However, thin or tightly adherent clothing may permit the partial transmission of UV radiation.

Diagnostic Pearls

- Consider an oral medication as a photosensitizer and take a complete medication history, including over-the-counter medications.
- Sunburns may trigger recurrences of other cutaneous disorders, such as herpes simplex, porphyria, or lupus erythematosus.

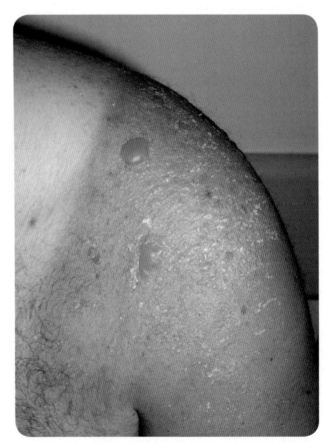

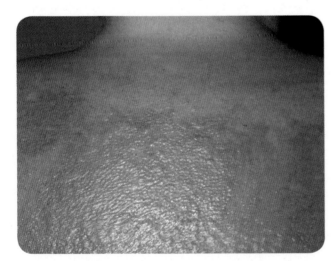

Figure 4-46 Vesicles and purpura can occur with acute sunburn.

Figure 4-47 Sharply bordered sunburn with some large vesicles.

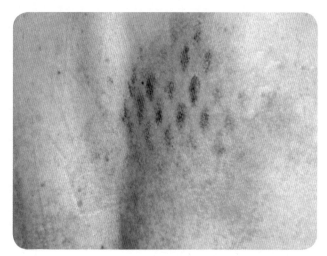

Figure 4-48 Patterned sunburn with purpura through straps of a lawn chair.

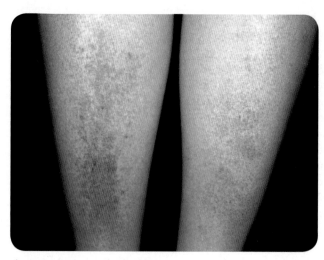

Figure 4-49 Purpura in a sunburn.

?? Differential Diagnosis and Pitfalls

- Many drugs that are phototoxic and cause exaggerated sunburn are active in the UVA spectrum. These can pass through window glass that stops UVB (the usual wavelength for inducing skin cancer).
- Photocontact dermatitis
- Photoallergic reaction
- Polymorphous light eruption
- Solar urticaria
- Chronic actinic dermatitis
- Cellulitis
- Exfoliative dermatitis
- Atopic dermatitis
- Chemical or thermal burns
- Lupus erythematosus
- Dermatomyositis
- Acute contact dermatitis
- Porphyria

✓ Best Tests

- This is a clinical diagnosis.

▲▲ Management Pearls

- Prevention is key!
- To prevent sunburn, impress upon patients to avoid sun exposure at midday (10:00 AM to 3:00 PM), use barrier protectants (tightly woven clothes and hats), and apply sunscreen (SPF 30 UVA and UVB block). A common cause of sunburn is the underapplication of sunscreen.

Approximately two tablespoons of sunscreen are required to appropriately cover the average-sized adult body.

Immunocompromised Patient Considerations

Patients on long-term immunosuppressive therapy, such as organ transplant recipients, are at significantly increased risk of skin cancer, owing to decreased cutaneous immune surveillance against tumorigenesis. Sunscreen and sun-protective practices are especially important in this population.

Therapy

Cool compresses will provide some symptomatic relief. Cool milk or Burow solution soaks are an alternative.

Nonsteroidal anti-inflammatory agents may help decrease the degree of erythema and will help with the discomfort. Topical corticosteroids may be of benefit in patients with moderate to severe sunburns.

For severe reactions, early administration of prednisone (40 to 60 mg per day for only a few days, no taper) may also help reduce the inflammation.

In very rare instances, patients may develop severe second-degree sunburns necessitating hospitalization with an aggressive skin care regimen, electrolyte management, and fluid replacement.

Suggested Readings

Centers for Disease Control and Prevention (CDC). Sunburn prevalence among adults—United States, 1999, 2003, and 2004. *MMWR Morb Mortal Wkly Rep.* 2007 Jun;56(21):524–528.

Driscoll MS, Wagner RF. Clinical management of the acute sunburn reaction. *Cutis.* 2000 Jul;66(1):53–58.

Han A, Maibach HI. Management of acute sunburn. *Am J Clin Dermatol.* 2004;5(1):39–47.

Rijken F, Bruijnzeel PL, van Weelden H, et al. Responses of black and white skin to solar-simulating radiation: differences in DNA photodamage, infiltrating neutrophils, proteolytic enzymes induced, keratinocyte activation, and IL-10 expression. *J Invest Dermatol.* 2004 Jun;122(6):1448–1455.

Rünger TM. Ultraviolet light. In: Bolognia J, Jorizzo JL, Rapini RP, eds. *Dermatology.* 2nd Ed. St. Louis, MO: Mosby; 2008:1322.

Verma GG, Dave D, Byrne E. Unusual presentation of sunburn. *Eur J Emerg Med.* 2008 Oct;15(5):279–280.

Diagnosis Synopsis

Urticaria, commonly known as welts or hives, refers to raised, erythematous wheals caused by the release of histamine and other vasoactive substances from mast cells. Urticaria can be triggered by a variety of mechanisms, both allergic and non-allergic. In half of cases, the inciting factor is never identified; 40% of cases are associated with an upper respiratory infection, 9% with drugs, and 1% with foods. Pruritus, prickling and stinging sensations, or pain may occur with urticaria.

Urticaria is defined as acute (new onset or recurring episodes of fewer than 6 weeks' duration) or chronic (recurring episodes of more than 6 weeks' duration). There is an increased incidence of positive thyroid autoantibodies in chronic cases. Chronic urticaria is more common in women and middle-aged individuals, whereas acute urticaria is more commonly seen in children. Disease resolves within 12 months in approximately 50% of adults with idiopathic urticaria.

Associated Factors:

- Systemic illnesses such as infections, collagen vascular diseases, neoplasia, endocrine disorders, and blood dyscrasias
- Environmental stimuli such as insect stings and inhalants (pollen, spores, animal dander, perfumes, and detergents)
- Pregnancy
- Foods such as strawberries, nuts, eggs, and shellfish
- Physical stimuli such as heat, cold, exertion, sunlight, water, vibration, or pressure are common causes of urticaria in adults.

- Drugs causing urticaria include aspirin, nonsteroidal anti-inflammatory agents, morphine and codeine, penicillin and its derivatives, cephalosporins, sulfa, streptomycin, tetracycline, griseofulvin, blood products, radiographic contrast media, angiotensin-converting enzyme inhibitors, and sulfonylureas.

Immunocompromised Patient Considerations

Cold urticaria may present as a paraneoplastic syndrome as a result of cryoglobulins associated with myeloma or lymphoma. Cold urticaria without cryoglobulins has been reported in HIV-infected individuals.

Look For

Well-circumscribed, erythematous, edematous papules, patches, or plaques, often with a pale center (Figs. 4-50–4-53). Individual urticarial lesions last less than 24 h versus urticarial vasculitis, where individual lesions are fixed and persist beyond 24 h.

Lesions vary in size from 2 to 5 mm to over 30 cm, are usually sharply marginated, and may be annular, serpiginous, or irregularly shaped. Edema of the mucous membranes may be present.

Urticaria may occur anywhere on the body but is more common on the trunk.

Angioedema, which manifests with swelling of the face, bowel, or part of an extremity, is seen in approximately 50% of urticaria cases.

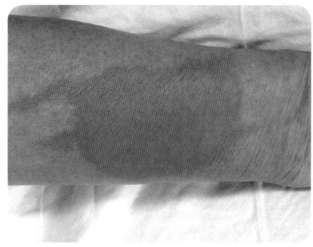

Figure 4-50 Urticaria can be induced by cold, defined as cold urticaria, and this form of urticaria can be reproduced by applying an ice cube to the skin.

Figure 4-51. Irregular discrete and confluent urticarial papules.

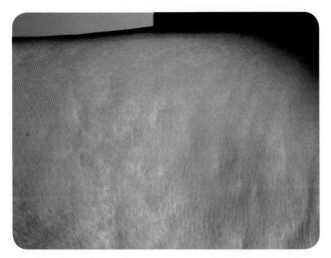

Figure 4-52 Confluent areas of very edematous skin from urticaria.

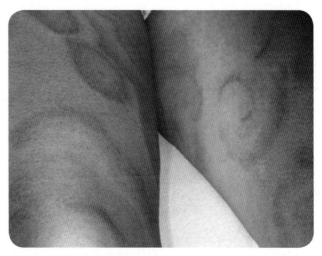

Figure 4-53 Giant hives with negative Lyme and lupus studies.

Dark Skin Considerations

Some authors suggest that black patients have an increased risk of ACE inhibitor–associated angioedema. While urticaria is characteristically pink in color in a lighter-skinned patient, the color may be obscured in darker skin.

Diagnostic Pearls

- Transient erythematous edematous pruritic plaques.
- Urticaria requires an extensive review of medications, supplements, and past medical history. Provocative tests (such as the ice cube test or strenuous exercise) may help establish a diagnosis of physical urticaria.

?? Differential Diagnosis and Pitfalls

- Urticarial vasculitis has lesions that persist over 24 h and may have associated purpura.
- Dermatographism may mimic urticaria and is induced by firmly stroking the skin. It lasts from 0.5 to 2 h.
- Contact dermatitis may have an unusual geometric shape correlating to the inciting irritant and often develops blisters.
- Drug reactions may be urticarial.
- Erythema multiforme typically presents with palmar and plantar targetoid plaques that last over 24 h.
- Bullous pemphigoid and dermatitis herpetiformis may present with urticarial lesions, but individual lesions last longer than 24 h and progress to vesicles or erosions. These are exceptionally pruritic as well.

- Herpes zoster may initially be urticarial but are painful and evolve into blisters and crusts.
- Insect bites (papular urticaria) last longer than 24 h.
- Serum sickness can be urticarial but is accompanied by arthralgias, fever, and malaise.
- Angioedema, edema of the subcutaneous or submucosal tissues, is not pruritic and commonly affects the face (eyelids, earlobes, and lips).
- In urticaria pigmentosa, hyperpigmented lesions will urticate when stroked (Darier sign) as histamine is released from the mast cells.

✓ Best Tests

- If lesions persist for more than 24 h, it is useful to biopsy a lesion to look for urticarial vasculitis. If a vasculitis is seen, further lab tests should include a CBC, erythrocyte sedimentation rate (ESR), urinalysis; renal and liver function tests; C3, C4, CH50 levels; hepatitis B and C serologies; ANA, cryoglobulins, immunoglobulin levels; and serum protein electrophoresis (SPEP)/urine protein electrophoresis (UPEP).
- Lab tests are not routinely indicated for acute urticaria. Occasionally, skin testing or radioallergosorbent assays are ordered if hypersensitivity to a particular allergen is suspected. In chronic urticaria, perform a CBC with differential, ESR, and thyroid function tests. Serologies for *Helicobacter pylori* may be ordered in cases of chronic urticaria as well.
- For patients with acquired cold urticaria, check cryoglobulins, a CBC with differential, and hepatitis serologies.

▲▲ Management Pearls

- Avoid common triggers such as aspirin, food additives, heat, and alcohol. Cooler temperatures and cooler bath water may be beneficial (except in cases of cold urticaria). Over-the-counter topical antipruritic lotions with menthol and phenol may provide relief.

- If features of anaphylaxis are present (hypotension, stridor or respiratory distress, etc.), immediate intervention is needed to secure the patient's airway and prevent circulatory collapse. Administer intramuscular or subcutaneous epinephrine 0.3 to 0.5 mg, repeated at 15 to 20 min intervals as needed.
- Reassure patients with acute urticaria that most cases resolve within 6 weeks spontaneously. Patients with chronic urticaria often experience resolution within 6 months, but the prognosis for resolution after 6 months is unclear.
- Make the patient an active participant in searching for agents inducing the disease. Exclusion diets may be helpful in determining potential food-related triggers.
- An allergist referral may be helpful in recurrent or chronic cases.

Therapy

Nonsedating H1 antagonists are first-line therapy:

- Cetirizine hydrochloride—10 mg p.o. nightly or twice daily
- Loratadine—10 mg p.o. daily or twice daily
- Fexofenadine—120 to 180 mg p.o. daily

First-generation (sedating) antihistamines may also be used:

- Diphenhydramine—10 to 25 mg p.o. four times daily
- Hydroxyzine—10 to 25 mg p.o. four times daily
- Chlorpheniramine—4 mg p.o. four times daily
- Cyproheptadine—4 mg p.o. three times daily
- Doxepin—10 to 25 mg p.o. nightly or 10 to 50 mg p.o. three times daily

Leukotriene inhibitors may be used in combination with antihistamines:

- Montelukast—10 mg p.o. daily
- Zafirlukast—20 mg p.o. twice daily
- Zileuton—600 mg p.o. four times daily

In severe cases, systemic corticosteroids (prednisone 0.5 to 1 mg/kg p.o. daily) can be used for 3 to 5 days while introducing antihistamine therapy.

Additional alternative therapies include nifedipine (up to 20 mg p.o. three times daily), psoralen plus UVA (PUVA), warfarin, cyclosporine (4 mg/kg p.o. daily), thyroid hormone replacement, plasmapheresis, intravenous immunoglobulin, acrivastine 8 mg and pseudoephedrine hydrochloride (60 mg p.o. four times daily), and H2-blocking antihistamines (famotidine, ranitidine).

If *H. pylori* serologies are positive, treatment of this chronic infection is warranted. The confirmation of eradication is important.

Suggested Readings

Baxi S, Dinakar C. Urticaria and angioedema. *Immunol Allergy Clin North Am.* 2005 May;25(2):353–367, vii.

Federman DG, Kirsner RS, Moriarty JP, et al. The effect of antibiotic therapy for patients infected with *Helicobacter pylori* who have chronic urticaria. *J Am Acad Dermatol.* 2003 Nov;49(5):861–864.

Grattan CE, Humphreys F; British Association of Dermatologists Therapy Guidelines and Audit Subcommittee. Guidelines for evaluation and management of urticaria in adults and children. *Br J Dermatol.* 2007 Dec;157(6):1116–1123.

Grattan C, Powell S, Humphreys F; British Association of Dermatologists. Management and diagnostic guidelines for urticaria and angio-oedema. *Br J Dermatol.* 2001 Apr;144(4):708–714.

Grattan CE, Sabroe RA, Greaves MW. Chronic urticaria. *J Am Acad Dermatol.* 2002 May;46(5):645–657; quiz 657–660.

Kaplan AP. Clinical practice. Chronic urticaria and angioedema. *N Engl J Med.* 2002 Jan;346(3):175–179.

Kaplan AP. Urticaria and angioedema. In: Fitzpatrick TB, Wolff K, eds. *Fitzpatrick's Dermatology in General Medicine.* 7th Ed. New York, NY: McGraw-Hill; 2008:330–343.

Kumar SA, Martin BL. Urticaria and angioedema: Diagnostic and treatment considerations. *J Am Osteopath Assoc.* 1999 Mar;99(3 Suppl.):S1–S4.

Powell RJ, Du Toit GL, Siddique N, et al.; British Society for Allergy and Clinical Immunology (BSACI). BSACI guidelines for the management of chronic urticaria and angio-oedema. *Clin Exp Allergy.* 2007 May;37(5):631–650.

Zuberbier T, Bindslev-Jensen C, Canonica W, et al. EAACI/GA2LEN/EDF guideline: Management of urticaria. *Allergy.* 2006 Mar;61(3):321–331.

◫ Diagnosis Synopsis

Basal cell carcinoma (BCC) is a neoplasm of basal keratinocytes and the most common skin cancer. It is largely a nonmetastasizing form of cancer. BCC is typically limited to areas on the head, neck, face, and nose but can occur at any location. BCC is primarily a disease of fair-skinned individuals and individuals with a lifetime of sun exposure, although other risk factors include arsenic exposure, basal cell nevus syndrome, Bazex syndrome, immunosuppression, xeroderma pigmentosum, and exposure to other sources of radiation. The incidence of BCC increases in older adults. Prognosis is excellent with prompt identification and treatment.

The four major subtypes of BCC are, nodular, superficial, infiltrating, and pigmented.

Nodular

Nodular BCC is the most common subtype and often presents as a pearly papule with a rolled border that may ulcerate and have superficial telangiectasias.

Superficial

Superficial BCC is the second most common subtype, and it tends to occur more often on the sun-exposed areas of the trunk and extremities and in slightly younger patients.

Infiltrating

Infiltrating, or morpheaform, BCCs often mimic scars and can be extensive, locally destructive, and require extensive plastic surgical repair if not treated early.

Pigmented

Pigmented BCCs contain dark-colored pigment and are considered a nodular BCC variant. The clinical differential diagnosis for this lesion includes melanoma.

Immunocompromised Patient Considerations

Nodular
Growth of BCC is slow, with progressive peripheral expansion with local tissue destruction. Metastasis is rare.

Some studies imply increased rates of BCC in immunocompromised patients, but other studies show that immunosuppressive therapy does not increase the risk of BCC, which is related to age, skin type, and UV exposure history.

◉ Look For

BCCs are most commonly found on sun-exposed areas: head and neck, upper chest and back, and upper extremities.

Nodular

Nodular BCCs have a pearly or lucent quality, with small telangiectasias and a rolled edge or border (Figs. 4-54 and 4-55). As the growth enlarges, crusting usually appears over the central depression, and bleeding with minor trauma is frequent. With time, a nonhealing erosion or ulcer may form.

Superficial

Superficial BCCs typically appear as dry, scaly, flat papules, or plaques that slowly enlarge and sometimes develop a raised

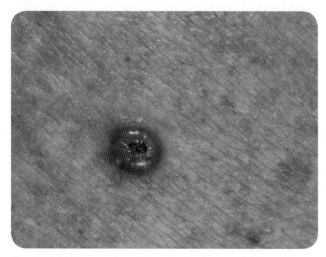

Figure 4-54 A single ulcerated papule with a shiny, translucent border and a telangiectatic blood vessel is typical of BCC.

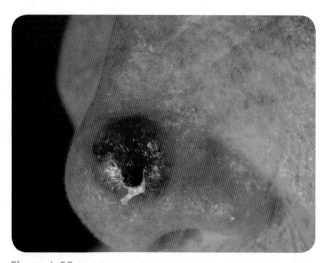

Figure 4-55 Nodular BCC with many prominent new blood vessels.

border. They are typically well defined and pink to red in color (Fig. 4-56).

Superficial BCC is encountered on the trunk more often than other subtypes of BCC. It may also occur on the head, neck, and extremities.

Infiltrating

A shiny or scar-like, indurated lesion sometimes with telangiectasias, erosions, or small crusts (Fig. 4-57). Infiltrating BCCs tend to be subtle. Some patients present with a hypopigmented or "white" area, which is found to be a firm plaque on palpation.

Examine the suspicious lesion from several angles, and redirect the lighting to see if you can appreciate a texture change in the skin. The abnormal area may be easier to appreciate by light touch (a firm, poorly defined plaque) than by the eye.

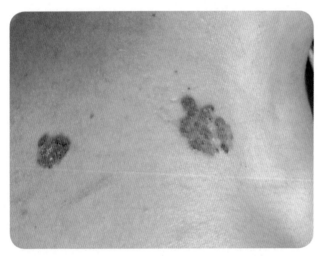

Figure 4-56 Two superficial BCCs with hyperpigmentation.

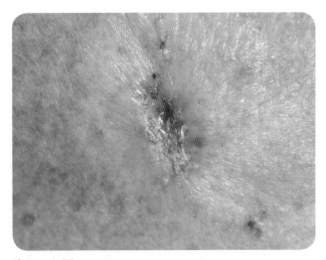

Figure 4-57 An infiltrated (or morpheaform) BCC has an irregular depressed or puckered appearance.

Pigmented

BCCs may be pigmented and present as brown papules with some of the other features of BCCs: pearly appearance, telangiectasias, and a rolled border (Figs. 4-58 and 4-59). Many BCCs have tiny specks of pigment when examined closely with a dermatoscope.

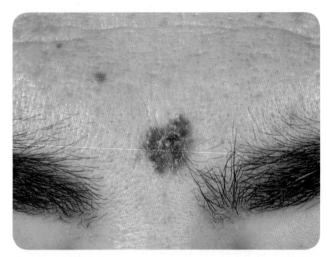

Figure 4-58 A deeply pigmented BCC can easily be confused with a malignant melanoma.

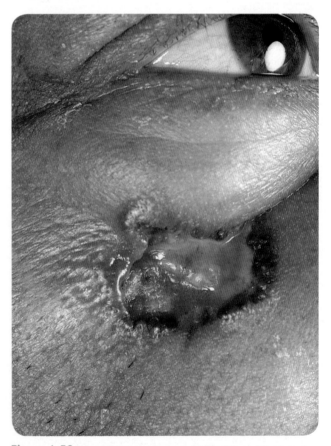

Figure 4-59 Ulceration in a pigmented BCC with eyelid edema in a patient with darkly pigmented skin.

Diagnostic Pearls

- The presence of more than one lesion of any of the subtypes before the age of 30 may suggest basal nevus syndrome or an exposure to therapeutic ionizing irradiation. Usually, these lesions are larger than they appear clinically.

 Differential Diagnosis and Pitfalls

Nodular

- Sebaceous hyperplasia can appear as yellow-white papules with a rolled edge.
- Molluscum contagiosum
- Amelanotic melanoma
- Melanocytic nevus
- Keratoacanthoma
- Squamous cell carcinoma (SCC)
- Merkel cell carcinoma
- Trichoepithelioma
- Seborrheic keratosis
- Bowen disease
- Fibrous papule of the face (angiofibroma)

Superficial

- Psoriasis
- SCC
- Bowen disease (SCC in situ)
- Paget disease
- Nummular dermatitis
- Actinic keratosis
- Amelanotic melanoma
- Tinea—This entity would be KOH positive.

Infiltrating

- A scar may present similarly to infiltrating BCC
- Merkel cell carcinoma
- Microcystic adnexal carcinoma
- Other adnexal neoplasms
- Amelanotic melanoma
- Dermatofibroma sarcoma protuberans
- Morphea, localized

Pigmented

- Melanocytic nevus
- Melanoma

 Best Tests

- Skin biopsy. If infiltrating BCC is suspected, perform a deep or large enough biopsy to allow for the dermatopathologist to adequately determine the subtype of the tumor.

Management Pearls

Nodular

- The diagnosis is made by initial biopsy.

Superficial

- If small and limited, consider cryosurgery or topical therapy (imiquimod, fluorouracil [5FU]) as an option. Electrodesiccation and curettage (ED&C) will often have excellent cosmetic results.

Infiltrating

- Proper care cannot be delivered if the specific subtype is not known and the treating physician does not understand the natural course of the disease. Infiltrating BCC is a subtype that must be treated with caution, as local tissue destruction and extensive reconstructive surgery are the results of delayed treatment. Small "strands" of tumor cells can infiltrate widely in the skin and be indistinct from normal skin (tip of the iceberg phenomenon). The diagnosis is made by initial biopsy, and if reports from the pathologist do not mention the subtype of BCC, then proceed with caution.

Superficial

Treatment must be individualized, but topical therapy (imiquimod, 5FU) or simple ED&C is often effective for superficial BCCs. In high-risk or cosmetically sensitive areas, consider Mohs micrographic surgery or simple excision.

Infiltrating

Infiltrative BCCs often extend beyond clinical margins and should, therefore, be referred for Mohs micrographic surgery. This technique will help establish clear margins intraoperatively by frozen section.

BCCs that are recurrent, primary BCCs occurring in the nasolabial fold areas, and BCCs with the morpheaform histopathology should be referred for Mohs micrographic surgery so that clear margins can be established intraoperatively by frozen section.

X-ray therapy is an accepted treatment modality for patients who are not good candidates for surgical removal.

Advise sun avoidance and sun protection with sunscreens and barrier clothing.

Patients with BCC should be followed by a dermatologist at regular intervals to assess for recurrence or the appearance of new lesions.

The following therapies may have lower cure rates than surgical removal, but when used correctly in selected patients, they can offer significant advantages:

- Topical imiquimod 5%
- Photodynamic therapy
- Topical 5FU has been used with some success, but penetration is an issue. It may not destroy malignant cells in the superficial dermis.
- Cryosurgery
- CO_2 laser

Immunocompromised Patient Considerations

Nodular

Topical agents such as imiquimod are sometimes used for small trunk or extremity lesions. X-ray therapy is an accepted treatment modality for patients who have inoperable or metastatic disease.

Suggested Readings

Aoyagi S, Nouri K. Difference between pigmented and nonpigmented basal cell carcinoma treated with Mohs micrographic surgery. *Dermatol Surg.* 2006 Nov;32(11):1375–1379.

Bath-Hextall FJ, Perkins W, Bong J, et al. Interventions for basal cell carcinoma of the skin. *Cochrane Database Syst Rev.* 2007 Oct;(4):CD005414.

Braathen LR, Szeimies RM, Basset-Seguin N, et al.; International Society for Photodynamic Therapy in Dermatology. Guidelines on the use of photodynamic therapy for nonmelanoma skin cancer: An international consensus. International Society for Photodynamic Therapy in Dermatology, 2005. *J Am Acad Dermatol.* 2007 Jan;56(1):125–143.

Carucci JA, Leffell DJ. Basal cell carcinoma. In: Fitzpatrick TB, Wolff K, eds. *Fitzpatrick's Dermatology in General Medicine.* 7th Ed. New York, NY: McGraw-Hill; 2008:1036–1042.

Geisse J, Caro I, Lindholm J, et al. Imiquimod 5% cream for the treatment of superficial basal cell carcinoma: Results from two phase III, randomized, vehicle-controlled studies. *J Am Acad Dermatol.* 2004 May;50(5): 722–733.

Pontén F, Lundeberg J, Asplund A. Principles of tumor biology and pathogenesis of BCCs and SCCs. In: Bolognia JL, Jorizzo JL, Rapini RP, eds. *Dermatology.* 2nd Ed. St. Louis, MO: Mosby; 2008:1635–1637, 1651–1652.

Richman T, Penneys NS. Analysis of morpheaform basal cell carcinoma. *J Cutan Pathol.* 1988 Dec;15(6):359–362.

Rubin AI, Chen EH, Ratner D. Basal-cell carcinoma. *N Engl J Med.* 2005 Nov;353(21):2262–2269.

Smucler R, Vlk M. Combination of Er:YAG laser and photodynamic therapy in the treatment of nodular basal cell carcinoma. *Lasers Surg Med.* 2008 Feb;40(2):153–158.

Wilkins K, Turner R, Dolev JC, et al. Cutaneous malignancy and human immunodeficiency virus disease. *J Am Acad Dermatol.* 2006 Feb;54(2): 189–206; quiz 207–210.

Drug Induced Pigmentation

Diagnosis Synopsis

Drug-induced pigmentation or hyperpigmentation may be caused by multiple drugs and through a number of differing mechanisms. Perhaps the most common reaction is postinflammatory hyperpigmentation as typically seen following inflammatory drug eruptions or fixed drug eruptions (considered separately). Other mechanisms include the cutaneous deposition of the drug or its metabolites, increased melanin synthesis, "pigment incontinence" from damage to melanocytes in the basal layer of the epidermis, or increased lipofuscin synthesis.

Increased melanin most often produces a brownish pigmentation. When drugs deposit in the dermis, however, there may be blue-black or blue-gray patches on the skin. Drugs known to have such an effect are metals (e.g., silver, gold, mercury, and bismuth), antimalarials, phenothiazines, amitriptyline, oral contraceptive pills, carbamazepine, gabapentin, lamotrigine, clozapine, amiodarone, clofazimine, and minocycline.

Immunocompromised Patient Considerations

Nail and skin hyperpigmentation have been observed in HIV/AIDS patients independent of HAART. Thus, pigmentary alteration in this population may be especially difficult to attribute to drugs. Newer agents used to treat HIV-infected patients have been shown to cause skin and nail hyperpigmentation, with nail hyperpigmentation being one of the most common cutaneous side effects of antiretroviral therapy (see below).

A number of chemotherapeutic agents are also associated with hyperpigmentation. Among them are carmustine, bleomycin, cisplatin, busulfan, doxorubicin, fluorouracil, hydroxyurea, mitoxantrone, vinorelbine, thiotepa, methotrexate, ifosfamide, cyclophosphamide, and docetaxel.

Look For

Blue-gray, brown, yellow, or red-brown macular skin discoloration is seen without any surface change (i.e., no scale) (Figs. 4-60–4-63). The pigmentation may be accentuated in certain areas (photodistributed, within scars, etc.) or may be widespread.

With a number of drugs, the pigmentary change also affects the nail unit (cyclophosphamide, doxorubicin, and nucleoside antiretroviral drugs) or the conjunctiva (phenothiazines, etc.). The nail matrix or nail bed may be darkened, and linear dark bands of varying width can occur.

Dark Skin Considerations

Antiretroviral- and diltiazem-induced skin hyperpigmentation occurs with higher frequency in blacks. In addition, periocular hyperpigmentation has been reported in black patients taking a prostaglandin F2-alpha derivative (latanoprost) for the treatment of glaucoma.

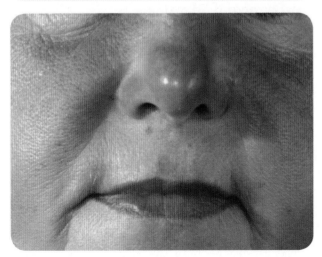

Figure 4-60 Amiodarone pigmentation in a characteristic location.

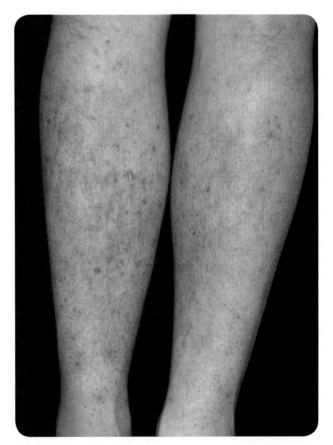

Figure 4-61 Bluish-black minocycline pigmentation is often on the legs, related to trauma.

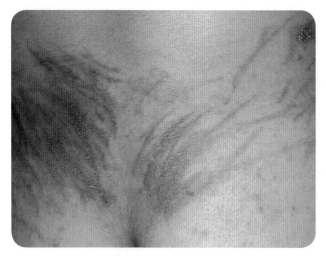

Figure 4-62 Flagellate hyperpigmentation is characteristic of systemic treatment with bleomycin.

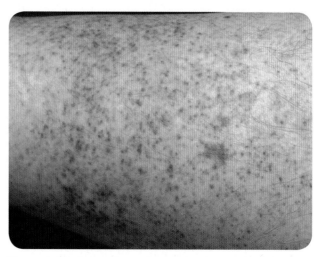

Figure 4-63 Punctate hyperpigmentation due to minocycline.

Immunocompromised Patient Considerations

Hyperpigmentation of the palms and soles can occur with emtricitabine, a nucleoside reverse transcriptase inhibitor used to treat HIV-infected individuals.

Diagnostic Pearls

- Diffuse hyperpigmentation may indicate drug-induced pigmentation or systemic disease.
- Some drugs and typical associated pigmentations:
- Yellow—quinacrine
- Blue-black—antimalarials, chloroquine, hydroxychloroquine, or hydroquinone
- Blue-gray—gold, silver
- Blue—minocycline, amiodarone
- Red-brown—clofazimine
- Brown streaks (flagellate or linear)—bleomycin
- Minocycline may cause pigmentation primarily within scars, especially acne scars.

Immunocompromised Patient Considerations

Emtricitabine—hyperpigmentation of palms and soles
Zidovudine—nail and oral hyperpigmentation

Generally, hyperpigmentation caused by these antiretroviral agents is dose dependent and reversible.

?? Differential Diagnosis and Pitfalls

- Jaundice causes a yellow cast to the skin.
- Carotenemia causes an orange color in the skin.
- Generalized hyperpigmentation is also seen in Addison disease, Cushing syndrome, scleroderma, Wilson disease, hemochromatosis, chronic renal failure, porphyria cutanea tarda, vitamin B_{12} deficiency, pellagra, ochronosis, Gaucher disease, and carcinoid.
- Melasma or chloasma
- Erythema ab igne
- Ashy dermatosis (erythema dyschromicum perstans)
- Confluent and reticulated papillomatosis (Gougerot-Carteaud syndrome)

Immunocompromised Patient Differential Diagnosis

Always have Kaposi sarcoma in the differential diagnosis of hyperpigmentation in HIV-infected individuals (have a low threshold to biopsy).

✓ Best Tests

- This diagnosis can usually be made clinically. Take a careful medication history.
- Antimalarials may fluoresce with a Wood light.
- Skin biopsy can often reveal the type of pigment within the skin and determine whether the pigmentation is dermal or epidermal.
- Other tests may be used to rule out systemic illnesses such as liver or renal function tests, iron studies, or ACTH, etc.

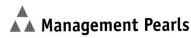

Management Pearls

- Discontinuing the responsible drug is the treatment of choice. Patients should be made aware that it may take months to years for the pigment to resolve or that it may never resolve.

Immunocompromised Patient Considerations

In some instances, antiretroviral-induced skin hyperpigmentation will resolve spontaneously without discontinuation of the offending drug. In most cases, however, the offending drug must be discontinued in order for the hyperpigmentation to resolve.

Therapy

Discontinue the medication if at all possible. Treatment is largely for aesthetic purposes. Consider the use of camouflage cosmetics.

Some forms of drug-induced pigmentation are worsened by sun exposure. Counsel the patient regarding sun avoidance and the use of barrier clothing and combined UVA/UVB sunscreens.

Topical corticosteroids, classes 3 and 4 to trunk and classes 6 and 7 to face, may help with some of the hyperpigmentation in the epidermis.

Mid-potency topical corticosteroids (classes 3 and 4)

- Triamcinolone cream, ointment—apply twice daily (15, 30, 60, 120, 240 g)
- Mometasone cream, ointment—apply twice daily (15, 45 g)
- Fluocinolone cream, ointment—apply twice daily (15, 30, 60 g)

Low-potency topical steroids (classes 6 and 7)

- Desonide cream, ointment—apply twice daily (15, 60, 90 g)
- Alclometasone cream, ointment—apply twice daily (15, 45, 60 g)

Immunocompromised Patient Considerations

Be aware of dermatophyte (tinea) infections in immunosuppressed patients treated with topical corticosteroids.

Suggested Readings

Borrás-Blasco J, Navarro-Ruiz A, Borrás C, et al. Adverse cutaneous reactions associated with the newest antiretroviral drugs in patients with human immunodeficiency virus infection. *J Antimicrob Chemother.* 2008 Nov;62(5):879–888. Epub 2008 Jul 23.

Dereure O. Drug-induced skin pigmentation. Epidemiology, diagnosis and treatment. *Am J Clin Dermatol.* 2001;2(4):253–262.

Granstein RD, Sober AJ. Drug- and heavy metal-induced hyperpigmentation. *J Am Acad Dermatol.* 1981 Jul;5(1):1–18.

Hendrix JD, Greer KE. Cutaneous hyperpigmentation caused by systemic drugs. *Int J Dermatol.* 1992 Jul;31(7):458–466.

Herndon LW, Williams RD, Wand M, et al. Increased periocular pigmentation with ocular hypotensive lipid use in African Americans. *Am J Ophthalmol.* 2003 May;135(5):713–715.

Nikolaou V, Stratigos AJ, Katsambas AD. Established treatments of skin hypermelanoses. *J Cosmet Dermatol.* 2006 Dec;5(4):303–308.

Saladi RN, Cohen SR, Phelps RG, et al. Diltiazem induces severe photodistributed hyperpigmentation: Case series, histoimmunopathology, management, and review of the literature. *Arch Dermatol.* 2006 Feb;142(2):206–210.

Vassallo P, Trohman RG. Prescribing amiodarone: An evidence-based review of clinical indications. *JAMA.* 2007 Sep;298(11):1312–1322.

Wiper A, Roberts DH, Schmitt M. Amiodarone-induced skin pigmentation: Q-switched laser therapy, an effective treatment option. *Heart.* 2007 Jan;93(1):15.

Erythema Dyschromicum Perstans

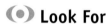 Diagnosis Synopsis

Erythema dyschromicum perstans (ashy dermatosis) is an acquired hypermelanosis of unknown etiology. It was originally described in Latin American individuals of intermediate skin tone but has subsequently been identified in other ethnicities and skin types. Recent studies suggest a cell-mediated immune reaction to antigens located in basal and mid-epidermal keratinocytes. Erythema dyschromicum perstans presents as asymptomatic or mildly pruritic gray-blue macules of various sizes on the trunk and proximal extremities. It is associated with lichen planus as well as with certain exposures, including ammonium nitrate, oral radiographic contrast media, cobalt, and parasitic whipworm infection. Erythema dyschromicum perstans is more common in women. Age of onset is usually in the second or third decade, but all age groups may be affected.

Look For

Blue-gray, "ashy" macules and patches of various sizes (0.5 to 3.0 cm), concentrated most commonly on the trunk, neck, and proximal extremities (Figs. 4-64–4-67).

Diagnostic Pearls

- Active lesions may have a narrow, difficult-to-discern, erythematous border.

?? Differential Diagnosis and Pitfalls

- Lichen planus (including the variant lichen planus pigmentosus)—pruritic
- Lichenoid drug eruptions—usually more erythematous
- Postinflammatory hyperpigmentation
- Fixed drug eruption—multiple
- Macular amyloidosis
- Maculae cerulea (arthropod bites)
- Macular urticaria pigmentosa
- Pinta—late
- Argyria
- Drug-induced pigmentation
- Addison disease
- Melasma
- Confluent and reticulated papillomatosis
- Dermal melanosis

✓ Best Tests

- Skin biopsy will demonstrate vacuolar degeneration of the basal layer with pigmentary incontinence and dermal macrophages laden with melanin.
- Serological tests for syphilis should be considered to exclude treponematosis.

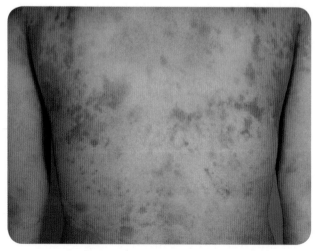

Figure 4-64 Bluish and brownish hyperpigmented lesions in a common location for erythema dyschromicum perstans.

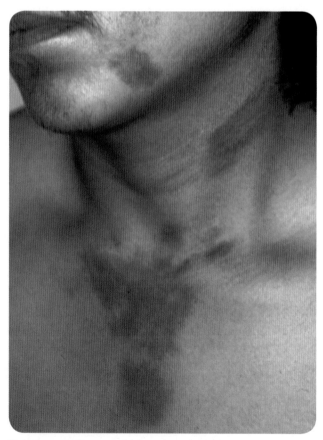

Figure 4-65 Bluish and brownish macules of erythema dyschromicum perstans.

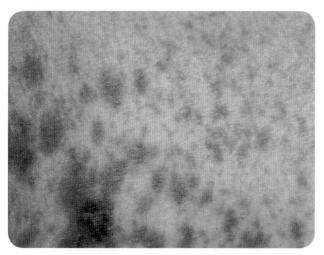

Figure 4-66 A 38-year-old male with multiple macular lesions consistent with erythema dyschromicum perstans.

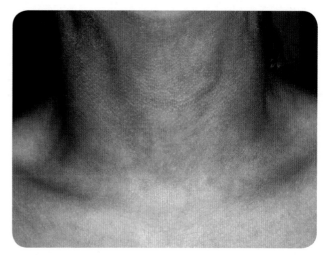

Figure 4-67 The neck is frequently involved with erythema dyschromicum perstans, with some sparing in the light-protected area in the midline of the neck.

▲▲ Management Pearls

- There have been reports of spontaneous resolution.
- Camouflage cosmetics may be used for cosmetic purposes.

Therapy

In some patients, no treatment may be a reasonable option.

In patients desiring treatment, the following have demonstrated variable success but may have serious cutaneous and systemic side effects:

- Clofazimine—100 mg p.o. daily for 3 months
- Vitamin A—100,000 U p.o. daily for 15 day pulses
- Dapsone—100 mg p.o. daily for 3 months

Suggested Readings

Bahadir S, Cobanoglu U, Cimsit G, et al. Erythema dyschromicum perstans: Response to dapsone therapy. *Int J Dermatol.* 2004 Mar;43(3):220–222.

Chang MW. Pigmentary disorders. In: Bolognia JL, Jorizzo JL, Rapini RP, eds. *Dermatology.* 2nd Ed. St. Louis, MO: Mosby; 2008:940–941.

Osswald SS, Proffer LH, Sartori CR. Erythema dyschromicum perstans: A case report and review. *Cutis.* 2001 Jul;68(1):25–28.

Schwartz RA. Erythema dyschromicum perstans: The continuing enigma of Cinderella or ashy dermatosis. *Int J Dermatol.* 2004 Mar;43(3):230–232.

Stratigos AJ, Katsambas AD. Optimal management of recalcitrant disorders of hyperpigmentation in dark-skinned patients. *Am J Clin Dermatol.* 2004;5(3):161–168.

Torrelo A, Zaballos P, Colmenero I, et al. Erythema dyschromicum perstans in children: A report of 14 cases. *J Eur Acad Dermatol Venereol.* 2005 Jul;19(4):422–426.

Vásquez-Ochoa LA, Isaza-Guzmán DM, Orozco-Mora B, et al. Immunopathologic study of erythema dyschromicum perstans (ashy dermatosis). *Int J Dermatol.* 2006 Aug;45(8):937–941.

Zaynoun S, Rubeiz N, Kibbi AG. Ashy dermatoses—a critical review of the literature and a proposed simplified clinical classification. *Int J Dermatol.* 2008 Jun;47(6):542–544.

Fixed Drug Eruption

Diagnosis Synopsis

Fixed drug eruption (FDE) is an adverse drug reaction manifested by skin lesions occurring at the same body site each time the individual is reexposed to the specific drug. It is most frequently solitary but may sometimes be multiple. Lesions are usually asymptomatic but may cause burning or pruritus. Sometimes these lesions will form blisters. Postinflammatory hyperpigmentation is common.

Trimethoprim-sulfamethoxazole is the most frequently associated drug, but other drugs known to cause the condition are analgesics/antipyretics (aspirin and NSAIDs), other antibiotics (ampicillin, metronidazole, and tetracycline), as well as barbiturates, oral contraceptives, and quinine. Phenolphthalein (historically, a component of laxatives, replaced in the United States largely by senna) was found to be a cause of fixed drug reactions.

Immunocompromised Patient Considerations

FDEs have been reported with the use of saquinavir in patients with HIV.

Look For

Solitary or multiple sharply demarcated, circular (almost a perfect circle), red or brown-red plaques recurring in exactly the same location(s) each time the drug is taken (Figs. 4-68–4-70). FDEs usually start as a red patch and frequently leave hyperpigmented patches between acute flares.

The most frequent location is the genitals, with the glans penis being a common location for a plaque (Fig. 4-71), but lesions can occur anywhere. Lesions on the hands and feet are also frequently seen.

Dark Skin Considerations

Solitary or multiple sharply demarcated deep red, brown, or black patches recurring in exactly the same location(s) each time the drug is taken. The darker the skin, the darker the fixed drug lesions.

Diagnostic Pearls

- Symptoms (e.g., itching and burning) and worsening of the plaques occur within 12 h of taking the drug.

Differential Diagnosis and Pitfalls

- Insect bite reaction can leave similar hyperpigmented patches.
- Postinflammatory pigmentation
- Contact dermatitis
- Lichen planus
- Erythema multiforme
- Recurrent herpes simplex virus
- Cellulitis or erysipelas
- Bullous impetigo
- Cicatricial pemphigoid

Best Tests

- Skin biopsy will be suggestive of the diagnosis.
- Rechallenge to the medication and observing for the characteristic change is possible but usually not recommended due to a risk of a more severe, generalized reaction.

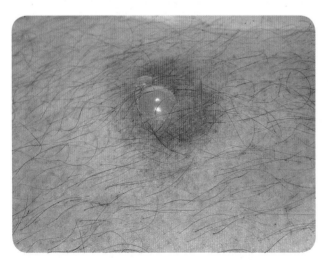

Figure 4-68 An early fixed drug eruption with two vesicles on a dusky red base.

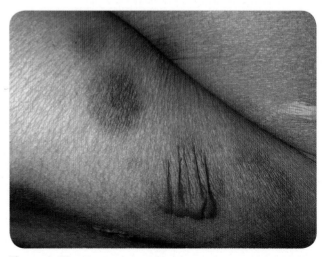

Figure 4-69 Bullae and hyperpigmentation in a fixed drug eruption.

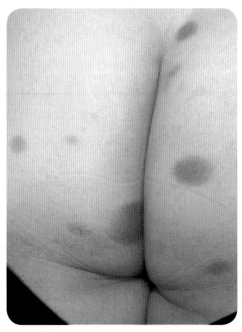

Figure 4-70 Multiple fixed drug eruption lesions due to a sulfa medication.

▲▲ Management Pearls

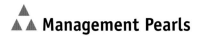

- It is important to explore anything ingested, including over-the-counter medications/preparations, health food supplements, and prescription medications. Discontinue the drug and any potential cross-reacting medications.

Therapy

The best therapy is watchful waiting and avoidance of the drug and its related compounds. The lesions will heal spontaneously; thus, treatment is only needed for any pain or secondary infection. Recovery usually takes 2 to 3 weeks. However, the secondary pigment alteration may be persistent.

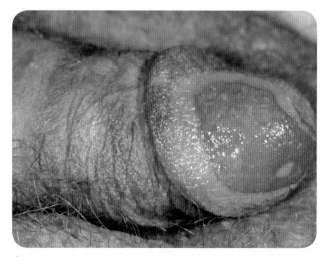

Figure 4-71 The penis is a common location for a fixed drug eruption.

Suggested Readings

Hughes BR, Holt PJ, Marks R. Trimethoprim associated fixed drug eruption. *Br J Dermatol.* 1987 Feb;116(2):241–242.

James WD, Berger TG, Elston DM. Contact dermatitis and drug eruptions. In: James WD, Berger TG, Elston DM, Odom RB, eds. *Andrews' Diseases of the Skin: Clinical Dermatology.* 10th Ed. Philadelphia, PA: Saunders Elsevier; 2006:127.

Lee AY. Fixed drug eruptions. Incidence, recognition, and avoidance. *Am J Clin Dermatol.* 2000 Sep–Oct;1(5):277–285.

Nigen S, Knowles SR, Shear NH. Drug eruptions: Approaching the diagnosis of drug-induced skin diseases. *J Drugs Dermatol.* 2003 Jun;2(3):278–299.

Pasricha JS. Drugs causing fixed eruptions. *Br J Dermatol.* 1979 Feb;100(2):183–185.

Sánchez-Borges M, Capriles-Hulett A, Caballero-Fonseca F. Risk of skin reactions when using ibuprofen-based medicines. *Expert Opin Drug Saf.* 2005 Sep;4(5):837–848.

Shear NH, Knowles SR, Shapiro L. Cutaneous reactions to drugs. In: Fitzpatrick TB, Wolff K, eds. *Fitzpatrick's Dermatology in General Medicine.* 7th Ed. New York, NY: McGraw-Hill; 2008:355–362.

Smith KJ, Yeager J, Skelton H. Fixed drug eruptions to human immunodeficiency virus-1 protease inhibitor. *Cutis.* 2000 Jul;66(1):29–32.

Thankappan TP, Zachariah J. Drug-specific clinical pattern in fixed drug eruptions. *Int J Dermatol.* 1991 Dec;30(12):867–870.

Wintroub BU, Stern R. Cutaneous drug reactions: Pathogenesis and clinical classification. *J Am Acad Dermatol.* 1985 Aug;13(2 Pt 1):167–179.

Lentigo Maligna and Lentigo Maligna Melanoma

Diagnosis Synopsis

Lentigo Maligna

Lentigo maligna is a noninvasive form of melanoma (melanoma in situ) found most commonly on sun-exposed areas of the head and neck in older patients. This precursor lesion has been likened to a "stain" on the skin and occurs most commonly in fair-skinned individuals with a history of significant UV radiation exposure. Histologically, lentigo maligna is characterized by confluent atypical melanocytes arranged along the dermal epidermal junction.

Lentigo maligna is difficult to distinguish from its invasive counterpart. The natural history of lentigo maligna is gradual horizontal growth with enlargement at the periphery of the lesion accompanied by a darkening of the lesion and the development of irregular edges. After several years to decades, a vertical growth phase may occur; at that point, the condition becomes lentigo maligna melanoma.

Lentigo Maligna Melanoma

Lentigo maligna melanoma develops when a lentigo maligna (melanoma in situ) enters a vertical growth phase and is no longer confined to the epidermis. Lifetime risk of a 45 year old with lentigo maligna progressing to lentigo maligna melanoma has been estimated at 5%. Elsewhere, progression rates have been estimated from 2% to 50%. Of patients initially diagnosed with lentigo maligna by biopsy, 8% to 16% will have lentigo maligna melanoma identified in the final excision specimen. Lentigo maligna melanomas may extend slightly above the surface of the skin and may be prone to bleeding. This condition generally occurs 5–20 years after the lentigo maligna first developed. It is most frequent on sun-damaged skin (usually facial) and is most frequently found on individuals aged 60 or older. Lentigo maligna melanoma represents between 10% and 26% of the head and neck melanomas.

Lentigo maligna and lentigo maligna melanoma have also been associated with light skin color, a history of severe sunburns, basal cell carcinoma, porphyria cutanea tarda, oculocutaneous albinism, xeroderma pigmentosum, and Werner syndrome (reported in Japanese patients).

Look For

Lentigo Maligna

Irregularly bordered, hyperpigmented (tan-brown), flat macule or patch, usually on the face of an elderly person (Figs. 4-72–4-74). There may be variations in pigmentation throughout. There is a particular predilection for the nose and the cheeks, but the arms, legs, and trunk may be affected.

Cutaneous lentigo maligna may spread to mucosal surfaces, in which case hyperpigmented areas may be observed on the conjunctiva and oral mucosa.

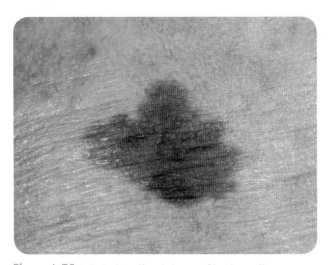

Figure 4-72 Relatively uniformly brown of lentigo maligna.

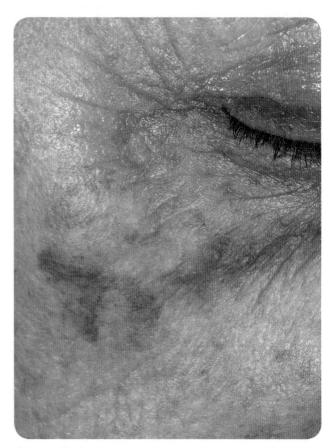

Figure 4-73 Uniformly brown lentigo maligna on sun-damaged skin.

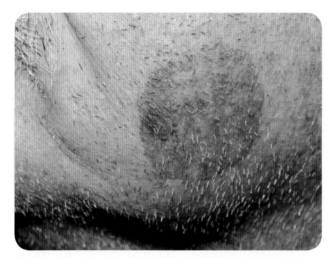

Figure 4-74 Mahogany brown plaque of lentigo maligna.

Lentigo Maligna Melanoma

An irregularly bordered, pigmented brown to black patch or plaque, typically on the head and neck regions, often on the nose and cheek, of an elderly patient (Figs. 4-75 and 4-76).

There may be palpable dermal induration or nodularity within the lesion.

Diagnostic Pearls

Lentigo Maligna

- Use a Wood lamp (UVA lamp) to examine the skin in a darkened room. This will often reveal more extensive disease, showing borders with more clarity than visible light.

Lentigo Maligna Melanoma

- Lesional borders are often very difficult to perceive. A Wood lamp is useful in clarifying the border.
- The discovery of a more deeply pigmented, irregular nodule within the lesion is often indicative of dermal invasion. Biopsy should be directed at such areas.

?? Differential Diagnosis and Pitfalls

Lentigo Maligna/Lentigo Maligna Melanoma

- Nevus
- Melanoma
- Lentigo maligna melanoma—in the case of lentigo maligna
- Melasma
- Seborrheic keratosis
- Pigmented basal cell carcinoma
- Pigmented actinic keratosis
- Solar lentigo
- Lentigo simplex
- Labial melanotic macules
- Café au lait spots
- Pigmented Bowen disease

✓ Best Tests

- Dermatoscopy may help distinguish benign from malignant pigmented lesions, but a full-thickness skin biopsy (i.e., a punch biopsy of at least 5 mm in diameter or an incisional biopsy) is indicated for all suspicious lesions. Multiple biopsies of larger or irregular lesions may be indicated as well.
- A metastatic workup is not indicated for lentigo maligna.

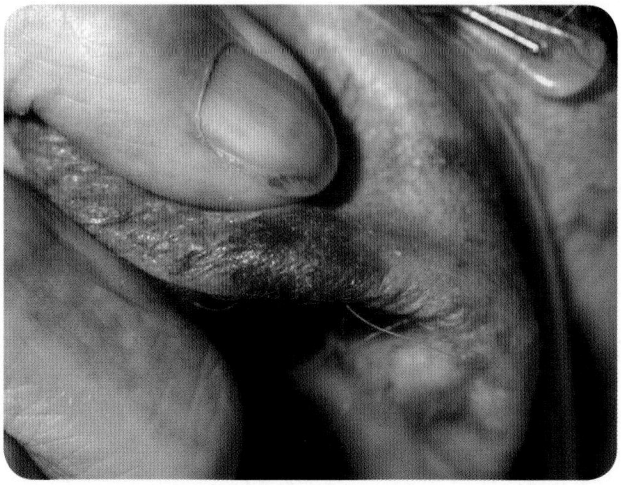

Figure 4-75 Lentigo maligna melanoma is an irregular black nodule on a brown macule on the helix.

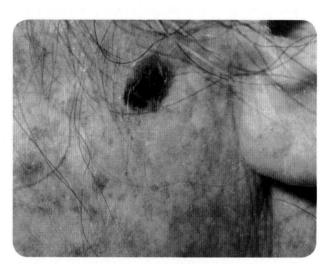

Figure 4-76 An irregular black nodule grows over a brown macule on the cheek as a lentigo maligna melanoma.

Lentigo Maligna Melanoma

- Full-thickness skin biopsy: Dermoscopy may help differentiate between benign and malignant pigmented lesions, but suspicious lesions should always be submitted for histopathologic examination.
- Because melanoma most often metastasizes to the lung, liver, and brain, the following studies may be considered as part of a metastatic or staging workup if symptoms are present:
  - Chest radiograph
  - Liver function tests and LDH
  - Proton emission tomography (PET) scan
  - MRI
  - CT scan(s)

▲▲ Management Pearls

Lentigo Maligna

- Lesional borders are often very difficult to perceive. A Wood lamp is useful in clarifying the border, and ample margins should be used in excisions.
- If there is a strong suspicion of invasive melanoma, the lesion should be excised fully at the time of the biopsy. Defer to the expertise of a dermatologist if one is available, and make sure that the specimen is interpreted by a dermatopathologist.
- Patients with lentigo maligna should have periodic (every 6 months) full-body skin examinations by a dermatologist.

Lentigo Maligna Melanoma

- Patients with suspicious, pigmented lesions and those with known melanoma should be referred to and followed by a dermatologist.
- Skin biopsy specimens should be interpreted by a dermatopathologist.
- All patients with melanoma *except* those with stage 0 or stage 1A disease (i.e., nonulcerated lesions less than or equal to 1.0 mm in thickness) should be considered for sentinel lymph node biopsy and possible formal lymph node dissection by a surgical oncologist. Medical oncology should be involved as well.
- Patients may ultimately require a plastic surgery consultation for reconstruction.

Therapy

Lentigo Maligna

Complete surgical excision is the treatment of choice. Staged excisions using delayed closure with rush permanent section confirmation of negative margins (so-called slow Mohs) is ideal. If staged excision is not practical, simple excision with *at least* 0.5 to 1.0 cm margins is advised with attention to one large retrospective study of staged excisions in which the mean total surgical margin required for margin-clear excision was 7.1 mm.

Mohs micrographic surgery in the hands of surgeons experienced with lentigo maligna is an alternative.

Treatment with topical imiquimod 5% for at least 12 weeks of nightly application is emerging as an alternative in patients who refuse surgery or for whom surgery is contraindicated or not feasible. Surgical excision is still considered the first-line therapy.

Although not recommended, in patients who are not candidates for surgery or who refuse surgery, successful use of the following modalities has also been reported:

- Radiotherapy
- Q-switched ruby laser
- Q-switched Nd:YAG laser
- Intralesional interferon-α
- Tazarotene 1% gel applied daily for 6 to 8 months
- Azelaic acid 15% to 20% applied twice daily for 2 weeks to 12 months

Lentigo Maligna Melanoma

Surgical excision is the treatment of choice. The margins required depend on the depth of invasion of the tumor determined by biopsy:

- Less than 1 mm—margins 1 cm
- 1 to 2 mm—margins 1 to 2 cm
- 2 to 4 mm—margins 2 cm
- Greater than 4 mm—margin at least 2 cm

Mohs micrographic surgery and staged excisions have also been used for lentigo maligna melanoma with low local recurrence rates.

In patients who are not surgical candidates, a number of nonsurgical therapies have been employed:

- Cryosurgery
- Radiation therapy
- Laser surgery
- Electrodesiccation
- Topical therapies such as imiquimod

All of the above options carry a significant rate of recurrence and metastasis.

Patients with nodal metastases will require a full lymph node dissection and adjuvant chemotherapy such as interferon-α 2b. Chemotherapy for patients with metastatic disease may also consist of temozolomide, interleukin-2 (IL-2), dacarbazine, or granulocyte macrophage-colony stimulating factor (GM-CSF).

Many vaccines against melanoma have been developed and are currently under development. As of yet, none has demonstrated an ability to impact survival.

Avoidance of sun and use of sun-protective clothing and sunscreens are strongly recommended.

Suggested Readings

Al-Niaimi F, Jury CS, McLaughlin S, et al. Review of management and outcome in 65 patients with lentigo maligna. *Br J Dermatol.* 2009 Jan;160(1):211–213.

Arlette JP, Trotter MJ, Trotter T, et al. Management of lentigo maligna and lentigo maligna melanoma: Seminars in surgical oncology. *J Surg Oncol.* 2004 Jul;86(4):179–186.

Bhardwaj SS, Tope WD, Lee PK. Mohs micrographic surgery for lentigo maligna and lentigo maligna melanoma using Mel-5 immunostaining: University of Minnesota experience. *Dermatol Surg.* 2006 May;32(5): 690–696; discussion 696–697.

Buettiker UV, Yawalkar NY, Braathen LR, et al. Imiquimod treatment of lentigo maligna: An open-label study of 34 primary lesions in 32 patients. *Arch Dermatol.* 2008 Jul;144(7):943–945.

Cohen LM. Lentigo maligna and lentigo maligna melanoma. *J Am Acad Dermatol.* 1995 Dec;33(6):923–936; quiz 937–940.

Hazan C, Dusza SW, Delgado R, et al. Staged excision for lentigo maligna and lentigo maligna melanoma: A retrospective analysis of 117 cases. *J Am Acad Dermatol.* 2008 Jan;58(1):142–148.

Huang CC. New approaches to surgery of lentigo maligna. *Skin Therapy Lett.* 2004 May;9(5):7–11.

Huilgol SC, Selva D, Chen C, et al. Surgical margins for lentigo maligna and lentigo maligna melanoma: The technique of mapped serial excision. *Arch Dermatol.* 2004 Sep;140(9):1087–1092.

McKenna JK, Florell SR, Goldman GD, et al. Lentigo maligna/lentigo maligna melanoma: Current state of diagnosis and treatment. *Dermatol Surg.* 2006 Apr;32(4):493–504.

Osborne JE, Hutchinson PE. A follow-up study to investigate the efficacy of initial treatment of lentigo maligna with surgical excision. *Br J Plast Surg.* 2002 Dec;55(8):611–615.

Rajpar SF, Marsden JR. Imiquimod in the treatment of lentigo maligna. *Br J Dermatol.* 2006 Oct;155(4):653–656.

Smalberger GJ, Siegel DM, Khachemoune A. Lentigo maligna. *Dermatol Ther.* 2008 Nov–Dec;21(6):439–446.

Stevenson O, Ahmed I. Lentigo maligna: Prognosis and treatment options. *Am J Clin Dermatol.* 2005;6(3):151–164.

Diagnosis Synopsis

A lentigo simplex is an extremely common hyperpigmented macule located anywhere on the body. They generally occur early in life (may be present at birth) and are not associated with sun exposure. They result from an increased number of normal melanocytes in the epidermis producing increased amounts of melanin.

Clinically, lesions are asymptomatic, well-circumscribed, symmetric, homogeneous light brown to black macules. They are usually smaller than 5 mm in size. They are distributed anywhere on the trunk, extremities, genitals, and mucous membranes. Lentigines found on mucous membranes can appear irregular with increased size, irregular borders, and heterogeneous pigmentation. They occasionally form in cutaneous scars and may be associated with psoralen/ultraviolet light therapy. Lentigo simplex may evolve into junctional nevi but are not thought to evolve into melanoma.

They differ from solar lentigines in that they appear earlier in life on non–sun-exposed skin.

Lentigo simplex may occur as single or multiple lesions. Occasionally, multiple lentigines are associated with rare genetic disorders. These include the following:

- LEOPARD syndrome—lentigines, EKG changes, ocular hypertelorism, pulmonary stenosis, abnormal genitalia, growth retardation, and deafness
- Carney complex—lentigines, atrial myxoma, mucocutaneous myxoma, and nevi
- Peutz-Jeghers syndrome—lentigines (perioral and oral), multiple gastrointestinal polyps, and visceral tumors (pancreas, ovary, and testes)
- Xeroderma pigmentosum—lentigines on sun-exposed skin and multiple skin cancers
- Cronkhite-Canada syndrome—lentigines (buccal mucosa, face, and palmoplantar), alopecia, nail dystrophy, and intestinal polyps

Other rare disorders associated with multiple lentigines include generalized lentigines, arterial dissection with lentiginosis, Laugier-Hunziker syndrome, Cantú (hyperkeratosis-hyperpigmentation) syndrome, Cowden disease, centrofacial lentiginosis, and Bannayan-Riley-Ruvalcaba syndrome.

Look For

Look for light brown to almost black, regular, oval or round, macules that are usually smaller than 5 mm in size (Figs. 4-77–4-80). The edge of the macule can be jagged or smooth.

Dark Skin Considerations

Lentigo simplex is the most common pigmented lesion found on the acral skin (palms and soles) of darkly pigmented patients.

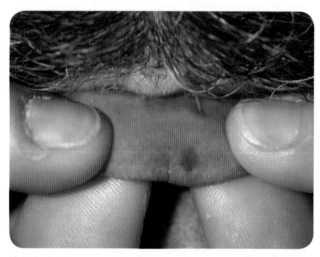

Figure 4-77 Lentigo simplex is not uncommon on the lower lip.

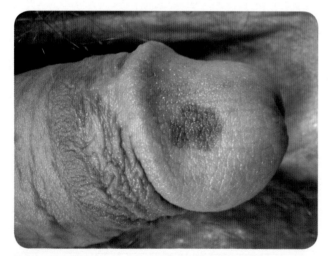

Figure 4-78 Uniform brown macule on the glans.

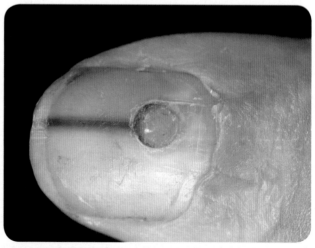

Figure 4-79 Biopsy-proven lentigo simplex of the nail bed.

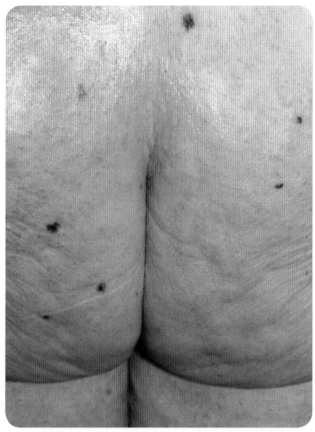

Figure 4-80 Very dark "black ink color" lentigines after psoralen plus UVA (PUVA) therapy for psoriasis.

Diagnostic Pearls

- Lentigo simplex is more regular than the sun-exposed variant (solar lentigo). Using, for example, an episcope allows closer appreciation of the pigment, which often seems to stream from the center of a lesion.
- Lentigo simplex lesions are typically darker than ephelides and do not darken or increase with sun exposure.

Differential Diagnosis and Pitfalls

- Blacks frequently have centrofacial lentigos that are autosomal dominant.
- Solar lentigo typically occurs on sun-exposed surfaces with increasing age and is less regular in appearance.

- A café au lait spot is macular and present from the time of infancy.
- An oral mucosal lesion may be difficult to distinguish from an amalgam tattoo and mucosal melanoma.
- Lentigo maligna
- Melanoma
- Ephelides
- Seborrheic keratoses
- Junctional and compound nevi
- Hemangioma

✓ Best Tests

- Episcopic examination may help differentiate lentigo simplex from a malignancy. If there is doubt, biopsy.

▲▲ Management Pearls

- Suspicious single lesions should be surgically removed because they may be difficult to distinguish from melanomas.

Therapy

Any suspicious lesions should be surgically excised and sent for histopathologic examination. It is appropriate to follow up on benign-appearing lesions periodically.

Cryosurgery or combination of tretinoin and hydroquinone cream applied once or twice daily may improve cosmetic appearance.

Suggested Readings

Buchner A, Merrell PW, Hansen LS, et al. Melanocytic hyperplasia of the oral mucosa. *Oral Surg Oral Med Oral Pathol.* 1991 Jan;71(1):58–62.

Erkek E, Erdogan S, Tuncez F, et al. Type I hereditary punctate keratoderma associated with widespread lentigo simplex and successfully treated with low-dose oral acitretin. *Arch Dermatol.* 2006 Aug;142(8):1076–1077.

Grichnik JM, Rhodes AR, Sober AJ. Benign neoplasms and hyperplasias of melanocytes. In: Fitzpatrick TB, Wolff K, eds. *Fitzpatrick's Dermatology in General Medicine.* 7th Ed. New York, NY: McGraw-Hill; 2008:1117–1119.

McCarthy DJ. Lentigo simplex. *J Am Podiatr Med Assoc.* 1987 Oct;77(10): 539–543.

Rhodes AR, Harrist TJ, Momtaz-T K. The PUVA-induced pigmented macule: A lentiginous proliferation of large, sometimes cytologically atypical, melanocytes. *J Am Acad Dermatol.* 1983 Jul;9(1):47–58.

Melanoma

Diagnosis Synopsis

Melanoma is a life-threatening malignancy of pigment-producing cells (melanocytes). There are 4 main subtypes: superficial spreading melanoma (the most-common type), nodular melanoma, lentigo maligna melanoma, and acral lentiginous melanoma (the least-common type, which tends to occur in dark-skinned individuals). There is also an amelanotic (i.e., nonpigmented) form of melanoma. Malignant melanoma may arise from a previously existing pigmented lesion or develop de novo. Prognosis is worse with an increasing depth of invasion, which is measured histologically in millimeters and referred to as Breslow thickness. Early diagnosis and treatment can lead to complete cure and survival, while advanced forms carry a poor prognosis. The most frequent sites of melanoma metastasis are the lungs, liver, and brain.

Predisposing factors for melanoma include a family history or prior personal history of melanoma, a history of severe sunburns, a changing mole, a giant congenital nevus (>20 cm), older age, fair skin, and multiple atypical nevi. Of these, the most powerful risk factor is having multiple atypical nevi. Men are more prone to developing melanoma on the head, neck, and trunk. Women tend to develop melanoma on the arms and legs. Mortality rates are higher among men than among women. Melanoma is most often diagnosed during middle age, and the incidence of melanoma has been increasing in recent years.

Melanomas may arise anywhere on the skin, on mucous membranes, around the nail apparatus, and in the eye.

Look For

Morphology will vary somewhat by subtype, but most melanomas share several common features as outlined in the

Immunocompromised Patient Considerations

While HIV-infected and immunocompromised patients have a slightly increased risk of melanoma (in contrast to a much higher risk of nonmelanoma skin cancers in these populations), the prognosis for melanoma in the HIV patient is markedly worse than in the immunocompetent patient. HIV patients have a significantly shorter life expectancy once diagnosed with melanoma.

ABCDEs of melanoma below. Ulceration and bleeding are universally late signs.

Superficial spreading melanoma—An asymmetric macule with brown variegated pigmentation and notched or ragged borders (Figs. 4-81 and 4-82). May occasionally be somewhat elevated. Usually seen on the trunk in men and the lower extremities in women. Melanomas are the second most common malignancy of the vulva; most are of the superficial spreading type (Fig. 4-83).

Nodular melanoma—A dark brown to bluish-black nodule that grows rapidly. This type of melanoma is most likely to ulcerate or bleed with minor trauma. Found commonly on the trunk, head, and neck.

Lentigo maligna melanoma—An asymmetric brown to black macule or patch with color variations and irregular borders. May have area(s) of dermal induration or nodularity. Usually seen on the face or other sun-exposed areas on an elderly individual. Also see separate write-up on lentigo maligna and lentigo maligna melanoma.

Acral lentiginous melanoma—Also an asymmetric brown to black macule with variegated pigmentation and irregular borders. Found on the palms, soles, or involving the nail apparatus (Fig. 4-84).

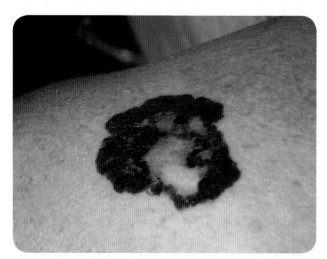

Figure 4-81 Superficial spreading melanoma with a large area of hypopigmented regression.

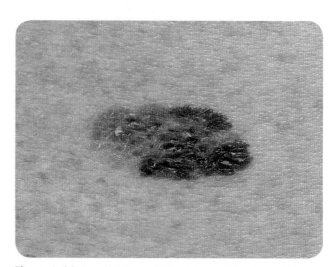

Figure 4-82 Superficial spreading melanoma with an area of pigment regression.

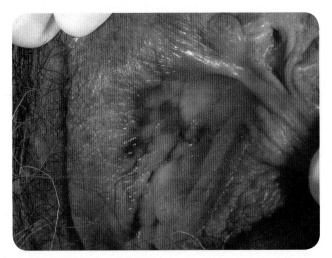

Figure 4-83 Melanoma of the vulva.

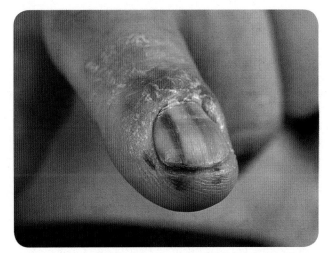

Figure 4-84 Melanoma of the nail extending to the distal digit.

Dark Skin Considerations

In black patients, subtle color variation can be difficult to see. Distal (hands and feet) melanomas are much more common in black patients than white patients. Ulceration and bleeding are very late signs.

Diagnostic Pearls

- Primary care physicians may play an important role in preventing mortality from melanoma. By identifying risk factors for melanoma (see Introduction) and by applying ABCDE criteria (see below) to lesions brought to clinical attention by patients or via a careful screening during physical exam, the generalist will make the proper decision on the need to refer to a dermatologist.
- Decision to biopsy should begin with a history and physical examination. Individual pigmented lesions are evaluated in the physical exam by applying "the ugly duckling rule" and the **ABCDEs** of melanoma:
  A—Asymmetry: One half of the lesion does not mirror the other half.
  B—Border: The borders are irregular, shaggy, or indistinct.
  C—Color: The color is variegated; the pigment is not uniform, and there may be varying shades and/or hues.
  D—Diameter: Classically, any pigmented lesion greater than 6 mm in diameter is concerning. Melanomas, however, are often detected at smaller sizes.
  E—Evolving: Notable change in a lesion over time raises suspicion for malignancy. Ulceration and bleeding are late signs and should certainly prompt biopsy.
- In a patient with multiple pigmented lesions, look for and strongly consider biopsy of "the ugly duckling" lesion, that is, one that strikes the examiner as unlike the others.

- Any new dark black lesion—irrespective of its size—should be considered a possible melanoma. However, being exophytic or raised does not make a pigmented papule more suspicious to be a melanoma. The presence of a depigmented "halo" is not a worrisome feature if the nevus in the center has no features of melanoma.
- Diagnostic aids such as magnifying glasses, serial photography, and dermoscopy (the latter in the hands of trained users) may increase diagnostic accuracy and minimize unnecessary biopsies.
- When suspicion for a melanoma is very high, the best biopsy technique is scalpel excision with 1 to 3 mm radial margins and a deep margin in the fatty subcutis. A deep shave biopsy with 1 to 2 mm margins (also called saucerization) is favored when suspicion for melanoma is lower but enough to warrant biopsy. Likewise, a punch excision is also acceptable in less suspicious lesions that are small enough to be completely removed in this manner. Incisional biopsies and other sampling approaches are less desirable, as they may miss the worst pathology.

?? Differential Diagnosis and Pitfalls

- Spitz nevus
- Compound nevus
- Seborrheic keratosis—the presence of pseudo horn cysts is typical
- Pigmented basal cell carcinoma—pearly quality
- Bowen disease (pagetoid or pigmented)
- Dysplastic nevus
- Congenital nevus
- Blue nevus
- Lentigo simplex
- Solar lentigo
- Pyogenic granuloma—friable, glistening surface
- Angiokeratoma

- Hemangioma—cherry, thrombosed
- Dermatofibroma—firm tan or brown papule with positive dimple sign
- Halo nevus—tan or brown papule with surrounding depigmented patch
- Metastatic carcinoma
- Paget disease
- Tinea nigra
- Subungual hematoma
- Pigmented actinic keratosis
- Talon noir (black heel)
- Longitudinal melanonychia (a pigmented line along the length of a nail plate) may be a benign finding or a sign of a nail matrix melanoma. Hutchinson sign—the presence of pigment in the proximal nail fold in a patient with longitudinal melanonychia should prompt the consideration of a nail matrix melanoma.

✓ Best Tests

- Full-thickness skin biopsy, preferably excisional or saucerization, as noted above. Dermatoscopy may help differentiate between benign and malignant pigmented lesions, but suspicious lesions should always be submitted for histopathologic examination.
- Because melanoma most often metastasizes to the lungs, liver, and brain, the following studies can be considered as part of a metastatic or staging workup once a diagnosis of melanoma is made if symptoms are present. However, in the absence of specific symptoms, these are not recommended as screening tools:
  - Chest radiograph
  - Liver function tests and LDH
  - PET scan
  - MRI
  - CT scan(s)

Management Pearls

- Patients with suspicious pigmented lesions and those with known melanoma should be referred to and followed regularly by a dermatologist. All skin biopsy specimens of pigmented lesions should be interpreted by a dermatopathologist.
- All patients with melanoma **except** those with stage 0 or stage 1A disease (i.e., nonulcerated lesions ≤1.0 mm and do not extend into or below the papillary dermis) should be offered a referral to an experienced surgical oncologist to consider sentinel lymph node biopsy and possible formal lymph node dissection. Medical oncology should be involved as well. The evaluation of a sentinel lymph

node for microscopic disease yields powerful prognostic information.
- Patients may ultimately require a plastic surgery consultation for reconstruction.

Therapy

Surgical excision is the treatment of choice. The margins required depend on the depth of invasion of the tumor. Guidelines vary, but the following are suggested:

- In situ—margins at least 0.5 cm (larger in the lentigo maligna form of melanoma in situ)
- Less than 1 mm—margins 1 cm
- 1 to 2 mm—margins 1 to 2 cm
- 2 to 4 mm—margins 2 cm
- Greater than 4 mm—margin at least 2 cm

Mohs micrographic surgery or staged excisions have been used for lentigo maligna melanoma with low local recurrence rates. This technique should only be performed by experienced surgeons.

Patients with nodal metastases will require a full lymph node dissection and adjuvant chemotherapy such as interferon-alpha-2b. Chemotherapy for patients with metastatic disease may also consist of temozolomide, interleukin-2 (IL-2), dacarbazine, or granulocyte macrophage-colony stimulating factor (GM-CSF). The treatment of advanced melanoma is difficult and often does not succeed. Patients with advanced disease stage should be referred to a center with expertise in the multidisciplinary care of melanoma and have access to participation in clinical trials. Immunotherapy, including the use of melanoma-specific therapeutic vaccines, is one exciting area of investigation but has yet to demonstrate improvements in survival.

Close clinical surveillance of patients after a diagnosis of melanoma is imperative as patients are at risk for local or systemic recurrence as well as for second primary melanomas. Published guidelines vary; one approach is to see patients four times a year in the first 2 years after a new diagnosis and then one to two times a year thereafter. First-degree family members of melanoma patients should also be screened and counseled as to their increased risk.

Suggested Readings

Bataille V, de Vries E. Melanoma—Part 1: Epidemiology, risk factors, and prevention. *BMJ.* 2008 Nov 20;337:a2249.

Coit D, Wallack M, Balch C. Society of Surgical Oncology practice guidelines. Melanoma surgical practice guidelines. *Oncology (Williston Park).* 1997 Sep;11(9):1317–1323.

Dummer R, Hauschild A, Jost L, ESMO Guidelines Working Group. Cutaneous alignant melanoma: ESMO clinical recommendations for diagnosis, treatment and follow-up. *Ann Oncol.* 2008 May;19(Suppl. 2):ii86–ii88.

Gogas H, Ioannovich J, Dafni U, et al. Prognostic significance of autoimmunity during treatment of melanoma with interferon. *N Engl J Med.* 2006 Feb;354(7):709–718.

Livestro DP, Kaine EM, Michaelson JS, et al. Melanoma in the young: Differences and similarities with adult melanoma: A case-matched controlled analysis. *Cancer.* 2007 Aug;110(3):614–624.

Lui P, Cashin R, Machado M, et al. Treatments for metastatic melanoma: Synthesis of evidence from randomized trials. *Cancer Treat Rev.* 2007 Dec;33(8):665–680.

Nestle FO, Halpern AC. Melanoma. In: Bolognia J, Jorizzo JL, Rapini RP, eds. *Dermatology.* 2nd Ed. St. Louis, MO: Mosby; 2008:1745–1769.

Schwartz JL, Wang TS, Hamilton TA, et al. Thin primary cutaneous melanomas: Associated detection patterns, lesion characteristics, and patient characteristics. *Cancer.* 2002 Oct;95(7):1562–1568.

Sober AJ, Chuang TY, Duvic M, et al; Guidelines/Outcomes Committee. Guidelines of care for primary cutaneous melanoma. *J Am Acad Dermatol.* 2001 Oct;45(4):579–586.

Swetter SM. Dermatological perspectives of malignant melanoma. *Surg Clin North Am.* 2003 Feb;83(1):77–95, vi.

Thirlwell C, Nathan P. Melanoma—part 2: Management. *BMJ.* 2008;337:a2488.

Tran KT, Wright NA, Cockerell CJ. Biopsy of the pigmented lesion—when and how. *J Am Acad Dermatol.* 2008 Nov;59(5):852–871.

Tsao H, Atkins MB, Sober AJ. Management of cutaneous melanoma. *N Engl J Med.* 2004 Sep;351(10):998–1012.

Melanotic Macule, Oral

Diagnosis Synopsis

An oral melanotic macule is a benign hyperpigmentation of the mucous membranes occurring in approximately 3% of the general population. There is an increase in focal melanin deposition without an increase in the number of melanocytes. Melanotic macules are most commonly found on the vermillion border of the lip, lower more often than upper. Lesions can also be found on the gingiva or palate, and they may be multiple. Although benign, biopsy may be needed to rule out a diagnosis of melanoma. Oral melanotic macule is common in patients of color and is seen more frequently in women than men. Average age at the time of presentation to the physician is at approximately 40 years, though these macules may appear at any age. In patients of darker skin types, onset typically occurs in adolescence. Some experts prefer to refer to lesions on the lip as "labial melanotic macules," although histopathology is identical to that at any other mucosal site.

Immunocompromised Patient Considerations

Oral melanotic macules have been reported to be more common in patients infected with HIV. However, a study of 217 HIV patients found no significant difference in incidence versus a control group.

Look For

A solitary, flat, brown or grayish-brown discoloration of the lip or an intraoral mucosal surface (Figs. 4-85–4-88). The macule appears slowly, and has a uniform color and border. Melanotic macules are typically 2 to 15 mm in diameter.

Dark Skin Considerations

Melanocytic pigmentation of the oral cavity is most common in black patients. In general, the darker the skin type, the more likely the patient is to develop mucosal melanotic macules.

Diagnostic Pearls

- Use diascopy (press on the lesion with a glass slide). The macule will appear purple and blanch if it is a vascular lesion such as a venous lake; if it does not blanche, it is a pigmented lesion. With an episcope, one sees a very dark linear pattern of pigmented streaks of a uniform width and pigmentation.
- Within the oral cavity, melanoma is most prevalent on the palate.

Differential Diagnosis and Pitfalls

- Nevus or blue nevus
- Melanoma
- Venous lake (purple rather than brown)
- Peutz-Jeghers syndrome
- Carney complex
- LEOPARD syndrome
- Drug induced pigmentation—e.g., antimalarials, tetracyclines, some chemotherapeutic agents
- Smoker melanosis
- Amalgam tattoo
- Heavy metal poisoning
- Addison disease
- Kaposi sarcoma

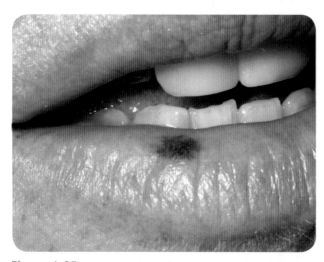

Figure 4-85 A 34 year old with a persistent brown, flat labial lesion.

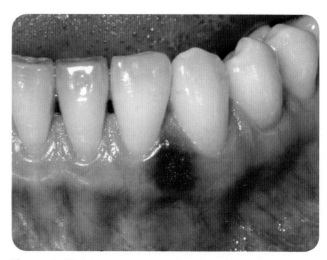

Figure 4-86 A 53 year old with a flat melanotic macule on the gingiva.

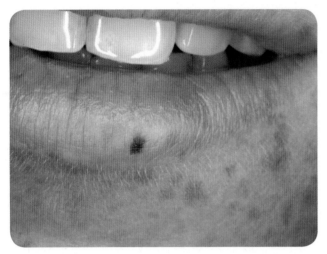

Figure 4-87 Flat, brown melanotic macule in a 21 year old.

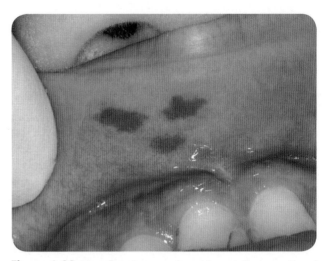

Figure 4-88 Three flat, brown oral macules on the upper buccal mucosa.

- Hematoma
- Melanoacanthoma
- Albright syndrome
- Laugier-Hunziker syndrome
- Acanthosis nigricans

✓ Best Tests

- Biopsy will confirm the diagnosis if there is any suspicion of melanoma.

▲▲ Management Pearls

- Measure the lesion or use photography to track change. Lesions that change significantly in size or character over time should be biopsied.

Therapy

Reassure the patient that the lesion is benign. Removal would be for cosmetic purposes only. The pigment is epidermal and would respond to laser treatment. Examples of lasers commonly used to treat pigmented lesions include the ruby, alexandrite, pulsed dye, and Q-switched Nd:YAG lasers.

Suggested Readings

Buchner A, Hansen LS. Melanotic macule of the oral mucosa. A clinicopathologic study of 105 cases. *Oral Surg Oral Med Oral Pathol.* 1979 Sep;48(3):244–249.

Carlos-Bregni R, Contreras E, Netto AC, et al. Oral melanoacanthoma and oral melanotic macule: a report of 8 cases, review of the literature, and immunohistochemical analysis. *Med Oral Patol Oral Cir Bucal.* 2007 Sep;12(5):E374–E379.

Cohen LM, Callen JP. Oral and labial melanotic macules in a patient infected with human immunodeficiency virus. *J Am Acad Dermatol.* 1992 Apr;26(4):653–654.

Ho KK, Dervan P, O'Loughlin S, Powell FC. Labial melanotic macule: A clinical, histopathologic, and ultrastructural study. *J Am Acad Dermatol.* 1993 Jan;28(1):33–39.

Horlick HP, Walther RR, Zegarelli DJ, et al. Mucosal melanotic macule, reactive type: a simulation of melanoma. *J Am Acad Dermatol.* 1988 Nov;19(5 Pt 1):786–791.

James WD, Berger TG, Elston DM. Disorders of the mucous membranes. In: James WD, Berger TG, Elston DM, Odom RB, eds. *Andrews' Diseases of the Skin: Clinical Dermatology.* 10th Ed. Philadelphia, PA: Saunders Elsevier; 2006:807.

Yeh CJ. Simple cryosurgical treatment of the oral melanotic macule. *Oral Surg Oral Med Oral Pathol Oral Radiol Endod.* 2000 Jul;90(1):12–13.

Melasma

▪▪ Diagnosis Synopsis

Melasma is a disorder of hyperpigmentation affecting sun-exposed areas, especially the face. The condition is much more common in women and is marked by brown patches that worsen in response to estrogen, such as with pregnancy (termed "chloasma") or the use of birth control pills. It is rare before puberty, and it occurs most commonly in the reproductive years. It also appears to be more common in individuals with a light brown skin color, especially Hispanics and Asians. An association between thyroid autoimmunity and melasma has been shown.

Melasma is a benign condition that is a cosmetic concern; treatment consists of sun avoidance and improving the skin's appearance through topical depigmenting agents, physical modalities, or chemical exfoliation.

◉ Look For

Hyperpigmented patches of the face and less commonly the forearms, typically involving the lateral cheeks, forehead, chin, and the superior lips (Figs. 4-89–4-92). The patches are usually symmetric and may have a "moth-eaten" appearance to their borders.

Dark Skin Considerations

Melasma can occur in all skin types, but it is most common in more deeply pigmented skin.

●● Diagnostic Pearls

- Pigment is epidermal and is markedly accentuated with a Wood lamp.

?? Differential Diagnosis and Pitfalls

- Postinflammatory pigmentation from acne or other inflammatory disease
- Lentigo
- Erythema dyschromicum perstans
- Drug-induced hyperpigmentation from medications such as tetracyclines, phenothiazines, and amiodarone
- Addison disease
- Poikiloderma of Civatte

✓ Best Tests

- This is primarily a clinical diagnosis.
- Consider checking thyroid function tests if the clinical situation warrants.

▲▲ Management Pearls

- Sun avoidance and protection are of primary importance in melasma management. The use of a broad-spectrum UVA/UVB sunscreen with SPF 30 or higher and long-acting broadband UVA protection is essential. Sunscreen should be used year-round because the skin is very sensitive to small amounts of ultraviolet light, and even penetration through window glass is relevant. To optimize

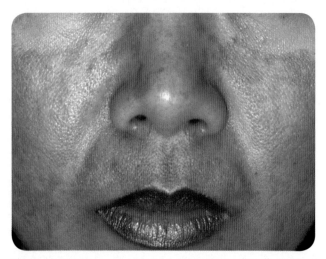

Figure 4-89 Melasma is composed of flat, brown, often symmetrical hyperpigmentation in sun-exposed locations on the face and neck.

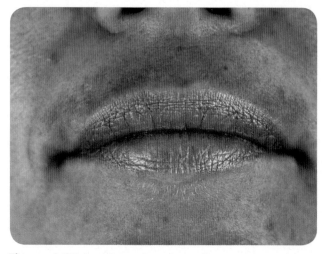

Figure 4-90 The upper lip is commonly hyperpigmented in melasma.

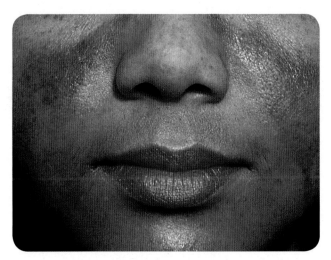

Figure 4-91 Butterfly-like pattern of melasma.

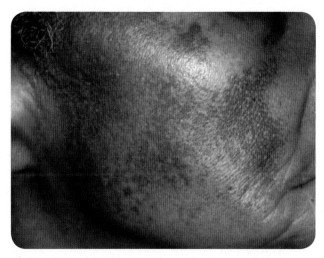

Figure 4-92 Melasma frequently occurs in heavily pigmented skin.

sun protection, protective clothing is also indicated. Sun exposure can also result in relapse of successfully treated melasma.

- If the patient is on oral contraceptive pills (OCPs) and needs to remain on the OCPs, improvement may be difficult. Even if OCPs are discontinued, OCP-induced melasma is challenging to treat and is easily stimulated by small amounts of sunlight.
- Reassure pregnant patients with melasma (chloasma) that the pigmentation will usually fade postpartum.

Therapy

Melasma should be treated in the early stages because increasing severity is accompanied by increasing treatment difficulty. In addition to limiting sun exposure, current treatments for melasma include hydroquinone alone or in combination with corticosteroids, tretinoin, retinol, or glycolic acid.

Bleaching agents (hydroquinone 4%) should be used carefully and not for the long term. A paradoxical effect of long-term or higher concentrations of hydroquinone (usually in concentrations above that in commercial preparations) is the occurrence of a bluish ochronosis-like pigmentation. Often, these agents are irritating and, thus, may require the concomitant use of 1% hydrocortisone cream, which will also help with the hyperpigmentation.

A combination formula of 4% hydroquinone, fluocinolone acetonide 0.01%, and 0.05% tretinoin in a cream formulation (Tri-Luma) has been used with good results.

Adjuvant procedures include superficial chemical peels and microdermabrasion, and laser and light sources may offer some additional help.

Suggested Readings

Abramovits W, Barzin S, Arrazola P. A practical comparison of hydroquinone-containing products for the treatment of melasma. *Skinmed*. 2005 Nov–Dec;4(6):371–376.

Gupta AK, Gover MD, Nouri K, et al. The treatment of melasma: A review of clinical trials. *J Am Acad Dermatol*. 2006 Dec;55(6):1048–1065.

Lynde CB, Kraft JN, Lynde CW. Topical treatments for melasma and postinflammatory hyperpigmentation. *Skin Therapy Lett*. 2006 Nov;11(9):1–6.

Rendon M, Berneburg M, Arellano I, et al. Treatment of melasma. *J Am Acad Dermatol*. 2006 May;54(5 Suppl. 2):S272–S281.

Resnik S. Melasma induced by oral contraceptive drugs. *JAMA*. 1967 Feb 27;199(9):601–605.

Rigopoulos D, Gregoriou S, Katsambas A. Hyperpigmentation and melasma. *J Cosmet Dermatol*. 2007 Sep;6(3):195–202.

Victor FC, Gelber J, Rao B. Melasma: A review. *J Cutan Med Surg*. 2004 Mar–Apr;8(2):97–102.

Nevus of Ito

Diagnosis Synopsis

Nevus of Ito is a unilateral dermal melanocyte hamartoma that is clinically differentiated from a nevus of Ota and a Mongolian spot by its speckled or mottled appearance and its location. A nevus of Ito presents as a blue to gray patch located over the supraclavicular, deltoid, or scapular area and is often present at birth or develops shortly thereafter. A Mongolian spot is typically over the buttocks or lumbosacral spine. A nevus of Ota is characteristically in a trigeminal distribution on the face. There may be associated sensory changes in the involved skin.

Look For

Blue to gray confluent or mottled patch in a supraclavicular, deltoid, or scapular location (Figs. 4-93–4-95).

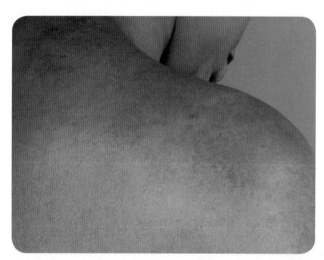

Figure 4-93 Nevus of Ito in a characteristic location on the posterior shoulder.

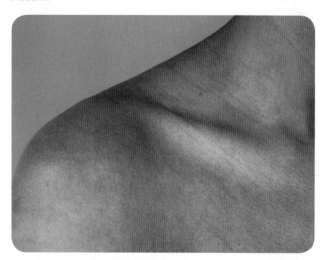

Figure 4-94 Nevus of Ito in a characteristic location on the anterior shoulder.

Diagnostic Pearls

- Patients are almost always of Asian, and in particular Japanese, descent. However, lesions have been reported in those of African and East Indian descent.

Differential Diagnosis and Pitfalls

- Blue nevus may have similar blue to grey pigmentation but is a smaller, well-demarcated macule or papule.
- Nevus of Ota is characteristically in the trigeminal distribution of the face.
- Tattoo from asphalt burns, gunpowder, or industrial accidents can be diagnosed by history.
- Mongolian spots typically overlie the buttocks or lumbosacral area.
- Melanoma can manifest with disseminated melanosis, but pigmentation will usually be less well demarcated and will present later in life.
- Lentigos or giant café au lait macules impart a tan to brown hue.
- Ochronosis is either focally on the face secondary to hydroquinone use or disseminated from congenital ochronosis.

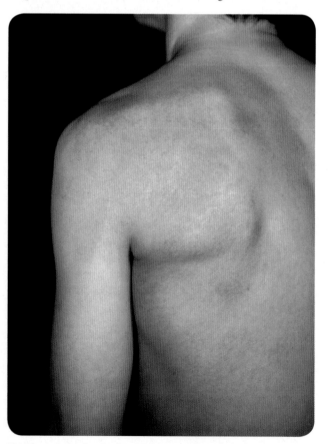

Figure 4-95 Nevus of Ito on the posterior shoulder.

- Phytophotodermatitis will usually have an acute onset and key history.
- Drug-induced hyperpigmentation can either be diffuse or photodistributed.
- Ecchymoses will have a history of trauma.
- Vascular malformations can range from blue to red.
- Nevus spilus presents with a tan to brown background patch with darker speckled pigmentation within.
- Becker nevus can be found in a similar distribution but is often tan or brown with coarse hair arising during adolescence.

✓ Best Tests

- Skin biopsy can be diagnostic.

▲▲ Management Pearls

- Cosmetic makeup can be used.
- If the lesion is extensive, evaluation for associated CNS involvement should be performed.

Therapy

Cosmetic coverage with opaque makeup.

Good cosmetic results can be achieved with pulsed Q-switched ruby, alexandrite, or Nd:YAG laser.

Suggested Readings

Burge SM, Ralfs IG. Nevus of Ito with sensory changes. *Int J Dermatol.* 1985 May;24(4):239–240.

Ferguson RE, Vasconez HC. Laser treatment of congenital nevi. *J Craniofac Surg.* 2005 Sep;16(5):908–914.

Lapeere H, Boone B, Schepper SD, et al. Hypomelanoses and hypermelanoses. In: Fitzpatrick TB, Wolff K, eds. *Fitzpatrick's Dermatology in General Medicine.* 7th Ed. New York, NY: McGraw-Hill; 2008:632.

Lee CS, Lim HW. Cutaneous diseases in Asians. *Dermatol Clin.* 2003 Oct;21(4):669–677.

Trindade F, Santonja C, Requena L. Bilateral nevus of Ito and nevus spilus in the same patient. *J Am Acad Dermatol.* 2008 Aug;59(2 Suppl. 1):S51–S52.

Diagnosis Synopsis

Nevus of Ota is a dermal melanocyte hamartoma located on the face in a trigeminal nerve distribution. It can be differentiated from a nevus of Ito, which is distributed over the supraclavicular, deltoid, or scapular area, and it can be differentiated from a Mongolian spot, which is commonly located over the buttocks or lumbosacral spine. Nevus of Ota is usually unilateral, but rare occurrences of a bilateral distribution have been reported. It may also involve the ocular and oral mucosal surfaces. The incidence is higher in Asians, in blacks, and in women. The lesion typically manifests at birth or infancy, but onset during adolescence has occurred. There are rare reports of melanoma arising in a nevus of Ota. Patients are also at risk of developing ipsilateral glaucoma.

Look For

Blue or brown, confluent or mottled pigmentation involving the forehead, temple, periorbital region, nose, and superior cheek, typically in a trigeminal distribution (Figs. 4-96–4-98). In females, the intensity of pigmentation can vary and increase during menstruation. The pigmentation may involve the sclera as well (Fig. 4-99). Lesions may also enlarge and darken over time.

Dark Skin Considerations

The lesion is more common in darker-skinned individuals, particularly Asians and blacks. The highest incidence is among Japanese women.

Diagnostic Pearls

- Look for ipsilateral, patchy blue discoloration of the sclera and conjunctiva in conjunction with a blue- to brown-pigmented lesion distributed within the first and second divisions of the trigeminal nerve.

?? Differential Diagnosis and Pitfalls

- Alkaptonuria (congenital ochronosis) or acquired ochronosis (occurring after high concentrations of hydroquinone) may have a similar hue, but may lack a trigeminal distribution.
- Melasma is characterized by tan- or brown-pigmented patches distributed bilaterally over the malar cheeks, temples, and forehead.
- Blue nevus may have similar blue-grey pigmentation but is a smaller well-demarcated macule or papule.
- Nevus of Ito is located over the supraclavicular, deltoid, or scapular region.
- Tattoo from gunpowder or industrial accidents can be diagnosed by history.
- Mongolian spots typically occur on the buttocks or lumbosacral area.

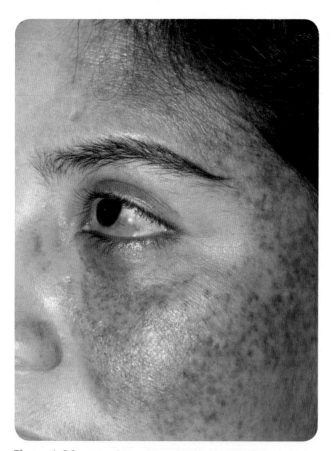

Figure 4-96 Nevus of Ota with periocular involvement.

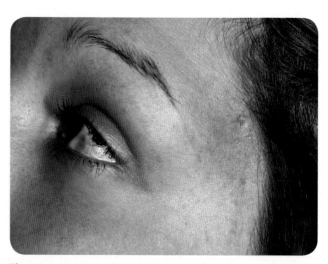

Figure 4-97 Nevus of Ota with moderate blue pigmentation.

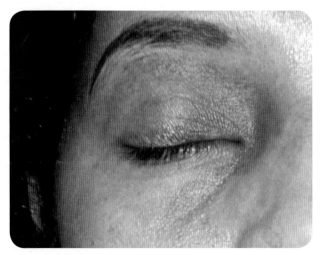

Figure 4-98 Nevus of Ota with periocular pigmentation.

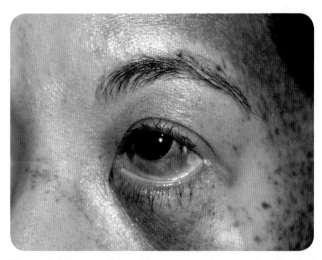

Figure 4-99 Nevus of Ota with punctate periocular and conjunctival pigmentation.

- Melanoma can manifest with disseminated melanosis, but pigmentation will usually be less well demarcated and will present later in life.
- Lentigos or giant café au lait macules are typically smaller and have a tan to brown hue.
- Phytophotodermatitis will usually have an acute onset and key history.
- Drug-induced hyperpigmentation can either be diffuse or photodistributed.
- Ecchymoses will have a history of trauma.
- Vascular malformations can range from blue to red.
- Nevus spilus presents with a tan to brown background patch with darker speckled pigmentation within.

✓ Best Tests

- The diagnosis can usually be made clinically, but skin biopsy is characteristic.

▲▲ Management Pearls

- Consider an ophthalmology referral due to the association of nevus of Ota with elevated intraocular pressure and glaucoma.
- If the lesion is extensive, an evaluation for associated CNS involvement should be performed. Skin biopsy is indicated if there is suspicion for malignant transformation.

Therapy

Cosmetic coverage with opaque makeup.

Pulsed Q-switched laser treatment with either the ruby, alexandrite, or Nd:YAG lasers has been effective in achieving good cosmetic results.

Suggested Readings

Chan HH, Kono T. Nevus of Ota: Clinical aspects and management. *Skinmed.* 2003 Mar–Apr;2(2):89–96; quiz 97–98.

Ferguson RE, Vasconez HC. Laser treatment of congenital nevi. *J Craniofac Surg.* 2005 Sep;16(5):908–914.

Grin JM, Grant-Kels JM, Grin CM, et al. Ocular melanomas and melanocytic lesions of the eye. *J Am Acad Dermatol.* 1998 May;38(5 Pt 1):716–730.

Lapeere H, Boone B, Schepper SD, et al. Hypomelanoses and hypermelanoses. In: Fitzpatrick TB, Wolff K, eds. *Fitzpatrick's Dermatology in General Medicine.* 7th Ed. New York, NY: McGraw Hill; 2008:632.

Lee CS, Lim HW. Cutaneous diseases in Asians. *Dermatol Clin.* 2003 Oct;21(4):669–677.

Mataix J, López N, Haro R, et al. Late-onset Ito's nevus: An uncommon acquired dermal melanocytosis. *J Cutan Pathol.* 2007 Aug;34(8):640–643.

Wang HW, Liu YH, Zhang GK, et al. Analysis of 602 Chinese cases of nevus of Ota and the treatment results treated by Q-switched alexandrite laser. *Dermatol Surg.* 2007 Apr;33(4):455–460.

Watanabe S, Takahashi H. Treatment of nevus of Ota with the Q-switched ruby laser. *N Engl J Med.* 1994 Dec 29;331(26):1745–1750.

Diagnosis Synopsis

Atypical nevi, also called dysplastic nevi or Clark nevi, are aggregates of melanocytes that display clinical and/or histologic features that distinguish them from common melanocytic nevi in concerning ways. Clinical features of atypical nevi include asymmetry, large size, irregular or ill-defined borders, and varied coloration. Histologically, they show abnormal architecture and cellular atypia. Atypical nevi are not malignant melanoma but share some of the same features, and atypical nevi may be a marker for the risk of developing a future melanoma. Atypical nevi typically arise de novo or may be due to a change in an existing nevus. They are more common in fair-skinned individuals.

The proclivity to developing atypical nevi may be inherited. An autosomal dominant mode of inheritance has been suggested. The risk of developing melanoma increases with a positive family history and an increasing number of lesions. Persons with a first- or second-degree relative with melanoma and a large number of nevi including atypical nevi are said to have the dysplastic nevus syndrome, also referred to as the familial atypical mole and melanoma syndrome. They are at an increased risk of developing malignant melanoma.

While there is some evidence that malignant melanomas may infrequently arise from an atypical nevus, it is incorrect to view any given atypical nevus as an incipient melanoma. Clinicians chiefly excise atypical nevi for one of the three reasons: to exclude the possibility of a current malignant melanoma, to relieve symptoms of physical irritation, or to satisfy a patient's request for cosmetic removal.

Look For

Atypical nevi can vary in size and/or color. They are often larger than common nevi. They may have variations in color within the lesion ranging from pink to reddish-brown to dark brown (Figs. 4-100–4-103). Borders are often irregular and/or ill defined. They may also have either a darker brown center or periphery. In the atypical nevus syndrome, hundreds of nevi of varying size and color are seen.

Common body sites include the trunk, the scalp, and areas under two layers of clothing (e.g., under undergarments).

Dark Skin Considerations

Flat or raised, deeply pigmented lesions in dark-skinned patients, possibly with an irregular border.

Diagnostic Pearls

Apply "the ugly duckling rule" and the **ABCDEs** of suspicious pigmented lesions:

A—Asymmetry: One half of the lesion does not mirror the other half.
B—Border: The borders are irregular or indistinct.
C—Color: The color is variegated; the pigment is not uniform, and there may be varying shades and/or hues.
D—Diameter: Classically, any pigmented lesion greater than 6 mm in diameter is concerning.
E—Evolving: Notable change in a lesion over time raises suspicion for malignancy. Ulceration and bleeding should certainly prompt biopsy.

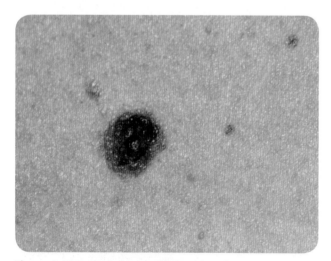

Figure 4-100 Atypical nevus with irregular, raised papules, irregular border, and complex pigmentary pattern.

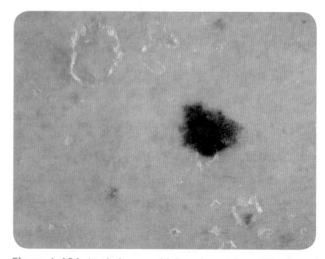

Figure 4-101 Atypical nevus with irregular notches and border and variegated pigmentation.

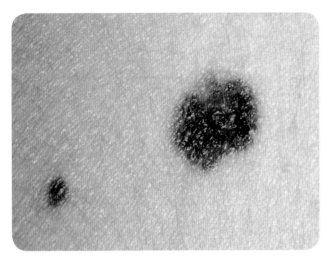

Figure 4-102 Atypical nevus with very irregular border and tiny pigmented papules.

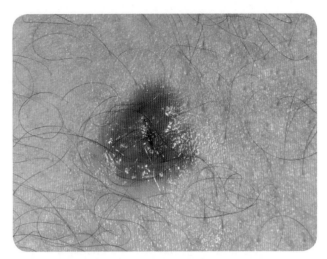

Figure 4-103 Spitz nevi are characteristically redder than common or atypical nevi.

In a patient with multiple pigmented lesions, look for and strongly consider biopsy of "the ugly duckling" lesion (i.e., one that strikes the examiner as unlike the others).

Any new dark black lesion—irrespective of its size—should be considered a possible melanoma. The occurrence of a new pigmented lesion in an adult aged older than 50 is unusual. Maintain a very low threshold of suspicion for new pigmented lesions in adults, and biopsy early to rule out melanoma.

?? Differential Diagnosis and Pitfalls

- Seborrheic keratosis—Many fulfill one or more of the ABCDE criteria; thus, the awareness of typical features of these exceedingly common skin lesions will prevent unnecessary biopsies. Notably, they are a "stuck on-" or waxy-appearing tan to dark brown papule.
- Pigmented basal cell carcinoma may be confused at times with a nevus.
- Melanoma
- Melanocytic nevus
- Blue nevus
- Combined nevus (blue nevus and compound nevus together)
- Dermatofibroma
- Lentigo simplex
- Solar lentigo
- Lentigo maligna
- Congenital nevus
- Ephelides (freckles)
- Recurrent melanocytic nevus
- Supernumerary nipple

✓ Best Tests

- Careful, complete skin examination in a fully disrobed patient that includes the scalp, the mouth, behind the ears, and between the toes. Dermatoscopy performed by a clinician experienced with this method may be useful.
- Skin biopsy—remove the entire lesion:
  - If suspicion for a melanoma is high, elliptical excision with 1 to 3 mm margins is recommended.
  - If the examiner favors an atypical nevus but concern for melanoma is non-negligible, complete removal by either a deep shave biopsy (also called "saucerization") or a punch biopsy is a common alternative. Saucerization yields less inadvertent sampling error than punch biopsy.

▲▲ Management Pearls

- Atypical nevi frequently run in families. Therefore, question the patient about the family history of melanoma and examine first-degree relatives.
- Use of a dermatoscope in experienced hands enhances the ability to discern normal from atypical pigment patterns.
- Patients with multiple nevi should be examined by a dermatologist every 3 to 12 months depending on their past medical and family history as well as the morphology of the lesions.
- Photography of lesions may be useful to track changes.

Therapy

Observation is a reasonable approach to a clinically atypical nevus that has remained unchanged for many years. Surgical removal is indicated for a changing or suspicious lesion or in the case of suspicious lesions that are difficult to follow or whose past behavior is unknown. It is unreasonable to remove all nevi as the increased proclivity for melanoma seems to be systemic rather than within each nevus.

Although controversial, the following is a common approach to patients for whom a pathology report indicates cellular atypia within the nevus:

- If "mildly atypical"—observation but no further treatment
- If "moderately atypical" and completely excised—observation but no further treatment
- If "moderately atypical" but incompletely excised—re-excision with negative margins (as unsampled portions may have areas with more concerning histology).
- If "severely atypical"—re-excision with a 5 mm margin given the difficulty in distinguishing severely atypical nevi from melanoma in situ. Re-excise whether or not the initial procedure resulted in "clear" margins.

Frequency of follow-up for persons with an atypical nevus ranges from every 3 months to every year.

Recommend sunscreens (SPF 30 at a minimum) on any days with sunlight. Follow the UV index listing in most local newspapers.

Suggested Readings

Barnhill RL, Rabinowitz H. Benign melanocytic neoplasms. In: Bolognia J, Jorizzo JL, Rapini RP, eds. *Dermatology.* 2nd Ed. St. Louis, MO: Mosby/Elsevier; 2008:1732–1735.

Chang YM, Newton-Bishop JA, Bishop DT, et al. A pooled analysis of melanocytic nevus phenotype and the risk of cutaneous melanoma at different latitudes. *Int J Cancer.* 2009 Jan;124(2):420–428.

Hofmann-Wellenhof R, Blum A, Wolf IH, et al. Dermoscopic classification of atypical melanocytic nevi (Clark nevi). *Arch Dermatol.* 2001 Dec;137(12):1575–1580.

Kmetz EC, Sanders H, Fisher G, et al. The role of observation in the management of atypical nevi. *South Med J.* 2009 Jan;102(1):45–48.

Naeyaert JM, Brochez L. Clinical practice. Dysplastic nevi. *N Engl J Med.* 2003 Dec;349(23):2233–2240.

Tran KT, Wright NA, Cockerell CJ. Biopsy of the pigmented lesion—when and how. *J Am Acad Dermatol.* 2008 Nov;59(5):852–871.

Tucker MA, Halpern A, Holly EA, et al. Clinically recognized dysplastic nevi. A central risk factor for cutaneous melanoma. *JAMA.* 1997 May;277(18):1439–1444.

Nevus, Becker

Diagnosis Synopsis

A Becker nevus (Becker melanosis) typically presents as a large, hyperpigmented patch with increased hair growth on the upper trunk in men. Lesions are usually present before puberty but often have increased coarse hair growth and a slightly raised texture during adolescence due to androgen stimulation. Rarely, there can be associated hypoplasia of the underlying tissues (e.g., breast hypoplasia, pectoralis hypoplasia, or limb hypoplasia). Most Becker nevi have no associated abnormalities. Treatment is only required in rare cases for severe cosmetic or psychosocial reasons. Other rare associated findings include acne, acanthosis nigricans, spina bifida, scoliosis, pectus carinatum, accessory scrotum, lipoatrophy, and congenital adrenal hyperplasia. A few cases of melanoma in association with a Becker nevus have been reported.

Look For

Becker nevi present as large, hyperpigmented, solitary patches with associated hypertrichosis typically distributed on the shoulder, upper chest, or back in men (Figs. 4-104–4-107). In women, however, they can present as multiple lesions. Becker nevi may have a distinct papular quality due to associated underlying smooth muscle hamartoma.

Dark Skin Considerations

Coarse, dark hairs can be evident within the lesion, especially in dark-skinned people.

Diagnostic Pearls

Large hyperpigmented hypertrichotic patch on the upper trunk in men.

?? Differential Diagnosis and Pitfalls

- Giant congenital nevi are darker and have a distorted hair pattern, often with coarse hair, unlike the regular but exuberant hair in a Becker nevus.
- Epidermal nevi frequently have more epidermal changes and lie in a dermatomal distribution.
- Tinea versicolor presents with small faintly hyperpigmented or hypopigmented scaly patches over the back and trunk.
- Ephelides (freckles) are small pigmented photodistributed macules.
- Lentigos are small nonpalpable pigmented macules and patches.
- Giant café au lait macules can clinically resemble a Becker nevus in preadolescent patients but can usually be distinguished later by the development of hypertrichosis and epidermal/dermal changes in a Becker nevus.

✓ Best Tests

- Biopsy can be used if there is any uncertainty about the diagnosis.

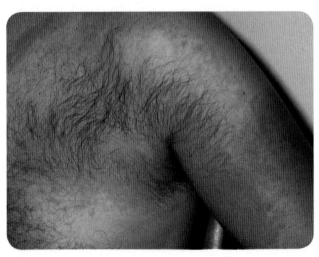

Figure 4-104 A Becker nevus typically has hypertrichosis and hyperpigmentation in the region of the shoulder.

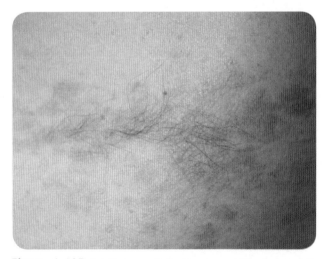

Figure 4-105 Relatively small Becker nevus with characteristic increased number and size of hairs and hyperpigmentation.

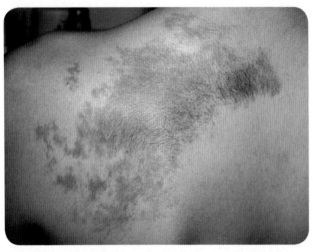

Figure 4-106 More hyperpigmentation than hypertrichosis in this Becker nevus.

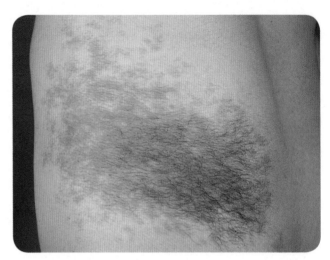

Figure 4-107 Becker nevus with much less hair in peripheral hyperpigmented macules.

 Management Pearls

- Observation is sufficient, as the risk for malignant degeneration is extremely low. For cosmetic reasons, associated hypertrichosis can be treated with laser therapy.

Therapy

Reassure the patient that the lesion is benign and no treatment is necessary. However, with insistent patients, the following can be offered for cosmetic or psychosocial reasons.

Treatments for hyperpigmentation
- Er:YAG laser
- Q-switched ruby laser
- Frequency-doubled QSNd:YAG laser

Treatment of hypertrichosis
- Ruby laser (normal mode)
- Electrolysis
- Depilatories

Suggested Readings

Angelo C, Grosso MG, Stella P, et al. Becker's nevus syndrome. *Cutis.* 2001 Aug;68(2):123–124.

Danarti R, König A, Salhi A, et al. Becker's nevus syndrome revisited. *J Am Acad Dermatol.* 2004 Dec;51(6):965–969.

Lapeere H, Boone B, Schepper SD, et al. Hypomelanoses and hypermelanoses. In: Fitzpatrick TB, Wolff K, eds. *Fitzpatrick's Dermatology in General Medicine.* 7th Ed. New York, NY: McGraw-Hill; 2008:639.

Santos-Juanes J, Galache C, Curto JR, et al. Acneiform lesions in Becker's nevus and breast hypoplasia. *Int J Dermatol.* 2002 Oct;41(10):699–700.

Trelles MA, Allones I, Vélez M, et al. Becker's nevus: Erbium:YAG versus Q-switched neodimium:YAG?. *Lasers Surg Med.* 2004;34(4):295–297.

Nevus, Benign and Common

■■ Diagnosis Synopsis

Nevi are aggregates of melanocytes that can extend from the epidermis into the deep dermis. They are considered benign neoplasms or hamartomas. Unlike junctional nevi, compound and intradermal nevi are usually papular (elevated relative to the surrounding skin). Nevi typically arise during childhood, adolescence, or very early adulthood. Their formation may be stimulated by sunlight. Compound nevi are more common in individuals with fair skin.

◉ Look For

Common nevi are usually elevated, pigmented growths that can be warty or smooth in appearance (Figs. 4-108–4-113). They may demonstrate an exophytic component combined with a flat component. These lesions vary in color from skin colored to dark brown and may have associated hair. They are generally 2 to 6 mm in diameter, nearly symmetric, and uniformly colored with a regular border.

They may occur anywhere on the body.

●● Diagnostic Pearls

The occurrence of a new pigmented lesion in an adult is unusual after the age of 50. Maintain a very low threshold of suspicion for new pigmented lesions in adults, and biopsy early to rule out melanoma.

Remember the ABCDEs of suspicious pigmented lesions:

A—Asymmetry: One half of the lesion does not mirror the other half.

B—Border: The borders are irregular or indistinct.

C—Color: The color is variegated; the pigment is not uniform, and there may be varying shades and/or hues.

D—Diameter: Classically, any pigmented lesion greater than 6 mm in diameter is concerning.

E—Evolving: Notable change over time is suspicious for malignancy. Bleeding or ulceration should prompt biopsy.

?? Differential Diagnosis and Pitfalls

- Atypical nevus
- Melanoma
- Blue nevus
- Combined nevus (blue nevus and compound nevus together)
- Pigment basal cell carcinoma—pearly, flesh-colored border
- Dermatofibroma—firm tan, bound-down papule
- Acrochordon
- Wart—more firm, verrucous papules
- Neurofibroma
- Congenital nevus
- Seborrheic keratosis—stuck-on appearing, warty

✓ Best Tests

- This diagnosis can often be made clinically, but suspicious lesions should be biopsied and examined by a dermatopathologist. If the suspicion for melanoma is relatively low, a deep shave biopsy (saucerization) of the lesion is sufficient. Complete excisional biopsy can also be considered in worrisome lesions.

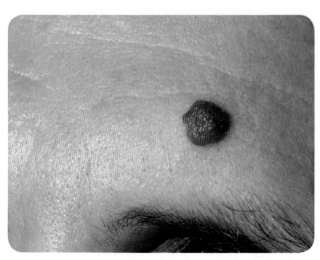

Figure 4-108 Dermal nevus with uniform reddish-brown color with small hairs growing from it.

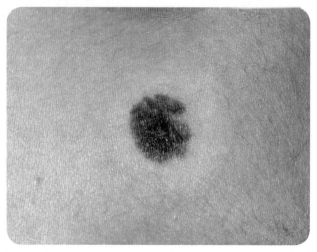

Figure 4-109 Compound nevus with darker area. A rim of hypopigmentation often surrounds nevi, as shown.

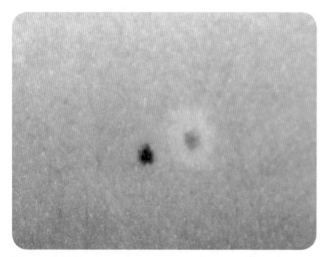

Figure 4-110 Junctional nevus with adjacent halo nevus.

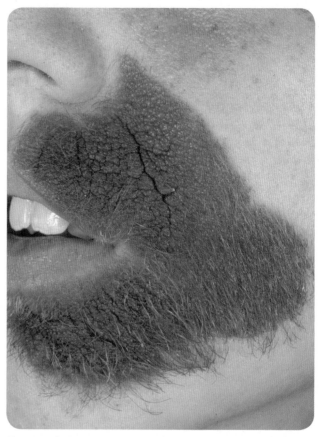

Figure 4-112 Congenital nevi often have dark pigment, epidermal thickening, and increased hair.

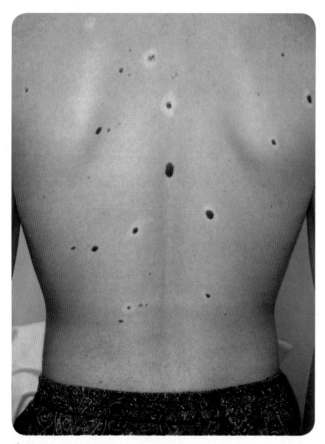

Figure 4-111 Multiple junctional and halo nevi.

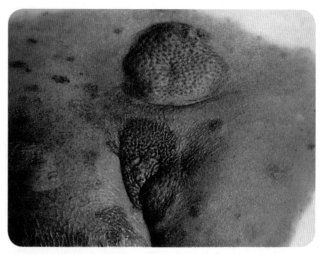

Figure 4-113 Large congenital nevus with very black areas and thickened epidermis. Giant congenital nevi have an increased potential for developing melanoma.

▲▲ Management Pearls

- Clearing the stratum corneum with oil and examining with magnification aids in the detection of irregular foci.
- Refer individuals with suspicious pigmented lesions to a dermatologist, and educate patients regarding the ABCDEs of melanoma (see "Diagnostic Pearls").

Therapy

No treatment is necessary. If the patient requests removal for cosmetic reasons, shave excision is often adequate.

Complete excision with histopathologic examination is indicated when the nevus becomes symptomatic or changes in shape or color. Deep shave removal with 1 to 2 mm margins is also useful.

Suggested Readings

Barnhill RL, Rabinowitz H. Benign melanocytic neoplasms. In: Bolognia J, Jorizzo JL, Rapini RP, eds. *Dermatology*. 2nd Ed. St. Louis, MO: Mosby; 2008:1723–1725.

Carmichael AJ, Tan CY. Speckled compound naevus. *Clin Exp Dermatol*. 1990 Mar;15(2):137–138.

Carrera C, Ferrer B, Mascaró JM, et al. Compound blue naevus: A potential simulator of melanoma. *Br J Dermatol*. 2006 Jul;155(1):207–208.

Jin ZH, Kumakiri M, Ishida H, et al. A case of combined nevus: Compound nevus and spindle cell Spitz nevus. *J Dermatol*. 2000 Apr;27(4):233–237.

Kmetz EC, Sanders H, Fisher G, et al. The role of observation in the management of atypical nevi. *South Med J*. 2009 Jan;102(1):45–48.

Sulit DJ, Guardiano RA, Krivda S. Classic and atypical Spitz nevi: Review of the literature. *Cutis*. 2007 Feb;79(2):141–146.

Nevus, Blue

Diagnosis Synopsis

Blue nevus is also known as a blue mole. These small blue-gray or blue-black papules are caused by an aggregate of melanocytes (pigment-producing cells) in the upper and mid dermis. Melanocytes originate embryologically in the neural crest and then migrate to the dermal epidermal junction or to the hair bulb. Blue nevi are hypothesized to arise from melanocytes that fail to complete their developmental journey and instead reside and proliferate in the dermis. Dermal melanocytes reflect low-wavelength blue light but absorb higher wavelength light, a phenomenon known as the Tyndall effect. This accounts for the characteristic blue hue of the lesion.

Blue nevi are more common in women and in those of Asian ancestry. They usually develop in young adulthood. Common blue nevi do not require excision, but a skin biopsy may be obtained to confirm the diagnosis. The clinical differential diagnosis of both common and cellular blue nevi is melanoma.

Look For

Blue-black or blue-gray nodules, papules, or plaques that may occur anywhere on the body but favor the hands, feet, face, and scalp (Figs. 4-114–4-117). They are typically 0.5 to 1.0 cm in diameter. The pigmentation is very uniform. Some lesions are a combination of blue nevi and compound nevi, and these may have a more complex clinical morphology.

A variant of blue nevus, called cellular blue nevus, has been described. Cellular blue nevi are typically larger than common blue nevi (1 to 3 cm in diameter), solitary, and although they may be found in similar locations as the common blue nevus, they also show a predilection for the buttocks or sacrococcygeal region.

Diagnostic Pearls

- Examine under bright light and look tangentially to see the definite blue hue. Rapid growth, size over 2 cm, or clinically atypical appearance (e.g., multinodularity) should prompt an excisional biopsy to assess for malignant transformation. A dermatoscope may facilitate the visualization of the dense color but does not demonstrate enough detail to avoid a biopsy of suspicious lesions in most instances.
- One variant, the epithelioid blue nevus, may be associated with other cutaneous and systemic abnormalities referred to as the Carney complex: endocrine abnormalities, myxomas, spotty skin pigmentation, and schwannomas.

Differential Diagnosis and Pitfalls

- Nodular melanoma is within the differential.
- Nevus of Ota and nevus of Ito are blue but macular and usually much larger.
- Tattoos (e.g., from a lead pencil or the mark used to locate X-ray therapy fields) are flat and usually not as regular as a blue nevus.
- Dermatofibroma
- Melanocytic nevus
- Venous lake
- Angiokeratoma
- Sclerosing hemangioma
- Pigmented basal cell carcinoma
- Glomus tumor
- Apocrine hidrocystoma

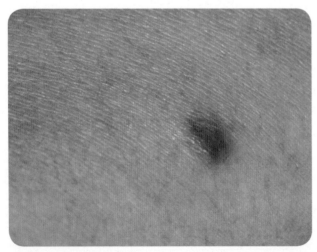

Figure 4-114 Darkly pigmented blue nevus slightly raised above the skin's surface.

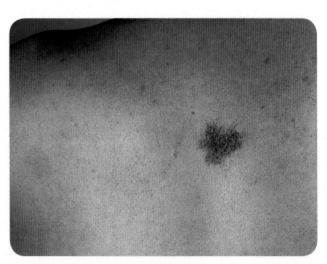

Figure 4-115 Relatively flat blue nevus.

108

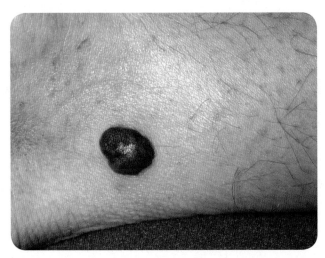

Figure 4-116 Blue nevus. A raised nodule that would not compress like a venous lake would.

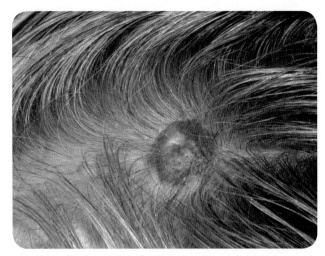

Figure 4-117 Blue nevi may be acquired after the age of 60, and the scalp is a common location.

✓ Best Tests

- Skin biopsy. If an adult patient complains of a growing pigmented lesion, excisional biopsy is recommended.

▲▲ Management Pearls

- Blue nevi are benign lesions, and no therapy is necessary. Melanoma has rarely been associated with cellular blue nevi, but this fact does not imply that these lesions should be preemptively excised.

Therapy

If removal is desired, a small elliptical excision is recommended.

Suggested Readings

Barnhill RL, Rabinowitz H. Benign melanocytic neoplasms. In: Bolognia J, Jorizzo JL, Rapini RP, eds. *Dermatology*. 2nd Ed. St. Louis, MO: Mosby; 2008:1722–1723.

Bogart MM, Bivens MM, Patterson JW, et al. Blue nevi: A case report and review of the literature. *Cutis*. 2007 Jul;80(1):42–44.

Busam KJ, Woodruff JM, Erlandson RA, et al. Large plaque-type blue nevus with subcutaneous cellular nodules. *Am J Surg Pathol*. 2000 Jan;24(1):92–99.

Ferrara G, Soyer HP, Malvehy J, et al. The many faces of blue nevus: A clinicopathologic study. *J Cutan Pathol*. 2007 Jul;34(7):543–551.

Fistarol SK, Itin PH. Plaque-type blue nevus of the oral cavity. *Dermatology*. 2005;211(3):224–233.

Grichnik JM, Rhodes AR, Sober AJ. Benign neoplasias and hyperplasias of melanocytes. In: Fitzpatrick TB, Wolff K, eds. *Fitzpatrick's Dermatology in General Medicine*. 7th Ed. New York, NY: McGraw-Hill; 2008:1109–1112.

Kasahara N, Kazama T, Sakamoto F, Ito M. Acquired multiple blue naevi scattered over the whole body. *Br J Dermatol*. 2001 Feb;144(2):440–442.

Knoell KA, Nelson KC, Patterson JW. Familial multiple blue nevi. *J Am Acad Dermatol*. 1998 Aug;39(2 Pt 2):322–325.

Ojha J, Akers JL, Akers JO, et al. Intraoral cellular blue nevus: Report of a unique histopathologic entity and review of the literature. *Cutis*. 2007 Sep;80(3):189–192.

◼◼ Diagnosis Synopsis

Notalgia paresthetica is the term for a condition of the skin of the upper back where the skin is extremely pruritic in a localized area just below or medial to the scapula. Notalgia paresthetica is felt to be secondary to spinal nerve impingement, causing the persistent itch. Pain, paresthesias, and hyperesthesias may coincide with itch. Hyperpigmented or lichenified skin changes, if present, are due to the chronic rubbing and scratching of the affected area.

Notalgia paresthetica can affect people of any age, any race, and either sex. However, it is thought to be most common in middle-aged adults to older adults. Women seem to develop notalgia paresthetica more frequently than men.

Though the etiology of notalgia paresthetica is not entirely certain, some studies have demonstrated, radiographically, vertebral spine disease correlating to the level of the nerve root affecting the pruritic skin, typically T2–6.

◉ Look For

Notalgia paresthetica most typically manifests with a unilateral, hyperpigmented patch just below the scapula at the upper back (Figs. 4-118–4-120). The patch is noninflammatory, usually not scaly, and follows the area of skin that the patient has constantly been rubbing.

●● Diagnostic Pearls

- Notalgia paresthetica is a clinical diagnosis, with localized macular pigmentation just below the scapula being almost pathognomonic for this condition.

?? Differential Diagnosis and Pitfalls

- Postinflammatory hyperpigmentation
- Nummular dermatitis
- Fixed drug eruption
- Macular amyloidosis
- Drug-related hyperpigmentation

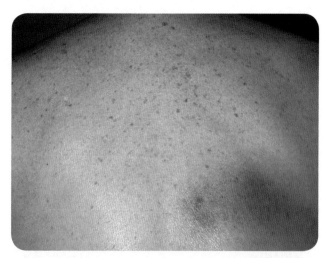

Figure 4-119 Hyperpigmented lesions of notalgia paresthetica may be sharply circumscribed or more diffuse.

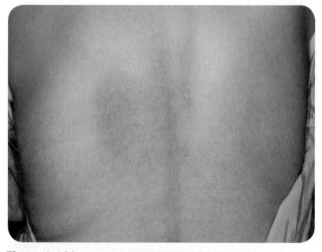

Figure 4-120 A subtle hyperpigmented patch over the upper back is a common finding in notalgia paresthetica.

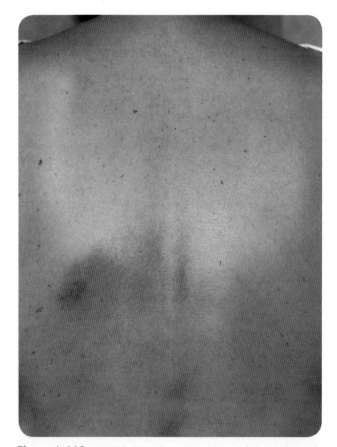

Figure 4-118 Hyperpigmented, very pruritic nodules near the angle of the scapula are characteristic of notalgia paresthetica.

✓ Best Tests

- Notalgia paresthetica is a clinical diagnosis. Laboratory studies and skin biopsy are not helpful.

▲▲▲ Management Pearls

- The management of notalgia paresthetica can be challenging. A low-cost therapy is treatment with topical capsaicin (topical extract of red pepper). Capsaicin depletes substance P in the cutaneous nerve endings, sometimes resulting in relief of the itch. Patients must be cautioned that the skin will burn and feel worse before it feels better. Patients must also be cautioned to wash their hands carefully after applying capsaicin.
- Understanding that the pathogenesis of the disease frequently involves the impingement of the posterior rami of spinal nerves T2–6 provides the rationale for therapies typically used for peripheral neuropathies (e.g., gabapentin or nerve blocks).

Therapy

- Capsaicin 0.025% cream five times daily for 1 week followed by three times daily for 3 to 6 weeks—may require long-term continuation of therapy
- Transcutaneous electrical nerve stimulation
- Gabapentin 300 to 900 mg daily
- Botulinum toxin A
- Topical anesthetics such as lidocaine, pramoxine, or EMLA cream
- Paravertebral local anesthetic block

Suggested Readings

Inaloz HS, Kirtak N, Erguven HG, et al. Notalgia paresthetica with a significant increase in the number of intradermal nerves. *J Dermatol.* 2002 Nov;29(11):739–743.

Loosemore MP, Bordeaux JS, Bernhard JD. Gabapentin treatment for notalgia paresthetica, a common isolated peripheral sensory neuropathy. *J Eur Acad Dermatol Venereol.* 2007 Nov;21(10):1440–1441.

Raison-Peyron N, Meunier L, Acevedo M, et al. Notalgia paresthetica: Clinical, physiopathological and therapeutic aspects. A study of 12 cases. *J Eur Acad Dermatol Venereol.* 1999 May;12(3):215–221.

Savk E, Savk SO. On brachioradial pruritus and notalgia paresthetica. *J Am Acad Dermatol.* 2004 May;50(5):800–801.

Savk O, Savk E. Investigation of spinal pathology in notalgia paresthetica. *J Am Acad Dermatol.* 2005 Jun;52(6):1085–1087.

Savk E, Savk O, Bolukbasi O, et al. Notalgia paresthetica: A study on pathogenesis. *Int J Dermatol.* 2000 Oct;39(10):754–759.

Weinfeld PK. Successful treatment of notalgia paresthetica with botulinum toxin type A. *Arch Dermatol.* 2007 Aug;143(8):980–982.

Weisshaar E, Fleischer AB, Bernhard JD. Pruritus and dysesthesia. In: Bolognia J, Jorizzo JL, Rapini RP, eds. *Dermatology.* 2nd Ed. St. Louis, MO: Mosby; 2008:100.

Yosipovitch G, Samuel LS. Neuropathic and psychogenic itch. *Dermatol Ther.* 2008 Jan–Feb;21(1):32–41.

Postinflammatory Hyperpigmentation

■ Diagnosis Synopsis

Postinflammatory hyperpigmentation describes localized darker skin areas as a consequence of trauma and/or inflammation. The inflammatory process may be incited by an infection, allergy, drug reaction, mechanical or thermal injury, phototoxic eruption, or an intrinsic skin disease. Although clinically benign, patches of postinflammatory hyperpigmentation can cause significant cosmetic and psychosocial distress.

Histologically, there is an increased production of melanin without an increase in the number of melanocytes. This increased pigment may be deposited in the epidermis or the dermis. This reaction is much more pronounced in individuals with dark skin and patients with lichenoid dermatoses (such as lichen planus). There is no age or gender predilection.

The lesions of postinflammatory hyperpigmentation may be accentuated by sunlight or exposure to certain chemicals or drugs, including tetracycline, antimalarial drugs, hormones, and some metals (silver and gold), and chemotherapeutic agents (doxorubicin, bleomycin, 5-fluorouracil, and busulfan).

◉ Look For

Asymptomatic, ill-defined, darkened macules or patches (Figs. 4-121–4-124). Lesions will often define an area of previous skin insult or inflammation of any kind. It can occur anywhere on the body (including the mucosa and within the nail unit).

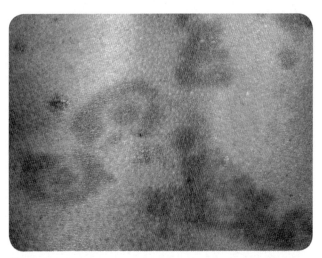

Figure 4-121 Postinflammatory hyperpigmentation due to pemphigus vulgaris.

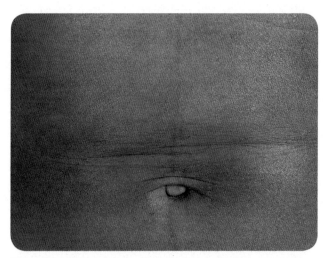

Figure 4-122 Postinflammatory hyperpigmentation consistent with previous atopic dermatitis.

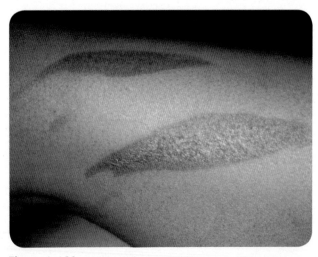

Figure 4-123 Hyperpigmentation secondary to a thermal burn.

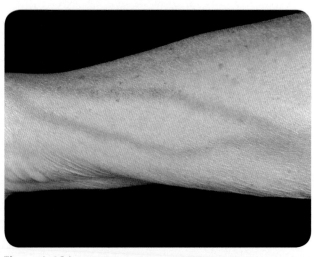

Figure 4-124 Hyperpigmentation in a venous pattern.

Pigment deposited in the epidermis is often light brown, while dermal pigment appears more blue-gray in color.

Dark Skin Considerations

This reaction is much more pronounced in individuals with dark skin. In dark skin, the resolution of hyperpigmentation can be prolonged, lasting for months to years. Postinflammatory hyperpigmentation secondary to acne is common in patients with dark skin and is often their major complaint.

Diagnostic Pearls

- Epidermal pigmentation is more accentuated with a Wood lamp and, thus, appears darker than the normal surrounding skin. In contrast, dermal pigmentation is not accentuated with a Wood lamp. This may have therapeutic implications, as epidermal pigmentation is more successfully treated with topical therapy (see below).

?? Differential Diagnosis and Pitfalls

- Melasma (if the pigmentation is facial)
- Drug-induced pigmentation
- Addison disease
- Acanthosis nigricans
- Tinea versicolor
- Lichen planus
- Lichen amyloidosis
- Erythema ab igne
- Solar lentigines
- Peutz-Jeghers syndrome
- Erythema dyschromicum perstans

✓ Best Tests

- This is usually a clinical diagnosis that is made based on the history of an antecedent inflammatory skin disease, trauma, or chronic rubbing in the area of pigmentation.
- Skin biopsy may be performed in equivocal cases. The biopsy specimen should be stained with Fontana-Masson silver stain to localize the melanin deposition.

▲▲ Management Pearls

- The prevention of the inciting dermatoses will help control the development of the condition. Conservative skin care is often best, with an emphasis placed on the importance of allowing the skin to heal itself. Discourage any picking, scratching, or rubbing by the patient.
- Advise the patient that they must photo-protect the area with clothes and/or sunscreens (with both UVB and UVA blockers) to prevent further darkening. Small amounts of UVA (even through window glass) can exacerbate the condition. In darker-pigmented individuals, postinflammatory hyperpigmentation may take many months to fade.
- Camouflage cosmetics may be helpful.

Therapy

Sun-protection measures and education as described above.

A variety of topical agents are available; these tend to work best on epidermal hyperpigmentation (as evidenced by Wood lamp). Oftentimes, a combination of various treatments is needed to achieve a significant result. The following regimens can be tried:

- 4% hydroquinone plus 1% hydrocortisone applied to lesions twice daily.
- 4% hydroquinone and tretinoin 0.025% applied to lesions twice daily.
- 4% hydroquinone, 1% hydrocortisone, and tretinoin 0.025% applied to lesions twice daily.
- Higher concentrations of tretinoin (0.05% and 0.1%) and more potent steroid preparations (betamethasone) may also be used, as tolerated. Use only low-potency topical corticosteroids on the face.

Azelaic acid applied to lesions twice daily may also have a bleaching effect.

It is recommended that topicals be applied to a cosmetically appropriate "test area" prior to large field treatment as pigmentary alteration induced by bleaching agents can vary widely among individuals.

Alpha hydroxy acid peels, gentle cryotherapy, and microdermabrasion have all been used with variable results. Caution should be exercised with these modalities because overly aggressive treatment may lead to depigmentation and/or scarring. Laser for these lesions is in the investigational phase. The Nd:YAG laser may be tried but is not recommended for dark skin because treatment can lead to depigmentation.

Suggested Readings

Bulengo-Ransby SM, Griffiths CE, Kimbrough-Green CK, et al. Topical tretinoin (retinoic acid) therapy for hyperpigmented lesions caused by inflammation of the skin in black patients. *N Engl J Med*. 1993 May 20;328(20):1438–1443.

Hexsel D, Arellano I, Rendon M. Ethnic considerations in the treatment of Hispanic and Latin-American patients with hyperpigmentation. *Br J Dermatol*. 2006 Dec;156(Suppl. 1):7–12.

Lacz NL, Vafaie J, Kihiczak NI, et al. Post-inflammatory hyperpigmentation: A common but troubling condition. *Int J Dermatol*. 2004 May;43(5):362–365.

Lerner EA, Sober AJ. Chemical and pharmacologic agents that cause hyperpigmentation or hypopigmentation of the skin. *Dermatol Clin*. 1988 Apr;6(2):327–337.

Lynde CB, Kraft JN, Lynde CW. Topical treatments for melasma and post-inflammatory hyperpigmentation. *Skin Therapy Lett*. 2006 Nov;11(9):1–6.

Ruiz-Maldonado R, Orozco-Covarrubias ML. Post-inflammatory hypopigmentation and hyperpigmentation. *Semin Cutan Med Surg*. 1997 Mar; 16(1):36–43.

Stratigos AJ, Katsambas AD. Optimal management of recalcitrant disorders of hyperpigmentation in dark-skinned patients. *Am J Clin Dermatol*. 2004; 5(3):161–168.

Taylor SC, Burgess CM, Callender VD, et al. Post-inflammatory hyperpigmentation: Evolving combination treatment strategies. *Cutis*. 2006 Aug; 78(2 Suppl. 2):6–19.

Speckled Lentiginous Nevus (Nevus Spilus)

■■ Diagnosis Synopsis

A speckled lentiginous nevus, or nevus spilus, is a lesion composed of small, dark "speckles," either macules or papules, superimposed on a lighter, but hyperpigmented, macular background. Some authorities consider these lesions to be subtypes of congenital melanocytic nevi. The speckles within the background patch are nevi, typically junctional or compound, and less often blue or Spitz nevi. The pathogenesis is thought to be related to a local defect in neural crest melanoblasts.

Speckled lentiginous nevi can be associated with a number of other conditions and findings, including but not limited to corneal dystrophy, scleral pigmentation, hearing loss, Ebstein anomaly, ichthyosis, neurofibromatosis type I, epidermal nevi, and a nevus sebaceus. Speckled lentiginous nevus is a component of certain subtypes of phakomatosis pigmentovascularis.

Speckled lentiginous nevi show no predilection to either sex but are slightly more common in whites than other ethnicities. The majority of lesions are present at birth or become evident during the first year of life. They are benign lesions with a rare incidence of malignant transformation. The risk of melanoma development appears to correlate with lesions greater than 4 cm, zosteriform or segmental subtypes, and lesions present at birth.

◉ Look For

A variety of brown, black, or reddish-brown macules and papules within a solitary patch of lighter tan hyperpigmentation (Figs. 4-125–4-128). Lesions are usually oval in shape, but they may follow a dermatome or be distributed along the lines of Blaschko.

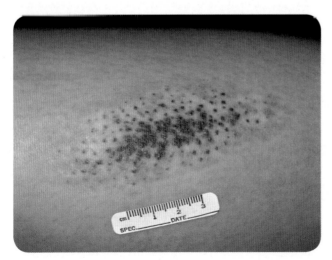

Figure 4-125 Complex macular, dark speckling on a large brown macule.

The trunk and extremities are the most common locations for a speckled lentiginous nevus, although they may occur at any body location.

The light brown background of most lesions is 1 to 4 cm in diameter (but ranges from 1 to 60 cm), with the speckles being 2 to 3 mm on an average. Giant or segmental nevus spilus may occupy an entire extremity or a significant portion of the trunk.

◉◉ Diagnostic Pearls

- Spitz nevi and blue nevi may also be present within the background-pigmented patch.
- Patients may notice a change in color or an increase in lesion size and number of speckles over time.

?? Differential Diagnosis and Pitfalls

- Café au lait macule
- Agminated nevus
- Blue nevus
- Partial (segmental) lentiginosis

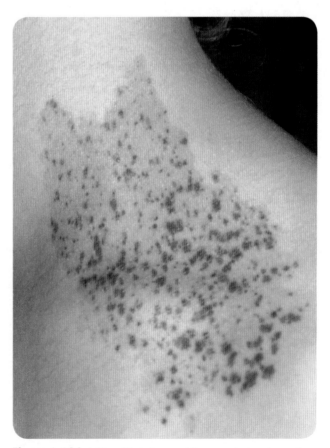

Figure 4-126 Axilla with darker speckling superimposed on a large brown macule.

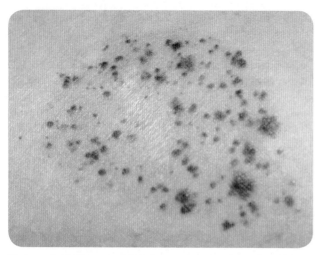

Figure 4-127 Large speckled nevus with minimal background pigmentation.

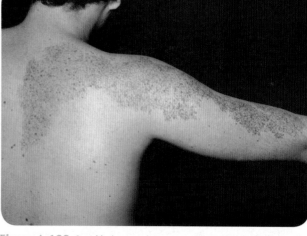

Figure 4-128 Speckled nevus in a zosteriform distribution. May be a variant of Becker nevus.

- Spitz nevus
- Lentigines/lentigo simplex
- Malignant melanoma
- Congenital nevus
- Mosaic hyperpigmentation

✓ Best Tests

This diagnosis can often be made clinically, although biopsy is often performed to rule out melanocytic atypia. All atypical lesions should be biopsied and submitted for histopathologic examination.

▲▲ Management Pearls

- Conservative management consists of observation with photography to assess for the development of atypical features and/or malignant change.
- Consider referral to a dermatologist if there is a question of the diagnosis.

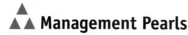

Therapy

Observation is a reasonable alternative for nevi that do not appear suspicious. Patients with nevi in cosmetically sensitive areas may wish to use a camouflage cosmetic. Encourage all patients to use sunscreen and wear sun-protective clothing.

Surgical removal may be undertaken, but the entire lesion must be excised to prevent recurrence. As some lesions are quite large, significant scarring may result.

The Q-switched ruby and Nd:YAG lasers have been used to treat the hyperpigmentation, often with equivocal or unsatisfactory results.

Suggested Readings

Barnhill RL, Rabinowitz H. Benign melanocytic neoplasms. In: Bolognia J, Jorizzo JL, Rapini RP, eds. *Dermatology*. 2nd Ed. St. Louis, MO: Mosby; 2008:1727.

Betti R, Inselvini E, Crosti C. Extensive unilateral speckled lentiginous nevus. *Am J Dermatopathol*. 1994 Oct;16(5):554–556.

McKee PH, Calonje E, Granter SR. Melanocytic nevi. In: McKee PH, Calonje E, Granter SR, eds. *Pathology of the Skin: With Clinical Correlations*. 3rd Ed. Edinburgh: Philadelphia, USA; 2005:1262.

Moreno-Arias GA, Bulla F, Vilata-Corell JJ, et al. Treatment of widespread segmental nevus spilus by Q-switched alexandrite laser (755 nm, 100 nsec). *Dermatol Surg*. 2001 Sep;27(9):841–843.

Piana S, Gelli MC, Grenzi L, et al. Multifocal melanoma arising on nevus spilus. *Int J Dermatol*. 2006 Nov;45(11):1380–1381.

Schaffer JV, Orlow SJ, Lazova R, et al. Speckled lentiginous nevus: Within the spectrum of congenital melanocytic nevi. *Arch Dermatol*. 2001 Feb;137(2):172–178.

Vente C, Neumann C, Bertsch H, et al. Speckled lentiginous nevus syndrome: Report of a further case. *Dermatology*. 2004;209(3):228–229.

Vidaurri-de la Cruz H, Happle R. Two distinct types of speckled lentiginous nevi characterized by macular versus papular speckles. *Dermatology*. 2006;212(1):53–58.

Vitiligo

Diagnosis Synopsis

Vitiligo is an acquired idiopathic type of leukoderma characterized by circumscribed depigmented macules or patches. The lesions are usually chalk-white in color and are surrounded by normal skin, creating well-demarcated margins. Vitiligo is usually asymptomatic, and lesions can range in size from millimeters to centimeters. While any part of the body can be affected, vitiligo often demonstrates distinct patterns including a symmetric involvement of the face, upper chest, hands, ankles, axillae, groin, and around orifices (eyes, nose, mouth, urethra, and anus).

Vitiligo occurs in all ages. It occurs in all ethnicities and in both sexes in equal proportions. The natural progression of the disease is unpredictable, ranging from insidious to rapid in onset. Years of stable, nonprogressive disease can be observed with the disease subsequently taking an unexpected rapid, exacerbated trajectory.

While the majority of vitiligo patients are otherwise healthy, an association with autoimmune thyroid dysfunction (hyperthyroidism or hypothyroidism) has been demonstrated. In new onset, for vitiligo patients with systemic symptoms, thyroid screening with anti-thyroid peroxidase (anti-TPO) antibody and a serum thyroid-stimulating hormone (TSH) is recommended. Additional endocrinopathy associations include diabetes mellitus, Addison disease, myasthenia gravis, and gonadal failure. It may exist as part of polyglandular autoimmune syndrome, particularly type III (Hashimoto thyroiditis, vitiligo or alopecia areata, and/or another organ-specific autoimmune disease).

Vitiligo has also been associated with ocular abnormalities. Pigmented cells reside in the uveal tract and epithelium of the retina. Patients with vitiligo can suffer from uveitis.

Variants of vitiligo include the following:

- Vitiligo with raised inflammatory borders—margins of vitiligo lesions have a raised, erythematous border
- Vitiligo ponctué—tiny punctate-like depigmented macules on a hyperpigmented macule or on normal skin
- Blue vitiligo—when vitiligo develops on a postinflammatory hyperpigmented lesion, giving a bluish tint
- Confetti type vitiligo—multiple small, depigmented macules resembling confetti

While the etiology of vitiligo remains unclear, several theories exist. These can be divided into host attack on normal melanocytes versus intrinsic melanocyte defects. The "host attack" theories are centered on the autoimmune destruction of melanocytes via autoantibodies or cytotoxic T-lymphocytes. The "intrinsic defects" theories include decreased melanocyte survival due to deficiencies in cellular maintenance proteins, an intrinsic defect in TYRP1 processing in melanocytes, and an intracellular metabolic disorder in affected melanocytes that results in the accumulation of oxidized pteridines and subsequent cell death.

Look For

Sharply demarcated, depigmented macules and/or patches (Figs. 4-129–4-132). There is no associated skin textural change, and erythema surrounding the lesions is rare.

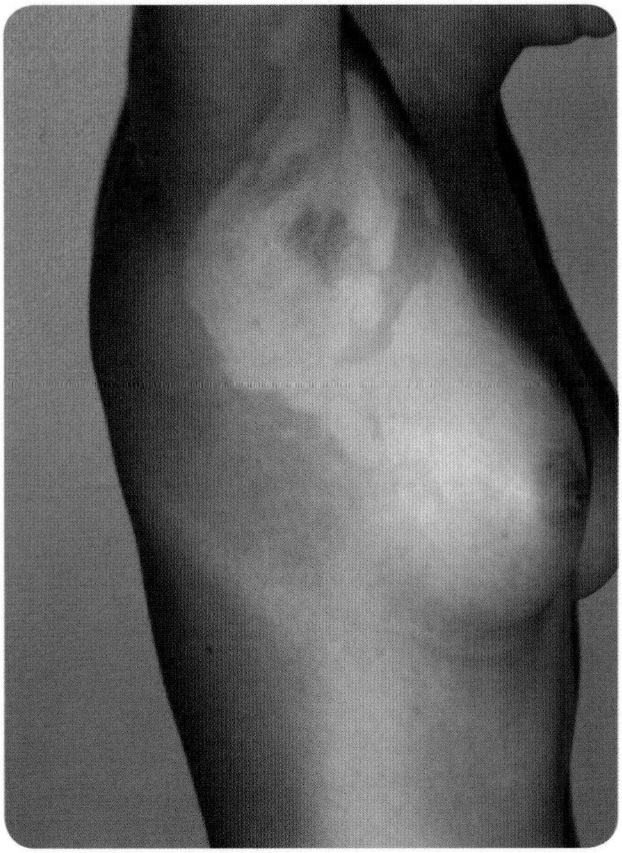

Figure 4-129 The macular hypopigmented areas of vitiligo may have a segmental distribution.

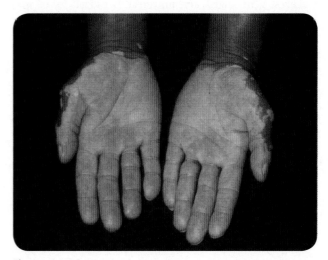

Figure 4-130 Vitiligo can affect the palms and may be difficult to ascertain.

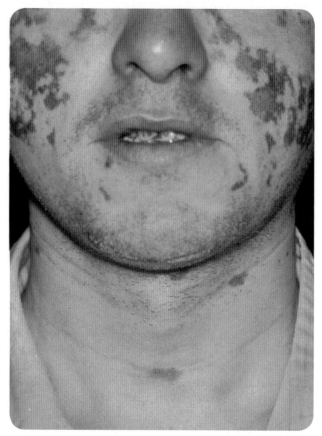

Figure 4-131 Extensive vitiligo can mimic small patches of hyper-pigmentation from the remaining normal skin color.

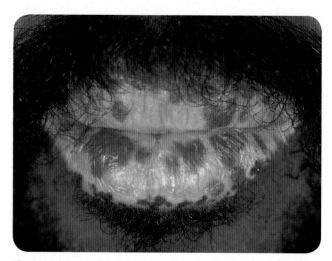

Figure 4-132 Extensive vitiligo affecting the vermillion border of the lips.

Hair may eventually turn white if the affected area is hair bearing.

Look for an occasional associated halo nevus, a nevus surrounded by depigmented skin.

Vitiligo can be classified into three general schemes: localized, generalized, and universal. Localized forms may be segmental or focal, neither crossing the midline. Areas of predilection include the face, neck, and scalp, as well as areas of repeated trauma (bony prominences, dorsal hands, extensor forearm, and fingers) and periorificial areas (around the lips, genitals, eyes, etc.). Mucous membrane involvement is not uncommon in generalized cases. Generalized forms include vulgaris (widely distributed, scattered macules and patches) and acrofacial (distal extremities and face). In the universal form, nearly 100% of the body surface area is depigmented.

Dark Skin Considerations

Trichrome vitiligo, containing a band of intermediate color separating normal skin and the typical depigmented patch, is more common in blacks.

Diagnostic Pearls

- Use a Wood lamp to demonstrate depigmentation as opposed to hypopigmentation, which will not be as pronounced under illumination. Under Wood lamp, vitiligo lesions give a yellow-green or blue fluorescence.
- In vitiligo, there is a notable absence of elevation, erythema, purpura, scale, or any textural changes to the skin.
- Some cases of vitiligo begin as halo nevi phenomenon.

?? Differential Diagnosis and Pitfalls

- Albinism, piebaldism, and other genetic disorders—Begin in infancy.
- Discoid lupus erythematosus—Presents with atrophy, telangiectasia, and follicular plugging, which are absent in vitiligo.
- Postinflammatory hypopigmentation
- Sarcoidosis—Look for indurated papules and plaques that are hypopigmented, not depigmented. Visual changes and shortness of breath on review of systems. Biopsy if needed.
- Leprosy—Lesions are usually hypopigmented, not depigmented. Some can have an erythematous border. Lesions are anesthetic. Patient must have recently lived in an endemic area.
- Nevus depigmentosus—Common on the trunk. Usually present since birth.
- Idiopathic guttate hypomelanosis—Characteristic pattern and shape of lesions different from vitiligo, including well-demarcated, 0.4 to 0.7 mm macules that do not coalesce, are symmetric, and involve the extensor forearms and shins; the face is rarely involved.
- Cutaneous T-cell lymphoma (mycosis fungoides)—Can have an associated scale. Lesions are usually hypopigmented, not depigmented.

- Scleroderma—Look for sclerotic skin; check ANA with nucleolar or speckled pattern, anti-centromere, anti-Scl-70 antibody, associated with Raynaud phenomenon, arthralgias, mat telangiectasias, and CREST.
- Morphea—Look for sclerotic plaques.
- Lichen sclerosus et atrophicus—Look for sclerotic plaques, often in the genital area; can be severely pruritic.
- Chemical leukoderma—Look for a history of chemical use and/or topical corticosteroids.
- Onchocerciasis—Shins are common site of involvement; suspect if patient is coming from endemic area (Africa, Central and South America).
- Tinea versicolor—KOH$^+$, mild scale noted, often seen in the shoulders, upper trunk.

✓ Best Tests

- Diagnosis can usually be made clinically, particularly when areas elsewhere on the body are affected. Skin biopsy specimens will reveal the absence of melanocytes.
- Consider the following tests to screen for autoimmune disorders:
  – Antinuclear antibodies
  – CBC with red blood cell indices
  – TSH level
  – Fasting blood glucose

▲▲ Management Pearls

- Take a detailed personal and family history of autoimmune disease, and consider a workup if the review of systems is suggestive.
- Sun avoidance and use of sunscreens are recommended so as not to enhance the contrast between the pigmented and nonpigmented areas.
- Spontaneous repigmentation occurs in a few patients but is usually incomplete.
- Check TSH and anti-TPO antibody to screen for thyroid involvement if symptoms are suggestive.

Therapy

The goals of treatment include halting the progression of disease and inducing repigmentation. There are many treatment options.

Steroid Therapy
Systemic steroids have been anecdotally reported to be efficacious in rapidly progressive vitiligo. A relatively short course may be useful in the setting of rapidly progressive vitiligo.

Oral Corticosteroids
Prednisone—Dosage and schedule guidelines have not been established. Consider a conservative dose (20 to 40 mg once daily), tapered over 2 weeks.

Topical Corticosteroids
Mid-potency topical corticosteroids (classes 3 and 4)
- Triamcinolone cream or ointment—apply twice daily (15, 30, 60, 120, 240 g)
- Mometasone cream or ointment—apply twice daily (15, 45 g)
- Fluocinolone cream and ointment—apply twice daily (15, 30, 60 g)

Low-potency topical steroids (classes 6 and 7)
- Desonide cream, ointment—apply twice daily (15, 60, 90 g)
- Alclometasone cream or ointment—apply twice daily (15, 45, 60 g)

Intralesional corticosteroids (triamcinolone acetonide 10 mg/mL) can also be tried for the most recalcitrant lesions. However, its use remains controversial due to the risk of skin atrophy and the pain associated with injection.

Phototherapy
Systemic phototherapy has demonstrated satisfactory repigmentation in a large percentage of patients with early disease.

The favored regimen is narrow-band UVB phototherapy. An emission spectrum of 310 to 315 nm and a maximum wavelength of 311 nm are used. Use two to three times weekly. This treatment can be used in children, pregnant women, and lactating women.

Photochemotherapy with 8 methoxypsoralen may be used with systemic PUVA (photochemotherapy) reserved for generalized cases. If no response to therapy is seen in 3 to 4 months, PUVA should be discontinued and tried again in 6 or 8 months. Narrow-band UVB may also be tried twice weekly for a maximum of 1 year.

Topical Calcipotriene
Can be used in combination with phototherapy or topical corticosteroids. Apply after phototherapy to affected areas twice daily; apply thin film, avoiding eyes and lips.

Laser Therapy
The 308-nm excimer laser and monochromatic excimer light treatments (twice weekly for 6 months) are newer treatment modalities with some promising results.

(Continued)

Immunomodulators

Tacrolimus ointment 0.03% or 0.1%—Apply to the affected area twice daily; can continue for 1 week after lesions repigment.

Pimecrolimus 1% cream—Apply to affected area twice daily.

Note that immunomodulators are often preferable to topical corticosteroids in the periocular and genital areas. Topical tacrolimus has been used in combination with the 308-nm excimer laser as well.

Depigmentation Therapy

For very extensive lesions in deeply pigmented patients, depigmentation of the normal skin with 20% monobenzyl ether of hydroquinone (applied twice daily for 9 to 12 months) is an option. This is not to be undertaken lightly, as it is permanent and easy sunburning is a consequence.

Surgical Therapy

Superficial autologous skin grafts (split-thickness and suction blister epidermal grafting) have successfully been used, especially in recalcitrant locations (e.g., over joints).

For patients with facial or other cosmetic regions involved, cosmetic tattooing or cosmetic cover-up makeup may be used.

Suggested Readings

Dell'Anna ML, Mastrofrancesco A, Sala R, et al. Antioxidants and narrow band-UVB in the treatment of vitiligo: A double-blind placebo controlled trial. *Clin Exp Dermatol*. 2007 Nov;32(6):631–636.

Grimes PE. New insights and new therapies in vitiligo. *JAMA*. 2005 Feb;293(6):730–735.

Handa S, Kaur I. Vitiligo: Clinical findings in 1436 patients. *J Dermatol*. 1999 Oct;26(10):653–657.

Mahmoud BH, Hexsel CL, Hamzavi IH. An update on new and emerging options for the treatment of vitiligo. *Skin Therapy Lett*. 2008 Mar;13(2):1–6.

Ortonne JP. Vitiligo and other disorders of hypopigmentation. In: Bolognia J, Jorizzo JL, Rapini RP, eds. *Dermatology*. 2nd Ed. St. Louis, MO: Mosby/Elsevier; 2008:913–920.

van Geel N, Ongenae K, De Mil M, et al. Double-blind placebo-controlled study of autologous transplanted epidermal cell suspensions for repigmenting vitiligo. *Arch Dermatol*. 2004 Oct;140(10):1203–1208.

Whitton ME, Ashcroft DM, Barrett CW, et al. Interventions for vitiligo. *Cochrane Database Syst Rev*. 2006 Jan;(1):CD003263.

Whitton ME, Ashcroft DM, González U. Therapeutic interventions for vitiligo. *J Am Acad Dermatol*. 2008 Oct;59(4):713–717.

Capillaritis

Diagnosis Synopsis

Leakage of red blood cells from the superficial post-capillary venules results in the cayenne pepper-like petechiae of capillaritis, also known as the "pigmented purpuric dermatoses." The precise etiology is unclear, but a cutaneous hypersensitivity reaction is believed most likely. Capillaritis is frequently seen in those who have long periods of extended standing related to their occupation. It is usually lifelong with intermittent exacerbations.

Several distinct clinical entities have been described and occur in people of all ages:

- Schamberg disease—may be related to medication use (salicylates and nonsteroidal anti-inflammatory drugs [NSAIDs])
- Purpura annularis telangiectodes of Majocchi
- Eczematid-like purpura of Doucas and Kapetanakis
- Lichenoid purpura of Gougerot and Blum
- Lichen aureus

There is no ethnic predilection. Men appear to be affected more commonly than women.

Look For

Petechiae and brown-red– or cayenne pepper–colored macules (represent hemosiderin) typically on the legs, but they can appear on the trunk and upper extremities (Figs. 4-133 and 4-134). Lesions never appear on the face. Schamberg disease has yellow-red-brown patches (hemosiderin) with petechiae and is mildly pruritic (Fig. 4-135).

Purpura annularis telangiectodes of Majocchi are annular lesions that occur on the lower legs of women, are reddish-brown in color, and may become atrophic.

Lichenoid purpura of Gougerot and Blum consists of symmetrical, purpuric, minimally elevated, flat-topped papules, and plaques on the distal legs. They may also be pruritic. Classically they occur in men aged 40 to 60 years.

Eczematid-like purpura of Doucas and Kapetanakis mimics eczema with erythema and scale as well as petechiae and hemosiderin.

Lichen aureus usually consists of a solitary lesion or group of lesions. The leg is the most commonly affected body location. Lichen aureus may also present in a linear or segmental configuration.

Diagnostic Pearls

- A tourniquet test may be done to assess for capillary fragility. Apply pressure to the arm at a value halfway between the systolic and diastolic pressures (approx. 100 mm Hg) for 5 min with a blood pressure cuff. Count the resultant petechiae within a 2.5 cm diameter area of the forearm. Any number between 10 and 20 is marginal; a number above 20 is considered abnormal.

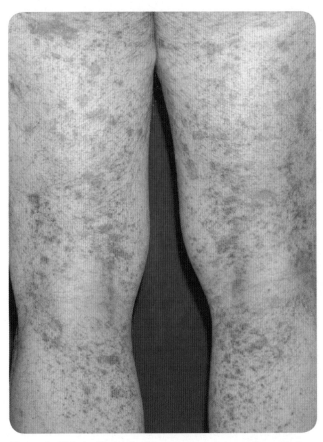

Figure 4-133 Capillaritis is often symmetrical, is usually on the legs, and differs from purpura and petechiae in that lesions persist for years, after the erythema has resolved, with yellow-orange cayenne-pepper pigmentation (hemosiderin).

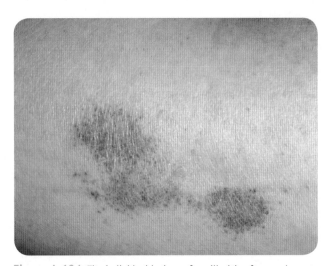

Figure 4-134 The individual lesions of capillaritis often coalesce to form plaque-like lesions.

121

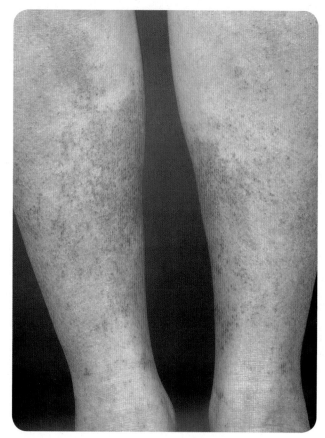

Figure 4-135 Capillaritis presenting bilaterally.

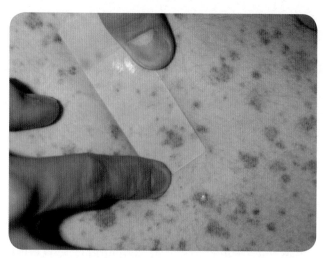

Figure 4-136 Cayenne-pepper lesions of capillaritis do not blanch with pressure from a glass slide, the procedure of diascopy.

?? Differential Diagnosis and Pitfalls

- Minute leakage of RBCs into an inflammatory rash, such as dermatitis, can sometimes cause similar skin lesions; however, the hemorrhage is epiphenomena to the primary dermatitis.
- Drug reaction
- Fixed drug reaction
- Kaposi sarcoma
- Lichen planus
- Mycosis fungoides/early cutaneous T-cell lymphoma
- Leukocytoclastic vasculitis
- Scurvy
- Thrombocytopenic purpura
- Trauma
- Venous stasis dermatitis
- Petechiae from other causes (thrombocytopenia, disseminated intravascular coagulation [DIC], etc.)

✓ Best Tests

- The diagnosis is typically made on clinical grounds, but a biopsy will be confirmatory if there is doubt. Be sure to take a careful medication history and look for signs of chronic venous insufficiency (e.g., leg edema, varicose veins, and stasis dermatitis).
- Press with a glass slide (diascopy) on the red or red-brown macules and they will not fully blanch, revealing that RBCs and hemosiderin have leaked from the venules into the dermis (Fig. 4-136).
- Additional studies may be obtained to rule out other disorders. In capillaritis, a CBC and coagulation profile will be normal. Consider checking serum IgA, IgG, and IgM to rule out a monoclonal gammopathy.

▲▲ Management Pearls

- Compression stockings are indicated if venous hypertension is present. Furthermore, encourage such patients to elevate their legs whenever they are at rest.

Therapy

There is no uniformly effective therapy, although topical steroids with or without occlusion may treat associated inflammation and pruritus and help resolve the discoloration.

Mid-potency topical corticosteroids (classes 3 and 4)

- Triamcinolone cream, ointment—apply twice daily (15, 30, 60, 120, 240 g)
- Mometasone cream, ointment—apply twice daily (15, 45 g)
- Fluocinolone ointment, cream—apply twice daily (15, 30, 60 g)

The discontinuation of asprin or NSAIDs may help prevent lesions of Schamberg disease.

Psoralen plus UVA (PUVA) has demonstrated efficacy in case series.

Vitamin C (500 to 1,000 mg per day) with or without bioflavonoids (rutoside 50 mg twice daily) is frequently used, but there is no robust evidence to support this practice.

Pentoxifylline (400 mg three times daily) helped resolve lesions in some patients.

Suggested Readings

Gupta G, Holmes SC, Spence E, et al. Capillaritis associated with interferon-alfa treatment of chronic hepatitis C infection. *J Am Acad Dermatol.* 2000 Nov;43(5 Pt 2):937–938.

Kwon SJ, Lee CW. Figurate purpuric eruptions on the trunk: Acetaminophen-induced rashes. *J Dermatol.* 1998 Nov;25(11):756–758.

Sardana K, Sarkar R, Sehgal VN. Pigmented purpuric dermatoses: An overview. *Int J Dermatol.* 2004 Jul;43(7):482–488.

Lymphangioma Circumscriptum

▪▪ Diagnosis Synopsis

Lymphangioma circumscriptum is a benign congenital vascular malformation of dilated superficial lymphatic channels. Subcutaneous lymphatic cisterns communicate through dilated channels with the skin surface. Clinically manifesting as localized clusters of translucent vesicles that contain clear or hemorrhagic lymphatic fluid, these malformations can be present at birth or appear early in childhood. Lymphangioma circumscriptum has a high rate of recurrence unless fully excised. Morbidity is due to pain, inflammatory flares, minor bleeding, and recurrent episodes of cellulitis.

Immunocompromised Patient Considerations

Lymphangioma circumscriptum may be mistaken for cutaneous viral infections such as herpes simplex, molluscum contagiosum, and human papillomavirus infections, which commonly present in immunocompromised patients. Anogenital lymphangiomas are relatively common and are frequently mistaken for condyloma acuminata.

◉ Look For

Multiple grouped or contiguous 2 to 4 mm pink/red translucent or hemorrhagic, thick-walled vesicles whose resemblance has been likened to that of "frog spawn" (Figs. 4-137–4-139). The lesions may also have a verrucous-appearing surface. Oral mucosal lesions may have thick walls and contain a milky-appearing fluid.

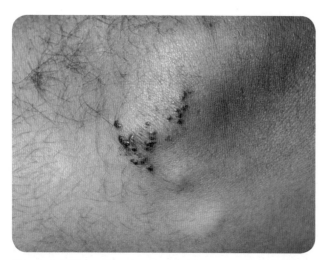

Figure 4-137 Lymphangioma circumscriptum may have connections to blood vessels and may appear hemorrhagic.

The lesions are most commonly encountered on the proximal extremities, trunk, axilla, and in the oral cavity. Anogenital lesions including the vulva and scrotum are frequently reported (Fig. 4-140).

Dark Skin Considerations

There does not appear to be any ethnic predilection to lymphangioma circumscriptum.

●● Diagnostic Pearls

- Though the lesions appear similar to vesicles, they do not break as easily as true vesicles. Lesions are generally longstanding with intermittent weeping of serosanguineous lymphatic fluid.
- The lesions of lymphangioma circumscriptum tend to expand and increase in number with age. Occasionally, ruptured vesicles may bleed or drain clear lymph.

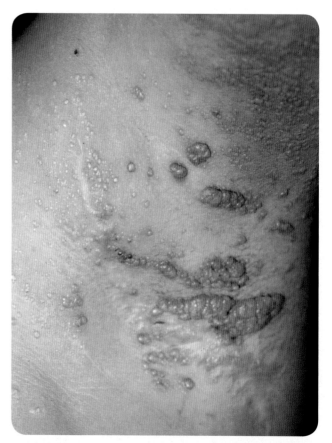

Figure 4-138 Discrete and grouped vesicopapules with the appearance of "frog spawn" in the axilla is typical of lymphangioma circumscriptum.

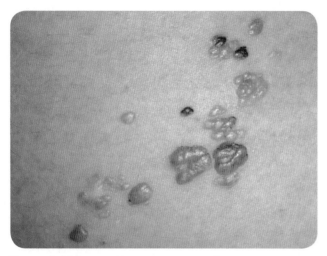

Figure 4-139 Clear discrete and grouped "frog spawn" lesions of lymphangioma circumscriptum.

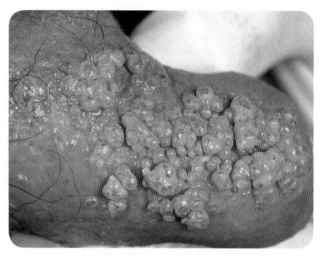

Figure 4-140 Lymphangioma circumscriptum of the penis.

?? Differential Diagnosis and Pitfalls

- Epidermal nevus
- Incontinentia pigmenti
- Venous ectasias
- Lymphangiectasia
- Metastatic carcinoma
- Melanoma
- Angiosarcoma
- Neurofibromatosis
- Hemangioma
- Verruca vulgaris
- Condyloma acuminata
- Molluscum contagiosum
- Irritant contact dermatitis
- Allergic contact dermatitis

Immunocompromised Patient Differential Diagnosis

- Verruca vulgaris
- Condyloma acuminata
- Molluscum contagiosum

✓ Best Tests

- Skin biopsy will demonstrate characteristic histopathology; the diagnosis can be made on clinical appearance alone.
- MRI and lymphangiography have been used to locate lymphatic cisterns in preparation for excision. MRI demonstrates hyperintensity in T2-weighted images.

▲▲ Management Pearls

- If the lesion is asymptomatic, adopting a "watch and wait" policy is reasonable.
- Surgical intervention is typically undertaken for cosmetic reasons, although other indications include pain, recurrent bleeding, and infections.
- Although lymphangioma circumscriptum is considered a benign entity, there are extremely rare case reports of malignant tumor appearance within this malformation. The risk of malignant change is greatest in malformations previously treated with irradiation.

Therapy

If treatment is desired for aesthetic reasons or symptomatic lesions (painful, bleeding, recurrent infections), wide local excision is the treatment of choice. At this time, all other therapies are considered noncurative but palliative for symptoms and cosmetic appearance. Therapies that have proven successful include electrocautery, cryotherapy, sclerotherapy, and laser vaporization (carbon dioxide laser). Pulsed dye laser has been reported as effective in treating smaller superficial cutaneous blebs. A good cosmetic outcome was also reported with intense pulsed light therapy. However, recurrence rates are high with all therapeutic modalities.

Complicating skin and soft tissue infections should be treated with the appropriate antibiotics.

125

Suggested Readings

Arpaia N, Cassano N, Vena GA. Dermoscopic features of cutaneous lymphangioma circumscriptum. *Dermatol Surg.* 2006 Jun;32(6):852–854.

Bardazzi F, Orlandi C, D'Antuono A, et al. Lymphangioma circumscriptum of the penis. *Sex Transm Infect.* 1998 Aug;74(4):303–304.

Bikowski JB, Dumont AM. Lymphangioma circumscriptum: Treatment with hypertonic saline sclerotherapy. *J Am Acad Dermatol.* 2005 Sep;53(3): 442–444.

Bond J, Basheer MH, Gordon D. Lymphangioma circumscriptum: Pitfalls and problems in definitive management. *Dermatol Surg.* 2008 Feb;34(2):271–275.

Emanuel PO, Lin R, Silver L, et al. Dabska tumor arising in lymphangioma circumscriptum. *J Cutan Pathol.* 2008 Jan;35(1):65–69.

Enjolras O. Vascular malformations. In: Bolognia J, Jorizzo JL, Rapini RP, eds. *Dermatology.* 2nd Ed. St. Louis, MO: Mosby; 2008:1589–1594.

James WD, Berger TG, Elston DM. Dermal and subcutaneous tumors. In: James WD, Berger TG, Elston DM, Odom RB, eds. *Andrews' Diseases of the Skin: Clinical Dermatology.* 10th Ed. Philadelphia, PA: Saunders Elsevier; 2006:586–587.

Maloudijan M, Stutz N, Hoerster S, et al. Lymphangioma circumscriptum of the penis. *Eur J Dermatol.* 2006 Jul–Aug;16(4):451–452.

Mendiratta V, Sarkar R, Sharma RC. Lymphangioma circumscriptum masquerading as irritant contact dermatitis. *J Dermatol.* 1999 Jul;26(7): 474–475.

Moss AL, Ibrahim NB. Lymphangiosarcoma of the hand arising in a pre-existing non-irradiated lymphangioma. *J Hand Surg [Br].* 1985 Jun;10(2):239–242.

Thissen CA, Sommer A. Treatment of lymphangioma circumscriptum with the intense pulsed light system. *Int J Dermatol.* 2007 Nov;46(Suppl. 3): 16–18.

Treharne LJ, Murison MS. CO_2 laser ablation of lymphangioma circumscriptum of the scrotum. *Lymphat Res Biol.* 2006;4(2):101–103.

Tulasi NR, John A, Chauhan I, et al. Lymphangioma circumscriptum. *Int J Gynecol Cancer.* 2004 May–Jun;14(3):564–566.

Diagnosis Synopsis

Port-wine stain is a congenital benign capillary malformation typically found on the head and neck. It is the most common type of vascular malformation, and it persists for life without involuting. In some individuals, a port-wine stain may become more violaceous and take on a cobblestoned texture with age. In addition to being cosmetically disturbing to the patient, these lesions may be associated with a number of other findings or conditions (e.g., glaucoma). They are more common in whites.

A port-wine stain may be isolated or may occur as part of a syndrome. The most common syndromes associated with such capillary malformations are as follows:

- Sturge-Weber (encephalotrigeminal angiomatosis)—There are cerebral and meningeal lesions in addition to a cutaneous lesion in the distribution of the ophthalmic branch of the trigeminal nerve. Patients may have seizures, glaucoma, mental retardation, hemiplegia, or subdural hemorrhages.
- Klippel-Trenaunay (angio-osteohypertrophy syndrome)—Consists of a triad of vascular stain, hemihypertrophy, and venous varicosities. In the past, the vascular stain has been thought to be a pure capillary malformation; however, it is now recognized that, more commonly, the vascular stain associated with Klippel-Trenaunay is a combined malformation of capillaries, lymphatics, and venous differentiation.

It is also important to note that lesions of the lower back may be associated with other skin findings such as dimples, sinuses, lipomas, and faun-tail deformities, but also with a possible underlying skeletal or neurologic abnormality such as a tethered cord.

Look For

At birth, a port-wine stain appears as a flat, irregular, unilateral patch. The color may vary from pink to red to purple (Figs. 4-141–4-144). With age, the lesion thickens and develops a rubbery, cobblestoned quality. The head and the neck are areas of predilection.

Diagnostic Pearls

- Pyogenic granulomas may develop within the lesion.
- Capillary malformations typically appear in a dermatomal/segmental distribution on the head and neck.
- Lesions in the V1 distribution are more likely to be associated with the Sturge-Weber syndrome.

?? Differential Diagnosis and Pitfalls

- Salmon patches—These are small capillary dilatations commonly occurring in the midline on the head (stork bites and angel kisses). They decrease in color with age (except for those on the nape of the neck, which tend to persist) and usually do not require treatment.

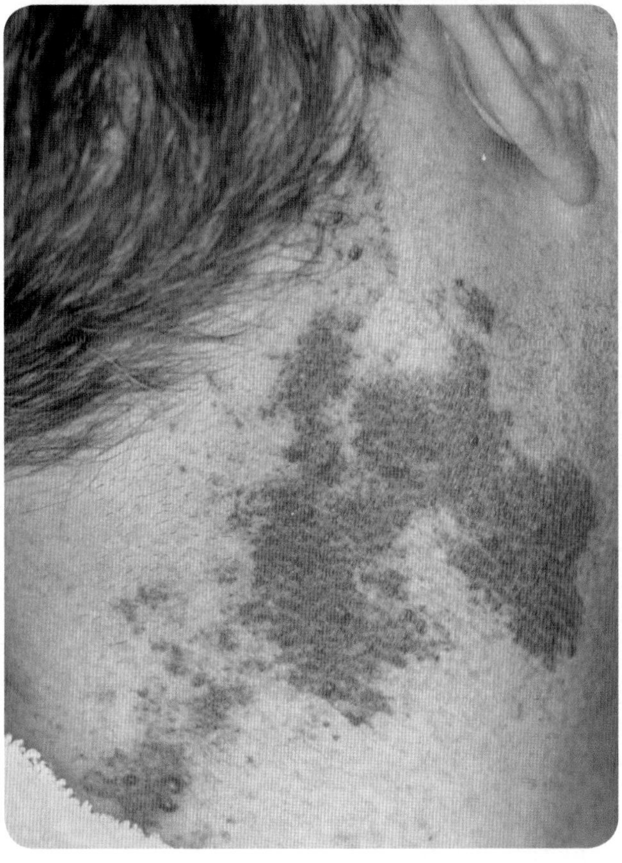

Figure 4-141 Purple plaque with satellite macules in a port-wine stain.

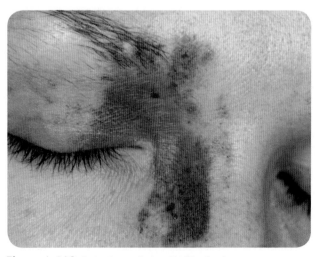

Figure 4-142 Port-wine stain in a V1 distribution.

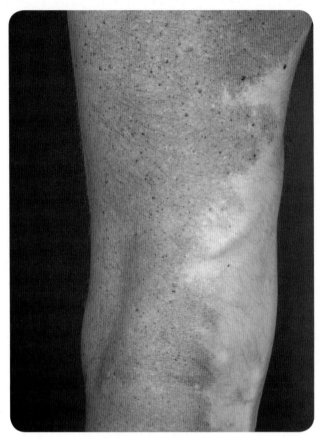

Figure 4-143 Large macular port-wine stain on a leg.

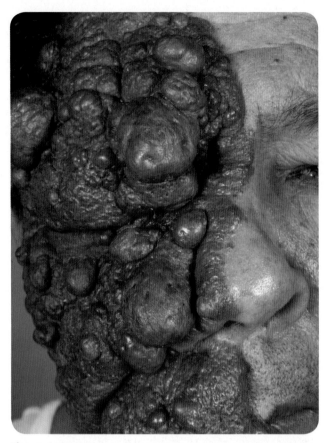

Figure 4-144 Hypertrophic vascular lesions can be a chronic feature of a port-wine stain.

- Early infantile hemangiomas in children
- Sturge-Weber syndrome
- Klippel-Trenaunay syndrome
- Cobb syndrome
- Proteus syndrome
- Rubinstein-Taybi syndrome
- Macrocephaly-capillary malformation syndrome

✓ Best Tests

- This is a clinical diagnosis.
- Perform an MRI of the head with gadolinium if Sturge-Weber syndrome is suspected. Consider an MRI or ultrasound in patients with lumbar lesions.
- An ophthalmologic examination with tonometry is indicated for patients with a port-wine stain that involves the periocular area (V1 distribution).

▲▲ Management Pearls

- Camouflage makeup can be used effectively (Dermablend or Covermark).

- Regular ophthalmologic examinations are recommended in patients with V1 port-wine stains.
- Consider a neurologic consultation for patients with suspected Sturge-Weber or those with lumbar lesions.

Therapy

Pulsed-dye laser (PDL, 585 to 595 nm) offers the most effective treatment of capillary malformations. Most families choose to initiate treatment with PDL prior to school age. This is typically performed in centers where brief general anesthetic is available in an outpatient setting. If performing without general anesthetic, consider locally anesthetizing the area with EMLA or 4% tetracaine gel prior to treatments.

Intense pulsed light and KTP (potassium-titanyl-phosphate, 532 nm) and long-pulsed Nd:YAG (1,064 nm) lasers have also been reported as useful.

Re-darkening of port-wine stains is reported to occur approximately 10 years after laser therapy; touch-up treatment may be necessary.

Suggested Readings

Huikeshoven M, Koster PH, de Borgie CA, et al. Redarkening of port-wine stains 10 years after pulsed-dye-laser treatment. *N Engl J Med.* 2007 Mar;356(12):1235–1240.

Jasim ZF, Handley JM. Treatment of pulsed dye laser-resistant port wine stain birthmarks. *J Am Acad Dermatol.* 2007 Oct;57(4):677–682.

Kelly KM, Choi B, McFarlane S, et al. Description and analysis of treatments for port-wine stain birthmarks. *Arch Facial Plast Surg.* 2005 Sep–Oct; 7(5):287–294.

Klapman MH, Yao JF. Thickening and nodules in port-wine stains. *J Am Acad Dermatol.* 2001 Feb;44(2):300–302.

Landthaler M, Hohenleutner U. Laser therapy of vascular lesions. *Photodermatol Photoimmunol Photomed.* 2006 Dec;22(6):324–332.

Pyogenic Granuloma

■■ Diagnosis Synopsis

Pyogenic granulomas are rapidly growing, benign, vascular growths of undetermined etiology. *Pyogenic granuloma* is a misnomer, as the lesion(s) are neither granulomatous nor infectious. Pyogenic granulomas usually present as a solitary red papule or nodule that grows rapidly and ulcerates or bleeds easily. Gingival lesions may arise during pregnancy (the so-called *pregnancy tumor* or *granuloma gravidarum*) or in the course of treatment with certain medications (protease inhibitors, retinoids, and some chemotherapeutic drugs). They are more common in children and women of childbearing potential. Treatment by removing the lesion is indicated in cases of bleeding, emotional distress, discomfort, or when the diagnosis is in doubt.

● Look For

A glistening, friable, bright red papule or nodule that bleeds spontaneously or after trauma (Figs. 4-145 and 4-146). There may be associated ulceration and/or crusting (Figs. 4-147 and 4-148). The base can have a well-circumscribed rim (collarette) of scale. They are usually solitary and frequently occur on the gingiva, the digits, and the face. There are reports of eruptive pyogenic granulomas. Oral mucosal lesions are most common in pregnant women. Occasionally, satellite lesions may develop near the site of a previously destroyed primary pyogenic granuloma. Pyogenic granulomas may be a complication of isotretinoin therapy and can arise in port-wine stains undergoing laser treatment. They may occur at sites of trauma as well. Size may range from several millimeters to a few centimeters; they tend to reach their maximum size in a matter of weeks.

Diagnostic Pearls

- There is sometimes a history of preceding trauma. Typically, a pyogenic granuloma forms quite rapidly over the course of several weeks.
- The pregnancy tumor variant most commonly arises during the second or third trimester and affects the oral mucosal surface.
- Drugs associated with pyogenic granulomas include isotretinoin, topical retinoids, indinavir, 5-fluorouracil, capecitabine, mitoxantrone, and anti–epidermal growth factor inhibitors (anti-EGFRs).

?? Differential Diagnosis and Pitfalls

- Melanoma
- Cherry hemangioma
- Glomus tumor
- Metastatic carcinoma
- Basal cell carcinoma
- Squamous cell carcinoma
- Spitz nevus
- Granulation tissue
- Angiosarcoma
- Atypical fibroxanthoma
- Venous lake
- Poroma
- Clear cell acanthoma

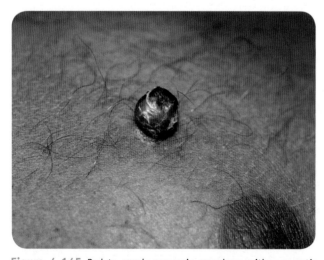

Figure 4-145 Red to purple pyogenic granuloma with a necrotic distal portion.

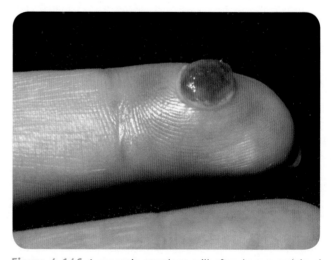

Figure 4-146 A pyogenic granuloma will often have a peripheral rim of compressed normal epidermis.

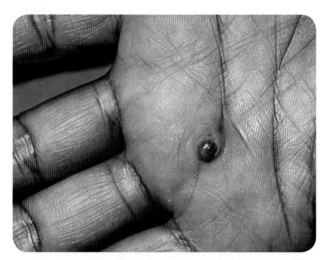

Figure 4-147 Pyogenic granuloma is often a hemorrhagic and crusted lesion. In a typical location on the palm.

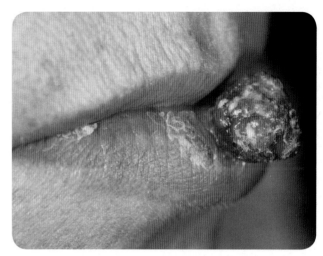

Figure 4-148 Heavily crusted pyogenic granuloma on the lower lip.

Immunocompromised Patient Differential Diagnosis

- In the immunocompromised or HIV-infected patient, consider bacillary angiomatosis and Kaposi sarcoma.

✓ Best Tests

- Dermatoscopy may assist in making a clinical diagnosis.
- Skin biopsy is confirmatory, and histopathology demonstrates an exophytic lobular proliferation of capillaries with an epidermal collarette and, commonly, overlying ulceration and hemorrhagic crust.

▲▲ Management Pearls

- Attempt to eliminate any potential inciting factor(s), such as trauma and offending medications, if possible.
- Recurrences are common regardless of the choice of treatment.
- Many lesions arising during pregnancy resolve after parturition.

Therapy

Shave excision with curettage and either electrodesiccation or application of silver nitrate to the base is a common treatment modality. Silver nitrate by itself may be used to treat smaller lesions.

Other modalities with reported success include sclerotherapy, cryotherapy, ligation, monoethanolamine oleate, and topically applied imiquimod. Systemic steroids have also been used for the management of giant and recurrent pyogenic granulomas. Pulsed dye laser may reduce the incidence of scarring.

Recurrences are common.

Suggested Readings

Blumental G. Paronychia and pyogenic granuloma-like lesions with isotretinoin. *J Am Acad Dermatol.* 1984 Apr;10(4):677–678.

Ghodsi SZ, Raziei M, Taheri A, Karami M, Mansoori P, Farnaghi F. Comparison of cryotherapy and curettage for the treatment of pyogenic granuloma: A randomized trial. *Br J Dermatol.* 2006 Apr;154(4):671–675.

Giblin AV, Clover AJ, Athanassopoulos A, Budny PG. Pyogenic granuloma—the quest for optimum treatment: Audit of treatment of 408 cases. *J Plast Reconstr Aesthet Surg.* 2007 Sep;60(9):1030–1035.

González S, Vibhagool C, Falo LD, Momtaz KT, Grevelink J, González E. Treatment of pyogenic granulomas with the 585 nm pulsed dye laser. *J Am Acad Dermatol.* 1996 Sep;35(3 Pt 1):428–431.

Jafarzadeh H, Sanatkhani M, Mohtasham N. Oral pyogenic granuloma: A review. *J Oral Sci.* 2006 Dec;48(4):167–175.

James WD, Berger TG, Elston DM. Dermal and subcutaneous tumors. In: James WD, Berger TG, Elston DM, Odom RB, eds. *Andrews' Diseases of the Skin: Clinical Dermatology.* 10th Ed. Philadelphia, PA: Saunders Elsevier; 2006:592.

Lin RL, Janniger CK. Pyogenic granuloma. *Cutis.* 2004 Oct;74(4):229–233.

North PE, Kincannon J. Vascular neoplasms and neoplastic-like proliferations. In: Bolognia JL, Jorizzo JL, Rapini RP, eds. *Dermatology.* 2nd Ed. St. Louis, MO: Mosby; 2008:1776–1777.

Scheinfeld NS. Pyogenic granuloma. *Skinmed.* 2008 Jan–Feb;7(1):37–39.

Spider Angioma

■■ Diagnosis Synopsis

A spider angioma, also known as a spider vein or spider nevus, is the most prevalent of the telangiectases. Clinically, there is a central arteriole from which numerous small, twisted vessels radiate. The ascending central arteriole appears as a spider's body, and the radiating vessels resemble the spider's legs, hence the spider appearance that is visible on the skin.

This common benign, acquired lesion usually appears spontaneously and is present in 40% of normal children up to age 8. Prevalence drops to about 10% to 15% of healthy adults. Many women develop lesions during pregnancy or while taking oral contraceptives, likely due to high estrogen levels in their blood. These lesions usually disappear following parturition or cessation of the contraceptives.

Spider angiomas may be indicative of underlying systemic disease, especially when found in large numbers. Liver dysfunction due to hepatic cirrhosis or hepatic tumors impair the metabolism of estrogen, which may play a role in increased nevus formation. In addition, elevated levels of serum vascular endothelial growth factor (VEGF) and young age are predictive of spider angioma formation in patients with cirrhosis. Patients with alcoholic cirrhosis are more likely to develop spider angioma than those with viral or idiopathic cirrhosis. In patients with diseases of the liver, a regression of the nevus may occur following an improvement of the underlying condition, although this is not usually so. They are also associated less frequently with thyrotoxicosis and in patients on estrogen therapy.

Spider angiomas usually appear on the upper half of the body, frequently on sun-exposed areas. It is very uncommon for lesions to occur below the level of the umbilicus. The lesion ranges in size from that of a pinhead to 2 cm.

Pyogenic granuloma developing within a large spider angioma is a possible complication of these benign vascular malformations.

◉ Look For

Spider angiomas occur most commonly on the face, neck, and upper part of the trunk and arms. Also look for lesions on the hands, forearms, and ears. Rarely, they may be visible in the mucous membrane of the nose, mouth, or pharynx.

Spider angiomas are bright red with a small central papule surrounded by small radiating vessels (**Figs. 4-149–4-152**).

Pressure applied to the angioma will lead to its disappearance. Blanching is quickly reversed when pressure is lifted, resulting in a rapid refill from the central arteriole. The refill pattern occurs from the center to the periphery due to the arteriolar origin of the spider nevus.

Dark Skin Considerations

Spider angiomas appear to be less frequent in patients with darker skin. However, epidemiologic studies are limited.

●● Diagnostic Pearls

- The typical spider appearance of the lesion is unmistakable. Pressure applied to the central arteriole causes the blanching of the entire lesion. When pressure is released, these vessels quickly refill with blood. This can be easily seen with diascopy using a glass slide.
- In patients who appear to have many spider angiomas, particularly on mucosal or acral sites, the diagnosis of hereditary hemorrhagic telangiectasia should be considered. Scleroderma (especially CREST syndrome) may also present with multiple mat-like telangiectasias on the face and acral sites.

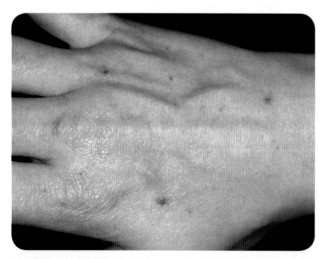

Figure 4-149 Spider angiomas on the dorsum of the hand with central papules and short legs.

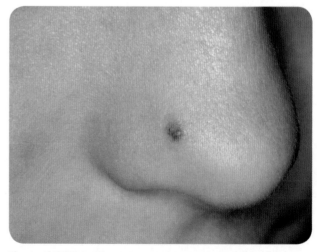

Figure 4-150 Spider angioma with red, shiny central papules and very short legs.

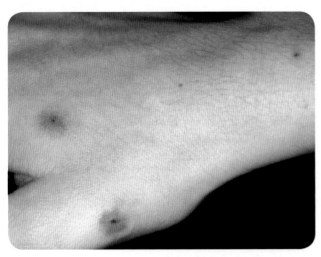

Figure 4-151 Spider angiomas on the hand with prominent central puncta and a red blush without prominent peripheral vessels.

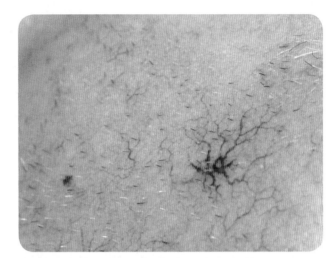

Figure 4-152 Spider angioma on sun-damaged skin.

?? Differential Diagnosis and Pitfalls

- Hereditary hemorrhagic telangiectasia
- Scleroderma (CREST syndrome)
- Cherry hemangioma
- Angiokeratoma corporis circumscriptum
- Ataxia telangiectatica
- Insect bites
- Essential telangiectasia
- Rosacea
- Pyogenic granuloma
- Capillary malformation—arteriovenous malformation syndrome

✓ Best Tests

- The classic refill pattern remains the diagnostic marker for the identification of spider angiomas. Press down on the lesion and watch for refill radiating from the central vessel outward.
- Liver function tests to assess the severity of liver disease, if present.

Management Pearls

- The treatment of spider angiomas is usually done for cosmetic purposes, especially when present on the face.

Therapy

Laser treatment and electrodesiccation are both effective methods, and the lesion is usually completely removed.

Electrodesiccation

The central arteriole can be ablated using fine needle electrodesiccation. This involves sealing of the blood vessels by monopolar high frequency electric current.

Laser Treatment

Treatment with lasers is very effective but may be more costly than electrodesiccation. KTP (potassium-titanyl-phosphate), pulsed dye, and argon lasers have all successfully been used in the treatment of spider angiomas. Local anesthesia may be used prior to the procedure. One must be careful not to blanch and obscure the spider vein when infiltrating the anesthesia.

Results are excellent with both types of treatment, and recurrence is infrequent.

Suggested Readings

Bernstein EF. The new-generation, high-energy, 595 nm, long pulse-duration, pulsed-dye laser effectively removes spider veins of the lower extremity. *Lasers Surg Med.* 2007 Mar;39(3):218–224.

Bernstein EF, Lee J, Lowery J, et al. Treatment of spider veins with the 595 nm pulsed-dye laser. *J Am Acad Dermatol.* 1998 Nov;39(5 Pt 1):746–750.

Goldman MP, Weiss RA, Brody HJ, et al. Treatment of facial telangiectasia with sclerotherapy, laser surgery, and/or electrodesiccation: A review. *J Dermatol Surg Oncol.* 1993 Oct;19(10):899–906; quiz 909–910.

Henry F, Quatresooz P, Valverde-Lopez JC, et al. Blood vessel changes during pregnancy: A review. *Am J Clin Dermatol.* 2006;7(1):65–69.

Okada N. Solitary giant spider angioma with an overlying pyogenic granuloma. *J Am Acad Dermatol.* 1987 May;16(5 Pt 1):1053–1054.

Requena L, Sangueza OP. Cutaneous vascular anomalies. Part I. Hamartomas, malformations, and dilation of preexisting vessels. *J Am Acad Dermatol.* 1997 Oct;37(4):523–549; quiz 549–552.

Witte CL, Hicks T, Renert W, et al. Vascular spider: A cutaneous manifestation of hyperdynamic blood flow in hepatic cirrhosis. *South Med J.* 1975 Feb;68(2):246–248.

Vasculitis, Leukocytoclastic

◼ Diagnosis Synopsis

Leukocytoclastic vasculitis (LCV), or cutaneous small vessel vasculitis, describes a heterogeneous group of disorders that are uniformly characterized by purpuric or erythematous papules, vesicles, urticarial lesions, or petechiae. The end-stage phenotype of LCV is an inflammatory process of small blood vessels due to a complex interplay of immune complex deposition, autoantibody production, complement activation, inflammatory cell activation, and mast cell degranulation. From a clinical perspective, different cutaneous features are seen in medium to large vessel vasculitis and include subcutaneous nodules, retiform purpura, ulcers, and livedo reticularis.

LCV can occur in all ages and in both sexes. It is more commonly found in adults, but up to 10% of cases are in the pediatric population. Clinical features include a single eruption of palpable purpuric papules or nodules, vesicles, urticarial plaques, or petechiae cropping up in dependant areas approximately 1 week after an inciting factor. A variety of inciting factors have been identified, including medications (especially antibiotics, nonsteroidal anti-inflammatory drugs [NSAIDs], and diuretics), pathogens (hepatitis viruses, HIV, and streptococci), foods or food additives, malignancy, inflammatory bowel disease, or collagen vascular diseases. Up to 50% of cases, however, have no identifiable cause and are considered idiopathic.

While the majority of cases are asymptomatic, LCV can be associated with pruritus, pain, or burning. A skin biopsy will greatly aid in confirming the diagnosis. Significantly, the physician will need to differentiate LCV from a systemic vasculitis and should suspect the latter if fever, myalgias, malaise, lymphadenopathy, abdominal pain, melena, hematochezia, diarrhea, hematuria, lower extremity swelling, or paresthesias are noted. The level of systemic involvement will largely influence the prognosis. Over 90% of patients with LCV limited to the skin will experience spontaneous resolution over several weeks to months.

Variants or subcategories of LCV include the following:

- Henoch-Schönlein purpura—Acute onset of palpable purpura usually seen in children aged younger than 10 years in the lower extremities/buttocks 1 to 2 weeks after a respiratory infection. Fever, arthralgias, and renal and gastrointestinal involvement are commonly seen. Can occur in adults.
- Urticarial vasculitis—Recurrent, painful eruptions of urticarial lesions that last for more than 24 h (assists in differentiating from chronic urticaria) with or without angioedema. Fever, malaise, myalgias, and arthritis are commonly associated. Urticarial vasculitis can be observed with systemic lupus erythematosus, Sjögren syndrome, and viral infections. Complement levels can predict systemic involvement; normal levels seen with cutaneous limited disease, hypocomplementemic levels seen with arthritis, and gastrointestinal and pulmonary involvement.
- Erythema elevatum diutinum—Rare; violaceous papules and plaques that favor the extensors symmetrically. Chronic course with spontaneous resolution after 5 to 10 years.

◉ Look For

Palpable purpura is the most common finding, consisting of nonblanching 1 to 3 mm violaceous, round papules, characteristically involving the lower extremities (Figs. 4-153–4-156). These may become larger over time and coalesce into nodules and plaques that may occasionally ulcerate. Older lesions may have brownish-red color.

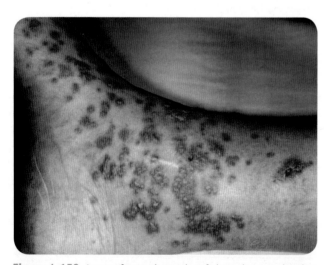

Figure 4-153 A crop of purpuric papules of about the same duration.

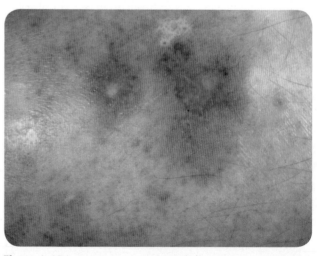

Figure 4-154 Vasculitic lesions may develop opaque, necrotic centers.

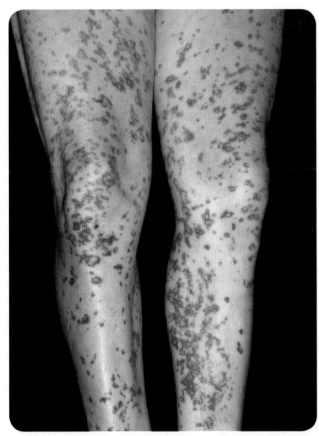

Figure 4-155 Vasculitic lesions are frequently symmetrically distributed on the legs.

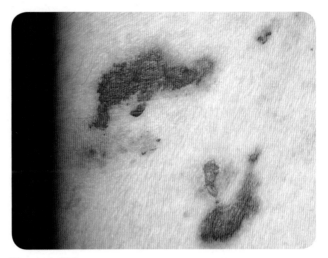

Figure 4-156 Vesicles developing within purpuric vasculitic papules.

Urticarial lesions may appear prior to the purpura in some patients. These tend to last longer than classic urticaria and may leave behind some hyperpigmentation as they resolve.

Dark Skin Considerations

Palpable purpura may resolve with atrophic scarring and/or hyperpigmentation, especially in black patients.

●● Diagnostic Pearls

- Diascopy is a simple and useful maneuver. It consists of pressing a glass slide over a purpuric papule and demonstrating the presence of red blood cells within the skin (nonvasculitic papules will blanch).
- Lesions are sometimes in a distinct linear arrangement due to external pressure or trauma.
- Take a careful history of medications and other supplements or alternative therapies.

Immunocompromised Patient Considerations

In the immunosuppressed patient or the patient with low polymorphonuclear leukocytes, the distribution of the lesions may be similar to that in the normal host, but there is a lesser degree of induration and purpura.

?? Differential Diagnosis and Pitfalls

The differential diagnosis for LCV is extensive. A skin biopsy will largely aid in the diagnosis. Secondary causes of LCV, such as infection, drug, neoplasms, and autoimmune connective tissue disorders, should be sought.

- Bacterial infections
- Viral infections—hepatitis A, B, or C; HIV; VZV; parvovirus B19; CMV
- Arthropod bites
- Erythema multiforme (EM)—Characteristic findings on histology will assist in differentiating EM from LCV. Systemic involvement is extremely rare. Also, in the center of targetoid lesions, look for epidermal damage including crust or bullae.
- Still disease—Look for high-spiking fevers (often greater than 38.88°C [102°F]) and a macular exanthem that is salmon pink in color and most commonly found on the trunk.
- Drug exposure—NSAIDs, penicillins, quinolones, antitumor, necrosis factor biologics, hydralazine, granulocyte colony stimulating factor (G-CSF), and ACE-inhibitors.
- Cryoglobulinemia—Check for serum IgM and IgG cryoglobulins and HCV infection.
- Microscopic polyangiitis—ANCA positive, palpable purpura, and constitutional symptoms; look for evidence of pulmonary and renal involvement.

- Wegener granulomatosis—ANCA positive, necrotizing granulomatous inflammation of the upper and lower respiratory tracts, and glomerulonephritis.
- Churg-Strauss syndrome—ANCA positive, associated with eosinophilia and asthma, and characteristic findings on histology.
- Polyarteritis nodosa—Medium vessel vasculitis with subcutaneous nodules, livido reticularis, ulcers, and gangrene as cutaneous manifestations.
- Behçet disease—Look for aphthous stomatitis, recurrent genital ulcerations, and ocular findings, particularly uveitis.
- Immune thrombocytopenic purpura—Look for isolated thrombocytopenia (anemia and neutropenia are more likely to be involved in other diseases).

Sometimes nonvasculitic purpura on the lower extremities may be palpable, such as those seen in

- Overanticoagulation with warfarin or heparin
- Early disseminated intravascular coagulation
- Pruritic insect bites
- Schamberg disease

✓ Best Tests

- The confirmation of LCV is achieved by skin biopsy.
- Testing to elucidate systemic involvement often includes a CBC with differential, ESR, urinalysis, chemistry panel, chest X-ray, and fecal occult blood testing.
- Further workup to rule out infectious or rheumatologic etiologies is indicated once vasculitis is confirmed. This is often accomplished with the following tests:
- ANA
- ANCA
- Rheumatoid factor
- Anti-Ro and anti-La
- Complement levels
- Cryoglobulins
- HIV and hepatitis B and C serologies
- Select patients may require echocardiography, angiography, direct immunofluorescence tests of skin biopsy samples, pulmonary function testing, and screening for malignancy (serum protein electrophoresis, bone marrow biopsy, etc.).

▲▲ Management Pearls

- Therapy is first directed at any underlying trigger, such as infection or withdrawal of a medication. Consider dietary restriction in patients in whom a food substance may be the inciting agent.

The following supportive/symptomatic measures may be taken:

- Rest with the elevation of the legs
- Graduated compression stockings
- NSAIDs for myalgias and arthralgias
- Antihistamines for pruritus, especially in urticarial forms:
  - Diphenhydramine (25, 50 mg tablets or capsules): 25 to 50 mg nightly or every 6 h as needed
  - Hydroxyzine (10, 25 mg tablets): 12.5 to 25 mg every 6 h as needed
  - Cetirizine (5,10 mg tablets): 5 to 10 mg per day
  - Loratadine (10 mg tablets): 10 mg tablet once daily
- Depending on the clinical scenario, the following consultations may be needed or helpful:
  - Dermatology
  - Gastroenterology
  - Rheumatology, allergy or immunology
  - Nephrology
  - Pulmonology

Therapy

The therapeutic management will depend on the level of systemic involvement. Patients without systemic involvement may be safely observed or managed with conservative, symptomatic measures as above.

Patients with visceral involvement will often need systemic corticosteroids (prednisone 0.5 to 2 mg/kg p.o. daily) with or without another immunomodulatory drug.

Corticosteroids
Prednisone: 1 mg/kg p.o. daily

Immunosuppressives
Methotrexate: 10 to 25 mg p.o. weekly
Mycophenolate mofetil: 1 to 2 g p.o. daily
Azathioprine: 2 to 3 mg/kg p.o. daily
Cyclophosphamide: 1 to 2 mg/kg p.o. daily
Rituximab: 375 mg/m^2 IV weekly for 4 weeks

Antimicrobials
Dapsone: 150 to 200 mg p.o. daily; check G6PD levels prior to starting medication

Anti-inflammatory
Colchicine (0.6 mg p.o. two to three times daily) or dapsone (100 to 150 mg p.o. daily) may be tried for patients in whom the disease is limited to the skin and/or joints. The two may also be used in combination.

Exclude infectious causes of LCV prior to instituting any of these therapies.

Other therapies such as plasmapheresis, interferon alpha, and intravenous immunoglobulin (IVIg) have also been used.

Treat any secondarily infected lesions with an appropriate topical or systemic antibiotic.

Suggested Readings

Carlson JA, Cavaliere LF, Grant-Kels JM. Cutaneous vasculitis: Diagnosis and management. *Clin Dermatol.* 2006 Sep–Oct;24(5):414–429.

Carlson JA, Chen KR. Cutaneous vasculitis update: Neutrophilic muscular vessel and eosinophilic, granulomatous, and lymphocytic vasculitis syndromes. *Am J Dermatopathol.* 2007 Feb;29(1):32–43.

Chen KR, Carlson JA. Clinical approach to cutaneous vasculitis. *Am J Clin Dermatol.* 2008;9(2):71–92.

Doyle MK, Cuellar ML. Drug-induced vasculitis. *Expert Opin Drug Saf.* 2003 Jul;2(4):401–409.

Iglesias-Gamarra A, Restrepo JF, Matteson EL. Small-vessel vasculitis. *Curr Rheumatol Rep.* 2007 Aug;9(4):304–311.

Russell JP, Weenig RH. Primary cutaneous small vessel vasculitis. *Curr Treat Options Cardiovasc Med.* 2004 Apr;6(2):139–149.

Schapira D, Balbir-Gurman A, Nahir AM. Naproxen-induced leukocytoclastic vasculitis. *Clin Rheumatol.* 2000;19(3):242–244.

Sunderkötter C, Bonsmann G, Sindrilaru A, et al. Management of leukocytoclastic vasculitis. *J Dermatolog Treat.* 2005;16(4):193–206.

Diagnosis Synopsis

Acne, or acne vulgaris (typical teenage acne), is an extremely common, usually self-limited chronic inflammatory condition of the pilosebaceous unit. The pathogenesis involves multiple factors, including (i) increased sebum production, (ii) follicular hyperkeratinization, (iii) proliferation of the bacterium *Propionibacterium acnes*, and (iv) inflammation. It typically begins at puberty as a result of the androgen stimulation of the pilosebaceous unit and changes in the keratinization at the follicular orifice.

There is a wide spectrum of clinical disease, ranging from a few comedones to many inflamed papules, pustules, and nodules. Acne vulgaris is most commonly found on areas of skin with the greatest density of sebaceous follicles, such as the face, back, and upper chest. Acne can last through the teenage years into adulthood. Women are more likely than men to have acne in adulthood. There is no racial predilection. While a benign condition, acne can lead to physical scarring and significant psychosocial distress; hence, the initiation of treatment in the earliest stages is preferable.

Immunocompromised Patient Considerations

Acne in HIV-infected patients is no different than in those without infection; the severity of the acne has no relationship to the severity of HIV infection. Age is the most important factor, with lesions usually developing in adolescence.

Look For

Open comedones (blackheads) and closed comedones (whiteheads), and erythematous papules and pustules

(Figs. 4-157–4-160). Nodules and cysts can result in pitted or hypertrophic scars. In adult women, deeper-seated, tender, red papules are common along the jaw line. Acne most frequently targets the face, neck, upper trunk, and upper arms.

Dark Skin Considerations

In darker-skinned individuals, open comedones (blackheads) and closed comedones (whiteheads) are subtle in comparison to white skin. Prolonged hyperpigmentation after the resolution of acute acne lesions commonly occurs.

Diagnostic Pearls

- In adult women, touching, rubbing, and overcleansing the face may exacerbate acne. In men, acne tends to be more severe on the trunk.
- Consider external agents, such as grease, from working in fast-food restaurants, occlusion from sports equipment, and drugs (e.g., progesterone-only birth control, steroids, some anticonvulsants, lithium, and isoniazid).
- Congenital adrenal hyperplasia, polycystic ovarian syndrome, and certain other endocrine disorders that cause hyperandrogenism may predispose to the development of acne.
- In women, if there is a perioral predilection, this may represent perioral dermatitis, not acne.

?? Differential Diagnosis and Pitfalls

- Perioral dermatitis
- Milia
- Folliculitis

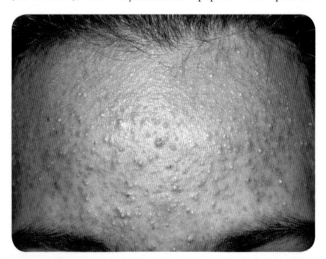

Figure 4-157 Multiple closed comedones on the forehead. Closed comedones (whiteheads) can occur with blackheads and conversely.

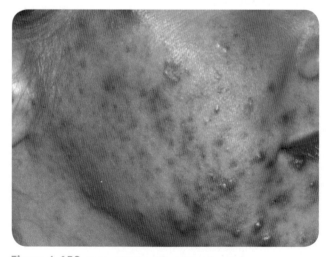

Figure 4-158 Acne vulgaris with cysts and pustules.

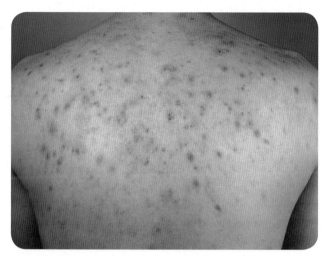

Figure 4-159 The upper back in males with acne vulgaris frequently has cystic and pustular lesions.

- *Pityrosporum* folliculitis
- Flat warts
- Molluscum contagiosum
- Rosacea
- Acne conglobata
- Sebaceous hyperplasia
- Syringomata

✓ Best Tests

- This is usually a clinical diagnosis, although a skin biopsy will define the process if there is any doubt.
- An assessment of acne severity is necessary for choosing the appropriate therapy.
- If the clinical scenario warrants (poor response to therapy, hirsutism, irregular menses, etc.), check sex hormone levels: testosterone, sex hormone–binding globulin, follicle stimulating hormone (FSH), luteinizing hormone (LH), prolactin, and dehydroepiandrosteone (DHEA).
- Late-onset congenital adrenal hyperplasia can be screened for using 9:00 AM levels of cortisol and 17-α-hydroxyprogesterone.
- Consider obtaining skin and nasal swabs to exclude Gramnegative folliculitis, if acne is not responding to traditional therapy.
- Several tests are indicated prior to initiating therapy with isotretinoin as well as monthly while on therapy: CBC, glucose, liver function tests, fasting lipids, and a pregnancy test in female patients.

▲▲ Management Pearls

- Acne often resolves after the teenage years. Severe cases of nodulocystic acne will require more aggressive treatment. Acne needs consistent, regular care that is administered

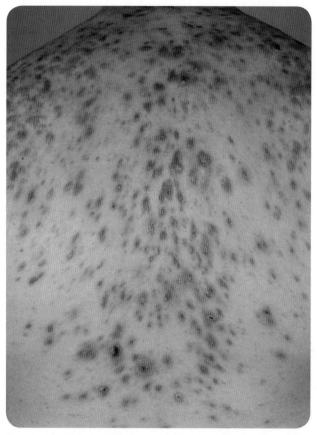

Figure 4-160 Acne vulgaris with cystic and pustular lesions.

over months. Make sure the patient has the correct expectation and applies topical medication to the entire area of potential acne involvement, not just on individual lesions.

- If there are cysts and scarring, consider timely referral to a dermatologist for isotretinoin therapy and to minimize permanent scarring. Referral to a dermatologist who regularly prescribes this medication is recommended, as a systematized method for monitoring patients for side effects and pregnancy avoidance in women is essential. Isotretinoin is teratogenic, and every effort must be made to monitor and manage these patients appropriately.
- Combination products with a topical antibiotic and benzoyl peroxide, if tolerated, are preferable to antibiotic preparations alone as they may discourage the development of antibiotic resistance and enhance compliance.

Immunocompromised Patient Considerations

Ensure that the patient is not taking exogenous hormones to increase his/her strength. Advise patients that the acne is not due to their drugs or the reason for the immunodeficiency.

Therapy

For mild comedonal acne (whiteheads and blackheads predominate), use a topical retinoid:

- Tretinoin (Retin-A 0.025% to 0.1% nightly)
- Tazarotene (Tazorac 0.05% to 0.1% cream or gel applied once daily)
- Adapalene gel (Differin gel 0.1% to 0.3% nightly)

For mild papular or pustular acne, use or add a topical antibiotic/benzoyl peroxide combination:

Erythromycin/benzoyl peroxide (Benzamycin gel) OR the following:

- 1% clindamycin/5% benzoyl peroxide (Duac topical gel 45 g or BenzaClin 50 g).
- Benzoyl peroxide gels can also be used without combination with an antibiotic: 2.5%, 4%, 5%, or 10% gel depending on skin dryness. (Use milder strengths when the skin is dry and higher concentrations on very oily skin.)

Topical antibiotics alone can be less costly than antibiotic-benzoyl peroxide combination products. To reduce the emergence of antibiotic resistance, they are best used with a benzoyl peroxide product. Examples are clindamycin 1% solution (Cleocin lotion) or 1% clindamycin phosphate (Clindets Pledgets), erythromycin 2% gel or solution, Akne-mycin 2% ointment (well tolerated by those with easily irritated skin), and sodium sulfacetamide 10% with 5% sulfur (Klaron, Novacet, Sulfacet-R, and Plexion).

Many exfoliant agents are available over the counter with sulfur, salicylic acid, or resorcinol; they are less effective than retinoids and, while sometimes helpful for mild acne, can add an irritant factor if used in addition to the above prescription agents.

When there are inflammatory papules or deeper-seated lesions, use or add an oral medication: Start with tetracycline 500 mg twice daily. If there is no response to tetracycline after 2 to 3 months, consider doxycycline 100 mg twice daily or minocycline 100 mg twice daily. Trimethoprim-sulfamethoxazole has also been used and is particularly useful if Gram-negative organisms evolve. Caution the patient regarding photosensitivity while taking tetracyclines, and advise patients to use sunscreens (SPF 30) when anticipating sun exposure.

Isotretinoin should be considered in cases of severe acne or moderate acne that has failed more conservative measures. Due to the drug's teratogenicity, patients and prescribers are required to be registered with the iPLEDGE program. Female patients should use two forms of birth control while taking isotretinoin and for 30 days after treatment has ended, and they need to have a documented negative pregnancy test prior to the initiation of therapy. Pregnancy testing continues monthly during therapy and at 1 month after the patient has stopped taking the drug. Patients are usually started on a dose of 0.5 mg/kg/day, which is increased to 1 mg/kg/day after 1 month. Blood work is required before and after the course of treatment.

For acne control in women, estrogen-containing oral conceptives are often used (e.g., Ortho Tri-Cyclen, Yasmin), as is spironolactone (100 to 200 mg per day) particularly in hirsute women with acne.

Note: Patients taking spironolactone will need their serum electrolytes monitored and should avoid becoming pregnant.

Other treatment modalities:

- Subpurpuric pulsed dye laser
- Red (660 nm) and blue (415 nm) light therapy

Suggested Readings

American Academy of Dermatology. Guidelines of care for acne vulgaris. *J Am Acad Dermatol.* 1990 Apr;22(4):676–680.

Campbell JL. A comparative review of the efficacy and tolerability of retinoid-containing combination regimens for the treatment of acne vulgaris. *J Drugs Dermatol.* 2007 Jun;6(6):625–629.

Gollnick H, Cunliffe W, Berson D, et al.; Global Alliance to Improve Outcomes in Acne. Management of acne: A report from a Global Alliance to Improve Outcomes in Acne. *J Am Acad Dermatol.* 2003 Jul;49(1 Suppl.):S1–S37.

Haider A, Shaw JC. Treatment of acne vulgaris. *JAMA.* 2004 Aug;292(6): 726–735.

Lai, KW, Mercurio MG. Update on the treatment of acne vulgaris: An evidence-based review. *J Clin Outcomes Manag.* 2009 Mar;16(3):115–126.

Leyden JJ. Therapy for acne vulgaris. *N Engl J Med.* 1997 Apr;336(16): 1156–1162.

Leyden JJ. A review of the use of combination therapies for the treatment of acne vulgaris. *J Am Acad Dermatol.* 2003 Sep;49(3 Suppl.):S200–S210.

Leyden JJ. Meta-analysis of topical tazarotene in the treatment of mild to moderate acne. *Cutis.* 2004 Oct;74(4 Suppl.):9–15.

Madden WS, Landells ID, Poulin Y, et al. Treatment of acne vulgaris and prevention of acne scarring: Canadian consensus guidelines. *J Cutan Med Surg.* 2000 Jun;4 (Suppl. 1):S2–S13.

Tanghetti E, Abramovits W, Solomon B, et al. Tazarotene versus tazarotene plus clindamycin/benzoyl peroxide in the treatment of acne vulgaris: a multicenter, double-blind, randomized parallel-group trial. *J Drugs Dermatol.* 2006 Mar;5(3):256–261.

Thiboutot DM. Overview of acne and its treatment. *Cutis.* 2008 Jan;81 (1 Suppl.):3–7.

Zaenglein AL, Graber EM, Thiboutot DM, et al. Acne vulgaris and acneiform eruptions. In: Fitzpatrick TB, Wolff K, eds. *Fitzpatrick's Dermatology in General Medicine.* 7th Ed. New York, NY: McGraw-Hill; 2008:690–701.

Acne, Steroid

Diagnosis Synopsis

Steroid acne is a form of acne resulting from the use of topical steroids, oral steroids, and even inhaled corticosteroids. Susceptible patients will experience the sudden onset of follicular papules and pustules approximately 2 to 5 weeks after starting the medication. The lesions of steroid acne, unlike acne vulgaris, are often of uniform size and symmetric distribution. The chest and back are sites of predilection after systemic steroid use. Steroid acne does not usually leave scars and clears with the withdrawal of the medication. It rarely occurs before puberty or in the elderly.

Look For

Numerous monomorphous 1 to 3 mm pink or red dome-shaped papules and pustules, all in the same stage of development (Figs. 4-161–4-164). Lesions are most common on the chest and back but may occur elsewhere, such as on the face and arms. A perioral distribution of the acne is most common with topical steroid use in that region. Comedones and nodules are rare.

Dark Skin Considerations

There is a greater tendency for postinflammatory hyperpigmentation after the resolution of primary lesions.

Diagnostic Pearls

- Lesions tend to be smaller papules and pustules and are not cystic.

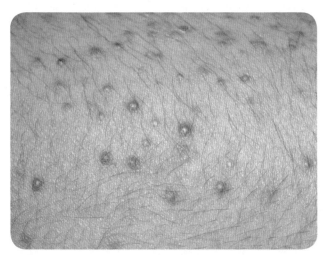

Figure 4-161 Monomorphic papules due to systemic corticosteroids.

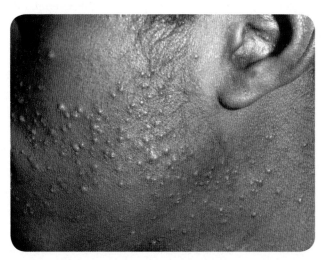

Figure 4-162 Monomorphic facial papules due to systemic corticosteroids.

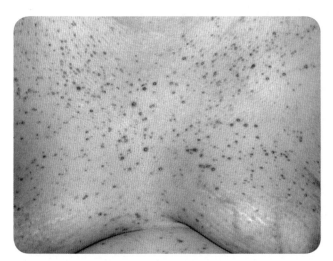

Figure 4-163 Chest with multiple inflammatory papules due to oral corticosteroids.

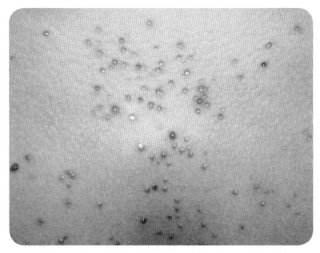

Figure 4-164 Discrete, monomorphic lesions in steroid-induced acne.

?? Differential Diagnosis and Pitfalls

- Consider *Pityrosporum* folliculitis, which is also triggered by oral corticosteroid use.
- Acne vulgaris
- Acne rosacea
- Perioral dermatitis
- Molluscum contagiosum

✓ Best Tests

- Clinical biopsy will confirm the diagnosis but is usually not necessary.

▲▲ Management Pearls

- Identify the illness and avoid calling it a drug eruption. Steroid acne is *not* a contraindication to the continued or future use of steroids if they are clinically indicated.

Therapy

The resolution of the lesions occurs with the discontinuation of the steroids and, in addition, may respond to the usual treatments for acne vulgaris.

Suggested Readings

Fung MA, Berger TG. A prospective study of acute-onset steroid acne associated with administration of intravenous corticosteroids. *Dermatology.* 2000;200(1):43–44.

Harlan SL. Steroid acne and rebound phenomenon. *J Drugs Dermatol.* 2008 Jun;7(6):547–550.

Hurwitz RM. Steroid acne. *J Am Acad Dermatol.* 1989 Dec;21(6): 1179–1181.

▗▖ Diagnosis Synopsis

An arthropod bite or sting may develop a localized inflammatory reaction manifested by localized swelling, redness, pain, burning, and pruritus.

Arthropods include insects (stinging or venomous hymenoptera [e.g., bees, wasps, and fire ants] and nonvenomous insects [e.g., mosquitos and fleas]) as well as ticks, mites, spiders, scabies, and body lice.

Arthropods may transmit human illness (including tick bite fever, Lyme disease, Rocky Mountain spotted fever, a variety of encephalitides, and malaria). Venomous bites may trigger systemic toxic or allergic reactions, including anaphylaxis. An ascending paralysis caused by a neurotoxin may occur after a tick bite.

Scabies, pediculosis capitis (head lice), and Lyme disease are discussed in detail under separate topics.

◉ Look For

A small central punctum with surrounding erythema and swelling (Figs. 4-165–4-166). Vesicles and bullae often occur (Fig. 4-167). Erosions are common (Fig. 4-168).

Immunocompromised Patient Considerations

Arthropod bite reactions may be more pronounced in the immunocompromised patient. An exaggerated, sometimes bullous reaction to an arthropod bite is characteristic of certain immunosuppressed states, especially a hematopoietic malignancy or HIV disease.

In HIV-positive patients, arthropod assaults may result in an extremely pruritic skin eruption, called "pruritic papular eruption."

Multiple papules and pustules may be seen in fire ant bites. Groupings of linear papules are seen with flea bites. Papular urticarial lesions may be seen with flea bites, chiggers, or bedbugs.

Multiple lesions just above the sock line can be due to chigger (harvest mite) bites, which are very common in the Southern United States. Lesions may resolve with residual postinflammatory pigment changes.

Although bites and stings can be found in any body location, in many instances, clothing has a protective effect.

In pediculosis corporis, the nits and adult organism are found on the seams of the clothing, not on the patient.

Dark Skin Considerations

The surrounding erythema may be less pronounced in darker skin types.

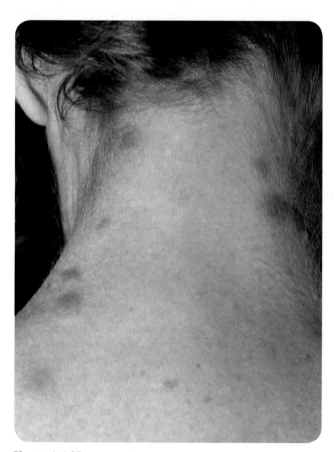

Figure 4-165 Urticarial insect bites.

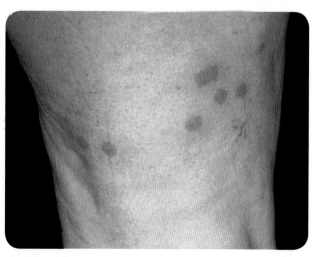

Figure 4-166 Grouped urticarial insect bites.

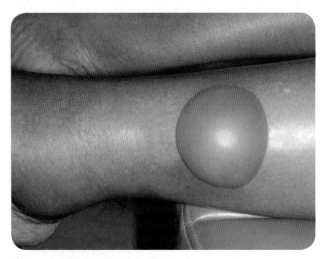

Figure 4-167 Bullous insect bite.

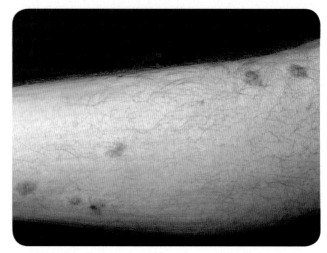

Figure 4-168 Eroded insect bites after travel to Alaska.

Immunocompromised Patient Considerations

A bullous or exaggerated response to an arthropod bite is more common in patients with hematopoietic malignancy and HIV infection.

Immunocompromised Patient Differential Diagnosis

- Herpes simplex virus
- Reactivated varicella-zoster virus
- When bullous, an autoimmune or acquired blistering disorder.

Diagnostic Pearls

- Do not discount the possibility of an arthropod bite or sting because other family members or close contacts do not have the same lesions. Some insects will bite one individual preferentially.
- Bedbugs and fleas often have several lesions in a row (breakfast, lunch, and dinner) from multiple meal samplings by the insect.

Best Tests

- High index of suspicion or patient recollection of a bite or sting.
- Skin scraping and microscopic examination for scabies mites.
- Recognition of nits in head lice (nits are firmly adherent to the hair shaft, whereas scale is easily removed).
- Recognition of nits and organisms in seams of clothing in pediculosis corporis.

Differential Diagnosis and Pitfalls

- Scabies, which is discussed in detail separately, should be identified by the microscopic examination of skin scrapings.
- Flea bites, in particular, can cause vesicles and bullae, which may mimic bullous pemphigoid, bullous impetigo, and linear IgA disease.
- Folliculitis
- Cellulitis
- Acne excoriée
- Pityriasis lichenoides et varioliformis acuta
- Lymphomatoid papulosis

Management Pearls

- Avoid the use of topical diphenhydramine and benzocaine as they may induce a secondary contact dermatitis.
- Cool compresses and baths are comforting, as are creams with 1/4% camphor and menthol or topical anesthetics such as pramoxine or lidocaine.
- To reduce insect bites, instruct patients to wear protective shoes and socks and to avoid bright-colored clothing, perfumes, and scented hair and body lotions.
- Other preventative measures include lotions or sprays containing N, N-Diethyl-3-methylbenzamide (DEET).

- Consult a veterinarian for eradicating flea infestations in pets. Consult an exterminator for bedbugs.
- Instruct children to not play near garbage or standing water during the summer or in areas where bees and wasp nests may be found.

Therapy

Symptomatic relief can be provided with anti-inflammatory agents and oral antihistamines designed to suppress the inflammatory reaction. An essential component of therapy is the reduction or elimination of further arthropod bites through measures as outlined above.

Oral antihistamines
- Hydroxyzine—25 mg three to four times daily, as needed
- Diphenhydramine hydrochloride—25 to 50 mg every 6 h, as needed

Nonsedating antihistamines
- Loratadine—10 mg daily
- Fexofenadine—60 mg twice daily
- Cetirizine hydrochloride—5 or 10 mg nightly

Psychotherapeutic agents
- Doxepin—25 mg nightly

For lesions on trunk and extremities, high potency (classes 1 and 2) topical steroids applied twice daily to individual insect bite reactions usually can control inflammation and itch. These agents should not be used on the face, genitals, or intertriginous areas.

For severe anaphylactic reactions, epinephrine and other vasoactive medications, fluids, and systemic glucocorticosteroids are required emergently.

Supportive treatment and hospitalization may be necessary for encephalitis and tick paralysis, as well as anaphylaxis.

Treatment summaries for the following conditions are discussed in other modules:

- Scabies (permethrin)
- Lice (permethrin, lindane, malathion, or others)
- Lyme disease (antibiotics [e.g., penicillin, cephalosporin, and tetracycline])
- Brown recluse spider bite, spider bite (dapsone and nonsteroidal anti-inflammatory agents [NSAIDs])

Suggested Readings

Ackerman AB, Metze D, Kutnzer H. Erythematous papules and nodules after tick bite. *Am J Dermatopathol.* 2002 Oct;24(5):427–428.

Dunlop K, Freeman S. Caterpillar dermatitis. *Australas J Dermatol.* 1997 Nov;38(4):193–195.

Goddard J, Jarratt J, de Castro FR. Evolution of the fire ant lesion. *JAMA.* 2000 Nov;284(17):2162–2163.

Greaves MW. Recent advances in pathophysiology and current management of itch. *Ann Acad Med Singapore.* 2007 Sep;36(9):788–792.

Hudson BJ, Parsons GA. Giant millipede 'burns' and the eye. *Trans R Soc Trop Med Hyg.* 1997 Mar–Apr;91(2):183–185.

Karppinen A, Kautiainen H, Petman L, et al. Comparison of cetirizine, ebastine and loratadine in the treatment of immediate mosquito-bite allergy. *Allergy.* 2002 Jun;57(6):534–537.

Krinsky WL. Dermatoses associated with the bites of mites and ticks (Arthropoda: Acari). *Int J Dermatol.* 1983 Mar;22(2):75–91.

Resneck JS Jr, Van Beek M, Furmanski L, et al. Etiology of pruritic papular eruption with HIV infection in Uganda. *JAMA.* 2004 Dec;292(21):2614–2621.

Steen CJ, Carbonaro PA, Schwartz RA. Arthropods in dermatology. *J Am Acad Dermatol.* 2004 Jun;50(6):819–842, quiz 842–844.

Steen CJ, Schwartz CA. Arthropod bites and stings. In: Fitzpatrick TB, Wolff K, eds. *Fitzpatrick's Dermatology in General Medicine.* 7th Ed. New York, NY: McGraw-Hill; 2008:2054–2063.

Dermatosis Papulosa Nigra

◧ Diagnosis Synopsis

Dermatosis papulosa nigra are benign epidermal growths similar to seborrheic keratoses. These lesions are typically asymptomatic and are most frequently seen on the cheeks. They are much more common in blacks and Asians. The onset is typically during adolescence, and women are affected more often than men. There may be a family history of similar lesions. The number of lesions typically increases with age; up to one-third of black adults have some of these lesions. Approximately 25% of patients with facial lesions will also have lesions at other body locations. They are a cosmetic concern only.

◉ Look For

The papules are small, round, skin colored or hyperpigmented, and typically located on the cheeks (Figs. 4-169–4-172). Over time, the lesions increase in size and number and spread from just below the eyes to the face, neck, and rarely the upper chest.

Dark Skin Considerations

Dermatosis papulosa nigra is more common in blacks and Asians.

●● Diagnostic Pearls

- Lesions are asymptomatic, frequently symmetric, and all of similar size.

?? Differential Diagnosis and Pitfalls

- Nevi
- Angiofibromas
- Benign appendageal tumors
- Warts
- Seborrheic keratoses
- Acrochordons (skin tags)

✓ Best Tests

- This is a clinical diagnosis. Biopsy is rarely needed but should be performed when the diagnosis is in doubt or if a pigmented lesion appears to be suspicious.

▲▲ Management Pearls

- Permanent scarring, pigmentation alteration, or keloid formation is a feature of aggressive treatment, so treatment must be extremely conservative.

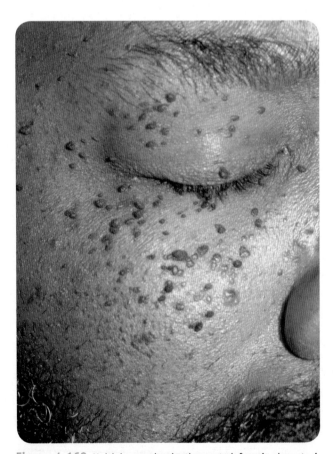

Figure 4-169 Multiple papules in the central face in dermatosis papulosa nigra.

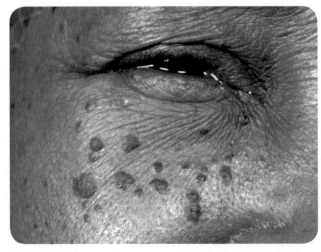

Figure 4-170 Individual lesions of dermatosis papulosa nigra may resemble typical seborrheic keratosis.

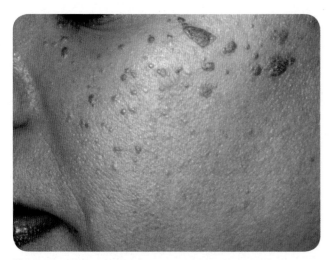

Figure 4-171 Individual lesions of dermatosis papulosa nigra may vary in size.

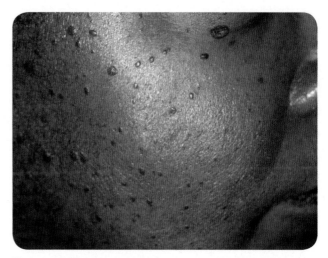

Figure 4-172 Typical distribution for dermatosis papulosa nigra.

Therapy

No treatment is necessary unless the patient requests it for cosmetic reasons.

Cryotherapy is often used. Before treating numerous lesions, test a few for postinflammatory dyspigmentation with very cautious use of liquid nitrogen.

Electrodesiccation and curettage are also effective. Both EMLA (mixture of lidocaine 2.5% and prilocaine 2.5%) and LMX (lidocaine) are reasonable methods of topical anesthesia, and either can be used, if desired, prior to this procedure.

Suggested Readings

Carter EL, Coppola CA, Barsanti FA. A randomized, double-blind comparison of two topical anesthetic formulations prior to electrodesiccation of dermatosis papulosa nigra. *Dermatol Surg.* 2006 Jan;32(1):1–6.

Dunwell P, Rose A. Study of the skin disease spectrum occurring in an Afro-Caribbean population. *Int J Dermatol.* 2003 Apr;42(4):287–289.

James WD, Berger TG, Elston DM. Epidermal nevi, neoplasms, and cysts. In: James WD, Berger TG, Elston DM, Odom RB, eds. *Andrews' Diseases of the Skin: Clinical Dermatology.* 10th Ed. Philadelphia, PA: Saunders Elsevier; 2006:638–639.

Kauh YC, McDonald JW, Rapaport JA, et al. A surgical approach for dermatosis papulosa nigra. *Int J Dermatol.* 1983 Dec;22(10):590–592.

Niang SO, Kane A, Diallo M, et al. Dermatosis papulosa nigra in Dakar, Senegal. *Int J Dermatol.* 2007 Oct;46(Suppl. 1):45–47.

Thomas VD, Swanson NA, Lee KK. Benign epithelial tumors, hamartomas, and hyperplasias. In: Fitzpatrick TB, Wolff K, eds. *Fitzpatrick's Dermatology in General Medicine.* 7th Ed. New York, NY: McGraw-Hill; 2008:1056.

Erythema Nodosum

■■ Diagnosis Synopsis

Erythema nodosum (EN) represents the most common type of inflammatory panniculitis (inflammation of the fat). It is an inflammatory process, typically symmetrical, and located on the pretibial region. It may be precipitated by endogenous or exogenous stimuli. Streptococcal infections are the most common etiologic factor in children. Sarcoidosis, inflammatory bowel disease, and drugs are more commonly implicated in adults. Most often a cause or trigger is never found. The eruption typically persists for 3 to 6 weeks and spontaneously regresses without scarring or atrophy.

Upper respiratory tract infection or flu-like symptoms may precede or accompany the development of the eruption. Arthralgias are reported by a majority of patients regardless of the etiology of EN.

EN can occur at any age, but most cases occur between the ages of 20 and 45, particularly in women. Oral contraceptives are the most common drug association, but EN has been associated with a number of other medications. Pregnancy may also be associated with EN. Bacterial, viral, fungal, and protozoal infections (e.g., *Streptococcus* spp., *Shigella*, *H. capsulatum*, HIV, *Giardia*) may cause EN. In addition to sarcoidosis and inflammatory bowel disease, patients with malignancies, patients undergoing radiation treatment for malignancies, and those with Behçet syndrome, reactive arthritis, Sweet syndrome, ulcerative acne conglobata, and Sjögren syndrome may develop EN. Recurrences are sometimes seen, especially with the repetition of the precipitating factors.

Löfgren syndrome is a benign variant of sarcoidosis with EN and bilateral enlargement of the hilar lymph nodes. It occurs more commonly in females, especially during pregnancy.

◉ Look For

Erythematous, tender nodules and plaques, usually 2 to 5 cm in diameter (Figs. 4-173–4-176). They are initially bright red and slightly elevated. After a week or two, the lesions become flatter and evolve into more purple/livid color or red-brown, somewhat indurated plaques that might appear to be bruised (contusiforme). Lesions never ulcerate (unlike nodular vasculitis).

The lesions are most commonly seen in a pretibial (anterior shin) distribution, but they can also occur on the legs, thighs, buttocks, extensor arms, and occasionally on the face and neck, predominantly in female patients.

Small nodules may also occur on the bulbar conjunctiva or other mucous membranes. Multiple nodules in a region may result in a large bruise called erythema contusiformis. In uncomplicated cases of EN, adenopathy, including hilar adenopathy on chest X-ray, may occur.

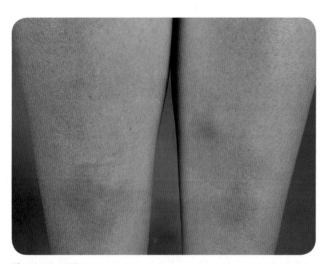

Figure 4-173 Several tender nodules on the shins are typical of EN.

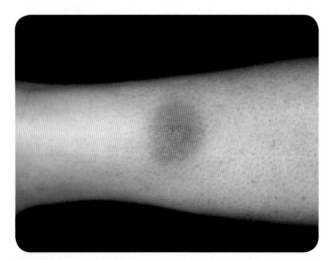

Figure 4-174 Lesions of EN often have a contusiforme (bruised) appearance.

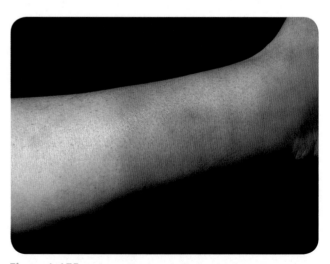

Figure 4-175 Lesions often have indistinct borders.

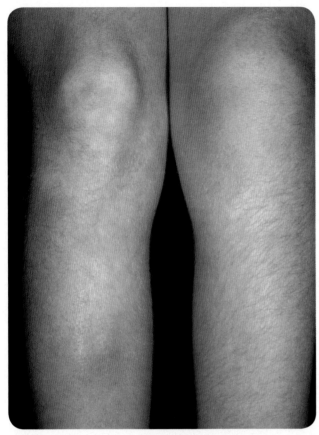

Figure 4-176 Bilateral lesions of EN on both lower legs.

Dark Skin Considerations

In people with darker skin, the lesions are more dusky red or violaceous.

●● Diagnostic Pearls

- The lesions usually occur bilaterally on the anterior shins and are distinguished by their tenderness and smooth, "deep-seated" appearance.

?? Differential Diagnosis and Pitfalls

- Other forms of panniculitis:
  - Subacute migratory panniculitis is often more focal, painless, and unilateral
  - Nodular vasculitis
  - Erythema induratum is typically on the posterior calves
- Some forms of lymphoma can mimic panniculitis
- Superficial migratory thrombophlebitis
- Sarcoidosis
- Insect bites
- Leprosy
- Erythema multiforme

- Trauma
- Erysipelas
- Urticaria
- Cutaneous polyarteritis

✓ Best Tests

- A skin biopsy will confirm a diagnosis of EN by demonstrating a septal panniculitis. The majority of other causes of panniculitis have a lobular inflammatory pattern.
- Investigations to identify the underlying etiology may include antistreptolysin O (ASO) titers, throat culture, tuberculin skin testing, and/or histoplasmin complement fixation. It is recommended that all patients have a CBC and chest X-ray to rule out associated pulmonary tuberculosis, coccidioidomycosis, or sarcoidosis.
- The need for further investigation will depend on the patient population (children versus adults) and history.

▲▲ Management Pearls

- Spontaneous resolution occurs in most cases.
- Bed rest and limb elevation are important alleviating measures.
- Identify and treat any underlying causes of the condition.

Therapy

Nonsteroidal anti-inflammatory drugs (NSAIDs) (aspirin 325 to 650 mg p.o. every 4 to 6 h, ibuprofen 400 to 800 mg p.o. every 6 to 8 h, naproxen 275 mg p.o. every 6 to 8 h, or indomethacin IR 25 to 50 mg p.o. three times daily) may be helpful.

Colchicine (0.6 mg twice daily) has been successful in acute lesions, as has hydroxychloroquine (200 mg twice daily). Intralesional corticosteroids have also been of some benefit. Applying topical corticosteroids with plastic cling wrap occlusion at night may help to reduce inflammation. Systemic corticosteroids have been used on rare occasion. Potassium iodide (400 to 900 mg daily) and antimalarials may be of some benefit in refractory cases.

Isolated case reports have touted the success of the following treatments: dapsone, erythromycin, infliximab, and mycophenolate mofetil.

Suggested Readings

González-Gay MA, García-Porrúa C, Pujol RM, et al. Erythema nodosum: A clinical approach. *Clin Exp Rheumatol.* 2001 Jul–Aug;19(4):365–368.

Mana J, Marcoval J. Erythema nodosum. *Clin Dermatol.* 2007 May–Jun; 25(3):288–294.

Requena L, Sánchez Yus E. Erythema nodosum. *Semin Cutan Med Surg.* 2007 Jun;26(2):114–125.

Favre-Racouchot Disease

Diagnosis Synopsis

Favre-Racouchot disease (FRD), also known as solar or senile comedones, is a disorder of the skin resulting from chronic exposure to the sun. The exact pathogenesis is unknown. After decades, small cysts and large blackheads form on the face and neck. Unlike the comedones of acne vulgaris, comedones in FRD do not become inflamed. The sebaceous glands may also atrophy. The lesions are most commonly seen on the face (in particular, on the temples, cheeks, and periorbital area) of elderly adults. It is more common in patients with a history of heavy smoking. Other types of radiation exposure also increase the risk. Males and whites are affected more commonly than females and darker-skinned individuals. Because the disease is benign, any treatment other than sun-protection measures is for cosmetic purposes only.

Look For

Multiple open comedones (pinpoint to larger blackheads) at the temples and cheeks appearing on a background of weathered-appearing skin (Figs. 4-177–4-180). There may be yellowish nodules of elastotic material present as well.

Occasionally, the lateral neck, forearms, and behind the ears are affected.

Diagnostic Pearls

- Look for other evidence of sun damage, such as solar lentigines, actinic keratoses, and dyspigmentation. Take a careful history of any outdoor occupations or recreational activities.

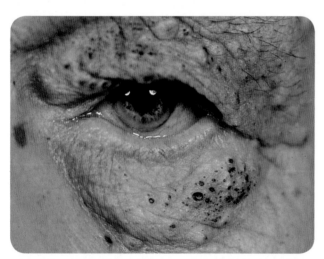

Figure 4-177 Periorbital large, open comedones (blackheads) and papules characterize FRD.

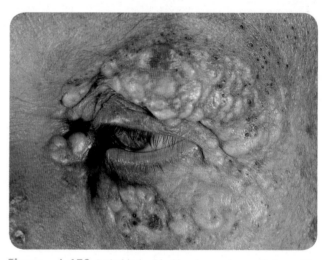

Figure 4-178 Periorbital blackheads and xanthelasma-like proliferations.

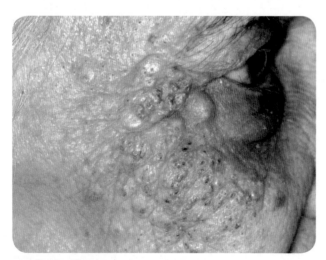

Figure 4-179 Comedones and papules with large variation in size in this patient with FRD.

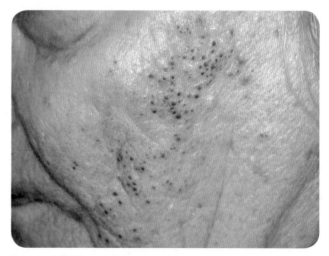

Figure 4-180 Favre-Racouchot lesions extending to the cheeks.

Differential Diagnosis and Pitfalls

- Colloid milia
- Milia
- Acne vulgaris
- Syringomas
- Chloracne
- Sebaceous hyperplasia
- Other adnexal tumors such as trichoepitheliomas and apocrine hidrocystomas
- In alkaptonuria, there may be blue or black pigmentation, but it does not present with the other signs of sun exposure seen in FRD.
- Cutis rhomboidalis nuchae

✓ Best Tests

- This is a clinical diagnosis. Biopsy is not necessary.

▲▲ Management Pearls

- The cobblestone appearance of skin is generally poorly responsive to treatment; however, consider tretinoin creams in 0.025%, 0.05%, or 0.1% strengths for the treatment of the comedones. Tazarotene gel (0.05%) has also been shown to be efficacious. Apply nightly for months. It is generally best to begin therapy at a concentration of .025% and attempt to increase the concentration over time (every 2 to 3 months) as the patient tolerates.

The patient should be made aware that it is a long course of treatment requiring months to years to work well.

Therapy

Topical retinoids as described above.

Simple office-based procedures include the manual expression of comedones with a comedone extractor or small curette while holding the skin taut. Retinoid use may facilitate the process.

Dermabrasion, chemical peels, and laser treatments have been used with variable results.

Implement preventive measures and risk factor modification via sun avoidance/protection with SPF 30 sunscreen and protective clothing. Advise smoking cessation.

Suggested Readings

Kaya TI, Tursen U, Yazici AC, et al. A simple open comedone extraction technique for Favre-Racouchot disease. *Photodermatol Photoimmunol Photomed.* 2005 Oct;21(5):275–277.

Keough GC, Laws RA, Elston DM. Favre-Racouchot syndrome: A case for smokers' comedones. *Arch Dermatol.* 1997 Jun;133(6):796–797.

Lewis KG, Bercovitch L, Dill SW, et al. Acquired disorders of elastic tissue: Part I. Increased elastic tissue and solar elastotic syndromes. *J Am Acad Dermatol.* 2004 Jul;51(1):1–21; quiz 22–24.

Patterson WM, Fox MD, Schwartz RA. Favre-Racouchot disease. *Int J Dermatol.* 2004 Mar;43(3):167–169.

Rallis E, Karanikola E, Verros C. Successful treatment of Favre-Racouchot disease with 0.05% tazarotene gel. *Arch Dermatol.* 2007 Jun;143(6):810–812.

Folliculitis

Diagnosis Synopsis

Folliculitis broadly refers to the inflammation of the pilosebaceous unit, clinically presenting as folliculocentric papules and pustules. There are many agents that can cause follicular inflammation. These include infectious pathogens (directly invading follicles), physical irritation, systemic drugs, and underlying disease states. This synopsis will primarily deal with bacterial folliculitis, namely that caused by *Staphylococcus*. Irritant- and drug-induced folliculitis will also briefly be discussed. Folliculitis caused by *Malassezia Pseudomonas* and underlying disease states (e.g., eosinophilic folliculitis and acne vulgaris) are unique cases of folliculitis and are considered separately.

One of the most common causes of folliculitis is infection with staphylococcal bacteria. Both methicillin-sensitive *Staphylococcus aureus* (MSSA) and methicillin-resistant *S. aureus* (MRSA) can cause folliculitis, which may be associated with the nasal carriage of the organism. Although MRSA skin infections most commonly present as erythematous abscesses and/or cellulitis, MRSA folliculitis is becoming increasingly prevalent. MRSA folliculitis may have a unique presentation. Whereas MSSA folliculitis is usually localized to the axillae, bearded area, buttocks, and extremities, MRSA folliculitis has been reported to present in the periumbilical area, chest, flank, and scrotum. Although the majority of cases of folliculitis are caused by staphylococcal bacteria, in many instances, bacterial cultures of pustules show no organisms. Those at increased risk of developing folliculitis include immunocompromised patients, individuals with nasal *Staphylococcus* carriage, hyperhidrosis, skin injury, and preexisting dermatitis.

Candida may cause folliculitis in diabetics, the immunocompromised, and those on antibiotics. Patients on chronic antibiotic therapy (e.g., taking a tetracycline for acne vulgaris) are at increased risk of developing Gram-negative folliculitis, which can have a more chronic and unremitting course. Gram-negative organisms that commonly cause folliculitis in this setting are *Klebsiella* species, *Escherichia coli*, *Enterobacter* species, and *Proteus* species. The eosinophilic folliculitis found in HIV-infected patients is not associated with an identified organism at present. Herpes simplex virus type 1 (HSV-1) and varicella-zoster virus (VZV) can primarily infect the hair follicle, inducing a folliculitis. These infections most commonly present as groups of infected follicles localized to the face and scalp that are resistant to conventional therapy and PCR-positive for HSV or VZV.

Not all cases of folliculitis are caused by infectious organisms. Physical irritation due to perspiration, friction, occlusion, or shaving may be associated with sterile folliculitis. This typically presents as pustules in sites of friction and irritation, such as areas that are shaved, in skin folds, or at places where clothing tends to rub (e.g., scalp, beard, buttocks, and extremities). Chemical irritants may cause a sterile folliculitis, particularly mineral oil and tar-based products.

Systemic medications have been shown to induce a sterile folliculitis. Corticosteroids, ACTH, androgens, iodides, bromides, lithium, isoniazid, and anticonvulsants have all been shown to induce a folliculitis-like cutaneous eruption. In addition, a folliculocentric papulopustular dermatitis is observed in almost all (approx. 90%) patients taking epidermal growth factor receptor inhibitors (e.g., erlotinib and cetuximab).

Regardless of the causative agent, individual lesions of folliculitis may be asymptomatic, painful, or pruritic. Lesions often heal spontaneously without scarring, although deep infection and excoriation may lead to scars. Folliculitis occurs in either sex as well as all ethnicities and age groups.

Immunocompromised Patient Considerations

Overall, folliculitis is more common in immunocompromised patients. Pruritic papular eruption of HIV, eosinophilic folliculitis, and *Pityrosporum* folliculitis are observed with relatively high frequency with HIV infection. In addition, uncommon causes of infectious folliculitis are seen in patients with HIV/AIDS. *Acinetobacter baumannii*, cryptococcosis, *Clostridium perfringens*, HSV, and VZV have all been reported in this population. *Pityrosporum* folliculitis has been reported in both solid organ and bone marrow transplant recipients.

Look For

Small erythematous papules and pustules pierced by a central hair (Figs. 4-181–4-184). They may be of varying size and will be in a follicular configuration. Deeper lesions are more nodular and may be fluctuant. Such lesions are frequently tender and may erupt to form crusts on the surface of the skin.

Sites of predilection include the face, scalp, axillae, thighs, and inguinal area. MRSA folliculitis can present in an atypical distribution such as the periumbilical area, chest, flank, and scrotum.

Dark Skin Considerations

In darker-skinned patients, the erythematous ("itis") portion of the lesions may be masked. Often there are hyperpigmented brown papules.

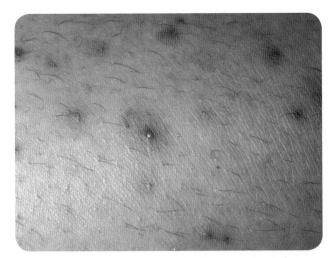

Figure 4-181 Lesions with central pustules and a rim of erythema characterize folliculitis.

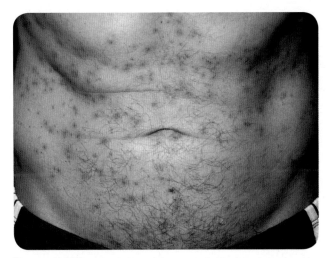

Figure 4-182 Increased sweating or occlusion in a hairy location may precipitate folliculitis.

Diagnostic Pearls

- Folliculitis occurs more frequently among people (especially males) who exercise daily. Shaving, occlusion, and chronic rubbing may incite or exacerbate the disease.
- Gram-negative folliculitis is more common among individuals taking long-term antibiotics (such as for the treatment of acne).

Immunocompromised Patient Considerations

HIV-infected patients pose a particular challenge, as differentiating between the infectious causes and an eosinophilic folliculitis may be difficult, and they may coexist.

Differential Diagnosis and Pitfalls

Consider alternative causes and organisms such as

- *Pseudomonas* folliculitis (hot tub folliculitis)
- *Pityrosporum* folliculitis
- *Demodex*
- Tinea barbae
- Folliculitis due to HSV, VZV, or molluscum contagiosum
- Pseudofolliculitis barbae
- Acne keloidalis nuchae
- Acute generalized exanthematous pustulosis
- Eosinophilic folliculitis
- Keratosis pilaris
- Perforating diseases
- Flat warts
- Milia

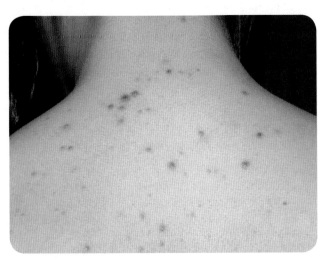

Figure 4-183 *Pityrosporum* folliculitis is more persistent than bacterial folliculitis and often requires a biopsy for diagnosis.

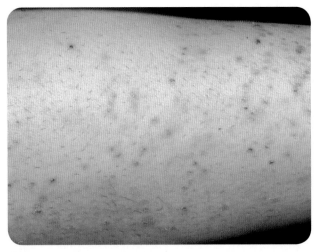

Figure 4-184 Multiple inflamed lesions with a characteristic follicular distribution.

- Perioral dermatitis
- Acne
- Rosacea
- Fox-Fordyce disease
- Candidiasis
- Seabather's eruption
- Insect bites
- Miliaria rubra

Immunocompromised Patient Differential Diagnosis

- Eosinophilic folliculitis of HIV
- Pruritic papular eruption of HIV
- *Pityrosporum* folliculitis
- *Demodex* folliculitis

✓ Best Tests

- Perform a Gram stain culture of lesions, especially in severe or recalcitrant cases. Incise the pustule with a no. 15 blade or small gauge needle to express the contents, if needed. Sensitivities should be performed on any *S. aureus* isolates to determine antibiotic resistance. Perform a KOH preparation if yeast or fungi is likely.
- Patients with recurrent infections should have their anterior nares swabbed to assess for colonization.
- Skin biopsy may be needed in cases that prove unresponsive to therapy.
- Any further workup will be dictated by the clinical scenario. Patients suspected of being immunosuppressed or having underlying systemic disease merit additional tests, such as a CBC, HIV testing, etc.

▲▲▲ Management Pearls

- Treatment directed at staphylococcal infection or avoidance of external irritants may be empiric initially, based on history and exam. Changing the patient's skin routine is often beneficial. Identify etiologic habits such as shaving. Often, patients are shaving in the wrong direction, creating irritation and breakdown of normal skin defense. Antibacterial soaps are sometimes helpful.
- Given the prevalence of MRSA, maintain a high index of suspicion for this diagnosis, and make the initial choice of any empiric antibiotic therapy accordingly. It is helpful to be aware of patterns of antimicrobial resistance within your community.
- The eradication of MRSA nasal carriage may be accomplished with an application of 2% mupirocin cream to the nares. The combination of rifampin plus trimethoprim-sulfamethoxazole (TMP-SMX) has also been shown to eradicate MRSA colonization.

Precautions: Standard and Contact. (Isolate patient, wear gloves and a gown, limit patient transport, and avoid sharing patient-care equipment.)

Immunocompromised Patient Considerations

Given the vast differential diagnosis of folliculitis in immunocompromised patients and the fact that this population has a predisposition to develop rare forms of infectious folliculitis, a biopsy of skin for histochemical analysis as well as culture is the rule. Although empiric therapy can be initiated at presentation for the most likely cause(s), skin pathology and biopsy cultures should guide definitive therapy.

Therapy

Mild cases of folliculitis may resolve spontaneously. Recommend the patient to use an antibacterial soap.

Possible topical regimens include mupirocin ointment three times daily to affected areas; alternatively, erythromycin solution 2%, clindamycin solution 2%, or Benzamycin cream twice daily to affected areas may be tried.

If there is no response to topical therapy after approximately 1 month or for widespread or deep-seated cases, use an anti-staphylococcal oral antibiotic:

- Dicloxacillin or cephalexin 500 mg p.o. four times daily for 10 to 14 days
- Azithromycin (Z-Pak) 500 mg the first day, then 250 mg daily for 5 days is an alternative

Standard cephalosporins and penicillins are of no benefit in treating MRSA. In recent studies, CA-MRSA has demonstrated a high degree of susceptibility to TMP-SMX and rifampin (100%), clindamycin (95%), and tetracycline (92%). Inducible resistance to clindamycin should be excluded by performing a D-zone disk-diffusion test.

Possible antibiotic regimens for MRSA include:

- Clindamycin 300 to 450 mg p.o. three times daily, TMP-SMX 1 to 2 double strength tabs p.o. twice daily, rifampin 300 mg p.o. twice daily

Pseudomonas may resolve spontaneously or with oral ciprofloxacin. *Pityrosporum* folliculitis responds to systemic antifungals and herpetic folliculitis to oral antivirals.

Suggested Readings

Böni R, Nehrhoff B. Treatment of Gram-negative folliculitis in patients with acne. *Am J Clin Dermatol.* 2003;4(4):273–276.

Budavari JM, Grayson W. Papular follicular eruptions in human immunodeficiency virus-positive patients in South Africa. *Int J Dermatol.* 2007 Jul;46(7):706–710.

Cohen PR. Community-acquired methicillin-resistant Staphylococcus aureus skin infection presenting as a periumbilical folliculitis. *Cutis.* 2006 Apr;77(4):229–232.

Fearfield LA, Rowe A, Francis N, et al. Itchy folliculitis and human immunodeficiency virus infection: Clinicopathological and immunological features, pathogenesis and treatment. *Br J Dermatol.* 1999 Jul;141(1):3–11.

Gisby J, Bryant J. Efficacy of a new cream formulation of mupirocin: Comparison with oral and topical agents in experimental skin infections. *Antimicrob Agents Chemother.* 2000 Feb;44(2):255–260.

Luelmo-Aguilar J, Santandreu MS. Folliculitis: Recognition and management. *Am J Clin Dermatol.* 2004;5(5):301–310.

Morrison VA, Weisdorf DJ. The spectrum of Malassezia infections in the bone marrow transplant population. *Bone Marrow Transplant.* 2000 Sep;26(6):645–648.

Weinberg JM, Turiansky GW, James WD. Viral folliculitis. *AIDS Patient Care STDS.* 1999 Sep;13(9):513–516.

Folliculitis, *Pseudomonas* (Hot Tub Folliculitis)

Diagnosis Synopsis

Pseudomonas folliculitis, or hot tub folliculitis, is a subset of folliculitis (an inflammation of the hair follicle) that requires special consideration. It is an infection of hair follicles with *Pseudomonas* bacteria. Outbreaks occur in people after bathing in a contaminated spa, swimming pool, or hot tub. It is also associated with the use of contaminated loofah sponges (that remain constantly wet in the shower) and contaminated water in the workplace. It also can be seen with higher incidence in patients on long-term antibiotic therapy for acne vulgaris.

Clinically, *Pseudomonas* folliculitis is characterized by tender or pruritic folliculocentric papules preferentially localized to the trunk, buttocks, and extremities. Symptoms typically develop within 1 to 4 days after exposure to the contaminated water source. Infection can be associated with mild fever, malaise, lymphadenopathy, and leukocytosis. The cutaneous eruption usually fades within 7 to 14 days without therapy.

Water sources contaminated with *Pseudomonas* are also associated with outbreaks of painful plantar nodules termed the "*Pseudomonas* hot-foot syndrome." These patients may or may not have a concomitant folliculitis.

Immunocompromised Patient Considerations

Pseudomonas folliculitis has been shown to evolve into ecthyma gangrenosum in immunocompromised patients. Ecthyma gangrenosum is a serious cutaneous manifestation of disseminated *Pseudomonas* infection, presenting as deep pustules, necrotic papules and plaques, and/or hemorrhagic bullae. It requires prompt antibacterial therapy.

Look For

Follicular, erythematous papules and pustules that may have crusts (Figs. 4-185–4-188). Pustules can be small with negligible pus, or large. Bright-red papules may also be present. Lesions are typically found in the trunk/bathing suit area and in intertriginous areas.

Pseudomonas folliculitis spares the palms, soles, and face.

Diagnostic Pearls

- In *Pseudomonas* folliculitis, there is more peripheral redness than the usual case of folliculitis.
- Breast tenderness is an occasional associated symptom in both men and women, as glands in the nipple may become infected.

?? Differential Diagnosis and Pitfalls

- Staphylococcal folliculitis
- *Pityrosporum* folliculitis
- *Demodex*
- Tinea barbae
- Folliculitis due to herpes simplex virus, varicella-zoster virus, or molluscum contagiosum
- Pseudofolliculitis barbae
- Acne keloidalis nuchae
- Acute generalized exanthematous pustulosis
- Eosinophilic folliculitis
- Keratosis pilaris
- Perforating diseases

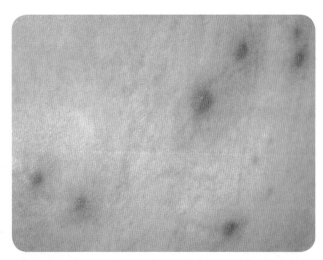

Figure 4-185 *Pseudomonas* folliculitis with a tiny pustule and large rim of erythema.

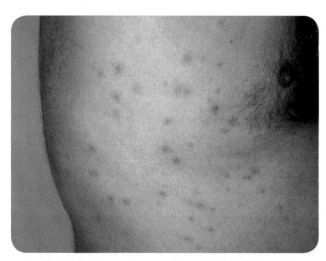

Figure 4-186 *Pseudomonas* folliculitis with multiple lesions in the same stage of development.

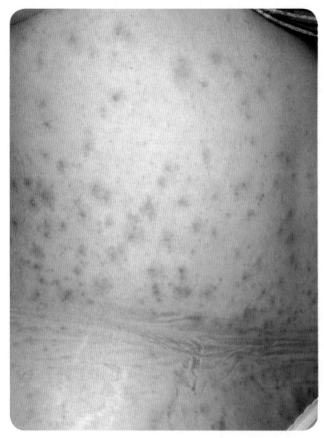

Figure 4-187 *Pseudomonas* folliculitis with multiple large lesions.

- Flat warts
- Milia
- Perioral dermatitis
- Acne
- Rosacea
- Fox-Fordyce disease
- Candidiasis
- Seabather's eruption
- Insect bites
- Miliaria rubra

Immunocompromised Patient Differential Diagnosis

- Eosinophilic folliculitis of HIV
- Pruritic papular eruption of HIV
- *Pityrosporum* folliculitis

✓ Best Tests

- Gram stain and culture of pustular lesions. It may be useful to perform cultures on any potential source of the infection (i.e., swimming pool water), if feasible.
- A biopsy is rarely required to make the diagnosis.

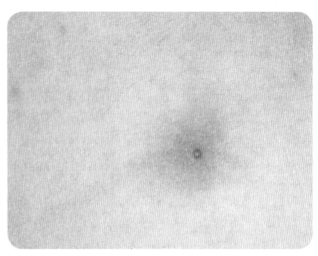

Figure 4-188 *Pseudomonas* folliculitis with a central pustule and large rim of erythema.

▲▲ Management Pearls

- The disease is self-limited. In severe symptomatic cases, ciprofloxacin can shorten the course of illness.
- The CDC recommends a free chlorine concentration of 1 to 3 mg/L and a pH of 7.2 to 7.8 for public spas and hot tubs.
- Sponges and loofahs should be thoroughly dried between uses.

Immunocompromised Patient Considerations

Prompt systemic anti-pseudomonal antibiotic therapy should be initiated in immunocompromised hosts.

Therapy

Ciprofloxacin 500 mg twice daily for 10 days should be prescribed for those who are immunosuppressed and patients with mastitis or persistent disease.

Topical therapies such as povidone-iodine, 1% acetic acid soaks, or gentamicin 0.1% cream may be helpful.

Suggested Readings

Berger RS, Seifert MR. Whirlpool folliculitis: A review of its cause, treatment, and prevention. *Cutis*. 1990 Feb;45(2):97–98.

Böni R, Nehrhoff B. Treatment of Gram-negative folliculitis in patients with acne. *Am J Clin Dermatol*. 2003;4(4):273–276.

Centers for Disease Control and Prevention (CDC). *Pseudomonas* dermatitis/folliculitis associated with pools and hot tubs—Colorado and Maine, 1999–2000. *MMWR Morb Mortal Wkly Rep*. 2000 Dec;49(48): 1087–1091.

El Baze P, Thyss A, Caldani C, et al. *Pseudomonas aeruginosa* O-11 folliculitis. Development into ecthyma gangrenosum in immunosuppressed patients. *Arch Dermatol*. 1985 Jul;121(7):873–876.

Fiorillo L, Zucker M, Sawyer D, et al. The *pseudomonas* hot-foot syndrome. *N Engl J Med*. 2001 Aug;345(5):335–338.

Gregory DW, Schaffner W. *Pseudomonas* infections associated with hot tubs and other environments. *Infect Dis Clin North Am*. 1987 Sep;1(3): 635–648.

Yu Y, Cheng AS, Wang L, et al. Hot tub folliculitis or hot hand-foot syndrome caused by *Pseudomonas aeruginosa*. *J Am Acad Dermatol*. 2007 Oct;57(4):596–600.

Zichichi L, Asta G, Noto G. *Pseudomonas aeruginosa* folliculitis after shower/bath exposure. *Int J Dermatol*. 2000 Apr;39(4):270–273.

Furunculosis

Diagnosis Synopsis

Furuncles (boils) are cutaneous abscesses associated with hair follicles. Carbuncles are a continuous collection of furuncles. By definition, furuncles are of infectious etiology, with the most common causative agent being *Staphylococcus aureus* (either methicillin-sensitive [MSSA] or methicillin-resistant [MRSA]). The infecting strain of *Staphylococcus* is usually colonizing the nares, umbilicus, or perineum. It most commonly affects adolescents and young adults and is rarely seen in childhood. Predisposing factors include *Staphylococcus* carriage, friction, malnutrition, poor hygiene, possibly diabetes, hyper-IgE syndrome, and HIV.

Clinically, lesions are painful (particularly when in the nose or ear canal). They often appear in crops, sometimes with fever. Patients may describe purulent drainage. They usually occur on the face, neck, axillae, buttocks, thighs, and perineum. When on the central face, cavernous sinus thrombosis is a rare complication. Lesions may continue for months to years, but individual lesions often heal spontaneously within 2 to 3 weeks.

Furuncles are one of the most frequent manifestations of cutaneous infection with MRSA. In the past, MRSA infection was thought to be primarily a nosocomial pathogen; however, community-acquired MRSA (CA-MRSA) is well established and quickly increasing in prevalence. It has been shown that the majority of purulent skin and soft tissue infections presenting to emergency rooms across the United States are caused by CA-MRSA.

Immunocompromised Patient Considerations

Immunocompromised patients have a significantly increased risk of developing both MSSA and MRSA furunculosis. HIV-infected patients are approximately 20 times more likely to develop skin and soft tissues infections caused by MRSA. Risk factors for MRSA infection in this population are low current CD4 cell count, recent beta-lactam antibiotic use, and high-risk sexual activity.

Look For

Perifollicular papule, pustule, or nodule with erythema (Figs. 4-189–4-192). Lesions may be single or multiple. Most common locations are the face, neck, arms, hands, buttocks, and anogenital region. The legs may be affected, particularly in women who shave their legs.

Diagnostic Pearls

- Furuncles caused by CA-MRSA can be necrotic and have been mistaken for spider bites.

Immunocompromised Patient Considerations

- In HIV disease, furuncles may coalesce into large plaques or progress to cellulitis with bacteremia.

Differential Diagnosis and Pitfalls

- Hidradenitis suppurativa—usually involves the axillae, groin, and submammary areas and has concomitant comedones
- Acne cysts—usually multiple on the upper trunk, neck, and face
- Halogenoderma
- Myiasis—usually not chronic and recurrent and only a single or few in number

Best Tests

- Skin culture and Gram stain—culture of nares, umbilicus, and perineum for carriage.
- Sensitivities should always be performed on any *S. aureus* isolates to determine antibiotic resistance.

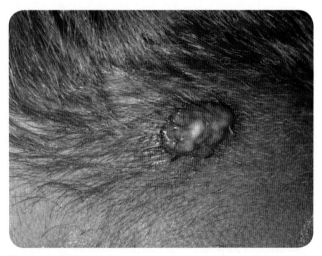

Figure 4-189 Deep furuncles are often at the base of the scalp.

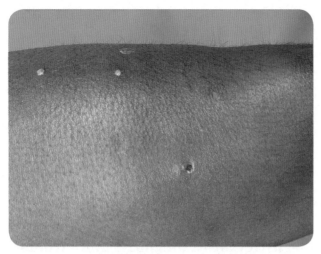

Figure 4-190 Furunculosis with an eroded papule with surrounding erythema, swelling, and opaque pustules.

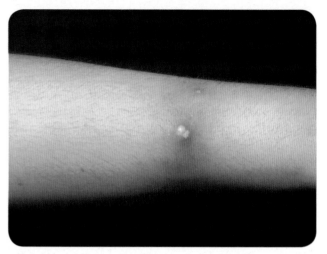

Figure 4-191 Groups of furuncles with deep erythema.

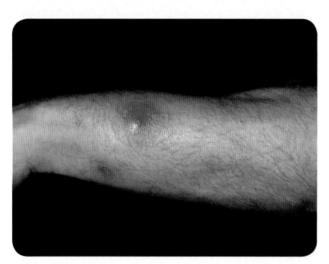

Figure 4-192 Furuncles are often warm and very tender.

▲▲ Management Pearls

- The mainstay of effective therapy is early and adequate drainage.
- If nasal or perineal carriage is documented, attempt to eradicate with 2% mupirocin ointment intranasal for 5 days and daily chlorhexidine for bathing and shampooing.
- Oral rifampin (300 mg twice daily for 7 to 10 days) or low-dose clindamycin (150 mg daily for 3 months) may be helpful in the temporary elimination of carriage (which is rarely achievable long term).
- Consider checking for carriage in family members.
- Given the prevalence of MRSA, maintain a high index of suspicion for this diagnosis, and make the initial choice of empiric antibiotic therapy accordingly. It is helpful to be aware of patterns of antimicrobial resistance within your community. The combination of rifampin plus

trimethoprim-sulfamethoxazole (TMP-SMX) has been shown to eradicate MRSA colonization.

Precautions: Standard and Contact. (Isolate patient, wear gloves and a gown, limit patient transport, and avoid sharing patient-care equipment.)

Therapy

If possible, adequate surgical drainage is the most effective therapy. Warm compresses and antibacterial washes with either chlorhexidine or triclosan can be utilized if surgery is not possible.

Systemic antibiotic therapy should be reserved for multiple, recurrent nose and ear canal lesions and lesions not responding to local care. Studies have shown that systemic antibiotic therapy is not necessary if adequate surgical drainage is achieved.

Suggested initial antibiotic regimens for MSSA include

- Dicloxacillin or cephalexin 500 mg p.o. four times daily for 10 to 14 days.
- Patients should be assessed frequently to determine appropriate response to therapy.

Standard cephalosporins and penicillins are of no benefit in treating MRSA. In recent studies, CA-MRSA has demonstrated a high degree of susceptibility to TMP-SMX and rifampin (100%), clindamycin (95%), and tetracycline (92%). Inducible resistance to clindamycin should be excluded by performing a D-zone disk-diffusion test on any isolates.

Possible antibiotic regimens for MRSA include the following:

- TMP-SMX 1 to 2 double strength tabs p.o. twice daily
- Clindamycin 300 to 450 mg four times daily
- Doxycycline 100 mg twice daily

Suggested Readings

Bernard P. Management of common bacterial infections of the skin. *Curr Opin Infect Dis*. 2008 Apr;21(2):122–128.

Crum-Cianflone NF, Burgi AA, Hale BR. Increasing rates of community-acquired methicillin-resistant Staphylococcus aureus infections among HIV-infected persons. *Int J STD AIDS*. 2007 Aug;18(8):521–526.

Elston DM. Community-acquired methicillin-resistant *Staphylococcus aureus*. *J Am Acad Dermatol*. 2007 Jan;56(1):1–16; quiz 17–20.

Gisby J, Bryant J. Efficacy of a new cream formulation of mupirocin: Comparison with oral and topical agents in experimental skin infections. *Antimicrob Agents Chemother*. 2000 Feb;44(2):255–260.

Gosbell IB. Epidemiology, clinical features and management of infections due to community methicillin-resistant *Staphylococcus aureus* (cMRSA). *Intern Med J*. 2005 Dec;35(Suppl. 2):S120–S135.

Rajendran PM, Young D, Maurer T, et al. Randomized, double-blind, placebo-controlled trial of cephalexin for treatment of uncomplicated skin abscesses in a population at risk for community-acquired methicillin-resistant *Staphylococcus aureus* infection. *Antimicrob Agents Chemother*. 2007 Nov;51(11):4044–4048.

Zetola N, Francis JS, Nuermberger EL, et al. Community-acquired meticillin-resistant *Staphylococcus aureus:* an emerging threat. *Lancet Infect Dis*. 2005 May;5(5):275–286.

Granuloma Annulare

Diagnosis Synopsis

Granuloma annulare is a benign granulomatous inflammatory disorder of the dermis or subcutis. Its cause is unknown. Small dermal papules may present in isolation or coalesce to form smooth annular plaques, often on extremities. Lesions are typically asymptomatic or only mildly pruritic, but the appearance may cause patients distress. The disease is more common in women (female-to-male ratio of 2:1), and two-thirds of patients are aged younger than 30. The disease usually resolves spontaneously with no adverse sequelae, though some cases prove to be persistent or recurrent.

A small amount of evidence points to granuloma annulare as being associated with certain systemic diseases, such as thyroid disease, diabetes mellitus, malignancy, and infections. "Actinic granuloma" presents with similar lesions but is regarded by many as a separate pathologic entity.

There are three principal variants of granuloma annulare: localized (75% of cases), disseminated (or generalized), and subcutaneous. A fourth variant—perforating granuloma annulare—refers to rare lesions that demonstrate histologic evidence of the transepidermal extrusion of degraded collagen.

Look For

Annular or arcuate, nonscaly, reddish-brown plaques or papules (Figs. 4-193 and 4-194). Plaque centers are often hypopigmented relative to the edges. They are commonly localized on the fingers, hands, elbows, dorsal feet, or ankles.

Patients with generalized or disseminated granuloma annulare typically have numerous smaller lesions (at least 10) in a widespread distribution that may include extremities, the trunk, and the neck (Fig. 4-195).

Subcutaneous granuloma annulare presents with a firm, skin-colored to slightly erythematous nodule, usually on the lower extremities (Fig. 4-196). It is more common in young children.

The lesions of perforating granuloma annulare also present as grouped 1 to 4 mm papules that may form annular plaques, but in some patients, these papules evolve into vesicular or pustular lesions that may umbilicate, ulcerate, or crust, leaving behind a scar as they heal.

Dark Skin Considerations

In dark skin, lesions can appear pigmented, skin-colored, grayish, hypopigmented, and noninflammatory.

Diagnostic Pearls

• The ring-shaped or arc-like lesions do not scale. The absence of scale or surface change is a crucial finding in differentiating granuloma annulare from other annular eruptions such as tinea corporis. When stretched, larger lesions show individual papules in a ring, and smaller annular lesions have a small central dell, or depression.

Differential Diagnosis and Pitfalls

• Granuloma annulare is often mistaken for dermatophyte infection (tinea corporis, or "ringworm"). The presence of definite scales in dermatophyte infection should allow the distinction.
• Sarcoidosis
• Erythema annulare centrifugum

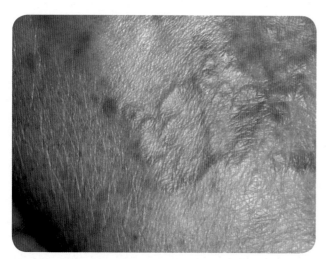

Figure 4-193 Discrete and confluent red papules and scales with a ringlike border of smaller papules characterize granuloma annulare.

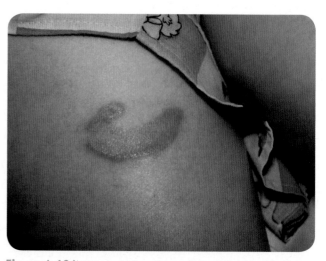

Figure 4-194 Arcuate lesion of granuloma annulare with discrete papules on the outer border.

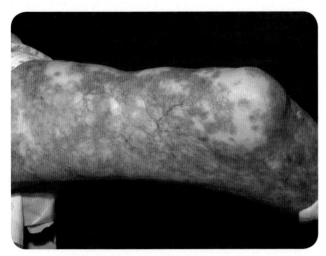

Figure 4-195 Disseminated granuloma annulare with multiple plaques has been weakly associated with diabetes.

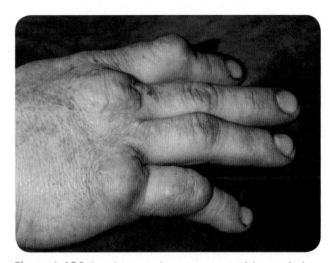

Figure 4-196 Granuloma annulare may present solely as a single or as few subcutaneous nodules.

- Lichen planus (especially the annular variant)—usually pruritic
- Leprosy—anesthetic lesions in endemic countries
- Erythema elevatum diutinum—over extensors, pruritic
- Actinic granuloma
- Necrobiosis lipoidica—atrophic plaques
- Perforating collagenosis
- Elastosis perforans serpiginosa
- Erythema migrans (Lyme disease)—slow growing, more erythematous
- Erythema gyratum repens
- Sweet syndrome
- Subacute cutaneous lupus erythematosus
- Annular elastolytic giant cell granuloma
- Pseudolymphoma
- Mycosis fungoides

✔ Best Tests

- Skin biopsy will confirm the diagnosis, but a clinical diagnosis is often made by lesional morphology and distribution.

▲▲ Management Pearls

- There are no clear-cut successful therapies, and large, well-designed trials are lacking.
- The plaques often resolve spontaneously, especially in localized disease; generalized granuloma annulare may prove more persistent.
- Patient reassurance and education about the benign nature of this disease is essential. Share images of the diagnosis with your patient to reinforce that this is a common process.

Therapy

For localized disease, some treatment success has been achieved with cryotherapy, topical corticosteroids with or without occlusion, topical calcineurin inhibitors, and careful use of intralesional corticosteroids (triamcinolone 3 to 5 mg/cc).

Note: Skin atrophy is a potential side effect with topical or intralesional steroids.

High-potency topical corticosteroids (classes 1 and 2)

- Clobetasol cream or ointment—apply twice daily
- Fluocinonide cream or ointment—apply twice daily
- Desoximetasone cream or ointment—apply twice daily
- Halcinonide cream or ointment—apply twice daily
- Amcinonide ointment—apply twice daily

Mid-potency topical corticosteroids (classes 3 and 4)

- Triamcinolone cream or ointment—apply twice daily
- Mometasone cream or ointment—apply twice daily
- Fluocinolone ointment or cream—apply twice daily

Topical Calcineurin Inhibitors

- Tacrolimus ointment 0.1%—apply twice daily
- Pimecrolimus cream 1%—apply twice daily

For generalized disease, psoralens plus UVA (PUVA), isotretinoin, dapsone, and hydroxychloroquine have been used:

- Isotretinoin—40 mg p.o. daily for 3 months
- Dapsone—100 mg p.o. daily for 8 weeks
- Hydroxychloroquine—200 mg p.o. twice daily for 3 months

Caution: Systemic therapies require careful patient screening and monitoring.

Suggested Readings

Blume-Peytavi U, Zouboulis CC, Jacobi H, et al. Successful outcome of cryosurgery in patients with granuloma annulare. *Br J Dermatol.* 1994 Apr;130(4):494–497.

Howard A, White CR. Non-infectious granulomas. In: Bolognia JL, Jorizzo JL, Rapini RP, eds. *Dermatology.* 2nd Ed. St. Louis, MO: Mosby; 2008: 1426–1429.

Kim YJ, Kang HY, Lee ES, et al. Successful treatment of granuloma annulare with topical 5-aminolaevulinic acid photodynamic therapy. *J Dermatol.* 2006 Sep;33(9):642–643.

Looney M, Smith KM. Isotretinoin in the treatment of granuloma annulare. *Ann Pharmacother.* 2004 Mar;38(3):494–497.

Muhlbauer JE. Granuloma annulare. *J Am Acad Dermatol.* 1980 Sep;3(3): 217–230.

Prendiville JS. Granuloma Annulare. In: Fitzpatrick TB, Wolff K, eds. *Fitzpatrick's Dermatology in General Medicine.* 7th Ed. New York, NY: McGraw-Hill; 2008:369–373.

Smith MD, Downie JB, DiCostanzo D. Granuloma annulare. *Int J Dermatol.* 1997 May;36(5):326–333.

Keratosis Pilaris

▪▪ Diagnosis Synopsis

Keratosis pilaris is an exceedingly common benign skin disorder of the follicular orifice. It is commonly referred to as "gooseflesh." It is characterized by small follicular papules on the extensor lateral extremities due to the retention of keratin at the follicular opening. It is frequently seen in adolescents and young adults, rarely in the elderly. Women are affected slightly more often than men. Dry weather often worsens the condition. Frequently, there is a family history of the condition. Autosomal dominant inheritance with variable penetrance has been described. Keratosis pilaris tends to be refractory to most treatments with complete cure highly unlikely; however, the condition tends to improve with age.

Keratosis pilaris most often occurs as described above but does have three main clinical variants: keratosis pilaris atrophicans faciei, atrophoderma vermiculatum, and keratosis follicularis spinulosa decalvans. All of these entities have hyperkeratotic follicular papules with varying degrees of atrophy. Keratosis pilaris atrophicans faciei is characterized by erythematous hyperkeratotic papules distributed on the lateral third of the eyebrows in young children. Atrophoderma vermiculatum (also termed honeycomb atrophy) is characterized by atrophic pits in a reticulate or worm-eaten array localized to the face of older children. Keratosis follicularis spinulosa decalvans is a disorder characterized by widespread keratosis pilaris, scarring alopecia, and eye abnormalities.

Keratosis pilaris is seen with an increased incidence in several syndromes and disease states. These include atopic dermatitis, ichthyosis vulgaris, erythromelanosis follicularis faciei et colli (erythema, brown pigmentation, and keratosis pilaris), Lassueur-Graham-Little-Piccardi syndrome (cicatricial alopecia of the scalp, loss of pubic and axillary hairs, and keratosis pilaris), cardiofaciocutaneous syndrome, Noonan syndrome, diabetes, Down syndrome, woolly hair, and obesity.

◉ Look For

In typical cases, monomorphic, tiny, 1 to 2 mm follicular papules giving the extensor arms or thighs the appearance of gooseflesh (Figs. 4-197 and 4-198). The facial cheeks (Figs. 4-199 and 4-200) and buttocks may be involved. There may be associated perifollicular erythema in lighter-skinned individuals.

●● Diagnostic Pearls

- The symmetry of follicular papules at the arms and/or legs (most often laterally distributed) is one clue to the diagnosis.

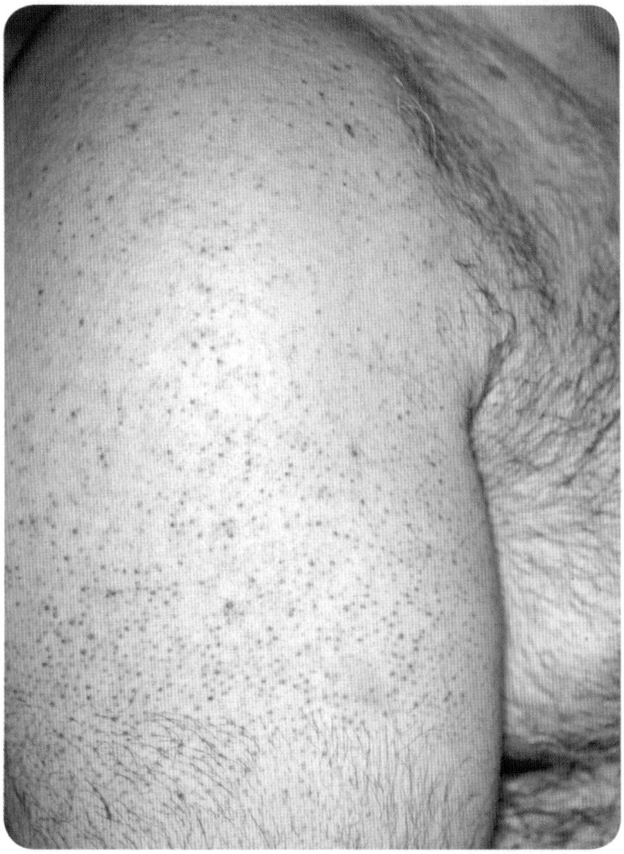

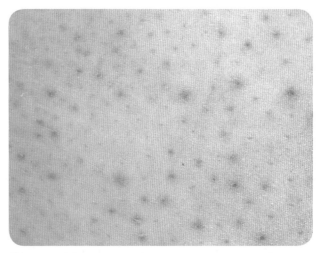

Figure 4-197 The discrete lesions of keratosis pilaris are often lifelong and lack the inflammation of folliculitis.

Figure 4-198 The lesions of keratosis pilaris have a regular pattern from their association with hair follicles.

165

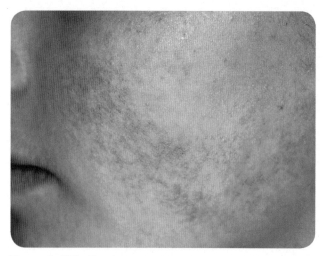

Figure 4-199 When keratosis pilaris involves the face, the lesions are frequently red, while lesions on the extremities typically are not.

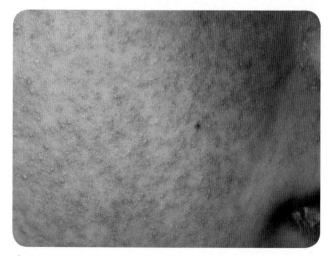

Figure 4-200 Inflamed facial lesions of keratosis pilaris in a 12 year old.

?? Differential Diagnosis and Pitfalls

- Folliculitis
- Milia
- Lichen spinulosus
- Acne vulgaris
- Atopic dermatitis
- Pityriasis rubra pilaris
- Darier disease
- Kyrle disease
- Scurvy
- Phrynoderma (vitamin A deficiency)
- Variants of keratosis pilaris (see above):
  – Keratosis pilaris atrophicans
  – Keratosis follicularis spinulosa decalvans
  – Atrophoderma vermiculatum

✓ Best Tests

- This is a clinical diagnosis, although a skin biopsy will confirm the diagnosis.

▲▲ Management Pearls

- Reinforce the need for a skin regimen by defining the process to your patient as a chronic, inherited skin condition and not a disease to be cured. Using a polyester sponge to exfoliate the skin may ameliorate symptoms.
- Preventing excessive dryness is also important. Harsh soaps (deodorant soaps) should be avoided in favor of a gentler, moisturizing soap, and emollients should be applied to damp skin after bathing.

Therapy

Keratolytics, such as lactic acid or salicylic acid 4% to 12% lotions or creams, applied twice daily may diminish the thickness of the papules.

Topical retinoids such as tazarotene 0.05% cream or tretinoin cream (0.1%) applied daily may be helpful.

If there is substantial erythema, consider brief use of topical steroids such as triamcinolone cream (0.1%) twice daily for 10 days.

Suggested Readings

Baden HP, Byers HR. Clinical findings, cutaneous pathology, and response to therapy in 21 patients with keratosis pilaris atrophicans. *Arch Dermatol.* 1994 Apr;130(4):469–475.

Chien AJ, Valentine MC, Sybert VP. Hereditary woolly hair and keratosis pilaris. *J Am Acad Dermatol.* 2006 Feb;54(2 Suppl.):S35–S39.

Gerbig AW. Treating keratosis pilaris. *J Am Acad Dermatol.* 2002 Sep;47(3):457.

Lateef A, Schwartz RA. Keratosis pilaris. *Cutis.* 1999 Apr;63(4):205–207.

Marqueling AL, Gilliam AE, Prendiville J, et al. Keratosis pilaris rubra: A common but underrecognized condition. *Arch Dermatol.* 2006 Dec;142(12):1611–1616.

Pavlović MD, Milenković T, Dinić M, et al. The prevalence of cutaneous manifestations in young patients with type 1 diabetes. *Diabetes Care.* 2007 Aug;30(8):1964–1967.

Poskitt L, Wilkinson JD. Natural history of keratosis pilaris. *Br J Dermatol.* 1994 Jun;130(6):711–713.

Yosipovitch G, DeVore A, Dawn A. Obesity and the skin: Skin physiology and skin manifestations of obesity. *J Am Acad Dermatol.* 2007 Jun;56(6): 901–916; quiz 917–920.

Lymphoma, Cutaneous T-cell (Mycosis Fungoides)

Diagnosis Synopsis

Primary cutaneous lymphomas can be divided into T-cell and B-cell lymphomas that involve the skin and various extracutaneous sites. Cutaneous T-cell lymphomas (CTCLs) account for 75% to 80% of these lymphomas and are a heterogeneous group of neoplasms that vary considerably in their clinical presentation, histology, immunophenotype, genetic landscape, and prognosis. The most recent classification scheme delineates the frequency and survival of patients with the varying types of cutaneous lymphomas and is outlined below (see Management Pearls). For physicians not specialized in treating CTCL, practical guidelines exist with respect to the diagnosis, classification, and staging of CTCL. They are outlined in Diagnostic Pearls and Management Pearls below. Most importantly, a clear diagnosis of CTCL must be made and may require large or multiple biopsies as well as specialized testing of the biopsy specimens. The typing of the CTCL and staging are important to determine the extent of disease and treatment strategy.

Mycosis fungoides (MF) and its variants, Sézary syndrome (SS), lymphomatoid papulosis (LyP), and cutaneous anaplastic large cell lymphoma (C-ALCL), make up 90% of all CTCL cases and will be discussed in this review. Note that for clinicians seeking additional information, CTCL has been the subject of several recent in-depth reviews.

Mycosis Fungoides

MF is the most common type of CTCL, accounting for 50% of all primary CTCL cases. Erythematous patches and plaques with fine scale and tumors that anatomically favor the buttocks and sun-protected areas of the trunk and limbs characterize this subtype. The etiology remains unclear. Current hypotheses propose that persistent antigenic stimulation occurs and that CD8+ T cells play a critical role. MF takes on an indolent course over years to decades. Associated features include pruritus, poikiloderma, and ulceration. Extracutaneous involvement correlates with generalized lesions and erythroderma. Neoplastic T cells demonstrate a memory T-cell phenotype: CD3+, CD4+, CD45RO+. MF staging requires CTCL physician specialists and is beyond the scope of this chapter.

Sézary Syndrome

SS is a rare type of CTCL accounting for less than 5% of all primary CTCL cases. Erythroderma, generalized lymphadenopathy, and neoplastic T-cells (Sézary cells) in the skin and peripheral lymph nodes classically characterize SS. Associated features include severe pruritus, palmoplantar hyperkeratosis, lichenification, edema, and exfoliation. The etiology remains largely unknown. Immunophenotyping demonstrating a CD4:CD8 ratio of more than 10, an absolute count of more than 1,000 Sézary cells per μL, and demonstration of T-cell clonality in the peripheral blood are diagnostic criteria.

Lymphomatoid Papulosis

LyP accounts for 15% of all primary CTCL cases and is characterized by CD30+ lymphoproliferation on histology and red to brown papules and nodules that take on a chronic, intermittently recurring, clinical course. It is unclear why some individuals experience spontaneous resolution and others have tumor progression. The etiology remains largely unknown. The papules and nodules may demonstrate crust, necrosis, and hemorrhage. LyP lesions are in varying stages of healing and can spontaneously resolve within 2 months of time. The cutaneous eruption may vary in number from few to more than 100. Lesions favor the trunk and extremities, are asymptomatic, and can vary in duration from months to decades. The prognosis is excellent.

Primary Cutaneous Anaplastic Large Cell Lymphoma

Primary C-ALCL accounts for 10% of all primary CTCL cases and is characterized by CD30+ lymphoproliferation on histology and solitary nodules or tumors that ulcerate on clinical exam. Microscopically, these cells have a characteristic morphology with anaplastic large cells with round or irregularly shaped nuclei. Similar to LyP, this condition demonstrates a chronic, intermittently recurring, clinical course. Approximately 10% of individuals will experience extracutaneous involvement. However, the prognosis remains excellent.

Look For

Mycosis Fungoides

- Erythematous patches and plaques with fine scale (usually from 2 to 20 cm) and papules and nodules that anatomically favor the buttocks and sun-protected areas of the trunk and limbs (Figs. 4-201–4-204).
- Associated features include pruritus, poikiloderma, and ulceration.

Sézary Syndrome

- Erythroderma and generalized lymphadenopathy.
- Associated features include extreme pruritus, palmoplantar hyperkeratosis, lichenification, edema, and exfoliation.

Lymphomatoid Papulosis

- Red to brown 5 to 15 mm papules and nodules on the trunk and extremities (Fig. 4-205).

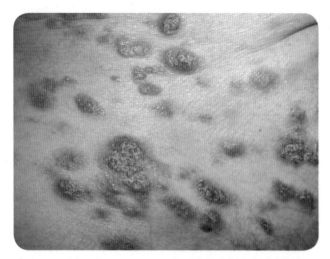

Figure 4-201 Infiltrated and scaly plaques of mycosis fungoides.

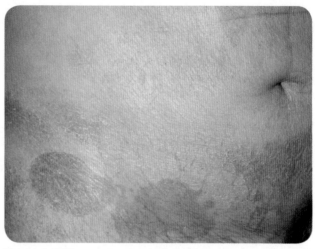

Figure 4-202 Large plaques with some scale and atrophy are characteristic of early mycosis fungoides.

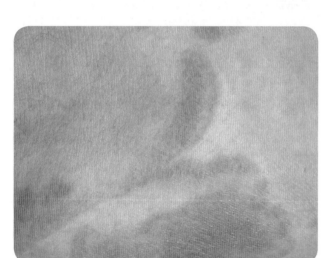

Figure 4-203 Red plaque of mycosis fungoides with an arcuate border. Such borders are common in this disease.

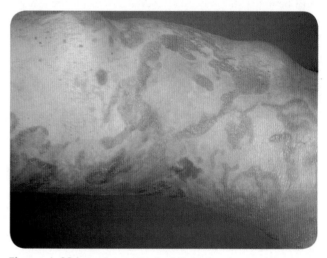

Figure 4-204 Arcuate and polycyclic lesions in complex patterns are very suggestive of mycosis fungoides.

- The papules and nodules may demonstrate crust, necrosis, and hemorrhage.
- Lesions are in varying stages of healing.

Primary Cutaneous Anaplastic Large Cell Lymphoma

- Solitary or localized nodules or plaques that ulcerate.

Diagnostic Pearls

Diagnosis

- The most important thing is to differentiate CTCL from a benign condition. This requires a strategy that incorporates clinical, histological, and immunophenotyping findings.

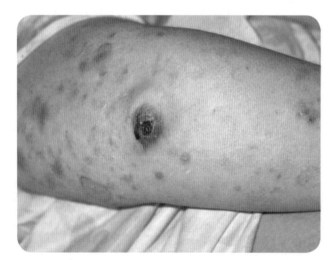

Figure 4-205 LyP with red-brown papules and an eroded ulcer with a hemorrhagic eschar.

- Ideal biopsy: 5 to 8 mm punch biopsy in previously untreated skin that is representative of the cutaneous lesions. Alternatively, an excisional biopsy can be performed.
- Because the conversion from premalignant phase to malignant phase often runs an indolent course, repeated biopsies may be necessary.
- Immunophenotyping utilizes fluorescently tagged antibodies that recognize cell surface markers. For example, the loss of CD3, CD4, or CD5 surface expression in neoplastic T cells assists in making the diagnosis.
- T-cell gene rearrangement analysis: This should be used in conjunction with the overlying clinical, histological, and immunophenotyping landscape. Note that clonal T cells can be found in benign inflammatory conditions such as lichen sclerosus, lichen planus, pityriasis lichenoides et varioliformis acuta and, hence, they support but never exclusively confirm a diagnosis of CTCL.

Classification

- Once a clinical-histological diagnosis is made, the type of T-cell lymphoma should be determined because varying CTCLs carry different prognoses and treatment strategies.
- See below for WHO-EORTC Classification.

Staging

- CT imaging, complete blood cell count with a differential, chemistry panel, peripheral blood cytology, immunophenotyping, gene rearrangement studies, and a bone marrow biopsy should all be considered when evaluating whether the T-cell lymphoma is a *primary* CTCL or a systemic T-cell lymphoma with associated secondary skin involvement. The number and types of staging studies will be largely determined by what is the suspected type of CTCL.

?? Differential Diagnosis and Pitfalls

Mycosis Fungoides

- Psoriasis—Look for erythematous silver-scaled plaques, nail oil-drop changes, and nail pitting. A family history of psoriasis is often noted. Psoriasis and CTCL are histologically different, and a biopsy will aid in the diagnosis.
- Atopic dermatitis—Patients are often aware of their atopic history, which commonly starts in childhood. Mild to moderate spongiosis is seen on histology. Look for lichenified plaques on the flexural surfaces and neck.
- Superficial fungal infections (e.g., tinea corporis)—Erythematous plaques with a raised, red scaling border. Central clearing is more common in tinea corporis. Check KOH.

- Drug eruption—Drug eruptions often present with urticarial, exanthematous, or vesicular/bullous lesions. Systemic symptoms include fever, lymphadenopathy, and facial edema. Eosinophilia on CBC and histology are often seen (but not an invariable finding). Look for nonsteroidal anti-inflammatory drugs (NSAIDs), sulfonamides, and penicillin medication history.
- Seborrheic dermatitis (PRP)—Sebaceous distribution of erythematous scaling plaques. Chronic history of mesio-labial, glabellar, auricular pruritus, erythema, and scale.
- Chronic contact dermatitis—Bright red erythematous or vesiculating plaques.
- Large plaque parapsoriasis
- Pityriasis rubra pilaris (PRP)—Look for orange-red, waxy-like keratoderma of the palms and soles. Islands of normal skin within larger plaques are characteristically seen in PRP. PRP and CTCL are histologically different, and a biopsy will aid in the diagnosis.
- Pityriasis lichenoides et varioliformis acuta—Papules and nodules in various stages of healing. Central necrosis can be noted in some papules, like LyP.
- Vasculitis—Purpuric or hemorrhagic papules and plaques. Check for rheumatoid factor (RF), ANA, anti-dsDNA, ANCA, cryoglobulins and C3, C4 levels.
- Varicella—Will have the prodrome of mild fever, malaise, and myalgia followed by pruritic erythematous papules. Lesions are pruritic. Varicella does not recur.
- Secondary syphilis—Generalized scaling papules and plaques. Can involve the palms and soles. Check RPR, history of chancre.
- Dermatitis herpetiformis—Pruritic papules and plaques over the extensor surfaces. Granular IgA deposition within the dermal papillae on direct immunofluorescence.
- Disseminated HSV—Crusted papules and erosions. Do viral culture and direct fluorescence antigen (DFA).
- Pityriasis rosea—Herald patch, scaly papules/plaques on trunk. Crusts/vesicles/bullae not a common finding.
- Lichen planus—Very pruritic, flat-toped violaceous papules with fine scale. Associated with hepatitis C.

Pitfalls

Previous treatment with phototherapy, topical steroids, and immunosuppressants can profoundly change the histology of the lesion. However, early CTCL, like many of the diseases in the differential diagnosis, will partially clear or completely clear with topical steroids or phototherapy.

✓ Best Tests

- Skin biopsy for basic histology, immunophenotyping, and T-cell receptor (TCR) gene analysis. Peripheral blood can be sent for TCR gene analysis.

- CBC with differential and buffy coat smear with Sézary cell count. Also, obtain CD4 and CD8 T-cell counts.
- Consider obtaining HTLV-1 serology, as this virus can cause lesions that appear similar to MF.
- Patients with clinically abnormal lymph nodes should have them biopsied, and the biopsy specimens should be examined by the same methods as the skin specimen(s).
- CT imaging, complete blood cell count with a differential, chemistry panel, peripheral blood cytology, immunophenotyping, gene rearrangement studies, and a bone marrow biopsy should all be considered when evaluating whether the T-cell lymphoma is a *primary* CTCL or a systemic T-cell lymphoma with associated secondary skin involvement. The number and types of staging studies will be largely determined by what is the suspected type of CTCL.

▲▲▲ Management Pearls

WHO-EORTC Classification	Frequency (%)	5-year survival rate (%)
Indolent Clinical Behavior		
Mycosis fungoides	54	88
MF Variants and Subtypes		
Folliculotropic	6	80
Pagetoid reticulosis	1	100
Granulomatous slack skin	<1	100
Primary Cutaneous CD30+ Lymphoproliferative Disorders		
Primary C-ALCL	10	95
LyP	16	100
Subcutaneous panniculitis-like T-cell lymphoma	1	82
Primary cutaneous CD4+ small/medium-sized pleomorphic T-cell lymphoma	3	75
Aggressive Clinical Behavior		
Sézary syndrome	4	24
Adult T-cell leukemia/lymphoma	NDA	NDA
Extranodal NK/T-cell lymphoma, nasal type	1	<5
Primary cutaneous aggressive epidermotropic CD8+ cytotoxic T-cell lymphoma	<1	18
Cutaneous γ/δ T-cell lymphoma	1	<5
Primary cutaneous peripheral T-cell lymphoma unspecified	3	16

Therapy

Mycosis Fungoides
Stage 1 disease:
Total body phototherapy—UVB or psoralens plus UVA (PUVA)

Topical corticosteroids may be used on limited lesions.

Superpotent corticosteroids (class 1)—use cautiously, on lesional skin only:

- Clobetasol propionate—apply twice daily (30, 60 g)
- Betamethasone dipropionate—apply twice daily (30, 60 g)
- Halobetasol—apply twice daily (20, 50 g)
- Diflorasone diacetate—apply twice daily (15, 30, 60 g)

High-potency topical corticosteroids (class 2)

- Fluocinonide cream or ointment—apply twice daily (15, 30, 60, 120 g)
- Desoximetasone cream or ointment—apply twice daily (15, 60, 120 g)
- Halcinonide cream or ointment—apply twice daily (15, 60, 240 g)
- Amcinonide ointment—apply twice daily (15, 30, 60 g)

Mid-potency topical corticosteroids (classes 3 and 4)

- Triamcinolone cream or ointment—apply twice daily (15, 30, 60, 120, 240 g)
- Mometasone cream or ointment—apply twice daily (15, 45 g)
- Fluocinolone ointment or cream—apply twice daily (15, 30, 60 g)

For localized disease unresponsive to the above treatments or more extensive disease, try the following topical therapies:

- Topical nitrogen mustard (mechlorethamine)—as an aqueous solution or in an ointment base; apply twice daily
- Topical carmustine (BCNU)—as an aqueous solution or in an ointment base; apply twice daily
- Topical bexarotene gel—apply twice daily
- Imiquimod 5% cream three to five times per week

Additional treatments
- Total skin electron-beam radiotherapy
- Interferon alpha—start at 3 MU three times per week and increase up to 12 MU three times per week, as tolerated

Stage 2 Disease

Therapies as for stage 1 disease (give more consideration to using interferon α or total skin electron beam therapy), plus local radiotherapy or low-dose methotrexate (5 to 12.5 mg p.o. weekly). Oral bexarotene (300 mg/m² daily) may also be tried. Chlorambucil 0.1 to 0.2 mg/kg/day p.o. or 3 to 6 mg/m²/day p.o. for 3 to 6 weeks. Vorinostat 400 mg p.o. daily. Prednisone 10 to 20 mg p.o. daily with low-dose chlorambucil and interferon α.

Caution: Bexarotene (a retinoid) can cause birth defects in pregnant females. It can also lead to increased triglycerides, pancreatitis, or central hypothyroidism requiring levothyroxine replacement. Bexarotene is modified by P4503A4 inhibitors.

Stage 3 Disease (Erythroderma)

- Interferon alpha (as above)
- Low-dose methotrexate (as above)
- Oral bexarotene (as above)
- Extracorporeal photopheresis
- PUVA
- Total skin electron beam therapy
- Radiation to lymph nodes
- Some oncologists may recommend single agent or reduced-dose combination chemotherapy such as etoposide 100 mg/m² IV for days 1 to 5

Stage 4 Disease

In addition to the treatments used for stage 2 and 3 disease, as above, stage 4 disease is often treated with combination chemotherapy. Agents that have had some treatment success include purine analogues (i.e., fludarabine), bleomycin, vincristine, etoposide, and cisplatin.

Denileukin diftitox (DAB-IL2) is a biologic agent that has recently been licensed for use in MF.

Oral bexarotene and allogeneic bone marrow transplantation have also been used for stage 4 disease.

Sézary Syndrome

Systemic treatment is required.

- Interferon alpha (as above)
- Methotrexate (as above)
- Oral bexarotene (as above)
- Vorinostat
- Depsipeptide
- Extracorporeal photopheresis and PUVA as adjuvants
- Some oncologists may recommend single agent or combination chemotherapy.

Lymphomatoid Papulosis

- Topical nitrogen mustard (mechlorethamine)—as an aqueous solution or in an ointment base; apply twice daily
- Topical carmustine (BCNU)—as an aqueous solution or in an ointment base; apply twice daily
- Methotrexate
- Body-wide phototherapy—UVB or PUVA

Primary Cutaneous Anaplastic Large Cell Lymphoma

- Radiation therapy
- Methotrexate (as above)

Suggested Readings

Assaf C, Sterry W. Cutaneous Lymphoma. In: Fitzpatrick TB, Wolff K, eds. *Fitzpatrick's Dermatology in General Medicine.* 7th Ed. New York, NY: McGraw-Hill; 2008:1386–1402.

Berthelot C, Rivera A, Duvic M. Skin directed therapy for mycosis fungoides: A review. *J Drugs Dermatol.* 2008 Jul;7(7):655–666.

Dummer R. Future perspectives in the treatment of cutaneous T-cell lymphoma (CTCL). *Semin Oncol.* 2006 Feb;33(1 Suppl. 3):S33–S36.

Girardi M, Heald PW, Wilson LD. The pathogenesis of mycosis fungoides. *N Engl J Med.* 2004 May;350(19):1978–1988.

Heald P, Mehlmauer M, Martin AG, et al.; Worldwide Bexarotene Study Group. Topical bexarotene therapy for patients with refractory or persistent early-stage cutaneous T-cell lymphoma: Results of the phase III clinical trial. *J Am Acad Dermatol.* 2003 Nov;49(5):801–815.

Horwitz SM, Olsen EA, Duvic M, et al. Review of the treatment of mycosis fungoides and sézary syndrome: a stage-based approach. *J Natl Compr Canc Netw.* 2008 Apr;6(4):436–442.

Hwang ST, Janik JE, Jaffe ES, et al. Mycosis fungoides and Sézary syndrome. *Lancet.* 2008 Mar;371(9616):945–957.

Kim EJ, Hess S, Richardson SK, et al. Immunopathogenesis and therapy of cutaneous T cell lymphoma. *J Clin Invest.* 2005 Apr;115(4):798–812.

Lansigan F, Choi J, Foss FM. Cutaneous T-cell lymphoma. *Hematol Oncol Clin North Am.* 2008 Oct;22(5):979–996, x.

Mestel DS, Assaf C, Steinhoff M, et al. Emerging drugs in cutaneous T cell lymphoma. *Expert Opin Emerg Drugs.* 2008 Jun;13(2):345–361.

Papadavid E, Antoniou C, Nikolaou V, et al. Safety and efficacy of low-dose bexarotene and PUVA in the treatment of patients with mycosis fungoides. *Am J Clin Dermatol.* 2008;9(3):169–173.

Stadler R. Optimal combination with PUVA: Rationale and clinical trial update. *Oncology (Williston Park).* 2007 Feb;21(2 Suppl. 1):29–32.

Stadler R, Otte HG, Luger T, et al. Prospective randomized multicenter clinical trial on the use of interferon-2a plus acitretin versus interferon-2a plus PUVA in patients with cutaneous T-cell lymphoma stages I and II. *Blood.* 1998 Nov;92(10):3578–3581.

Vonderheid EC, Bernengo MG, Burg G, et al.; ISCL. Update on erythrodermic cutaneous T-cell lymphoma: Report of the International Society for cutaneous lymphomas. *J Am Acad Dermatol.* 2002 Jan;46(1):95–106.

Vose JM. Update on T-cell lymphoma. *Ann Oncol.* 2008 Jun;19(Suppl. 4):iv74–iv76.

Willemze R, Jaffe ES, Burg G, et al. WHO-EORTC classification for cutaneous lymphomas. *Blood.* 2005 May;105(10):3768–3785.

Diagnosis Synopsis

Milia (singular, milium) are minute epidermoid cysts (also known as infundibular cysts) that present as small white or yellow papules, usually on the face. They are typically smaller than 3 mm in diameter. Primary milia affect 40% to 50% of newborns but may be found in patients of all ages. Secondary milia often occur after cosmetic procedures (dermabrasion, chemical peels, and ablative laser therapy) or trauma, or in conjunction with a number of blistering disorders. Milia have also been known to occur in areas of topical steroid-induced atrophy. Persistent or widespread milia are associated with a number of syndromes. There is no predilection for either sex or for any ethnicity.

Immunocompromised Patient Considerations

There is no reported association between immunocompromised status and increased milia formation.

Look For

White to yellow 1 to 2 mm papules typically seen on the cheeks and eyelids, also commonly on the nose and chin areas (Figs. 4-206 and 4-207). Milia are also well described as occurring on genital skin.

Milia en plaque has recently been described and refers to a rare entity with multiple milia within an erythematous, edematous plaque. It most commonly occurs in the postauricular area but may be found anterior to the ear.

Diagnostic Pearls

- Milia on the hands, in particular, may be a sign that there is a subepidermal bullous disease such as porphyria cutanea tarda or epidermolysis bullosa acquisita (Figs. 4-208 and 4-209). Ask the patient about preceding lesions.

Immunocompromised Patient Considerations

Porphyria cutanea tarda should be considered in patients with viral hepatitis and milia in sun-exposed areas.

?? Differential Diagnosis and Pitfalls

- Milia are sometimes confused with closed comedones.
- Pustular acne
- Molluscum contagiosum
- Sebaceous hyperplasia
- Trichoepitheliomas
- Syringomas

Some syndromes associated with milia are as follows:

- Hereditary trichodysplasia
- Oral-facial-digital syndrome type 1
- Rombo syndrome
- Bazex syndrome
- Pachyonychia congenita

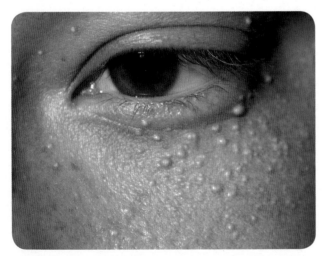

Figure 4-206 Extensive fields of milia are not rare.

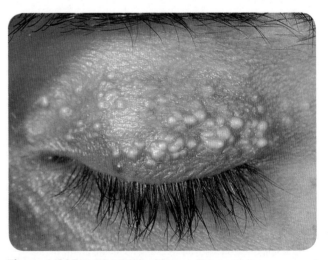

Figure 4-207 Multiple milia with some larger papules may suggest a benign appendageal tumor.

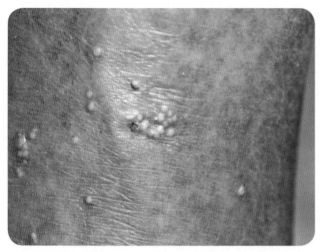

Figure 4-208 Noninflammatory white papules characterize milia.

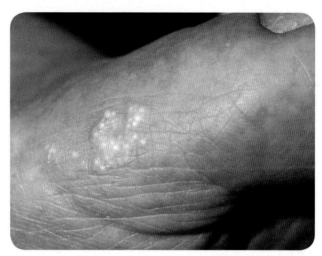

Figure 4-209 Milia in nonfacial locations are often the consequence of a blistering disorder.

Blistering disorders that may heal with milia and scarring are as follows:

- Epidermolysis bullosa
- Porphyrias, including porphyria cutanea tarda
- Bullous pemphigoid
- Herpes zoster
- Contact dermatitis
- Bullous lupus erythematosus
- Dermatitis herpetiformis

✓ Best Tests

- Primarily, a clinical diagnosis based on appearance. The clinical impression can be confirmed by the removal of the keratin core.

▲▲ Management Pearls

- Make a minute incision or "nick" in the skin overlying the milia with a fine-gauge needle or scalpel. They will express easily with a comedone extractor.

Therapy

Milia do not require treatment. For patients who request it, the extraction technique as above is appropriate for patients with few lesions.

Retin-A (0.1% cream or 0.025% gel nightly) used chronically may prevent the formation of new lesions in a patient with multiple recurring milia.

The use of laser vaporization and electrodesiccation has been reported.

Milia en plaque has been treated with cryosurgery, electrodesiccation, the carbon dioxide laser, and oral minocycline.

Suggested Readings

Berk DR, Bayliss SJ. Milia: A review and classification. *J Am Acad Dermatol.* 2008 Dec;59(6):1050–1063.

Diba VC, Al-Izzi M, Green T. A case of eruptive milia. *Clin Exp Dermatol.* 2005 Nov;30(6):677–678.

Hisa T, Goto Y, Taniguchi S, et al. Post-bullous milia. *Australas J Dermatol.* 1996 Aug;37(3):153–154.

Seabury Stone M. Cysts. In: Bolognia J, Jorizzo JL, Rapini RP, eds. *Dermatology.* 2nd Ed. St. Louis, MO: Mosby; 2008:1682–1683.

Stefanidou MP, Panayotides JG, Tosca AD. Milia en plaque: A case report and review of the literature. *Dermatol Surg.* 2002 Mar;28(3):291–295.

◼◼ Diagnosis Synopsis

Miliaria rubra, also known as heat rash or prickly heat, consists of erythematous papules caused by the blockage of the eccrine sweat duct. The pathogenesis is often related to conditions of high fever and/or heavy sweating, and it is more prevalent in hot, humid conditions and tropical climates. Resident bacteria (*Staphylococci spp.*) on the skin may also play a role. It is a benign disease characterized by intense pruritus and a stinging or "prickly"-type sensation. It is a common phenomenon post-operatively and in bedridden and febrile patients.

◉ Look For

Small erythematous and uniform papulovesicles are present and can be widely distributed with background erythema (Fig. 4-210). Miliaria rubra is most prominent in occluded areas, such as on the back of hospitalized or bedridden patients (Fig. 4-211). Other sites of predilection in adults include intertriginous and flexural areas and elsewhere on the trunk.

●● Diagnostic Pearls

- The palms, soles, and acral areas are spared.
- There is often anhidrosis in the affected site(s).

?? Differential Diagnosis and Pitfalls

- Miliaria rubra is often mistaken for a drug eruption, especially after a new antibiotic is started in a febrile patient.
- Candidiasis often has some pustules.
- Scabies, unlike miliaria, often involves acral sites, especially the presence of borrows in the finger webs.
- Varicella presents as vesicles on an erythematous base ("dewdrops on a rose petal") and are in different stages of development.
- Folliculitis has follicular-based pustules.
- Acne can also be worsened by occlusion but usually lacks pruritus and is less acute.
- Acute generalized exanthematous pustulosis is more diffuse with widespread pustules.

✓ Best Tests

- This is a clinical diagnosis that could be confirmed by skin biopsy if absolutely necessary.
- Consider bacterial or fungal culture if there is concern for infection.

▲▲ Management Pearls

- Patient should be placed in a cool and dry environment. Reassure the patient that the problem is self-limited. Lesions rarely become infected.

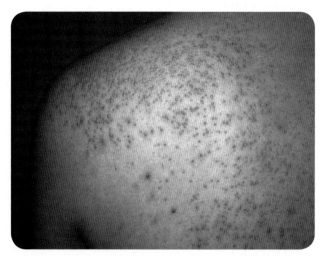

Figure 4-210 Multiple closely grouped red papules of malaria rubra.

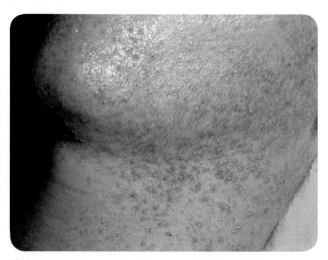

Figure 4-211 Multiple areas of miliaria rubra—some with pustules—in a hospitalized patient.

Therapy

Instruct the patient to avoid conditions of excessive heat and sweating. Place the patient in a cool environment if possible, and encourage him/her to wear loose-fitting clothing. Exertion in hot weather should be minimized.

Treat the underlying cause of any fever and administer antipyretics. Talcum powder or cornstarch may be applied to the skin, but patients should avoid heavy emollients.

Symptomatic relief may be achieved with cool oatmeal baths or showers, cool compresses, and the application of calamine lotion. Mid-potency steroid lotions can reduce inflammation.

Mid-potency topical corticosteroids (classes 3 and 4)

- Triamcinolone cream, ointment—apply twice daily (15, 30, 60, 120, 240 g)
- Mometasone cream, ointment—apply twice daily (15, 45 g)
- Fluocinolone ointment, cream—apply twice daily (15, 30, 60 g)

Suggested Readings

Donoghue AM, Sinclair MJ. Miliaria rubra of the lower limbs in underground miners. *Occup Med* (*Lond*). 2000 Aug;50(6):430–433.

Koh D. An outbreak of occupational dermatosis in an electronics store. *Contact Dermatitis*. 1995 Jun;32(6):327–330.

Pandolf KB, Griffin TB, Munro EH, et al. Heat intolerance as a function of percent of body surface involved with miliaria rubra. *Am J Physiol*. 1980 Sep;239(3):R233–R240.

Molluscum Contagiosum

Diagnosis Synopsis

Molluscum contagiosum is a contagious disease caused by infection with a DNA poxvirus. It manifests as smooth, firm papules with a central umbilication. Molluscum contagiosum may be spread by direct contact (most often in children) or via sexual transmission in adults. Molluscum contagiosum infections have also been associated with swimming pools. Many cases are asymptomatic, but there can be surrounding irritation in association with pruritus. The disease is relatively chronic and may persist for several months and up to 2 years before disappearing. Auto-inoculation allows the spread of lesions prior to resolution. In the immunocompetent host, the disease tends to be self-limited.

Immunocompromised Patient Considerations

Immunosuppressed patients and those with HIV/AIDS are at particular risk of molluscum contagiosum infection, with a prevalence of 5% to 18%. The number of lesions is inversely correlated with the CD4 count, and the presence of molluscum contagiosum lesions can actually indicate an AIDS diagnosis. Molluscum contagiosum has also been reported in several immunosuppressed states including malignancies, severe combined immune deficiency (SCID), transplant patients, and in those receiving chemotherapy. Sarcoidosis and atopic dermatitis also predispose patients to molluscum contagiosum infections, most likely due to abnormal T-cell immunity.

Look For

Presents with smooth, whitish or skin-colored, 2 to 6 mm pearly papules with a central umbilication (depression), often clustered together. With excoriation, lesions can be spread directly, forming a linear array of mollusca.

In adults, molluscum contagiosum is usually sexually transmitted, and lesions are, therefore, more commonly distributed on the mons pubis, the genitalia, perineum, inner thighs, and lower abdomen (Figs. 4-212–4-215). This is not true in children.

Lesions are rarely found in the mouth or on the palms or soles. As lesions resolve, they may become more inflamed and erythematous, causing a characteristic "molluscum dermatitis."

Dark Skin Considerations

Mollusca can be hyperpigmented in black patients.

Immunocompromised Patient Considerations

Giant molluscum, with lesions up to 1.5 cm in size, is a variant that can be seen in AIDS and in other immunosuppressed patients. Molluscum contagiosum lesions can be spread by shaving and are common in the beard area of men with AIDS. Reports of cyst-like lesions have been reported in immunocompromised patients as well. In atopic dermatitis, lesions tend to be limited to skin affected by the dermatitis.

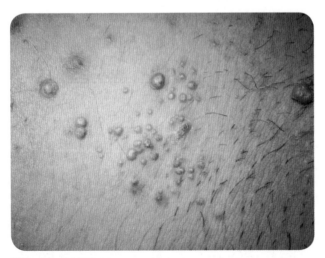

Figure 4-212 Multiple papules with hyperkeratotic centers are characteristic of molluscum contagiosum.

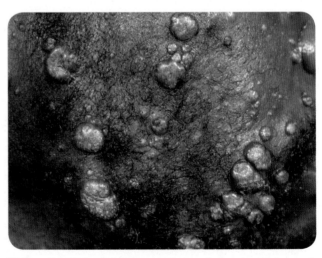

Figure 4-213 Small and giant molluscum lesions are often seen in HIV-infected patients with low CD4 counts.

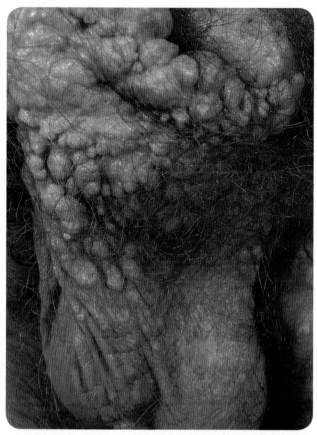

Figure 4-214 Genitals are a common location for molluscum.

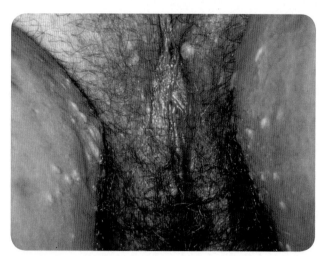

Figure 4-215 Molluscum on the thighs and genitals.

- Warts tend to have a verrucous or jagged surface, whereas molluscum contagiosum lesions are smooth.
- Milia tend to be whiter in color and more concentrated on the face.
- Nevi
- Pyogenic granuloma is obviously vascular with frequent ulceration.
- Lichen planus lesions are purple, pruritic planar papules that can also spread in a linear pattern.
- Basal cell carcinoma tends to be solitary.
- Keratoacanthomas have a central keratin core and grow rapidly.
- Sebaceous hyperplasia primarily occurs on the face and has a whiter, lobular appearance.

Immunocompromised Patient Differential Diagnosis

- In AIDS/HIV patients, cutaneous deep fungal infections with cryptococcus, blastomycoses, or coccidioidomycoses can resemble molluscum contagiosum lesions.

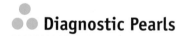

Diagnostic Pearls

- The central umbilication within a firm papule is highly suggestive of molluscum contagiosum. The umbilication may be difficult to see but becomes more obvious when the lesion is gently frozen with liquid nitrogen. Larger lesions will frequently have more than one umbilication.

Immunocompromised Patient Considerations

When there are multiple molluscum contagiosum lesions in the beard area, they tend to be flatter with a larger umbilication, almost resembling acne scarring or sebaceous hyperplasia. If this is observed in a patient, HIV testing is indicated.

?? Differential Diagnosis and Pitfalls

- Herpes simplex lesions can resemble molluscum with a central umbilication, but lesions are fluid filled rather than solid as in molluscum contagiosum.

✓ Best Tests

- This diagnosis can often be made clinically based on the characteristic clinical appearance.
- Extracting the central core of the molluscum and viewing with light microscopy can confirm molluscum bodies (appearing red using Wright stain). Methylene blue may also be used to stain smears made from lesions.
- The skin biopsy of a lesion can confirm the diagnosis when in doubt and should certainly be used in immunocompromised patients to rule out deep fungal infections.

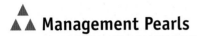

Management Pearls

- The condition is self-limited in immunocompetent patients. However, treatment is often desirable and will help to prevent autoinoculation and further spread.
- In cases of sexually transmitted molluscum contagiosum, consider the possibility of other concomitant STDs.
- Instruct patients to avoid communal bathing, sharing of bath towels, and shaving if lesions are present on the face of men or legs of women.

Immunocompromised Patient Considerations

Even if there are just a few molluscum contagiosum lesions, it is important to treat early to prevent autoinoculation and further spread.

Therapy

Cryotherapy with liquid nitrogen. Use with caution in darker-skinned patients.

Curettage of central core/umbilication followed by gentle hyfrecation.

Imiquimod cream—Apply to affected area three to seven times per week for 4 to 12 weeks.

Cantharidin solution, commonly known as "beetle juice," can be applied to individual lesions with a cotton-tipped applicator and washed off after 4 h. Be sure to inform patients that the lesions will later blister. Protect unaffected areas with petroleum jelly.

Tazarotene 0.05% cream or ointment—Apply daily to affected area for 4 to 12 weeks.

Other topical therapies:

- 5% sodium nitrate co-applied with 5% salicylic acid nightly
- 40% silver nitrate paste (after topical anesthetization with 2% lidocaine jelly)—can pigment the skin permanently
- 0.5% podophyllotoxin once daily
- 10% povidone-iodine and 50% salicylic acid plaster applied once daily

Immunocompromised Patient Considerations

Longer treatment durations and more frequent interventions may be required in the immunosuppressed host. In HIV-infected individuals, an initiation of highly active antiretroviral therapy (HAART) therapy can lead to the rapid resolution of lesions.

Suggested Readings

Bikowski JB. Molluscum contagiosum: The need for physician intervention and new treatment options. *Cutis.* 2004 Mar;73(3):202–206.

Cribier B, Scrivener Y, Grosshans E. Molluscum contagiosum: Histologic patterns and associated lesions. A study of 578 cases. *Am J Dermatopathol.* 2001 Apr;23(2):99–103.

Gottlieb SL, Myskowski PL. Molluscum contagiosum. *Int J Dermatol.* 1994 Jul;33(7):453–61.

Husar K, Skerlev M. Molluscum contagiosum from infancy to maturity. *Clin Dermatol.* 2002 Mar–Apr;20(2):170–172.

James WD, Berger TG, Elston DM. Viral diseases. In: James WD, Berger TG, Elston DM, Odom RB, eds. *Andrews' Diseases of the Skin: Clinical Dermatology.* 10th Ed. Philadelphia, PA: Saunders Elsevier; 2006:394–397.

National guideline for the management of molluscum contagiosum. Clinical Effectiveness Group (Association of Genitourinary Medicine and the Medical Society for the Study of Venereal Diseases). *Sex Transm Infect.* 1999 Aug;75(Suppl. 1):S80–S81.

Schornack MM, Siemsen DW, Bradley EA, et al. Ocular manifestations of molluscum contagiosum. *Clin Exp Optom.* 2006 Nov;89(6):390–393.

Schwartz JJ, Myskowski PL. Molluscum contagiosum in patients with human immunodeficiency virus infection. A review of twenty-seven patients. *J Am Acad Dermatol.* 1992 Oct;27(4):583–588.

Skinner RB. Treatment of molluscum contagiosum with imiquimod 5% cream. *J Am Acad Dermatol.* 2002 Oct;47(4 Suppl.):S221–S224.

Strauss RM, Doyle EL, Mohsen AH, et al. Successful treatment of molluscum contagiosum with topical imiquimod in a severely immunocompromised HIV-positive patient. *Int J STD AIDS.* 2001 Apr;12(4):264–266.

Syed TA, Goswami J, Ahmadpour OA, et al. Treatment of molluscum contagiosum in males with an analog of imiquimod 1% in cream: A placebo-controlled, double-blind study. *J Dermatol.* 1998 May;25(5):309–313.

Tyring SK. Molluscum contagiosum: The importance of early diagnosis and treatment. *Am J Obstet Gynecol.* 2003 Sep;189(3 Suppl.):S12–S16.

van der Wouden JC, Menke J, Gajadin S, et al. Interventions for cutaneous molluscum contagiosum. *Cochrane Database Syst Rev.* 2006 Apr;(2):CD004767.

Morphea

Diagnosis Synopsis

Morphea is a rare connective tissue disease of excess collagen production in the dermis and/or subcutaneous tissues. It represents a localized form of scleroderma (systemic sclerosis). Both diseases present with spontaneous sclerosis or thickening of the skin, but morphea lacks such findings as Raynaud phenomenon, sclerodactyly, and internal organ involvement. The etiology is largely unknown, but in certain cases, morphea has been noted to develop after trauma, radiation, vaccination, and certain infections such as *Borrelia burgdorferi*. It has been postulated that localized injury to cutaneous microvasculature is the inciting event. Morphea is usually divided into plaque, generalized, and linear subcategories, but other forms have been described (guttate, bullous, nodular, subcutaneous). In the linear variant, underlying muscles, fascia, and joints can be affected, leading to deformity and disability. Growth restriction and/or joint contractures may be present in up to 10% of patients. However, there is no significant difference in survival between patients affected with morphea and the general population. The condition occurs in both children and adults; the linear form of morphea typically presents in childhood. It is more common in whites, and women are affected more commonly than men (2.6:1).

Immunocompromised Patient Considerations

Chronic, sclerodermoid graft-versus-host disease is indistinguishable from morphea, both clinically and histologically.

Look For

The most common manifestation is that of firm, indurated, sometimes waxy or "shiny" oval plaques, a few to 10 cm or greater in diameter with a surrounding violaceous ring (Figs. 4-216–4-218). The red to violet rim may fade with time. Early on, the most common findings are that of a bruise or hyperpigmentation. In well-developed lesions, there is loss of hair follicles and sweat glands. The lesions remain localized. The trunk and extremities are commonly affected.

When linear morphea affects the mid-line or paramedian forehead, it is known as *en coup de sabre* (blow of the sword) (Fig. 4-219). This variant can be severe and may affect underlying bone and muscle. Linear morphea in other locations, such as the limbs, can compromise the range of motion and affect the growth of the underlying structures.

Parry-Romberg syndrome (progressive hemifacial atrophy) refers to a severe segmental form of craniofacial linear morphea in the distribution of the trigeminal nerve. The neurologic and ophthalmologic manifestations (headache, seizures, visual changes, and cranial nerve palsies) may occur.

Dark Skin Considerations

The plaques can be hyperpigmented in blacks or with central atrophic hypopigmentation in mature lesions. Moreover, in late lesions, the border may appear hyperpigmented rather than violaceous or erythematous.

Keloidal (or nodular) forms of both morphea and scleroderma have been described and are more common in patients of African descent.

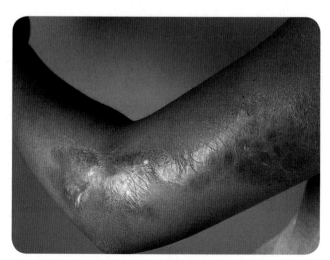

Figure 4-216 Linear plaques on the extremities is one presentation of linear scleroderma.

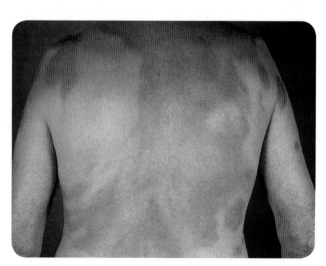

Figure 4-217 Multiple indurated truncal plaques are common in morphea.

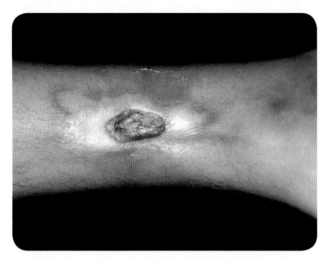

Figure 4-218 Ivory white sclerotic plaques of morphea may ulcerate.

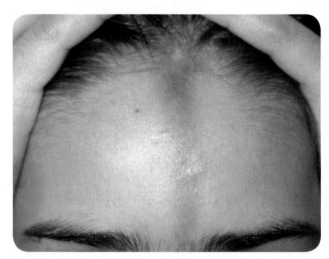

Figure 4-219 Midline localized morphea on the scalp defines the *en coup de sabre* localized form of morphea.

Diagnostic Pearls

- Individual plaques tend to progress for 3 to 5 years and then arrest. Progression can be expected to cease when the violaceous or lilac appearance to plaque borders disappears.
- When linear or deep morphea crosses joint lines, the lesions may affect joint mobility and impair muscle growth and development.
- Patients with craniofacial morphea may have concomitant ocular and/or oral complaints.
- Epileptic seizures have been reported with *en coup de sabre.*
- Carpal tunnel syndrome is a complication of morphea at the wrist.

?? Differential Diagnosis and Pitfalls

- Morphea and lichen sclerosus et atrophicus may present together. This presentation is known as LS&A/morphea overlap, complicating the diagnosis and therapy plan.
- Systemic sclerosis (scleroderma)
- Stasis dermatitis with fibrosis/lipodermatosclerosis
- Lipoatrophy
- Amyloidosis
- Porphyria cutanea tarda with sclerodermoid features
- Keloid or hypertrophic scar
- Carcinoid syndrome
- Phenylketonuria
- Panniculitis
- Scleredema
- Scleromyxedema
- Progeria or Werner syndrome
- Drug/chemical-induced sclerodermoid lesions (some chemotherapeutic agents, polyvinyl chloride (PVC), injection site reactions from vitamin K, enfuvirtide, silicone, paraffin, and many other compounds)
- Nephrogenic systemic fibrosis
- Acrodermatitis chronic atrophicans
- Chronic graft-versus-host disease
- Radiation fibrosis
- Cutaneous metastases
- Reflex sympathetic dystrophy
- Atrophoderma of Pasini and Pierini and eosinophilic fasciitis are considered to be a part of the morphea spectrum.

✓ Best Tests

- This diagnosis may be made clinically, but skin biopsy is confirmatory.
- X-rays may be useful for linear or deep morphea if the involvement of underlying bone is suspected.
- Magnetic resonance imaging (MRI) can be used to rule out the involvement of the underlying tissues, and ultrasound can be used to assess skin thickness (which correlates with disease severity).
- Electroencephalography (EEG) abnormalities may be demonstrated in some patients with craniofacial morphea.
- Various autoantibodies may be present in all types of morphea, but, as a diagnostic test, they lack specificity. Procollagen type I carboxy-terminal propeptide is increased in approximately 30% of patients. Serum levels have been shown to correlate with the degree of skin involvement.

▲▲ Management Pearls

- Patients should be assured that morphea lesions are usually not a sign of systemic sclerosis and that there is no increased risk of death with morphea. Lesions may spontaneously become inactive.

- In Europe, *B. burgdorferi* is an associated etiologic agent. This finding may make antibiotic usage seem reasonable, but clinical trials usually have not proven efficacy.
- Consider consultation with an orthopedic or plastic surgeon in cases with marked deformity affecting function or appearance. The involvement of the following disciplines may also be warranted: ophthalmology, dermatology, neurology, dentistry, and physical therapy.

Therapy

High potency topical steroids (classes 1 and 2) twice daily to involved areas have been shown to be of modest benefit. This treatment is probably most helpful during the initial inflammatory stage.

Intralesional corticosteroids (triamcinolone 5 mg/mL every 4 weeks for 3 months) may be of help in cases of linear morphea involving the forehead.

Calcipotriol cream or ointment 0.005% twice daily under occlusion for 3 months has been used successfully in some cases.

Phototherapy (UVA, UVA1, PUVA [psoralen plus UVA], and PUVA bath photochemotherapy) are all effective treatments.

For rapidly progressive disease and cases with potential disability:

- Prednisone 30 to 40 mg per day tapered over 3 weeks
- Methotrexate 15 to 25 mg per week
- Methotrexate has also been administered with prednisone for its steroid-sparing effect.
- Phototherapy with UVA, with or without psoralens, has produced marked improvement in many reports.

Physical therapy is an essential component of therapy for any cases involving joints, muscle, bone, or other functional structures.

Suggested Readings

Bielsa I, Ariza A. Deep morphea. *Semin Cutan Med Surg*. 2007 Jun;26(2):90–95.

Jacobson L, Palazij R, Jaworsky C. Superficial morphea. *J Am Acad Dermatol*. 2003 Aug;49(2):323–325.

Man J, Dytoc MT. Use of imiquimod cream 5% in the treatment of localized morphea. *J Cutan Med Surg*. 2004 May–Jun;8(3):166–169.

Peterson LS, Nelson AM, Su WP. Classification of morphea (localized scleroderma). *Mayo Clin Proc*. 1995 Nov;70(11):1068–1076.

Rencic A, Brinster N, Nousari CH. Keloid morphea and nodular scleroderma: Two distinct clinical variants of scleroderma? *J Cutan Med Surg*. 2003 Jan–Feb;7(1):20–24.

Röchen M, Ghoreschi K. Morphea and lichen slerosus. In: Bolognia J, Jorizzo JL, Rapini RP, eds. *Dermatology*. 2nd Ed. St. Louis, MO: Mosby; 2008: 1469–1476.

Shetty G, Lewis F, Thrush S. Morphea of the breast: Case reports and review of literature. *Breast J*. 2007 May–Jun;13(3):302–304.

Diagnosis Synopsis

Mycobacterium marinum, the causative agent of fish tank or swimming pool granuloma, is an atypical mycobacterial skin infection often contracted from contaminated fish tanks, swimming pools, and, occasionally, ocean or lake water. Minor trauma is a predisposing factor. Aquarium enthusiasts are usually not aware of the risk of infection. Because of occupational risks (e.g., fisherman), men are more commonly affected than women. The typical skin lesion consists of a pustule or nodule and develops on the exposed extremity 2 to 3 weeks after exposure. Constitutional symptoms are rare and fever, if present, is typically low grade. The disease is usually self-limited, and lesions tend to heal over a period of 1 to 2 years if left untreated.

Immunocompromised Patient Considerations

Patients with AIDS, organ transplant recipients, and patients on chronic steroids may occasionally develop disseminated infections on the skin, bone marrow, and joints, leading to synovitis and arthritis.

Look For

A pustule or nodule typically begins distally on an exposed extremity (usually the arm), which can later ulcerate and spread in a lymphangitic (sporotrichoid) fashion up the affected extremity (Figs. 4-220–4-223). Plaques or nodules can become verrucous and multiply, thus mimicking the lesions of sporotrichosis. They may also become purulent.

Immunocompromised Patient Considerations

Lesions can become disseminated in immunocompromised patients, resulting in larger crusted plaques and ulcers as well as tenosynovitis, septic arthritis, or even osteomyelitis in underlying tissue.

Diagnostic Pearls

- This condition may be seen in an exaggerated fashion in immunosuppressed patients. Bone, synovial, and even systemic involvements may occur.
- Take a careful history of relevant exposures.

Immunocompromised Patient Considerations

Ascending nodules along the lymphatic chain ("sporotrichoid spread") are the typical distribution of *M. marinum*. In the immunocompromised patient, there may be larger crusted plaques and ulcers as well as tenosynovitis, septic arthritis, or even osteomyelitis in underlying tissue.

Differential Diagnosis and Pitfalls

- Other infections (sporotrichosis, blastomycosis, coccidiomycosis, nocardiosis, tularemia, cutaneous tuberculosis, leishmaniasis, and actinomycosis) may have a similar lymphangitic spread from cutaneous inoculation. Exposure and travel history are key for diagnosis.
- Sarcoidosis rarely ulcerates or spreads along lymphatics.

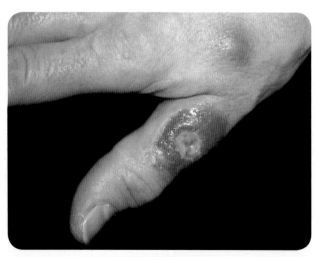

Figure 4-220 Papules and ulcers characterize *M. marinum* infection.

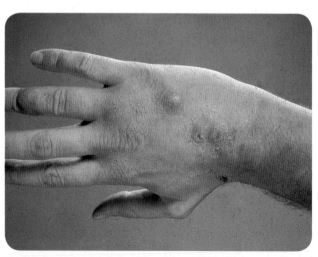

Figure 4-221 Linear papules strongly suggest *M. marinum* infection.

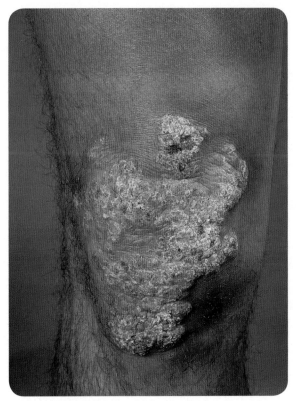

Figure 4-222 Large papules with ulcerations are common in *M. marinum* infection.

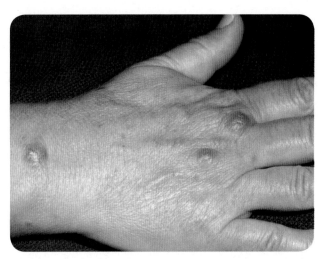

Figure 4-223 Multiple nodules and ulcerative nodules in a fish tank owner with *M. marinum* infection.

- Cellulitis has a background of erythema and a more rapid onset and spread.
- Cutaneous lymphoma may have associated fevers and weight loss.
- Sarcoma may have associated fevers and weight loss.
- Bacterial abscess has an acute onset.
- Pyoderma gangrenosum bleeds easily and appears vascular.
- Vasculitis does not usually have an exophytic growth pattern.
- Superficial thrombophlebitis
- Granuloma annulare rarely ulcerates.
- Hypertrophic lichen planus is highly pruritic and usually located on the shins.
- Foreign body reaction to sea urchin spines or barnacles

Immunocompromised Patient Considerations

- Immunocompromised patients are more susceptible to the deep fungal, bacterial, and atypical mycobacterial infections listed above.
- Bacillary angiomatosis can be seen in HIV/AIDS patients with low CD4 counts.
- Kaposi sarcoma is a consideration in this population as well.

✓ Best Tests

- Skin biopsy with tissue culture. The culture results will identify the type of *Mycobacterium* to help direct therapy. Cultures may grow organisms by 7 to 14 days but may often be negative. Care must be taken to inform the microbiology lab of the suspicion for atypical mycobacteria.
- PCR can be used to detect mycobacterial DNA.
- Consider imaging studies if tenosynovitis or osteomyelitis is suspected.

▲▲▲ Management Pearls

- Heat treatment of the infected area (gloves, hot water, or a heated arm band) may have an adjunctive role in therapy.

Therapy

Treatment is typically continued for 4 to 6 weeks after clinical resolution. The WHO recommends at least 8 weeks of treatment, and though treatment may rarely last 18 months or more, it averages around 3 months duration.

Several antibiotic regimens have reported efficacy:

- Clarithromycin (500 mg p.o. twice daily)
- Minocycline or doxycycline therapy (100 mg p.o. twice daily)
- Rifampin (600 mg p.o. daily) plus ethambutol (1.2 g p.o. daily)

- Other effective antibiotics include trimethoprim-sulfamethoxazole (TMP-SMX) and levofloxacin

Surgical methods (simple excision, incision and drainage, or electrodesiccation and curettage) may be employed for resistant solitary lesions.

Immunocompromised Patient Considerations

Three months of clarithromycin 500 mg p.o. twice daily, minocycline or doxycycline therapy (100 to 200 mg p.o. daily), or TMP/SMX 160/800 p.o. twice daily.

More extensive lesions may be treated with a combination of the above or ethambutol 25 mg/kg p.o. daily plus rifampin 600 mg p.o. daily.

For immunocompromised patients, therapy should be extended for 6 to 9 months.

Suggested Readings

Aubry A, Chosidow O, Caumes E, et al. Sixty-three cases of *Mycobacterium marinum* infection: Clinical features, treatment, and antibiotic susceptibility of causative isolates. *Arch Intern Med.* 2002 Aug;162(15):1746–1752.

Beran V, Matlova L, Dvorska L, et al. Distribution of mycobacteria in clinically healthy ornamental fish and their aquarium environment. *J Fish Dis.* 2006 Jul;29(7):383–393.

Dodiuk-Gad R, Dyachenko P, Ziv M, et al. Nontuberculous mycobacterial infections of the skin: A retrospective study of 25 cases. *J Am Acad Dermatol.* 2007 Sep;57(3):413–420.

Jernigan JA, Farr BM. Incubation period and sources of exposure for cutaneous *Mycobacterium marinum* infection: Case report and review of the literature. *Clin Infect Dis.* 2000 Aug;31(2):439–443.

Jogi R, Tyring SK. Therapy of nontuberculous mycobacterial infections. *Dermatol Ther.* 2004;17(6):491–498.

Liao CH, Lai CC, Ding LW, et al. Skin and soft tissue infection caused by nontuberculous mycobacteria. *Int J Tuberc Lung Dis.* 2007 Jan;11(1):96–102.

Peters DH, Clissold SP. Clarithromycin. A review of its antimicrobial activity, pharmacokinetic properties and therapeutic potential. *Drugs.* 1992 Jul;44(1):117–164.

Petrini B. *Mycobacterium marinum*: Ubiquitous agent of waterborne granulomatous skin infections. *Eur J Clin Microbiol Infect Dis.* 2006 Oct;25(10):609–613.

Rallis E, Koumantaki-Mathioudaki E. Treatment of *Mycobacterium marinum* cutaneous infections. *Expert Opin Pharmacother.* 2007 Dec;8(17):2965–2978.

Neurofibroma, Solitary

Diagnosis Synopsis

Solitary neurofibromas are benign tumors of neuromesenchymal tissue (Schwann cells, perineural cells, fibroblasts, and mast cells) with nerve axons. They present as asymptomatic, flesh-colored or violaceous, rubbery papules or nodules. Solitary neurofibromas occur primarily in adulthood and late adolescence and are not an indication of neurofibromatosis. There is no sex predilection.

Look For

Firm, 0.2 to 2.0 cm, skin-colored papules, nodules, or large pedunculated papules (Figs. 4-224 and 4-225).

The head, neck, and upper trunk are the most common sites of involvement.

Diagnostic Pearls

- Lesions may exhibit the "button hole" sign. That is, when they are compressed from above, lesions invaginate, or feel as if they are being pushed deeper into the skin.
- Up to 10% of patients may have multiple neurofibromas. Further workup for neurofibromatosis should be considered in this population.

Differential Diagnosis and Pitfalls

- Neurofibromatosis (should be ruled out with a complete cutaneous exam)

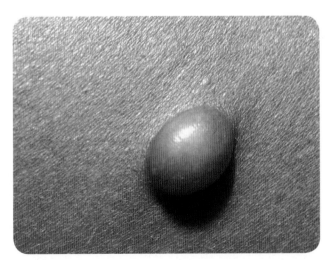

Figure 4-224 A solitary neurofibroma is a soft lesion that is often compressible.

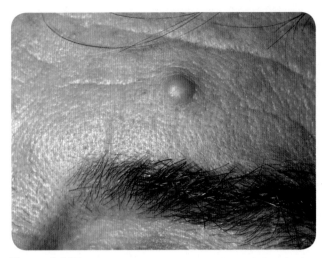

Figure 4-225 This solitary neurofibroma could easily be mistaken for a nevus.

- Dermal melanocytic nevi
- Neuromas
- Soft fibromas
- Acrochordons
- Lipomas
- Dermatofibromas

Best Tests

- The diagnosis can often be made clinically. Perform a biopsy if there is doubt.

Management Pearls

- Reassure the patient. Do not do an extensive neurofibromatosis workup on the basis of a solitary neurofibroma if there are no other signs (such as multiple nodules, café au lait spots, or axillary freckling).

Therapy

Simple excision is the treatment of choice. Rates of recurrence are low.

Suggested Readings

Argenyi ZB. Neural and neuroendocrine neoplasms (other than neurofibromatosis). In: Bolognia J, Jorizzo JL, Rapini RP, eds. *Dermatology*. 2nd Ed. St. Louis, MO: Mosby; 2008:1801–1802.

Chopra R, Morris CG, Friedman WA, et al. Radiotherapy and radiosurgery for benign neurofibromas. *Am J Clin Oncol*. 2005 Jun;28(3):317–320.

Ferner RE, O'Doherty MJ. Neurofibroma and schwannoma. *Curr Opin Neurol*. 2002 Dec;15(6):679–684.

Gottfried ON, Viskochil DH, Fults DW, et al. Molecular, genetic, and cellular pathogenesis of neurofibromas and surgical implications. *Neurosurgery*. 2006 Jan;58(1):1–16; discussion 1–16.

Rapini RP. Neural neoplasms. In: Rapini RP. *Practical Dermatopathology*. Philadelphia, PA: Elsevier Mosby; 2005:333–334.

Weedon D. Neural and endocrine tumors. In: Weedon D, Strutton G. *Skin Pathology*. 2nd Ed. London: Churchill Livingstone; 2002:983.

Zhu Y, Ghosh P, Charnay P, et al. Neurofibromas in NF1: Schwann cell origin and role of tumor environment. *Science*. 2002 May;296(5569):920–922.

Neurofibromatosis

▪️ Diagnosis Synopsis

Neurofibromatosis type 1 (von Recklinghausen disease or NF1) is a multisystem genetic disorder with hallmark cutaneous findings, including café au lait macules, neurofibromas, and axillary freckling. NF1 may affect the skin, nervous system, eyes, bone, and soft tissue. It is the most common autosomal dominant genetic disorder, affecting approximately 1 in 3,000 human beings and occurring as either an inherited defect or, frequently, as a spontaneous (i.e., de novo) mutation.

NF1 occurs equally in all ethnicities and among both sexes and is often identified in childhood with the appearance of café au lait macules. The genetic defect is in a tumor suppressor gene on chromosome 17, which codes for neurofibromin, a RAS GTPase–activating protein. Patients are at increased risk of developing benign and malignant neoplasms. Benign neoplasms include neurofibromas—complex tumors of admixed Schwann cells, fibroblasts, myelinated and unmyelinated nerve axons, endothelial cells, and mast cells—that occur in 1 of 4 forms: cutaneous, subcutaneous, nodular, and deep. Plexiform neurofibromas (present in 25% of patients) are a variant of neurofibroma that are typically deeper, more anatomically complex, and more likely to be symptomatic. Deep plexiform neurofibromas may degenerate into malignant peripheral nerve sheath tumors. Other malignancies and tumors associated with neurofibromatosis include gliomas (especially optic pathway gliomas in 10% to 15% of patients), pheochromocytomas, meningiomas, sarcomas, gastrointestinal tumors of neuroendocrine origin such as duodenal carcinoid tumors, and juvenile myelomonocytic leukemia. In addition to tumors and skin findings, patients may also have learning disabilities (30% to 50%), skeletal anomalies, vasculopathies, and endocrinologic abnormalities.

The diagnosis of NF1 is made on clinical grounds, based on two or more of the following features:

- Six or more café au lait macules greater than 5 mm in prepubertal individuals and greater than 15 mm in diameter in postpubertal patients
- Two or more Lisch nodules (iris hamartomas) in older patients
- Sphenoid dysplasia or thinning of a long bone's cortex, with or without pseudoarthrosis
- Two or more neurofibromas of any type or a single plexiform neurofibroma
- Freckling in the axillary or inguinal region
- Optic glioma (in early childhood)
- First degree relative with NF1 (although new mutations are frequent)

Patients with neurofibromatosis type 2 (NF2) present primarily with acoustic neuromas (schwannomas of the eighth cranial nerve). NF2, which is ten times less common than NF1, is associated with the mutation of a different tumor suppressor gene that is located on chromosome 22 and codes for a protein called merlin. Patients have fewer café au lait macules than those with NF1, and they do not form Lisch nodules in the iris.

👁 Look For

Multiple (six or more) café au lait macules (flat, uniformly darker patches with sharp borders) in postpubertal patients (Fig. 4-226). The macules are typically larger than 15 mm in diameter.

Also, look for axillary freckling or freckling in other intertriginous areas.

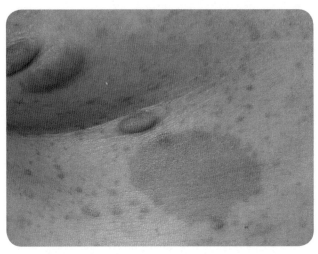

Figure 4-226 Large and small café au lait macules and two neurofibromas in neurofibromatosis.

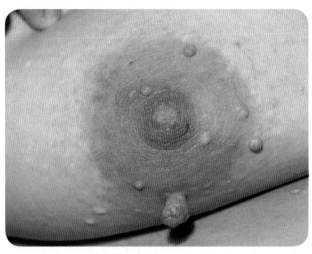

Figure 4-227 Multiple flesh-colored neurofibromas are common in the areola of the breast.

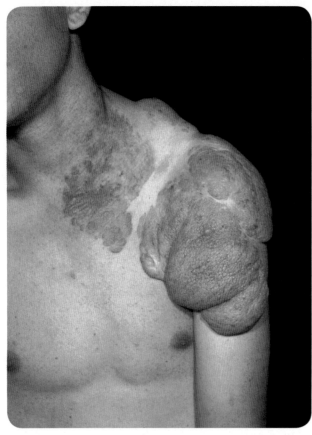

Figure 4-228 Large multinodular plexiform neurofibromas.

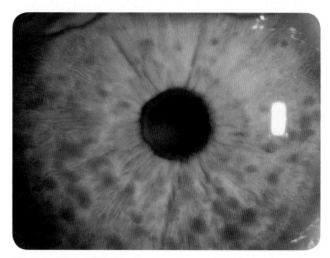

Figure 4-229 Iris with multiple Lesch nodules in neurofibromatosis.

Neurofibromas will increase with age and appear as pink, brown, or skin-colored soft tumors and nodules (Fig. 4-227). Cutaneous neurofibromas are soft and will descend into the underlying dermis with direct pressure (the "button hole" sign). Subcutaneous neurofibromas are tender (often painful) and can be up to several centimeters in size. Plexiform neurofibromas are deep, sometimes involving all layers of the skin to the fascia. They are thick and irregular and may infiltrate or disfigure nearby structures (Fig. 4-228). Plexiform neurofibromas may also cause the hyperpigmentation and/or hypertrichosis of overlying skin.

Iris hamartomas (Lisch nodules) are also associated with the disease and are ultimately identifiable in 90% of patients (Fig. 4-229).

Dark Skin Considerations

At least 1 café au lait macule has been found in 0.3% of white and 18.3% of black infants, and in 13% of white and 27% of black older children, respectively.

Café au lait macules may appear lighter than the surrounding skin in heavily pigmented individuals.

⬤⬤ Diagnostic Pearls

- Café au lait macules may appear lighter than the surrounding skin in heavily pigmented individuals.

?? Differential Diagnosis and Pitfalls

The differential diagnosis of NF1 includes

- Other forms of neurofibromatosis
- Segmental/mosaic NF1
- Watson syndrome
- Autosomal dominant multiple café au lait macules alone (some allelic with NF1)
- Neurofibromatosis type 2
- Schwannomatosis (recently distinguished disorder associated with mutation in the gene *INI1*)

Other conditions with café au lait macules are the following:

- McCune-Albright syndrome (premature puberty, bony abnormalities, and a few large café au lait macules with an irregular outline). In NF1, the outline of the café au lait macule is smooth.
- Genetic disorders of DNA repair or chromosomal instability
- Homozygosity for one of the genes causing hereditary nonpolyposis cancer of the colon
- Noonan syndrome

Conditions with pigmented macules confused with NF1 are the following:

- LEOPARD syndrome
- Neurocutaneous melanosis
- Peutz-Jeghers syndrome
- Piebaldism

Localized overgrowth syndromes:

- Klippel-Trenaunay-Weber syndrome
- Proteus syndrome

Conditions causing tumors confused with those seen in NF1 are the following:

- Lipomatosis
- Bannayan-Riley-Ruvalcaba syndrome
- Fibromatoses
- Multiple endocrine neoplasia types 1 and 2B

Note

- One or two café au lait macules may commonly be seen in patients unaffected by NF1.
- Isolated neurofibromas without neurofibromatosis are also common.

✓ Best Tests

- See above for the clinical diagnostic criteria. It may be helpful to examine family members.
- Check for Lisch nodules with a slit-lamp examination.
- If the patient is having neurologic symptoms, obtain an MRI of the brain, orbits, and/or spinal cord. It may also be useful to perform an MRI of any particularly deep or changing plexiform neurofibromas.
- Genetic testing is possible in equivocal cases.
- Plain radiographs may be obtained if bony involvement is suspected.

▲▲ Management Pearls

- A multidisciplinary approach is essential to the management of an NF1.
- Genetic counseling is an important aspect of proper care because children have a 50% chance of inheriting this disorder.
- Neurofibromas are sex hormone sensitive, and can be expected to develop and grow during adolescent years and pregnancy.
- Children should have comprehensive vision exams performed by an ophthalmologist annually to age 8 and then every other year to age 18 to look for signs of optic glioma. Adults should have only routine vision screening. Routine MRIs to look for optic gliomas in asymptomatic patients are controversial and generally not indicated.
- Orthopedic surgeons may be consulted in the management of bony abnormalities such as scoliosis or tibial bowing.
- Psychological or psychiatric assessment may be necessary for those with learning disabilities.
- Plastic surgery may be indicated to correct deformities.
- Screening for pheochromocytoma with urine catecholamine measurement is indicated for any NF1 patient who will undergo general anesthesia.

- Blood pressure should be measured annually in all patients, including children, to screen for pheochromocytoma or renovascular hypertension.
- Excise or biopsy any lesion suspected of undergoing malignant transformation. Five to ten percent of patients will develop malignant peripheral nerve sheath tumors, which can be highly aggressive.

Therapy

Excision of tumors is palliative and should be reserved for symptomatic or grossly disfiguring lesions. Surgery is not practical for patients with a large burden of disease. Simple excision is often performed when there are few or symptomatic neurofibromas. Many small lesions can be treated at once using monopolar diathermy with a wire loop. Healing is by secondary intention.

Vaporization with the carbon dioxide laser has also been used to treat neurofibromas.

Methods for treating plexiform neurofibromas and malignant peripheral nerve sheath tumors with angiogenesis inhibitors and anti-inflammatory agents are largely experimental. Thalidomide and 3-D conformal radiotherapy have also been used.

Symptomatic or growing optic gliomas in children are treated with a combination of carboplatin and vincristine.

Ketotifen has been used with success to treat pain and pruritus: 2 to 4 mg p.o. daily. Common antihistamines typically do not work for pruritus in NF1.

Café au lait macules can be treated cosmetically with the Nd:YAG, ruby, or pulsed dye laser.

Suggested Readings

Drappier JC, Khosrotehrani K, Zeller J, et al. Medical management of neurofibromatosis 1: A cross-sectional study of 383 patients. *J Am Acad Dermatol*. 2003 Sep;49(3):440–444.

Eichenfield LF, Levy ML, Paller AS, et al. Guidelines of care for neurofibromatosis type 1. American Academy of Dermatology Guidelines/Outcomes Committee. *J Am Acad Dermatol*. 1997 Oct;37(4):625–630.

Ferner RE, Huson SM, Thomas N, et al. Guidelines for the diagnosis and management of individuals with neurofibromatosis 1. *J Med Genet*. 2007 Feb;44(2):81–88.

Listernick R, Charrow J. The neurofibromatoses. In: Fitzpatrick TB, Wolff K, eds. *Fitzpatrick's Dermatology in General Medicine*. 7th Ed. New York, NY: McGraw-Hill; 2008:1331–1338.

Parsons CM, Canter RJ, Khatri VP. Surgical management of neurofibromatosis. *Surg Oncol Clin N Am*. 2009 Jan;18(1):175–196, x.

Yohay K. Neurofibromatosis types 1 and 2. *Neurologist*. 2006 Mar;12(2):86–93.

Pseudofolliculitis Barbae

Diagnosis Synopsis

Pseudofolliculitis barbae, commonly known as "shaving bumps," is an inflammatory disease of hair-bearing areas incited by shaving. The close shaving of curly hair causes the hair to penetrate the wall of the follicle and extend into the dermis as it grows back or to curve back on itself and pierce the skin, such as with an ingrown hair. The condition is common among black men, particularly black policemen and military personnel, who are required to be clean shaven.

Methods of close shaving that predispose to the development of pseudofolliculitis barbae include using razors with multiple blades, plucking hairs with tweezers, shaving against the grain of hair growth, and pulling the skin taut while shaving. Pseudofolliculitis barbae is primarily a cosmetic concern, but it can lead to scarring, infection, hyperpigmentation, and keloid formation.

Pseudofolliculitis pubis is a similar condition that occurs in the genital area after pubic hair is shaved. The shaving of the axillae may cause a similar condition.

Look For

Multiple flesh-colored to erythematous papules with a hair shaft in the center on areas of the skin that are shaved (typically the beard area) **(Figs. 4-230–4-232)**. Pustules and abscess formation can occur if the lesions become infected. In chronic cases, postinflammatory hyperpigmentation, scarring, and/or keloid formation may be seen. Chronic lesions may cause the grooving of the skin, particularly in the anterior neck and submandibular areas **(Fig. 4-233)**.

The mustache area is often spared.

Hirsute women who shave may present with pseudofolliculitis barbae; evaluation for an endocrine disorder, such as polycystic ovarian syndrome, is indicated in these cases.

Dark Skin Considerations

Multiple moderately inflamed lesions concentrated on the facial and neck areas with prominent hairs. The eruption is papular and/or pustular, especially in acute lesions that may easily bleed with shaving. Hyperpigmentation is common in black patients.

Diagnostic Pearls

- Examine for curved hairs that can be lifted from the papules with a fine needle.
- Patients with acne keloidalis nuchae may also have pseudofolliculitis barbae.

Differential Diagnosis and Pitfalls

- Tinea barbae
- Acne
- Bacterial folliculitis
- Sarcoidosis (usually develops into larger papules and plaques)

Immunocompromised Patient Differential Diagnosis

- Molluscum contagiosum (umbilicated papules)
- Verruca vulgaris
- Cryptococcus
- Histoplasmosis

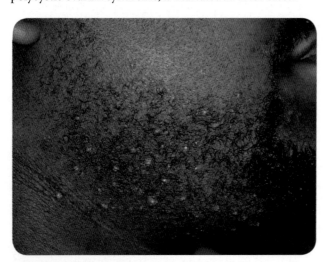

Figure 4-230 The neck is a common location for an inflammatory reaction to ingrown hairs.

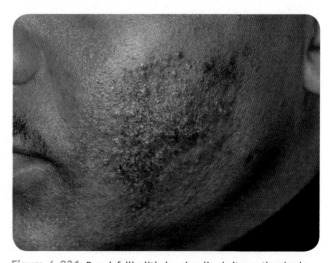

Figure 4-231 Pseudofolliculitis in a localized site on the cheek.

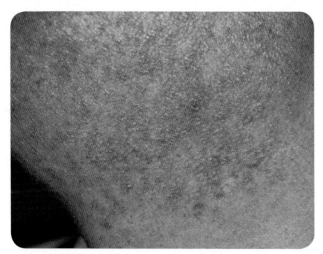

Figure 4-232 Multiple small papules of pseudofolliculitis barbae.

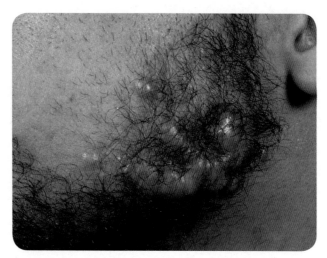

Figure 4-233 Extensive keloidal reaction associated with ingrown hairs.

✓ Best Tests

- This is largely a clinical diagnosis. If the diagnosis is in doubt, biopsy will be confirmatory. Bacterial and/or fungal culture can rule out infectious etiologies if the diagnosis is not certain.

▲▲ Management Pearls

- If possible, stop shaving.
- There are specialized razors that allow for a less close shave and, thereby, prevent the hairs from growing inward. Shaving should be done in the direction of hair growth and without pulling the skin taut. A sharp razor is recommended, and care should be taken to avoid shaving over the same area more than twice. Shave with either a single-blade razor or an electric razor on the highest setting (i.e., minimize close shaving). Alternatively, hair clippers or a safety razor can also be used on its gentlest setting.
- Instruct the patient on how to extract the "foreign body" by lifting the embedded distal end of the ingrown hair from the papule with a pair of tweezers or a needle. The patient should not pluck the hair out.
- Treat any secondary infection with the appropriate antibiotics.

Therapy

The best way to treat the condition is to stop shaving either permanently or temporarily until inflammatory papules and pustules have cleared and no ingrown hairs remain (1 to 2 months for mild cases, 2 to 3 months for moderate cases, and 6 to 12 months for severe cases).

Beards may be kept trimmed to 0.5 cm in length during a period of temporary shaving cessation.

If stopping shaving is not possible, instruct the patient to soak face with a warm, wet cloth prior to shaving and to use shaving gels. Institute other modifications to the shaving regimen as above.

1% hydrocortisone cream or lotion or a combination of clioquinol 3%/hydrocortisone 1% may be used after shaving.

Consider clindamycin 1% lotion or benzoyl peroxide 5%/clindamycin 1% gel applied once daily (after shaving, when applicable) or twice daily.

Topical retinoids such as tretinoin (0.025% to 0.1%) applied nightly and/or doxycycline 100 mg once or twice daily might be helpful.

Chemical depilatory lotions or pastes such as calcium thioglycolate or barium sulfide may be used, approximately every 2 or 3 days. Care must be taken to carefully rinse these agents off: calcium thioglycolate after 10 to 15 min and barium sulfide after 3 to 5 min. Irritant contact dermatitis is a possible side effect.

Eflornithine hydrochloride cream 1% twice daily might be useful in men and women.

Electrolysis, laser, chemical peels, and surgical depilation techniques have been used; laser treatment is particularly effective. The long pulsed diode and Nd:YAG lasers may be best for pigmented skin types.

Tretinoin or hydroquinone 4% may be useful to treat hyperpigmentation associated with pseudofolliculitis barbae.

Suggested Readings

Bridgeman-Shah S. The medical and surgical therapy of pseudofolliculitis barbae. *Dermatol Ther*. 2004;17(2):158–163.

Cook-Bolden FE, Barba A, Halder R, et al. Twice-daily applications of benzoyl peroxide 5%/clindamycin 1% gel versus vehicle in the treatment of pseudofolliculitis barbae. *Cutis*. 2004 Jun;73(6 Suppl.):18–24.

Garcia-Zuazaga J. Pseudofolliculitis barbae: Review and update on new treatment modalities. *Mil Med*. 2003 Jul;168(7):561–564.

McMichael A, Guzman Sanchez D, Kelly P. Folliculitis and the follicular occlusion tetrad. In: Bolognia J, Jorizzo JL, Rapini RP, eds. *Dermatology*. 2nd Ed. St. Louis, MO: Mosby; 2008:524–526.

Quarles FN, Brody H, Johnson BA, et al. Pseudofolliculitis barbae. *Dermatol Ther*. 2007 May–Jun;20(3):133–136.

Ross EV, Cooke LM, Timko AL, et al. Treatment of pseudofolliculitis barbae in skin types IV, V, and VI with a long-pulsed neodymium:yttrium aluminum garnet laser. *J Am Acad Dermatol*. 2002 Aug;47(2):263–270.

Scheinfeld NS. Pseudofolliculitis barbae. *Skinmed*. 2004 May–Jun;3(3): 165–166.

Smith EP, Winstanley D, Ross EV. Modified superlong pulse 810 nm diode laser in the treatment of pseudofolliculitis barbae in skin types V and VI. *Dermatol Surg*. 2005 Mar;31(3):297–301.

Weaver SM, Sagaral EC. Treatment of pseudofolliculitis barbae using the long-pulse Nd:YAG laser on skin types V and VI. *Dermatol Surg*. 2003 Dec;29(12):1187–1191.

Pseudoxanthoma Elasticum

Diagnosis Synopsis

Pseudoxanthoma elasticum (PXE) is an inherited disorder of abnormal calcification affecting elastic fibers in the dermis, retina, and cardiovascular system. PXE is inherited in autosomal recessive fashion. The basic defect is in the ABCC6 gene, which codes for a cellular transport protein. However, the exact relation between the genetic defect and the phenotype remains to be determined. A correlation of the severity of PXE with high calcium intake has been suggested.

Cutaneous lesions often begin in childhood as "leathery" skin at flexural sites but may not be noted until adolescence due to their asymptomatic nature. The disorder is frequently undiagnosed until the third or fourth decade of life. A retinal elastic lamina change, called the angioid streak, is a characteristic of the condition. It appears later than the skin changes but is present in nearly 100% of patients by age 30. Retinal hemorrhages, leading to central vision loss, and gastrointestinal (GI) hemorrhages are potential complications of the disease. Patients may also have hypertension, mitral valve prolapse, and accelerated arthrosclerosis. For unknown reasons, PXE is more common in women. There is no known predilection for any ethnicity.

Look For

Small, yellowish papules and plaques that cover the sides of the neck, axillae, the antecubital and popliteal spaces as well as the inguinal and periumbilical areas in a linear or reticular pattern; these papules frequently clinically resemble "plucked chicken skin" (Figs. 4-234 and 4-235). Lesions tend to be symmetrical. Mucous membranes, such as the inner lip, rectum, and vagina, may demonstrate yellowish papules.

Patients may have perforating lesions such as elastosis perforans serpiginosa, which presents with multiple papules with an irregular, protruding core that represents elastic tissue being eliminated from the skin. The late laxity of skin is typical, especially in flexural areas (Fig. 4-236).

Retinal angioid streaks can be seen as slate gray to reddish brown, curved bands radiating from the optic disk on funduscopic exam (Fig. 4-237). Blood vessels can become calcified and may cause symptoms related to decreased blood flow (Fig. 4-238).

Diagnostic Pearls

- As the disease process continues, the skin of the neck, axillae, and groin may become soft, lax, wrinkled, and hang in folds.

Differential Diagnosis and Pitfalls

- Severe photodamage (solar elastosis)
- Poikiloderma
- Cutis laxa
- Ehlers-Danlos syndrome
- Elastosis perforans serpiginosa
- Dermatofibrosis lenticularis (Buschke-Ollendorf syndrome)
- Marfan syndrome
- Acquired PXE
- Focal dermal elastosis
- Elastoderma
- Xanthomas
- White fibrous papulosis of the neck
- Granulomatous slack skin/Cutaneous T-cell lymphoma

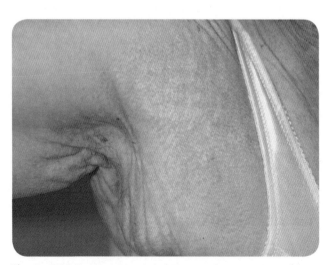

Figure 4-234 Yellowish streaks due to calcified elastic tissue in PXE.

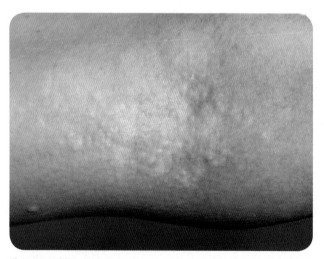

Figure 4-235 Yellowish papules, "plucked chicken skin," of PXE in a typical location.

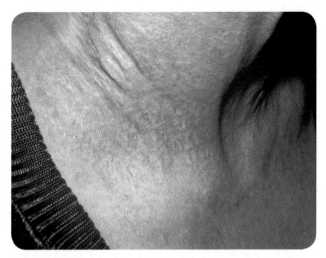

Figure 4-236 Redundant neck dermis of PXE.

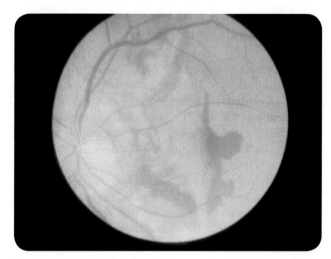

Figure 4-237 Typical retinal angioid streaks of PXE.

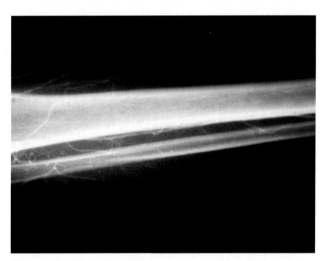

Figure 4-238 Calcified blood vessels are commonly seen in advanced PXE.

✓ Best Tests

- A skin biopsy for histopathology with an elastic (von Kossa) stain is the gold standard for diagnosis. A biopsy of a scar or normal-appearing skin may be diagnostic in patients without typical skin findings.
- Further workup and preventative measures are as follows:
  - Blood pressure assessment and monitoring.
  - Hematology and complete fasting lipid profile.
  - Fecal occult blood test.
  - Serum chemistries, including complete liver and kidney profiles.
  - Funduscopic exam with retinal photos. Patients should regularly test themselves using an Amsler grid. Repeat funduscopic exam annually or biannually.

  - Doppler ankle-brachial index measurements are indicated in patients with claudication.
  - Perform echocardiography for patients with a heart murmur.

▲▲ Management Pearls

- Because of the eye lesions, contact sports and heavy lifting/straining are not recommended for patients with PXE.
- Advise smoking cessation, when applicable. Tobacco may exacerbate the disease course. Optimize the management of any concomitant hypertension or lipid abnormalities. Patients should also be advised to avoid excess alcohol use.
- Diet and exercise are also important. Patients should follow a heart-healthy diet and restrict their dietary calcium intake to 800 mg per day.
- PXE patients *must* be routinely followed by an ophthalmologist. The viewing of wavy lines on an Amsler grid should prompt immediate ophthalmologic evaluation.
- Offer genetic counseling to patients and their family members. Patients with GI hemorrhage should be seen by a gastroenterologist; likewise, patients with cardiovascular manifestations should be followed by a cardiologist.

Therapy

Risk factor modification and preventative measures as above.

A low-calcium and phosphorus diet may be beneficial (800 mg calcium per day).

Patients should avoid the use of any anticoagulants or antiplatelet agents on a long-term basis.

Pentoxifylline (400 mg p.o. before each meal) is occasionally prescribed to patients with claudication.

Patients with mitral valve insufficiency require prophylactic antibiotics prior to the dental and surgical procedures.

There is no specific treatment for the skin findings of PXE. Plastic surgery to remove lax skin often achieves good cosmetic results.

There is anecdotal evidence that certain vitamin and mineral supplements may be advantageous in retinal disease (vitamins A, C, E, zinc, selenium, and copper).

Suggested Readings

Bercovitch L, Terry P. Pseudoxanthoma elasticum 2004. *J Am Acad Dermatol.* 2004 Jul;51(1 Suppl.):S13–S14.

Lacouture ME, Paller AS. Heritable disorders of connective tissue with skin changes. In: Fitzpatrick TB, Wolff K, eds. *Fitzpatrick's Dermatology in General Medicine.* 7th Ed. New York, NY: McGraw-Hill; 2008:1304–1308.

Ng AB, O'Sullivan ST, Sharpe DT. Plastic surgery and pseudoxanthoma elasticum. *Br J Plast Surg.* 1999 Oct;52(7):594–596.

Ohtani T, Furukawa F. Pseudoxanthoma elasticum. *J Dermatol.* 2002 Oct;29(10):615–620.

Ringpfeil F, Lebwohl MG, Christiano AM, et al. Pseudoxanthoma elasticum: Mutations in the MRP6 gene encoding a transmembrane ATP-binding cassette (ABC) transporter. *Proc Natl Acad Sci U S A.* 2000 May;97(11):6001–6006.

Ringpfeil F, Uitto J. Heritable disorders of connective tissue. In: Bolognia J, Jorizzo JL, Rapini RP, eds. *Dermatology.* 2nd Ed. St. Louis, MO: Mosby; 2008:1490–1493.

Uitto J, Frieden I, Hirschhorn K, et al. Disorders of connective tissue. In: Spitz JL, ed. *Genodermatoses: A Clinical Guide to Genetic Skin Disorders.* 2nd Ed. Philadelphia, PA: Lippincott Williams & Wilkins; 2005:145–147.

Viljoen DL, Bloch C, Beighton P. Plastic surgery in pseudoxanthoma elasticum: experience in nine patients. *Plast Reconstr Surg.* 1990 Feb;85(2):233–238.

Diagnosis Synopsis

Rosacea is a common, chronic inflammatory condition of unknown etiology. It presents with facial flushing and localized erythema, telangiectasia, papules, and pustules on the nose, cheeks, brow, and chin. There are four main subtypes of the disease: erythematotelangiectatic, papulopustular, phymatous, and ocular rosacea.

Erythematotelangiectatic rosacea presents with flushing and prolonged erythema and redness of the central portion of the face. Patients often complain of stinging or burning sensations on the skin.

In papulopustular rosacea, acneiform papules and pustules predominate; there is also erythema and edema of the central face with relative sparing of the periocular areas. In papulopustular rosacea, dramatic swelling can result in lymphedematous changes manifesting as solid facial edema or lead to phymatous changes.

In patients with the phymatous subtype of rosacea, chronic inflammation and edema result in a marked thickening of the skin with sebaceous hyperplasia, resulting in an enlarged, cobblestoned appearance of affected skin, most commonly on the nose. Men are more often affected.

Ocular rosacea presents with conjunctivitis, blepharitis, and hyperemia. Patients complain of dry, irritated, itchy eyes. Keratitis, scleritis, and iritis are potential but infrequent complications.

The etiology and pathogenesis of rosacea are poorly understood, but cutaneous vascular changes and environmental exposures, such as infectious agents, sunlight, and certain foods or drugs, may play a role.

Rosacea commonly develops in individuals aged 30 to 50. Females tend to present at a younger age than males; however, overall prevalence is equal in men and women. Fair-skinned individuals are primarily affected, though the disease is seen in Mediterranean skin types as well. Rosacea fulminans (pyoderma faciale) refers to the sudden onset of severe facial pustulation with abscess and sinus tract formation. Systemic signs and symptoms are present.

Dark Skin Considerations

Rosacea is thought to be rare in blacks, although mild cases limited to erythema and/or telangiectasia may simply remain overlooked.

Immunocompromised Patient Considerations

Acne rosacea has been reported as a manifestation of immune reconstitution syndrome in HIV patients starting antiretroviral treatment.

Look For

Rosacea is one of the classic causes of the "red face." Erythema and edema in the central portion of the face are common in almost all of the rosacea subtypes (Figs. 4-239 and 4-240). In papulopustular rosacea, erythematous papules and pustules located on the nose and cheeks are most prominent. There is often a varying amount of background erythema and telangiectasia (Fig. 4-241). Some individuals present with erythema alone and/or telangiectasias (erythematotelangiectasia variant). In patients with ocular involvement, conjunctival injection and chalazia may be seen. Rhinophyma (hypertrophy of the distal nose) is more common in men (Fig. 4-242). Facial edema may also be present.

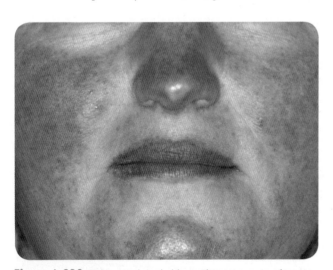

Figure 4-239 Malar, nasal, and chin erythemas are very characteristic of rosacea.

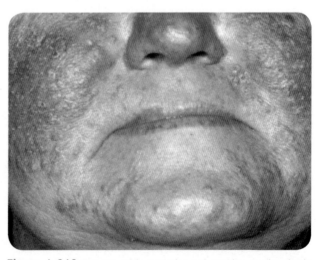

Figure 4-240 Rosacea with extensive red papules on the cheeks and chin and sparing the upper lip.

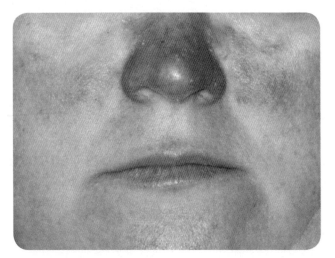

Figure 4-241 Malar and nasal red papules on background of telangiectasias in rosacea.

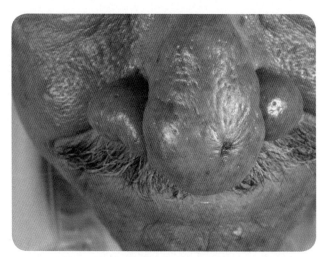

Figure 4-242 Marked hypertrophy of nasal soft tissues (rhinophyma) is one of the late complications of rosacea.

Extrafascial involvement is rare, but the disease may involve the neck and superior chest.

Rosacea fulminans presents with pustules, nodules, and abscesses with sinus tract formation.

Dark Skin Considerations

Most presenting cases in blacks are of the papulopustular variety.

Diagnostic Pearls

- Ask the patient about ocular symptoms; many patients experience a gritty sensation in their eyes and have evidence of conjunctivitis, episcleritis, iritis, and keratitis.
- Rosacea patients do not have comedones, which are frequently seen in acne.
- Seborrheic dermatitis is commonly observed in patients who also have rosacea.

?? Differential Diagnosis and Pitfalls

Papulopustular Rosacea

- Acne vulgaris
- Perioral dermatitis (periorificial dermatitis)
- Bromoderma
- Folliculitis
- Gram-negative folliculitis
- Sarcoidosis
- Demodicidosis
- Pyoderma faciale

Erythematotelangiectatic Rosacea

- Menopause, "hot flashes"
- Carcinoid syndrome
- Pheochromocytoma
- Medullary thyroid carcinoma
- VIPoma
- Lupus erythematosus
- Seborrheic dermatitis
- Photodermatitis
- Mastocytosis

Dark Skin Considerations

- Sarcoidosis
- Systemic lupus erythematosus
- Mycosis fungoides

✓ Best Tests

- This is a clinical diagnosis. If the situation warrants, testing for urinary 5-HIAA may be performed to rule out carcinoid syndrome and serology to rule out lupus erythematosus.
- There is no substantial evidence that testing for *Helicobacter pylori* in the stomach (and treating it specifically) has any value in rosacea.

▲▲ Management Pearls

- In severe cases, use of both an oral therapy and a topical therapy is often warranted.

- Advise patients to avoid triggers that aggravate vasodilation (e.g., coffee, tea, hot drinks in general, spicy foods, chocolate, and alcohol). Encourage the use of sunscreens and sun-protective clothing.
- Patients with long-standing or severe rosacea should be seen by an ophthalmologist.

Therapy

Conservative Therapy
Individuals with rosacea should be counseled on avoidance of known triggers, including spicy foods, alcohol, emotional stress, extremes of temperature, etc. An appropriate use of broad-spectrum sunscreens and sun avoidance are also important. Camouflage makeups with green- or yellow-based preparations are helpful in masking underlying redness.

Topical Therapies
There are many topical medications that are reported effective in the treatment of rosacea. These topical agents are used most effectively in papulopustular rosacea. Only specific metronidazole preparations and 15% azelaic acid gel have an FDA indication for rosacea.

Topical therapies for rosacea include the following:

- Metronidazole cream, gel
- Sodium sulfacetamide lotion, wash
- Azelaic acid 15% gel
- Erythromycin and clindamycin lotion, solution
- Benzoyl peroxide 5% to 10% cream, lotion, gel, or wash
- Calcineurin inhibitors such as tacrolimus ointment and pimecrolimus cream
- Tretinoin cream and gel

Systemic Therapies
Tetracyclines are a mainstay of therapy in rosacea and are first line: tetracycline 500 to 1,000 mg twice daily OR doxycycline 100 to 200 mg daily OR minocycline 50 mg twice daily for at least 2 to 3 months, then taper to 1 pill daily. Oral erythromycin is also a good choice: 250 to 500 mg twice daily. Low dose doxycycline (20 mg twice daily or 40 mg slow release form daily) has also shown effectiveness for rosacea.

Alternative Regimens

- Oral metronidazole 200 mg twice daily
- Azithromycin 250 to 500 mg daily three times weekly

Isotretinoin is also effective in treating severe papulopustular rosacea and rosacea fulminans.

Therapies aimed at specific disease manifestations and subtypes include the following:

- Telangiectasias/erythematotelangiectasia rosacea—vascular lasers (pulsed dye, KTP (potassium-titanyl-phosphate), etc), intense pulsed light therapy, and camouflage cosmetics
- Flushing—clonidine 0.05 mg twice daily, intense pulsed light, pulsed dye laser, and beta blockers (nadolol 40 mg daily)
- Rhinophyma—surgical paring/sculpting, electrosurgery, and laser (argon, carbon dioxide, Nd:YAG [neodymium-yttrium-aluminum-garnet])
- Rosacea fulminans—prednisolone 1 mg/kg daily is usually required while isotretinoin is being initiated and then tapered over several weeks. Isotretinoin therapy is continued for several months.

Suggested Readings

Baldwin HE. Systemic therapy for rosacea. *Skin Therapy Lett*. 2007 Mar;12(2):1–5, 9.

Crawford GH, Pelle MT, James WD. Rosacea: I. Etiology, pathogenesis, and subtype classification. *J Am Acad Dermatol*. 2004 Sep;51(3):327–341; quiz 342–344.

Kyriakis KP, Palamaras I, Terzoudi S, et al. Epidemiologic aspects of rosacea. *J Am Acad Dermatol*. 2005 Nov;53(5):918–919.

Laube S, Lanigan SW. Laser treatment of rosacea. *J Cosmet Dermatol*. 2002 Dec;1(4):188–195.

Pelle MT, Crawford GH, James WD. Rosacea: II. Therapy. *J Am Acad Dermatol*. 2004 Oct;51(4):499–512; quiz 513–514.

Pelle MT. Rosacea. In: Fitzpatrick TB, Wolff K, eds. *Fitzpatrick's Dermatology in General Medicine*. 7th Ed. New York, NY: McGraw-Hill; 2008: 703–709.

Powell FC. Clinical practice. Rosacea. *N Engl J Med*. 2005 Feb;352(8): 793–803.

Quarterman MJ, Johnson DW, Abele DC, et al. Ocular rosacea. Signs, symptoms, and tear studies before and after treatment with doxycycline. *Arch Dermatol*. 1997 Jan;133(1):49–54.

Scott C, Staughton RC, Bunker CJ, et al. Acne vulgaris and acne rosacea as part of immune reconstitution disease in HIV-1 infected patients starting antiretroviral therapy. *Int J STD AIDS*. 2008 Jul;19(7):493–495.

Stone DU, Chodosh J. Ocular rosacea: An update on pathogenesis and therapy. *Curr Opin Ophthalmol*. 2004 Dec;15(6):499–502.

Thiboutot D, Thieroff-Ekerdt R, Graupe K. Efficacy and safety of azelaic acid (15%) gel as a new treatment for papulopustular rosacea: Results from two vehicle-controlled, randomized phase III studies. *J Am Acad Dermatol*. 2003 Jun;48(6):836–845.

van Zuuren EJ, Graber MA, Hollis S, et al. Interventions for rosacea. *Cochrane Database Syst Rev*. 2005 Jul;(3):CD003262.

van Zuuren EJ, Gupta AK, Gover MD, et al. Systematic review of rosacea treatments. *J Am Acad Dermatol*. 2007 Jan;56(1):107–115.

Wilkin J, Dahl M, Detmar M, et al. Standard classification of rosacea: Report of the National Rosacea Society Expert Committee on the Classification and Staging of Rosacea. *J Am Acad Dermatol*. 2002 Apr;46(4):584–587.

Sarcoidosis

■■ Diagnosis Synopsis

Sarcoidosis is an immune-mediated systemic disorder that is typified by the granuloma formation of the lung parenchyma and the skin, but it can affect any other organs. The inciting immune-activating agent remains unknown (autoimmune versus infectious versus environmental). The disease affects all ages, ethnicities, and both sexes, with peak incidence demonstrating a bimodal age distribution: ages 25 to 35 and 45 to 65. It is most commonly observed in black women in their fourth decade.

The clinical manifestations of sarcoidosis can be divided into cutaneous and systemic. Approximately 25% of patients will have cutaneous involvement and, commonly, many patients have skin-limited disease. Asymptomatic red-brown dermal papules and/or plaques that favor the face, neck, upper extremities, and upper trunk are the most common specific cutaneous sarcoid lesions. Less common manifestations include sarcoid lesions with epidermal change such as scale, hypopigmentation, subcutaneous nodules, cicatricial alopecia, ulceration, and scar.

Erythema nodosum (EN) is associated with sarcoidosis and is a common nonspecific cutaneous finding. It follows a subacute, self-limiting course that is characterized by multiple well-demarcated, tender, bruise-like, or erythematous subcutaneous nodules that are present on the lower extremities (most commonly on the shins). EN due to sarcoidosis usually spontaneously remits and does not require systemic treatment.

Systemic manifestations of sarcoidosis are profound and can affect the lungs, peripheral lymph nodes, heart, kidneys, gastrointestinal tract, nervous system, liver, spleen, bone, muscle, and endocrine glands. Approximately 90% of patients will have lung involvement. Pulmonary fibrosis and bronchiolectasis result in "honeycombing" of the lung and represent end-stage lung disease due to chronic granulomatous inflammation. Hilar lymphadenopathy is asymptomatic and affects 90% of patients. Approximately 10% of patients have hypercalcemia.

The clinical course of sarcoidosis is variable, ranging from an acute, self-limiting disease that spontaneously remits to a chronic progressive course resulting in death. Approximately two-thirds of patients experience spontaneous remission, and 15% to 30% of patients experience a chronic progressive course. Mortality is most commonly due to significant granulomatous disease in the lungs and heart, leading to respiratory failure, cardiac arrhythmias, and heart failure. Central nervous system (CNS), liver, and renal diseases are also well-known causes of morbidity and mortality.

The pathogenesis of sarcoidosis is poorly understood. However, it is characterized by noncaseating epithelioid granulomas made up mostly of CD4+ helper T cells, a predominantly Th1 type immune response, and elevated levels of IFN-γ and IL-2.

Variants

- Lupus pernio—Violaceous papules and plaques that are most commonly found on areas affected by the cold (hence, the name pernio): nose, ears, and cheeks. Approximately 75% of patients with lupus pernio have chronic sarcoidosis of the lungs, and approximately 50% of patients will have upper respiratory tract involvement. Cystic lesions in the distal portion of the phalanges can be seen. In contrast to other cutaneous sarcoid lesions, lupus pernio can result in scarring.
- Löfgren syndrome—EN with fever, hilar adenopathy, anterior uveitis, and migrating polyarthritis.
- Darier-Roussy disease—Also known as subcutaneous nodular sarcoidosis, this disease is characterized by asymptomatic, firm, mobile subcutaneous nodules without epidermal involvement.
- Heerfordt syndrome—Fever, uveitis, parotid gland enlargement, and cranial nerve palsies. The facial nerve is often affected.

◉ Look For

There is a wide range of cutaneous findings.

Specific Sarcoidosis Findings

- Red-brown macules and papules seen on extensor surfaces or on the face, particularly the nasolabial folds and the periorbital areas (Fig. 4-243).
- Red-brown or violaceous infiltrated plaques on the face, scalp, extremities, buttocks, and back. These plaques can have peripheral elevation and central hypopigmentation.

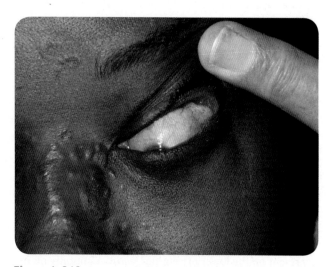

Figure 4-243 Enlargement of lacrimal glands and small flesh-colored facial papules are characteristics of sarcoidosis.

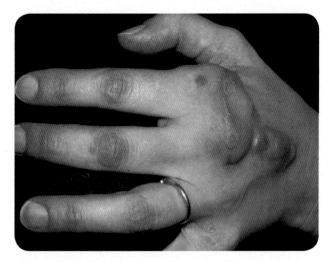

Figure 4-244 Cutaneous papules and subcutaneous nodules are common in sarcoidosis.

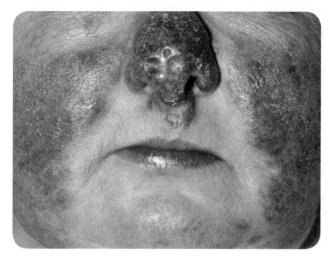

Figure 4-245 Lupus pernio characteristic of sarcoidosis with infiltration and atrophy of the nose.

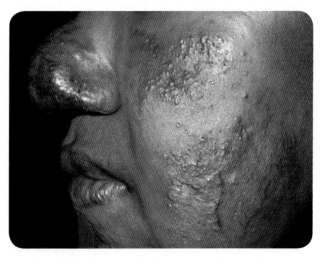

Figure 4-246 Infiltrated and atrophic plaques on the face and on the nose (lupus pernio).

- Firm, oval, flesh-colored, or violaceous subcutaneous nodules may be present on the trunk or the extremities (Fig. 4-244).
- Lupus pernio consists of violaceous, firm nodules and plaques. They are most often seen on the distal nose but are also seen on the ears, lips, and face. Hands, fingers, and toes are less affected sites (Figs. 4-245 and 4-246).

Nonspecific Findings

- EN—Multiple well-demarcated, tender, bruise-like or erythematous, red-brown subcutaneous nodules that are present on the lower extremities (most commonly on the shins).

Note that preexisting scars or prior sites of trauma are common sites for cutaneous lesions to form.

Dark Skin Considerations

The following clinical forms of cutaneous sarcoidosis are noted almost exclusively in darkly pigmented skin:

- Ichthyosiform sarcoidosis—The skin is parched, scaly, and ashy white, without the presence of papules or nodules.
- Hypopigmented macular form—Hypopigmented macules without the presence of papules or nodules.
- Annular configurations of violaceous papules and/or nodules.

Diagnostic Pearls

- Check for enlarged lacrimal glands by everting the upper eyelid.
- Some lesions of sarcoidosis can have significant atrophy in addition to infiltration.

?? Differential Diagnosis and Pitfalls

Sarcoidosis is a diagnosis of exclusion, on a clinical and histological level. Clinically, sarcoid papules, nodules, and plaques are not unique, and a histologic evaluation is often required. The histological differential is broad, and detailed histological findings are beyond the scope of this text. Special stains for acid-fast and fungal organisms and tissue cultures should be obtained when necessary.

The following is a clinical differential.

Papules

- Leprosy—Skin lesions are anesthetic. Look for inflamed nerve and acid-fast bacilli on skin biopsy.
- Tuberculosis—Tuberculin skin testing (Mantoux test); submit sputum for smear and culture of acid-fast bacilli.
- Lichen planus—Violaceous, flat-topped papules that are pruritic. Biopsy will differentiate.
- Trichoepitheliomas
- Adenoma sebaceum
- Lupus erythematosus—Check ANA, anti-ds DNA.
- Secondary syphilis—Check RPR, fluorescent treponemal antibody (FTA), look for systemic symptoms, history of primary chancre.
- Acne rosacea
- Granuloma annulare—Biopsy will assist in differentiation.

Nodules

- Leukemia/lymphoma cutis
- Cutaneous lymphoid hyperplasia
- Tertiary syphilis—Check RPR, FTA, look for systemic symptoms, history of primary chancre.

Plaques

- Tuberculosis—Tuberculin skin testing (Mantoux test); submit sputum for smear and culture of acid-fast bacilli.
- Necrobiosis lipoidica
- Psoriasis—Pruritic, characteristic silvery, and scaly plaques.
- Tinea corporis—Check KOH.
- Morphea—Look for shiny, taut appearance. Biopsy will assist in differentiation.
- Ichthyosis
- Leprosy—Lesions are anesthetic; look for inflamed nerve and acid-fast bacilli on skin biopsy.
- Leishmaniasis—Usually develop into plaques with central ulceration. Microscopy or biopsy should reveal the parasite in majority of cases.
- Wegener granulomatosis
- Rhinoscleroma

✔ Best Tests

- A punch biopsy should show sarcoidal granulomas. Similar granulomas can be found in other body tissues. Various specialized techniques, stains, and cultures may be performed to rule out other diagnoses.
- Approximately 30% of patients have elevated ANA titers. There is cutaneous anergy in sarcoidosis; more than 60% of patients have a blunted immune response to the tuberculin skin test. In about 60% of patients, serum angiotensin-converting enzyme (ACE) level is also elevated. However, it has a false-positive rate of 10%. ACE level has been more appropriately used for monitoring disease progression.
- Routine laboratory investigations are aimed at determining the extent of internal organ involvement. A CBC with differential, a comprehensive electrolyte panel, and liver and renal function tests should be ordered. Perform a serum calcium and 24-h urine calcium determination, as many patients have hypercalcemia and hypercalciuria.
- Chest radiography should be performed and will often reveal bilateral hilar adenopathy with or without pulmonary infiltrates. A CT scan of the chest will provide similar information. Pulmonary function tests may show decreased vital capacity, diffusion capacity, and total lung capacity. An ECG should be performed, as patients may experience arrhythmias or heart block.

▲▲▲ Management Pearls

- Even limited lesions of sarcoidosis warrant a systemic evaluation with radiography and blood tests.
- The cutaneous lesions of sarcoidosis respond to systemic corticosteroid therapy; however, in the absence of other systemic involvement, this long-term therapy is difficult to justify. Likewise, therapy for internal involvement often takes precedence over that of the skin lesions, and response to treatment is often variable depending on the type of tissue involved.
- Patients should be assessed by a dermatologist and may need other specialty consultations in fields such as ophthalmology, pulmonology, cardiology, neurology, and nephrology.

Therapy

Corticosteroids remain the mainstay of therapy. Therapeutic strategy should be dictated by the severity and level of systemic involvement.

Corticosteroid Therapy
- Prednisone—0.5 to 1 mg/kg p.o. daily for 4 to 6 weeks with slow taper. Initiation, taper, and maintenance doses should be determined by the activity of lung disease or for recalcitrant or deforming skin disease.
- Triamcinolone—3 to 20 mg/mL intralesional injection once monthly until lesions flatten (for mild cutaneous limited disease).

(Continued)

- Clobetasol—Apply topically with or without occlusion to affected areas twice daily until lesions resolve (for mild cutaneous limited disease).

Steroid Sparing Therapy

This type of therapy should be instituted in steroid-resistant sarcoidosis or in patients who are unable to tolerate steroids.

- Methotrexate—7.5 to 25 mg weekly for at least 4 to 6 months
- Thalidomide—50 to 300 mg per day
- Minocycline—200 mg per day
- Isotretinoin—0.5 to 2.0 mg/kg/day for 3 to 8 months
- Allopurinol—100 to 300 mg per day
- Chloroquine or hydroxychloroquine—250 to 750 mg p.o. daily or every other day for 6 to 9 months. (**Note:** max 3.5 mg/kg daily for chloroquine, and max 6.5 mg/kg daily for hydroxychloroquine.)
- Pentoxifylline—400 mg p.o. three times daily
- Cyclophosphamide—Start at 25 to 50 mg p.o. daily, increase by increments of 25 mg; not to exceed 150 mg per day.

Biologics

- Infliximab—IV infusion at doses of 3 to 10 mg/kg at 0, 2, and 6 weeks and as indicated thereafter
- Adalimumab—40 mg subcutaneously (SC) either weekly or every 2 weeks

Suggested Readings

Asukata Y, Ishihara M, Hasumi Y, et al. Guidelines for the diagnosis of ocular sarcoidosis. *Ocul Immunol Inflamm*. 2008 May–Jun;16(3):77–81.

Badgwell C, Rosen T. Cutaneous sarcoidosis therapy updated. *J Am Acad Dermatol*. 2007 Jan;56(1):69–83.

Baughman RP, Lower EE. Evidence-based therapy for cutaneous sarcoidosis. *Clin Dermatol*. 2007 May–Jun;25(3):334–340.

Bonfioli AA, Orefice F. Sarcoidosis. *Semin Ophthalmol*. 2005 Jul–Sep;20(3): 177–182.

Costabel U, Ohshimo S, Guzman J. Diagnosis of sarcoidosis. *Curr Opin Pulm Med*. 2008 Sep;14(5):455–461.

Doherty CB, Rosen T. Evidence-based therapy for cutaneous sarcoidosis. *Drugs*. 2008;68(10):1361–1383.

Fernandez-Faith E, McDonnell J. Cutaneous sarcoidosis: differential diagnosis. *Clin Dermatol*. 2007 May–Jun;25(3):276–287.

Heffernan MP, Anadkat MJ. Recalcitrant cutaneous sarcoidosis responding to infliximab. *Arch Dermatol*. 2005 Jul;141(7):910–911.

Iannuzzi MC, Rybicki BA, Teirstein AS. Sarcoidosis. *N Engl J Med*. 2007 Nov;357(21):2153–2165.

Marchell RM, Judson MA. Chronic cutaneous lesions of sarcoidosis. *Clin Dermatol*. 2007 May–Jun;25(3):295–302.

Margolis R, Lowder CY. Sarcoidosis. *Curr Opin Ophthalmol*. 2007 Nov;18(6):470–475.

Rose AS, Tielker MA, Knox KS. Hepatic, ocular, and cutaneous sarcoidosis. *Clin Chest Med*. 2008 Sep;29(3):509–524, ix.

Tchernev G. Cutaneous sarcoidosis: The "great imitator": etiopathogenesis, morphology, differential diagnosis, and clinical management. *Am J Clin Dermatol*. 2006;7(6):375–382.

Sebaceous Hyperplasia

Diagnosis Synopsis

Sebaceous gland hyperplasia refers to the localized hypertrophy of the sebaceous glands, usually on the central face and forehead. Sebaceous hyperplasia may also be present on the nipples, where it is referred to as Montgomery tubercles, and on anogenital skin. Generally, this hyperplasia does not appear until after 40 years of age, but it may arise in immunocompromised patients; typically, those treated with cyclosporine. The condition is benign, and treatment is for cosmetic purposes, though in rare cases eruptions can be severe and disfiguring.

Immunocompromised Patient Considerations

Organ transplant recipients, typically those receiving cyclosporine, have a higher incidence of sebaceous hyperplasia. Extensive, rapid onset sebaceous hyperplasia has also been reported in an HIV-positive patient receiving highly active antiretroviral therapy.

Look For

Small yellow papules, often with a central dell, tend to localize on the forehead, temples, and below the eyes (Figs. 4-247–4-250). Less commonly, they may also be seen on the chest, areolae, mouth, and genitals. Lesions may be solitary, grouped, annular, or linearly arrayed.

Diagnostic Pearls

- There may be a very small dilated blood vessel (telangiectasia) visible over the rim of yellow papules.

Differential Diagnosis and Pitfalls

- Sometimes there is a central umbilication, with papules being confused with basal cell carcinoma.
- Xanthoma
- Xanthelasma
- Calcifying epithelioma of Malherbe
- Lupus miliaris disseminatus faciei
- Milia
- Rosacea/rhinophyma
- Dermal nevus
- Flat wart
- Molluscum contagiosum
- Syringoma
- Fibrous papule
- Acne vulgaris
- Colloid milium
- Trichoepithelioma

Best Tests

- This is largely a clinical exam. Perform a biopsy if the diagnosis is in doubt, typically done to rule out basal cell carcinoma.

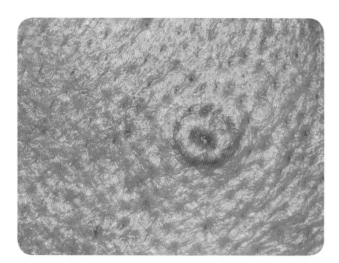

Figure 4-247 Sebaceous hyperplasia with an annular configuration of small yellow-pink papules with telangiectasias surrounding a central dell.

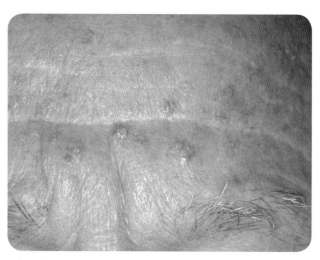

Figure 4-248 Multiple lesions of sebaceous hyperplasia are common on the forehead.

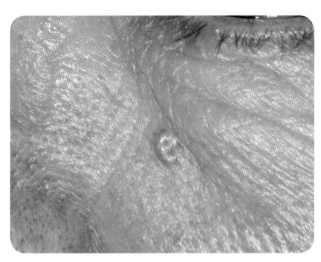

Figure 4-249 Sebaceous hyperplasia, as in this case, may so closely resemble a basal cell carcinoma that a biopsy is necessary.

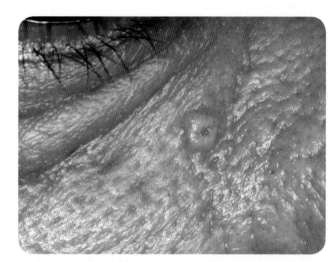

Figure 4-250 The papules on the rim of a lesion of sebaceous hyperplasia may have dilated vessels suggesting a basal cell carcinoma.

▲▲ Management Pearls
▲▲

- Sebaceous hyperplasia is a benign condition; patients requesting treatment for cosmetic purposes should be made aware that there is a risk of scarring.
- Cosmetic camouflage provides an acceptable treatment alternative for many patients.

Therapy

If treatment is desired, first-line treatments include the following:

- Low-voltage electrodesiccation with an epilating needle on the hyfrecator
- Cryosurgery

Additional options include the following:

- Isotretinoin—typically reserved only for severe or extensive involvement refractory to other therapies
- Laser therapy—pulsed dye, argon, carbon dioxide, and Er:YAG
- Bichloracetic acid crystals
- Photodynamic therapy
- Retin-A.25% cream—must be used for 6 to 18 months before seeing improvement
- Surgery/curettage

Suggested Readings

Bader RS, Scarborough DA. Surgical pearl: intralesional electrodesiccation of sebaceous hyperplasia. *J Am Acad Dermatol.* 2000 Jan;42(1 Pt 1): 127–128.

de Berker DA, Taylor AE, Quinn AG, et al. Sebaceous hyperplasia in organ transplant recipients: shared aspects of hyperplastic and dysplastic processes? *J Am Acad Dermatol.* 1996 Nov;35(5 Pt 1):696–699.

Iezzi G, Rubini C, Fioroni M, et al. Sebaceous adenoma of the cheek. *Oral Oncol.* 2002 Jan;38(1):111–113.

Kato N, Yasuoka A. "Giant" senile sebaceous hyperplasia. *J Dermatol.* 1992 Apr;19(4):238–241.

McCalmont TH. Adnexal neoplasms. In: Bolognia J, Jorizzo JL, Rapini RP, eds. *Dermatology.* 2nd Ed. St. Louis, MO: Mosby; 2008:1702.

No D, McClaren M, Chotzen V, et al. Sebaceous hyperplasia treated with a 1450-nm diode laser. *Dermatol Surg.* 2004 Mar;30(3):382–384.

Salim A, Reece SM, Smith AG, et al. Sebaceous hyperplasia and skin cancer in patients undergoing renal transplant. *J Am Acad Dermatol.* 2006 Nov;55(5):878–881.

Short KA, Williams A, Creamer D, et al. Sebaceous gland hyperplasia, human immunodeficiency virus and highly active anti-retroviral therapy. *Clin Exp Dermatol.* 2008 May;33(3):354–355.

Terrell S, Wetter R, Fraga G, et al. Penile sebaceous adenoma. *J Am Acad Dermatol.* 2007 Aug;57(2 Suppl.):S42–S43.

Sporotrichosis

■ Diagnosis Synopsis

Sporotrichosis is caused by the dimorphic fungus *Sporothrix schenckii,* found worldwide, but more commonly in the tropical and subtropical climates. The organism resides in decaying vegetation, plants, and soil. Cutaneous infection usually results from traumatic inoculation.

The lesions of sporotrichosis may present in three different patterns:

- Lymphocutaneous or sporotrichoid pattern—80% of cases
- Fixed cutaneous—occurs in endemic areas with prior exposure
- Disseminated cutaneous—occurs with systemic involvement

Extracutaneous disease is rare but manifests with osteoarticular involvement in immunocompetent individuals, whereas immunocompromised patients typically present with multisystem involvement. Pulmonary sporotrichosis is associated with alcoholism, tuberculosis, diabetes mellitus, sarcoidosis, and steroid use.

Thorny plants, such as barberry and rose bushes, are the most common source of cutaneous inoculation of sporotrichosis. Other plant exposures include sphagnum moss, straw, hay, soil, and mine timbers. Occupational exposures include farmers, florists, gardeners, and forestry workers. Outside the United States, sporotrichosis outbreaks have been associated with infected cats. Untreated cutaneous sporotrichosis usually waxes and wanes over months to years without systemic manifestations.

Immunocompromised Patient Considerations

In immunocompromised patients, multisystem disease can occur after hematogenous spread with pulmonary, central nervous system (CNS), and urogenital involvement, eventually resulting in disseminated cutaneous sporotrichosis.

◉ Look For

Lymphocutaneous

The lymphatic distribution of painless nodules on distal extremities, typically the forearm (Figs. 4-251–4-254). Initially, an erythematous papule, pustule, or nodule is seen on the distal extremity at the site of inoculation. New lesions appear along the lymphatics over several weeks. Lesions may eventually ulcerate.

Fixed Cutaneous

Absence of lymphangitic spread. Fixed lesions present as verrucous or gummatous plaques and are more commonly seen on the face.

Disseminated Cutaneous

Manifests as multiple diffusely distributed papules, nodules, ulcers, or plaques.

Immunocompromised Patient Considerations

Disseminated cutaneous sporotrichosis usually occurs in the setting of immunocompromised patients with underlying systemic involvement.

●● Diagnostic Pearls

- For lesions presenting with a lymphangitic pattern, a very careful occupational and exposure history is essential.

Immunocompromised Patient Considerations

- For immunocompromised patients presenting with disseminated cutaneous disease, it is important to search for underlying systemic involvement.

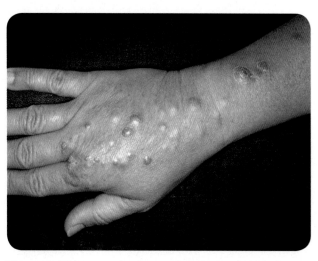

Figure 4-251 Typical lymphatic spread of sporotrichosis nodules on the arm.

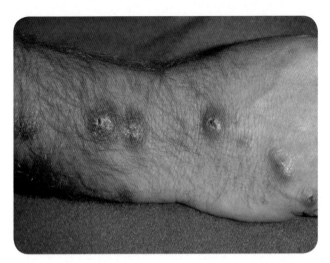

Figure 4-252 Sporotrichosis nodules frequently have ulcerations and a red halo.

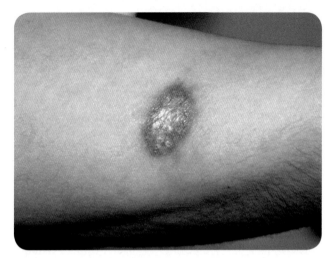

Figure 4-253 Sporotrichosis may initially be a well-delimited plaque with reddish and brown pigmentation.

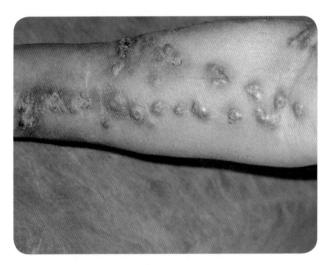

Figure 4-254 Extensive sporotrichosis on a forearm.

?? Differential Diagnosis and Pitfalls

- *Microbacterium marinum* infection may also present with a lymphocutaneous pattern on the extremity in the setting of exposure to contaminated water.
- Cellulitis has ill-defined erythema but lacks well-formed nodules.
- Furunculosis is marked by indurated tender nodules expressing purulent material.
- Thrombophlebitis is tender and erythematous but has a more rapid onset.
- Anthrax typically presents as a black, necrotic eschar.
- Tularemia may also have lymphocutaneous spread but with exposure to infected animals.
- Nocardia may also present with lymphocutaneous spread.

- Majocchi granuloma is usually a solitary plaque on the lower extremity.
- Leishmaniasis has painless, clean-based ulcerations on exposed skin but can also have a sporotrichoid pattern of spread. Travel to endemic areas is required.
- Secondary syphilis has a characteristic palm and sole rash.
- Cat-scratch disease presents with proximal lymphadenopathy on the affected extremity.
- Foreign body granulomas lack lymphocutaneous spread.
- Panniculitis is characterized by deeper indurated plaques.
- Pyoderma gangrenosum has a characteristic ulcer with an undermined border.
- Sarcoidosis is classically violaceous and uncommonly presents with a sporotrichoid pattern.
- Halogenoderma will have a history of exposure to iodine or bromine.

Immunocompromised Patient Considerations

- Other deep fungal infections (cryptococcus, coccidiomycosis, blastomycoses, and histoplasmosis)
- Cutaneous tuberculosis
- Other disseminated mycobacterial infections

✓ Best Tests

- A skin biopsy may not readily show the organisms for sporotrichosis. Fluorescent-labeled antibodies can improve the visualization of organisms.
- Diagnosis is confirmed by tissue culture. *S. schenckii* grows on most media in 3 to 5 days.

- It is important to rule out mycobacterial infections with tissue culture and stains for acid fast bacilli (AFB-Fite stain or Ziehl-Neelsen stain). Other deep fungal infections can be ruled out with mathenamine-silver stains (GMS) or tissue culture.

▲▲▲ Management Pearls

- Consultation with an infectious disease specialist is recommended.

Immunocompromised Patient Considerations

- For disseminated cutaneous sporotrichosis, it is necessary to perform additional investigational studies to rule out systemic involvement.

Therapy

Localized Cutaneous (Fixed Cutaneous or Lymphocutaneous)
Topical therapy is not sufficient.

- Itraconazole 100 to 200 mg p.o. daily for 3 to 6 months is the treatment of choice
- Oral potassium iodide solution, 5 drops three times daily gradually increased to 30 to 50 drops three times daily is also effective but has multiple side-effects
- Terbinafine 1,000 mg p.o. daily

Disseminated Cutaneous
- Amphotericin B IV 0.5 mg/kg/day up to a total of 1 to 2 g

Immunocompromised Patient Considerations
Disseminated cutaneous disease in immunocompromised patients requires IV amphotericin B.

Suggested Readings

Bustamante B, Campos PE. Endemic sporotrichosis. *Curr Opin Infect Dis.* 2001 Apr;14(2):145–149.

Chapman SW, Pappas P, Kauffmann C, et al. Comparative evaluation of the efficacy and safety of two doses of terbinafine (500 and 1000 mg day(-1)) in the treatment of cutaneous or lymphocutaneous sporotrichosis. *Mycoses.* 2004 Feb;47(1–2):62–68.

da Rosa AC, Scroferneker ML, Vettorato R, et al. Epidemiology of sporotrichosis: a study of 304 cases in Brazil. *J Am Acad Dermatol.* 2005 Mar;52(3 Pt 1):451–459.

Kauffman CA, Hajjeh R, Chapman SW; For the Mycoses Study Group. Infectious Diseases Society of America. Practice guidelines for the management of patients with sporotrichosis. *Clin Infect Dis.* 2000 Apr;30(4):684–687.

Morris-Jones R. Sporotrichosis. *Clin Exp Dermatol.* 2002 Sep;27(6): 427–431.

Rafal ES, Rasmussen JE. An unusual presentation of fixed cutaneous sporotrichosis: A case report and review of the literature. *J Am Acad Dermatol.* 1991 Nov;25(5 Pt 2):928–932.

Ramos-e-Silva M, Vasconcelos C, Carneiro S, et al. Sporotrichosis. *Clin Dermatol.* 2007 Mar–Apr;25(2):181–187.

Stalkup JR, Bell K, Rosen T. Disseminated cutaneous sporotrichosis treated with itraconazole. *Cutis.* 2002 May;69(5):371–374.

Syringomas

▪ Diagnosis Synopsis

Syringomas are benign skin-adnexal tumors that present as small, dome-shaped papules, often in a periorbital distribution; they may, however, occur at any site on the body. Syringomas likely arise from luminal cells of eccrine sweat ducts. The tumors are asymptomatic but do persist over time. They are more common in women. They occur with an increased frequency in Down syndrome patients. Treatment is for cosmetic purposes.

◉ Look For

Multiple discrete, flesh-colored papules, 2 to 4 mm in diameter, distributed periorbitall (Figs. 4-255–4-258).

They are usually more common on the lower lid and are asymptomatic. The firm papules may be skin-colored, yellow, brown, or pink, and they have also been found to occur on the eyelids, cheeks, axilla, abdomen, forehead, penis, and vulva.

In eruptive syringoma, multiple lesions appear in childhood or early adulthood on the anterior neck, chest, shoulders, abdomen, and pubic area and may regress spontaneously later in life.

Dark Skin Considerations

Multiple discrete, pink/yellowish papules and skin-colored or reddish-brown papules in patients with darker skin.

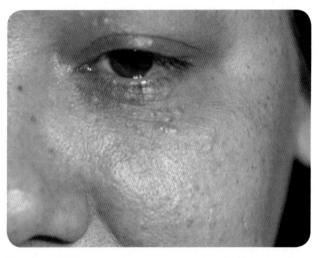

Figure 4-255 Multiple flesh-colored papules of syringomas around both eyes.

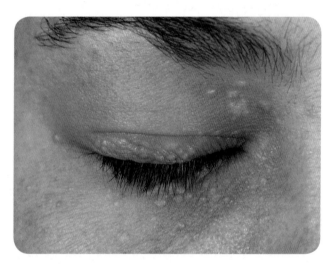

Figure 4-256 Discrete, flesh-colored syringomas around eyes and on the lids, which are not as yellow as xanthelasma.

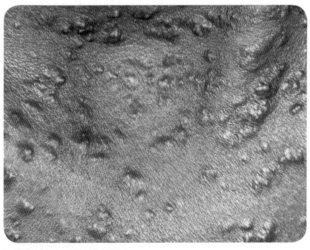

Figure 4-257 Syringomas can be in locations other than periorbitally.

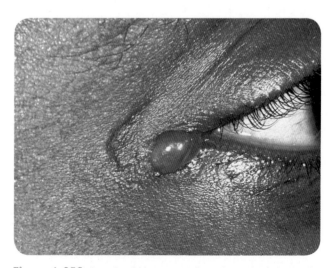

Figure 4-258 Apocrine hidrocystoma is more cystic than a syringoma, usually single, and close to the eyelids.

Diagnostic Pearls

- Small (2 to 4 mm in diameter) monomorphic papules that are slightly firm to palpation.
- Syringomas often first appear during puberty and may be eruptive.

Differential Diagnosis and Pitfalls

- Basal cell carcinoma—pearly papule with telangiectasia
- Sarcoidosis—more infiltrative plaques
- Flat warts—more flat-topped papules
- Milia—white center
- Xanthelasma—favor upper eyelids, white to yellow plaques
- Trichoepitheliomas—favor alar creases; flesh-colored and rubbery papules
- Sebaceous hyperplasia—white umbilicated papules
- Steatocystoma multiplex—white to yellow smooth papules and nodules

Best Tests

- This is often a clinical diagnosis. If the diagnosis is in doubt, skin biopsy will demonstrate characteristic histopathology.

Management Pearls

- Clear cell syringomas may be associated with diabetes. They should be ruled out.
- Laser ablation may be the optimal choice when multiple syringomata are present.

Therapy

As these are benign neoplasms, removal is for cosmetic reasons.

The following techniques are suitable:

- Simple excision with primary closure (best reserved for those with few lesions or larger lesions)—a punch excision is often sufficient
- Snip excision with healing by secondary intention

- Electrocautery
- Intralesional electrodesiccation
- CO_2 laser
- Cryotherapy
- Dermabrasion

Because these are dermal neoplasms, the patient should be warned that there is a risk of scarring or recurrence with any therapy.

Suggested Readings

Chao PZ, Lee FP. Pleomorphic adenoma (chondroid syringoma) on the face. *Otolaryngol Head Neck Surg.* 2004 Apr;130(4):499–500.

Frazier CC, Camacho AP, Cockerell CJ. The treatment of eruptive syringomas in an African American patient with a combination of trichloroacetic acid and CO_2 laser destruction. *Dermatol Surg.* 2001 May;27(5):489–492.

Karam P, Benedetto AV, Karma P. Intralesional electrodesiccation of syringomas. *Dermatol Surg.* 1997 Oct;23(10):921–924.

Langbein L, Cribier B, Schirmacher P, et al. New concepts on the histogenesis of eccrine neoplasia from keratin expression in the normal eccrine gland, syringoma and poroma. *Br J Dermatol.* 2008 Sep;159(3):633–645.

Lee JH, Chang JY, Lee KH. Syringoma: A clinicopathologic and immunohistologic study and results of treatment. *Yonsei Med J.* 2007 Feb;48(1):35–40.

McCalmont TH. Adnexal neoplasms. In: Bolognia JL, Jorizzo JL, Rapini RP, eds. *Dermatology.* 2nd Ed. St. Louis, MO: Mosby; 2008:1704.

Miranda JJ, Shahabi S, Salih S, et al. Vulvar syringoma, report of a case and review of the literature. *Yale J Biol Med.* 2002 Jul–Aug;75(4):207–210.

Park HJ, Lee DY, Lee JH, et al. The treatment of syringomas by CO(2) laser using a multiple-drilling method. *Dermatol Surg.* 2007 Mar;33(3): 310–313.

Powell CL, Smith EP, Graham BS. Eruptive syringomas: An unusual presentation on the buttocks. *Cutis.* 2005 Oct;76(4):267–269.

Schulhof Z, Anastassov GE, Lumerman H, et al. Giant benign chondroid syringoma of the cheek: case report and review of the literature. *J Oral Maxillofac Surg.* 2007 Sep;65(9):1836–1839.

Soler-Carrillo J, Estrach T, et al. Eruptive syringoma: 27 new cases and review of the literature. *J Eur Acad Dermatol Venereol.* 2001 May;15(3):242–246.

Diagnosis Synopsis

Trichoepitheliomas are benign neoplasms derived from the hair follicles. They usually present as asymptomatic smooth, skin-colored papules or small nodules on the face or the trunk. They may occur singly and sporadically, but multiple trichoepitheliomas are often inherited as an autosomal dominant trait. This heritable form (multiple familial trichoepithelioma) may be caused by a mutation in a tumor suppressor gene on chromosome 9. Due to decreased penetrance of this gene in men, trichoepitheliomas are seen more commonly in women. They arise most often during childhood or early adolescence. Treatment is for cosmetic purposes, as malignant transformation of trichoepitheliomas is quite rare.

Look For

Most often, they appear as multiple smooth, rounded papules on the face, scalp, neck, and upper trunk, though solitary lesions may appear on any hair-bearing part of the body (Figs. 4-259–4-262). The lesions can be skin-colored or slightly red in color. They are often symmetrical and occur in a grouped distribution when multiple. Ulceration is rarely seen.

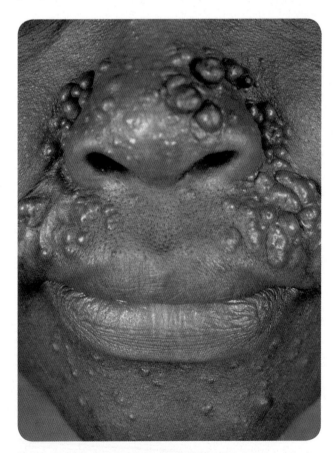

Figure 4-259 Flesh-colored papules on the distal nose and the lateral lips is a characteristic distribution for trichoepitheliomas.

The density is often greatest in the midface with a particular predilection for the nose and nasolabial folds.

Diagnostic Pearls

- Trichoepitheliomas are sometimes associated with cylindromas, which are large turban tumors on the scalp.
- Trichoepitheliomas may be a part of the Rombo syndrome, which also includes milia, hypertrichosis, basal cell carcinoma, vermiculate atrophoderma, and peripheral vasodilation.

Differential Diagnosis and Pitfalls

- Sarcoidosis
- Sebaceous hyperplasia
- Molluscum contagiosum
- Small epidermoid cysts
- Basal cell carcinoma
- Colloid milium
- Cylindroma
- Syringoma
- Milia
- Steatocystoma multiplex
- Trichilemmoma
- Trichofolliculoma

Heritable conditions with multiple facial papules:

- Follicular hamartomas including basaloid follicular hamartomas
- Trichilemmomas (Cowden syndrome)
- Pilomatrixomas
- Fibrofolliculomas/fibrodiscomas (Birt-Hogg-Dubé syndrome)
- Sebaceous tumors (Muir-Torré syndrome)

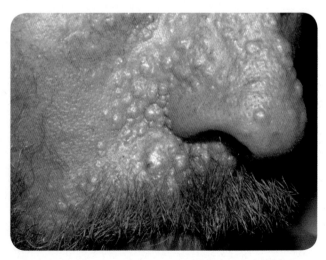

Figure 4-260 The papules of trichoepithelioma may vary in size and be anywhere on the face.

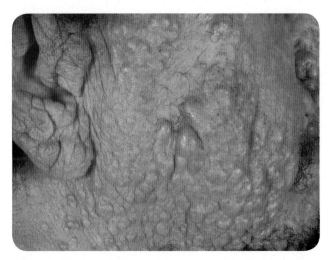

Figure 4-261 Rarely, trichoepitheliomas may involve most of the face.

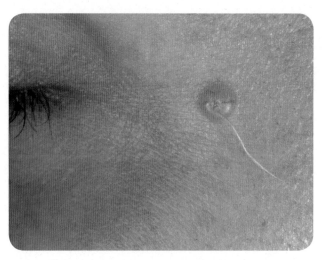

Figure 4-262 Trichofolliculomas are characteristic of Cowden syndrome and have a thin, wispy, hair-like protrusion.

- Cylindromas
- Basal cell carcinomas (basal cell nevus syndrome)
- Epidermal cysts (Gardner syndrome)
- Neurofibromas (neurofibromatosis)
- Angiofibromas (tuberous sclerosis)—Note: Trichoepitheliomas favor the upper lip, which is typically spared in the setting of multiple angiofibromas in tuberous sclerosis.

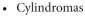 ## Best Tests

- Biopsy is necessary to exclude other skin adnexal tumors and the basal cell nevus syndrome.
- Ask for family history of similar lesions.

Management Pearls

- This is primarily a cosmetic issue. Rarely do trichoepitheliomas undergo malignant transformation.

Therapy

Growths respond to excision (often impractical with many lesions). Ablative therapy with electrosurgery and the CO_2 laser has proven effective in case reports.

Patients should be warned that treatment may result in scarring and that more lesions often develop over time.

Suggested Readings

Alsaad KO, Obaidat NA, Ghazarian D. Skin adnexal neoplasms—part 1: An approach to tumours of the pilosebaceous unit. *J Clin Pathol.* 2007 Feb;60(2):129–144.

Ashinoff R, Jacobson M, Belsito DV. Rombo syndrome: A second case report and review. *J Am Acad Dermatol.* 1993 Jun;28(6):1011–1014.

Bettencourt MS, Prieto VG, Shea CR. Trichoepithelioma: A 19-year clinico-pathologic re-evaluation. *J Cutan Pathol.* 1999 Sep;26(8):398–404.

Martinez CA, Priolli DG, Piovesan H, et al. Nonsolitary giant perianal trichoepithelioma with malignant transformation into basal cell carcinoma: Report of a case and review of the literature. *Dis Colon Rectum.* 2004 May;47(5):773–777.

McCalmont TH. Adnexal neoplasms. In: Bolognia J, Jorizzo JL, Rapini RP, eds. *Dermatology.* 2nd Ed. St. Louis, MO: Mosby; 2008:1697–1698.

Shehan JM, Huerter CJ. Desmoplastic trichoepithelioma: Report of a case illustrating its natural history. *Cutis.* 2008 Mar;81(3):236–238.

Stan Taylor R, Perone JB, Kaddu S, et al. Appendage tumors and hamartomas of the skin. In: Fitzpatrick TB, Wolff K, eds. *Fitzpatrick's Dermatology in General Medicine.* 7th Ed. New York, NY: McGraw-Hill; 2008:1083–1084.

Wang SH, Tsai RY, Chi CC. Familial desmoplastic trichoepithelioma, *Int J Dermatol.* 2006 Jun;45(6):756–758.

Diagnosis Synopsis

Flat warts (plane warts, verruca plana) are benign skin growths caused by human papillomavirus (HPV) types 3, 10, and 28. As the name implies, flat warts are flatter and smoother than common warts. They may be numerous and arranged in groups. Flat warts may be transmitted by direct or indirect contact; autoinoculation is common. Warts can be spread from person to person via contact or within an individual via trauma (Koebnerization) or via shaving. They are most frequently observed in young adults, children, and immunosuppressed patients. They often spontaneously regress, and treatment is, therefore, mainly for cosmetic purposes.

Immunocompromised Patient Considerations

Widespread or extensive warts are often a presenting sign of an immunocompromised state. Warts, in general, tend to be more numerous in immunosuppressed patients and have a higher potential for malignant transformation.

Look For

Minimally elevated, flat-topped papules that may be skin-colored or hyperpigmented, with a tendency to occur in groups or in a linear distribution secondary to Koebnerization

(Figs. 4-263–4-266). Warts are most commonly seen on the face, neck, wrists, and legs.

Diagnostic Pearls

- Flat warts can be both discrete and confluent and have a flat surface. The warts may occur in a linear distribution secondary to Koebnerization.

?? Differential Diagnosis and Pitfalls

- Lichen planus also presents with flat lesions, which are typically more violaceous and pruritic.
- Epidermodysplasia verruciformis is a genetic disease characterized by diffuse flat warts and a high potential for squamous cell carcinoma transformation. Common warts have a more verrucous surface.
- Lichen nitidus is characterized by discrete, dome-shaped papules.
- Molluscum contagiosum lesions are smooth, dome-shaped papules with a central umbilication.
- Follicular eczema or keratosis pilaris is located over the posterior arms and thighs.
- Actinic keratoses tend to be scaly, erythematous papules in sun-exposed areas of elderly individuals.

✓ Best Tests

- This is largely a clinical diagnosis. However, a skin biopsy is diagnostic, when in doubt.

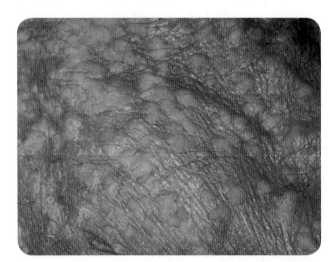

Figure 4-263 Flat warts may be large fields of confluent papules and plaques.

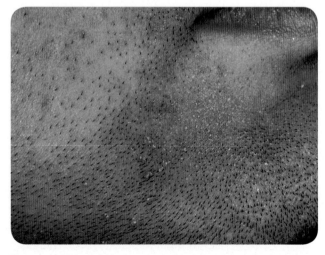

Figure 4-264 Flat warts as multiple small, nonkeratotic papules in the beard.

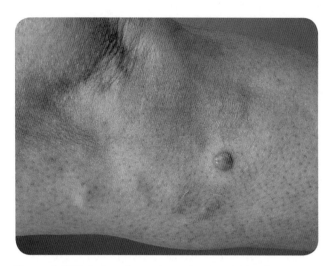

Figure 4-265 Red, nonkeratotic papules, some with a linear grouping from autoinoculation, are typical of flat warts.

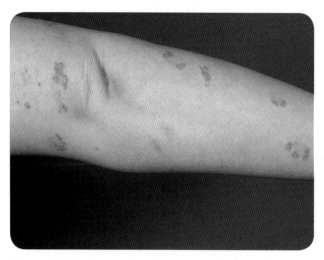

Figure 4-266 Linear papules typical of autoinoculation. Flat warts are frequently lighter than surrounding heavily pigmented skin.

▲▲▲ Management Pearls

- Flat warts typically remit spontaneously. Therefore, medical intervention is usually instituted for cosmetic reasons when the warts are located on the face or hands, or in immunosuppressed patients to decrease the spread of new lesions.
- Aggressive home therapy with 40% salicylic acid plaster available over the counter (OTC) applied daily or twice daily and taped on with strong adhesive tape (e.g., duct tape). Have the patient pare the wart down with a file or pumice stone between applications of each patch.

Immunocompromised Patient Considerations

Warts in immunosuppressed patients can be quite resistant to traditional therapies.

All therapies for warts can be used in immunosuppressed patients.

Dark Skin Considerations

Use caution with liquid nitrogen treatment in darkly pigmented individuals, as there is a risk of hyper- and hypopigmentation.

Therapy

Warts are benign and usually self-limited. Therefore, it is reasonable to not treat them. Patients often request treatment, however, in which case therapeutic options include the following:

- Destructive therapy: Cryotherapy using liquid nitrogen applied for 3 to 5 s with 1 to 3 freeze/thaw cycles; trichloroacetic acid applied topically; electrodesiccation (with caution to avoid scarring); CO_2 laser therapy in extreme cases.
- Topical medications: 5-fluorouracil (1% or 5% cream) applied daily or twice daily; or imiquimod 5% cream can be applied three to five times per week for 6 weeks or longer until lesions disappear. An irritation of the lesions is expected. 0.1% Tretinoin cream or gel daily or twice daily as tolerated. Tretinoin can be combined with imiquimod as well.
- Intralesional immunotherapy: Topical diphenylcyclopropenone, topical squaric acid, intralesional candida antigen, mumps antigen, and trichophyton antigens can sensitize patients to HPV. This is normally reserved for extreme cases.
- Salicylic acid plasters/ointments (OTC) with therapy as described above. Alternatives include silver nitrate and glutaraldehyde solution.

Suggested Readings

Androphy EJ, Lowy DR. Warts. In: Fitzpatrick TB, Wolff K, eds. *Fitzpatrick's Dermatology in General Medicine*. 7th Ed. New York, NY: McGraw-Hill; 2008:1914–1923.

Gibbs S, Harvey I. Topical treatments for cutaneous warts. *Cochrane Database Syst Rev*. 2006 Jul;(3):CD001781.

Gibbs S, Harvey I, Sterling J, Stark R. Local treatments for cutaneous warts: Systematic review. *BMJ*. 2002 Aug;325(7362):461.

Kirnbauer R, Lenz P, Okun MM. Human papillomavirus. In: Bolognia J, Jorizzo JL, Rapini RP, eds. *Dermatology*. 2nd Ed. St. Louis, MO: Mosby; 2008:1183–1198.

Lee S, Kim JG, Chun SI. Treatment of verruca plana with 5% 5-fluorouracil ointment. *Dermatologica*. 1980;160(6):383–389.

Lipke MM. An armamentarium of wart treatments. *Clin Med Res*. 2006 Dec;4(4):273–293.

Micali G, Dall'Oglio F, Nasca MR, et al. Management of cutaneous warts: An evidence-based approach. *Am J Clin Dermatol*. 2004;5(5):311–317.

Prose NS, von Knebel-Doeberitz C, Miller S, et al. Widespread flat warts associated with human papillomavirus type 5: A cutaneous manifestation of human immunodeficiency virus infection. *J Am Acad Dermatol*. 1990 Nov;23(5 Pt 2):978–981.

Ritter SE, Meffert J. Successful treatment of flat warts using intralesional Candida antigen. *Arch Dermatol*. 2003 Apr;139(4):541–542.

Xanthelasma Palpebrarum

▪ Diagnosis Synopsis

Xanthelasma palpebrarum is a type of plane xanthoma of the eyelids, and it is the most common type of xanthoma, in general. Xanthomas are yellow to orange macules, plaques, and papules containing lipid-rich deposits. Histologically, they represent the accumulation of lipid-containing, foamy macrophages in the dermis. Approximately half of patients with xanthomas have a lipid disorder; the remainder are normolipemic patients. Women are affected more than men. Although xanthomas themselves are often asymptomatic, investigations into and treatment of any underlying cause(s) are warranted to prevent morbidity from lipid disorders and to prevent xanthelasma from progressing.

⊙ Look For

Soft, yellow-to-orange macules, papules, and plaques, primarily on the superior eyelids near the medial canthus (Figs. 4-267–4-270). They frequently occur symmetrically and may be present on all four eyelids.

⊙⊙ Diagnostic Pearls

- Check for other visible signs of hyperlipidemia, such as cutaneous xanthomas, over joints and in intertriginous locations and arcus senilis in the cornea.
- Plane xanthomas may be seen in individuals with monoclonal gammopathy.

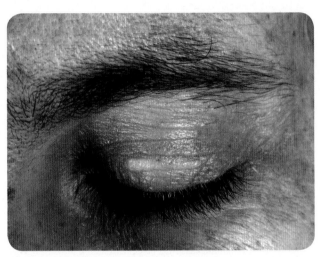

Figure 4-267 Yellow plaques in the mid upper lid.

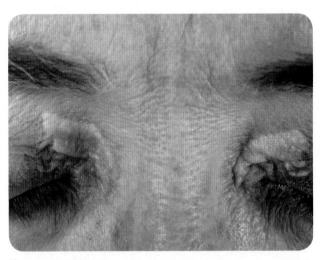

Figure 4-268 Yellow plaques are typically more medial in xanthelasma palpebrarum.

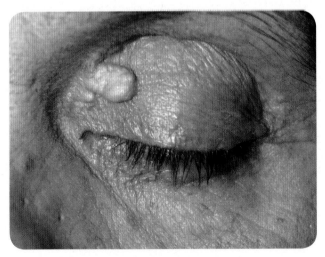

Figure 4-269 Papular-nodular plaques on xanthelasma palpebrarum.

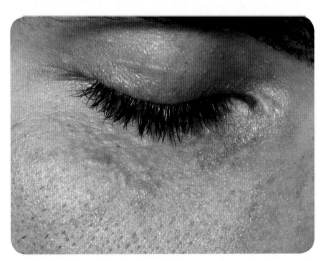

Figure 4-270 Subtle plaques of xanthelasma palpebrarum may be difficult to detect.

Differential Diagnosis and Pitfalls

- Epidermoid cysts are typically unilateral and not as yellow or orange in color.
- Basal cell carcinoma typically has telangiectasias and a central umbilication.
- Appendageal tumors are less obviously yellow.
- Molluscum contagiosum
- Milia
- Sebaceous hyperplasia
- Amyloidosis
- Lipoid proteinosis

 Best Tests

- This is usually a clinical diagnosis. However, if necessary, biopsy will confirm it.
- Fasting serum lipid panel including total cholesterol, triglycerides, VLDL, LDL, and HDL.

Management Pearls

- Exercise and dietary modifications should be recommended to all patients with lipid abnormalities. Many will also require systemic lipid-lowering therapy as well.
- Recurrence is common after surgical excision.

Therapy

Dietary modifications and exercise for hyperlipidemic patients. Many will need systemic lipid-lowering therapy in the form of statins, fibrates, nicotinic acid, or bile-acid–binding resins. While these measures are important in the treatment of hyperlipidemia, they typically do not cure the xanthelasma.

For the cosmetic treatment of the lesions themselves, the following treatments are options:

- Surgical excision
- Laser ablation – carbon dioxide, argon, Er:YAG, Nd:YAG, or pulsed dye
- Chemical cauterization with topical di- or trichloroacetic acid (TCA). For TCA: clean area with alcohol, apply petroleum jelly to the areas surrounding the xanthelasma, apply 100% TCA on thicker papular lesions, 70% TCA to flat plaques, or 50% TCA to macular lesions. Apply wet cotton balls to treated areas. In some cases, a single treatment is sufficient, and in some cases, one to three treatments at intervals of 2 weeks is necessary. Pigmentary changes and scarring (uncommonly) are possible side effects of TCA treatment.
- Cryosurgery
- Light electrodesiccation

Patients should be advised that there is a risk of scarring and recurrence after definitive treatment.

Suggested Readings

Bergman R. The pathogenesis and clinical significance of xanthelasma palpebrarum. *J Am Acad Dermatol.* 1994 Feb;30(2 Pt 1):236–242.

Fusade T. Treatment of xanthelasma palpebrarum by 1064-nm Q-switched Nd:YAG laser: A study of 11 cases. *Br J Dermatol.* 2008 Jan;158(1):84–87.

Haque MU, Ramesh V. Evaluation of three different strengths of trichloroacetic acid in xanthelasma palpebrarum. *J Dermatolog Treat.* 2006;17(1):48–50.

Raulin C, Schoenermark MP, Werner S, et al. Xanthelasma palpebrarum: treatment with the ultrapulsed CO$_2$ laser. *Lasers Surg Med.* 1999;24(2): 122–127.

Rohrich RJ, Janis JE, Pownell PH. Xanthelasma palpebrarum: A review and current management principles. *Plast Reconstr Surg.* 2002 Oct; 110(5):1310–1314.

White LE. Xanthomatoses and lipoprotein disorders. In: Fitzpatrick TB, Wolff K, eds. *Fitzpatrick's Dermatology in General Medicine.* 7th Ed. New York, NY: McGraw-Hill; 2008:1272.

■■ Diagnosis Synopsis

Xanthomas are cutaneous accumulations of lipid-laden macrophages in the skin. There are multiple varieties including tuberous xanthomas, plane xanthomas, tendinous xanthomas, eruptive xanthomas, palmar xanthomas, and xanthelasma. Each variety is associated with a particular underlying lipid abnormality.

Eruptive xanthomas are a cutaneous consequence of severe chylomicronemia and hypertriglyceridemia. They present with crops of small, pruritic, yellow-orange papules scattered over the buttocks and extremities. They are occasionally erythematous. Primary hypertriglyceridemia may result from hereditary conditions such as lipoprotein lipase deficiency, familial deficiency of apoprotein CII, or endogenous familial hypertriglyceridemia. Secondary causes include excessive alcohol intake, pancreatitis, obesity, hypothyroidism, renal failure, or diabetes mellitus. Certain medications, such as systemic retinoids and estrogens, can cause hypertriglyceridemia and manifest with eruptive xanthomas. Triglyceridemia in these patients can exceed 3,000 to 4,000 mg/dL. Higher triglycerides can also lead to pancreatitis. Treatment is aimed at correcting the underlying dyslipidemia through pharmacological and/or behavioral means. The skin lesions usually resolve within 6 months with appropriate treatment.

◉ Look For

Dome-shaped 1 to 4 mm yellow-orange, firm papules with an erythematous halo, most commonly located over the buttocks and extensor surfaces of extremities (Figs. 4-271–4-275). There can be crops of several dozen to hundreds of lesions,

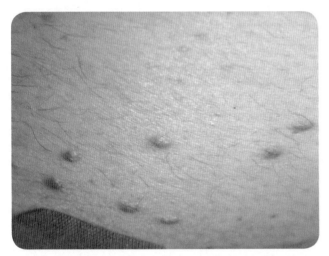

Figure 4-271 Discrete yellow-red papules of eruptive xanthomas.

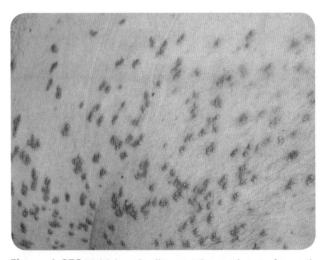

Figure 4-272 Multiple red-yellow eruptive xanthomas, frequently with an opaque center.

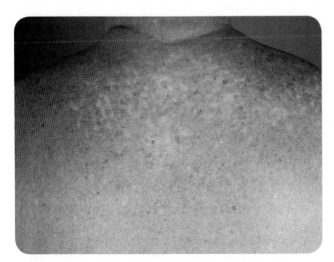

Figure 4-273 An 80 year old with a 3-year history of progressive, generalized yellow discoloration and small papules with increased histiocytes.

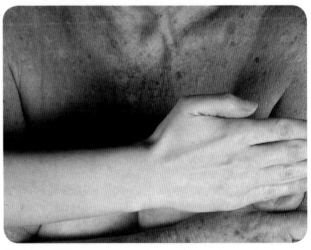

Figure 4-274 Patient with plane xanthomas with a normal arm for comparison.

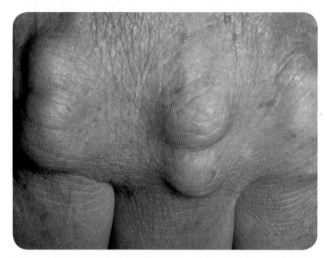

Figure 4-275 Tendon xanthomas are large nodules localized to tendons.

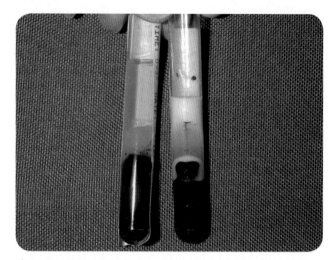

Figure 4-276 Serum on the right with triglycerides greater than 5,000 mg/dL, giving a milky appearance.

and Koebnerization (spread of lesions in traumatized skin) is known to occur.

Diagnostic Pearls

- Eruptive xanthomas occur with a rapid onset in the presence of hypertriglyceridemia (Fig. 4-276) and are characteristically yellow-orange papules.

Differential Diagnosis and Pitfalls

- Tuberous xanthomas are yellow to orange nodules—typically over joints, in particular the elbows and knees—that are associated with primary hyperlipoproteinemias, myxedema, and biliary cirrhosis.
- Tendinous xanthomas are yellow to orange nodules distributed over tendons, most commonly over the dorsal hand, dorsal feet, and Achilles tendons.
- Plane xanthomas are large yellow-orange, minimally elevated plaques distributed near the eyelids and on the trunk, neck, axilla, and flexors. They are commonly associated with an underlying monoclonal gammopathy such as multiple myeloma or monoclonal gammopathy of undetermined significance.

- Xanthelasma is the most common xanthoma, and it consists of yellow-orange papules distributed around the eyelids, seen in patients with either abnormal or normal lipid profiles.
- Granuloma annulare is typically annular but can present as discrete papules when disseminated.
- Xanthoma disseminatum tends to present in flexural and intertriginous regions, has a normal lipid profile, and can be associated with diabetes insipidus.
- Papular xanthoma
- Sarcoidosis typically has a purplish hue but can be more difficult to distinguish in darkly pigmented skin.
- Leukemia cutis
- Drug eruption
- Generalized eruptive histiocytomas
- Rosai-Dorfman disease has associated massive cervical lymphadenopathy.
- Indeterminate cell histiocytosis
- Langerhans cell histiocytosis
- Juvenile xanthogranuloma tends to present in infants and young children.
- Multicentric reticulohistiocytosis has associated mutilating arthritis.
- Lichen amyloidosis typically presents on the anterior shins.

✓ Best Tests

Fasting serum lipid panel consisting of cholesterol, triglycerides, VLDL, LDL, and HDL.

A skin biopsy can confirm the diagnosis.

▲▲ Management Pearls

- A reduction of the fat content to less than 30% of daily caloric intake is extremely important. Medium-chain triglycerides can be substituted for dietary fat. Triglyceride levels should be maintained below 1,500 mg/dL.
- Consider consultation with a dietician.
- Avoidance of alcohol and other contributing factors and medications should be strongly encouraged.

Therapy

Patients will require dietary modifications and exercise in addition to systemic therapy. Fibrates and niacin work best to lower triglycerides. Avoid bile acid sequestrants, as these drugs may actually worsen hypertriglyceridemia.

Fibrates
- Clofibrate—1 g p.o. twice daily
- Fenofibrate—48 to 145 mg p.o. daily

- Gemfibrozil—600 mg p.o. 30 min prior to morning and evening meals

Niacin
Sustained release niacin—begin with 500 mg p.o. at bedtime and increase by 500 mg every 8 weeks up to a maximum dose of 2,000 mg daily. Patients should be warned of potential side effects, including flushing and pruritus.

Suggested Readings

Crowe MJ, Gross DJ. Eruptive xanthoma. *Cutis.* 1992 Jul;50(1):31–32.

Eeckhout I, Vogelaers D, Geerts ML, Naeyaert JM. Xanthomas due to generalized oedema. *Br J Dermatol.* 1997 Apr;136(4):601–603.

Geyer AS, MacGregor JL, Fox LP, et al. Eruptive xanthomas associated with protease inhibitor therapy. *Arch Dermatol.* 2004 May;140(5):617–618.

Köstler E, Porst H, Wollina U. Cutaneous manifestations of metabolic diseases: uncommon presentations. *Clin Dermatol.* 2005 Sep–Oct;23(5):457–464.

Massengale WT, Nesbitt LT Jr. Xanthomas. In: Bolognia J, Jorizzo JL, Rapini RP, eds. *Dermatology.* 2nd Ed. St. Louis, MO: Mosby; 2008:1413–1419.

Merola JF, Mengden SJ, Soldano A, et al. Eruptive xanthomas. *Dermatol Online J.* 2008 May 15;14(5):10.

Parker F. Xanthomas and hyperlipidemias. *J Am Acad Dermatol.* 1985 Jul;13(1):1–30.

White LE. Xanthomatoses and lipoprotein disorders. In: Fitzpatrick TB, Wolff K, eds. *Fitzpatrick's Dermatology in General Medicine.* 7th Ed. New York, NY: McGraw-Hill; 2008:1272–1275.

Acanthosis Nigricans

Diagnosis Synopsis

Acanthosis nigricans is a localized skin disorder manifesting with hyperpigmented, velvety plaques located in the flexural and intertriginous regions. The precise pathogenesis is unknown but is speculated to involve the stimulation of growth factor receptors on keratinocytes and fibroblasts. Acanthosis nigricans has various subtypes relating to cause and/or location: obesity-associated, syndromic, acral, unilateral, familial, drug-induced, and malignant. Associated conditions include obesity, diabetes, polycystic ovarian syndrome (PCOS), Cushing syndrome, HAIR-AN (hyperandrogenism, insulin resistance, and acanthosis nigricans) syndrome, and acromegaly. Atypical (palmar or mucosal) distributions or acute onset acanthosis nigricans may also be associated with malignancy (usually gastrointestinal adenocarcinoma). Certain drugs, such as niacin, insulin, folate, estrogens, protease inhibitors, and triamcinolone, have been associated with the condition as well. The treatment of the underlying condition may help resolve the associated skin findings.

◉ Look For

Symmetrical hyperpigmentation and velvety thickening of the skin are typically seen in the axillae, inguinal, and inframammary folds (Fig. 4-277), as well as in the folds of the neck (Fig. 4-278). Severe forms may show velvety plaques on the knuckles (Fig. 4-279), palms (tripe palm), soles, or near mucosal surfaces (Fig. 4-280). Acrochordons (skin tags) are frequently present in involved areas.

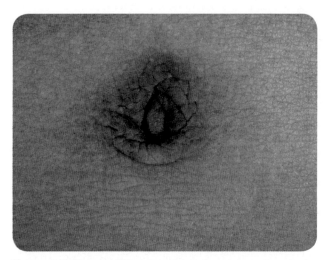

Figure 4-277 Periumbilical hyperkeratosis and hyperpigmentation are not uncommon in acanthosis nigricans.

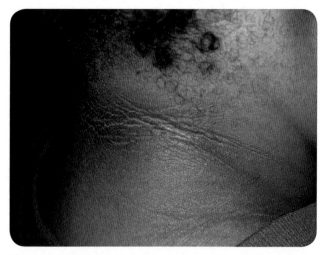

Figure 4-278 Hyperkeratosis, hyperpigmentation, and deep furrows in acanthosis nigricans.

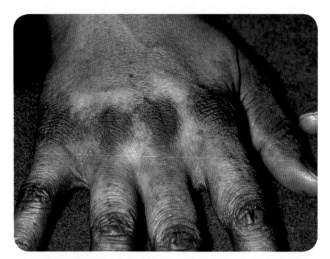

Figure 4-279 Symmetrical hyperpigmented and hyperkeratotic plaques on dorsum of hand and fingers.

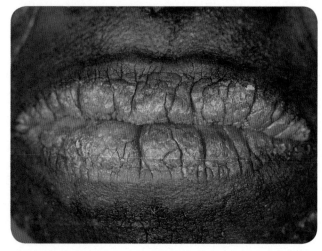

Figure 4-280 Acanthosis nigricans of mucosal surfaces is suggestive of internal gastrointestinal malignancy.

Diagnostic Pearls

- Oral and other mucosal lesions as well as extensive palmar involvement (tripe palm) are suggestive of associated malignancies, typically gastrointestinal.
- Acanthosis nigricans may also coexist with other cutaneous signs of internal malignancy, such as the acute appearance of multiple seborrheic keratoses (the sign of Leser-Trélat), tylosis, and florid cutaneous papillomatosis.

?? Differential Diagnosis and Pitfalls

- Confluent and reticulated papillomatosis of Gougerot-Carteaud (CARP) presents with reticulated, pigmented patches on the trunk.
- Epidermal and Becker nevi are usually not symmetric and often have associated hypertrichosis.
- Hemochromatosis has skin darkening without epidermal thickening.
- Localized plaques of epidermolytic hyperkeratosis have more corrugated surfaces.
- Pellagra presents with photodistributed dermatitis (Casal necklace) as well as diarrhea and dementia (the 3 Ds).
- Addison disease has skin darkening without epidermal thickening.
- Parapsoriasis en plaque tends to have scaly plaques diffusely distributed.
- Pemphigus vegetans has verrucous ulcerated plaques.
- Erythema dyschromicum perstans usually has diffuse hyperpigmentation over the trunk.

✓ Best Tests

- This is usually a clinical diagnosis. However, perform a complete history (including a medication history) and physical examination. Pertinent findings include obesity, masculinization, weight loss, lymphadenopathy, or organomegaly. Calculate the patient's body mass index.
- Skin biopsy is rarely needed to confirm the diagnosis.

- Concurrent fasting plasma insulin and glucose, as diabetes and obesity are the most common associations.
- Plasma testosterone and dehydroepiandrosterone sulfate test in women with signs of hyperandrogenism to rule out PCOS.
- Antinuclear and anti-insulin receptor autoantibodies for patients with rheumatic symptoms.
- Depending on the clinical scenario, a more extensive search for visceral malignancy may be warranted (fecal occult blood testing, imaging, endoscopy, etc).

Management Pearls

- The management of patients with acanthosis nigricans may be multidisciplinary depending on the underlying cause and can include specialists in endocrinology, oncology, and nutrition.

Therapy

The correction of the underlying condition often leads to very slow resolution or improvement of the acanthosis nigricans. Counsel patients with obesity-associated acanthosis nigricans regarding healthy diet and exercise, or enlist the aid of a dietician.

The treatment of the skin lesions of acanthosis nigricans is for cosmetic purposes only.

Keratolytic agents have achieved modest success in reducing the thickness of the lesions:

- Lactic acid (12% lotion or cream—apply twice daily 5 or 12 oz)
- Urea (10, 20, or 40% creams—6 oz)
- Topical retinoids (tretinoin cream 0.05%, tazarotene 0.05%, and retinoic acid ointment 0.1%)
- 6% Salicylic acid in propylene glycol twice daily may be beneficial
- A combination of a topical retinoid (tretinoin 0.05% nightly) with 12% ammonium lactate cream twice daily

Other therapies:

- Oral metformin 500 mg p.o. twice daily
  (**Note:** For patients with insulin resistance, check serum creatinine prior to initiation of therapy.)
- Topical calcipotriol 0.005% twice daily
- Laser therapy—long-pulsed alexandrite and continuous wave carbon dioxide lasers

Suggested Readings

Hermanns-Lê T, Scheen A, Piérard GE. Acanthosis nigricans associated with insulin resistance: Pathophysiology and management. *Am J Clin Dermatol.* 2004;5(3):199–203.

Romo A, Benavides S. Treatment options in insulin resistance obesity-related acanthosis nigricans. *Ann Pharmacother.* 2008 Jul;42(7):1090–1094.

Rosenbach A, Ram R. Treatment of Acanthosis nigricans of the axillae using a long-pulsed (5-msec) alexandrite laser. *Dermatol Surg.* 2004 Aug;30(8):1158–1160.

Schwartz RA. Acanthosis nigricans. *J Am Acad Dermatol.* 1994 Jul;31(1):1–19; quiz 20–22.

Torley D, Bellus GA, Munro CS. Genes, growth factors and acanthosis nigricans. *Br J Dermatol.* 2002 Dec;147(6):1096–1101.

Diagnosis Synopsis

Actinic, or solar, keratosis is a neoplastic condition in which precancerous epithelial lesions are found on sun-exposed areas of the body. This is a very common condition in fair-skinned individuals (e.g., northern European descent) and virtually unseen in people of darker skin types. They are commonly seen on sun-exposed skin of the face, neck, upper chest, forearms, and dorsal hands. These flat, scaly papules are of varying sizes and usually begin as "rough" localized skin lesions that the patient feels but are difficult to see. Actinic keratoses have the potential to evolve into squamous cell carcinoma. They are usually asymptomatic but may be pruritic or painful. The frequency of actinic keratoses increases with increasing age and cumulative lifetime sun exposure. They are also more common in immunosuppressed individuals. They may resolve with protection from UV light. Patients with actinic keratoses are also at higher risk for developing nonmelanoma skin cancer.

Immunocompromised Patient Considerations

Actinic keratoses are more common in immunosuppressed patients, especially after solid organ transplantation.

Look For

Subtle, barely elevated to thicker, hypertrophic, rough papules with ill-defined borders (Figs. 4-281–4-283). There may be adherent scale with color variation from whites to yellows and, more rarely, a reddish-brown or gray-colored scale. The papules usually have an underlying red base. Size varies. When large in number, actinic keratoses may coalesce to form plaques (Fig. 4-284). Lower lip involvement with actinic keratoses is considered actinic cheilitis.

Diagnostic Pearls

- Actinic keratoses are often more easily palpated (with light touch) than seen.

Immunocompromised Patient Considerations

There is an increased occurrence in transplant patients and other immunosuppressed patients.

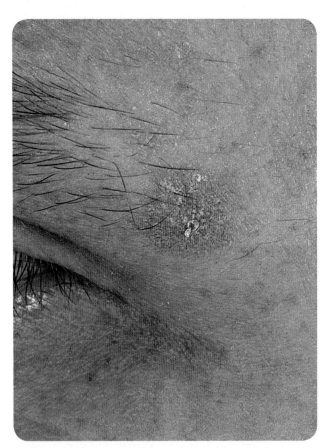

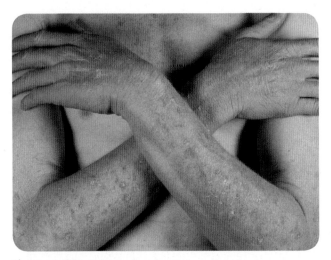

Figure 4-281 Multiple hyperkeratotic actinic keratoses on sun-exposed extensor arms.

Figure 4-282 Actinic keratoses may range in size from a few millimeters in diameter to 1 to 2 cm.

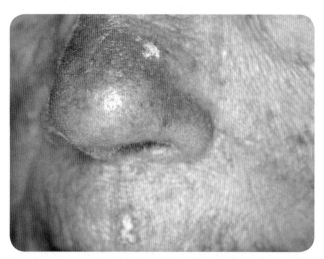

Figure 4-283 Hypertrophic actinic keratoses on nose and upper lip.

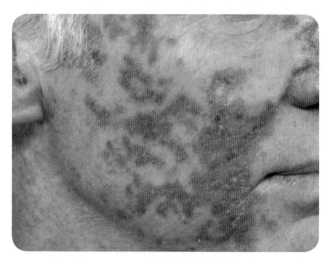

Figure 4-284 Inflamed actinic keratosis during topical therapy with 5-fluorouracil.

?? Differential Diagnosis and Pitfalls

- Actinic keratoses are usually smaller and more irregular than flat warts, common warts, and superficial basal cell carcinomas.
- Bowen disease
- Psoriasis
- Seborrheic dermatitis
- Squamous cell carcinoma
- Seborrheic keratosis
- Porokeratosis
- Discoid lupus erythematosus

✓ Best Tests

- This is a clinical diagnosis. If necessary, confirm with a skin biopsy. Biopsies should be performed on recurrent, hyperkeratotic, large (>6 mm), or indurated lesions to rule out invasive carcinoma.

▲▲ Management Pearls

- Aggressive sun avoidance/sun-protective measures should be instituted. Patients should wear protective clothing, broad-brimmed hats, and a broad-spectrum (UVA and UVB blocking) sunscreen with sun-protecting factor 30 or higher when exposed to the sun.
- If patient does not respond to therapy, perform a biopsy to rule out squamous cell carcinoma.

Therapy

Treat individual lesions with liquid nitrogen cryotherapy or superficial curettage and cautery.

5-Fluorouracil 5% cream can be applied twice daily to areas of more extensive involvement for about 2 weeks. It will cause a vigorous reaction (redness and hemorrhagic crusting). Have the patient apply an emollient, such as petroleum jelly, to aid in crust dissolution.

Other treatments that may be tried include:

- Topical imiquimod 5% cream applied to affected areas two to three times per week for 12 weeks
- Photodynamic therapy with methyl aminolevulinate
- 0.3% Topical adapalene gel applied to affected areas one to two times daily
- Topical 3.0% diclofenac in 2.5% hyaluronan gel applied to affected areas twice daily

A low-fat diet (<21% of calories from fat) has been shown to reduce the incidence of actinic keratoses. Actinic keratoses will decrease and sometimes resolve with sunscreen use.

Immunocompromised Patient Considerations

Extensive areas have also been treated with the CO_2 laser.

In the immunosuppressed population, one should maintain a low threshold to biopsy actinic keratoses that do not respond to appropriate treatment to rule out non-melanoma skin cancer.

Suggested Readings

Ben M'barek L, Mebazaa A, Euvrard S, et al. 5% topical imiquimod tolerance in transplant recipients. *Dermatology*. 2007;215(2):130–133.

Black HS, Herd JA, Goldberg LH, et al. Effect of a low-fat diet on the incidence of actinic keratosis. *N Engl J Med*. 1994 May;330(18):1272–1275.

Braathen LR, Szeimies RM, Basset-Seguin N, et al.; International Society for Photodynamic Therapy in Dermatology. Guidelines on the use of photodynamic therapy for nonmelanoma skin cancer: an international consensus. International Society for Photodynamic Therapy in Dermatology, 2005. *J Am Acad Dermatol*. 2007 Jan;56(1):125–1243.

Cockerell CJ. Histopathology of incipient intraepidermal squamous cell carcinoma ("actinic keratosis"). *J Am Acad Dermatol*. 2000 Jan;42(1 Pt 2): 11–17.

Duncan KO, Geisse JK, Leffell DJ. Epithelial precancerous lesions. In: Fitzpatrick TB, Wolff K, eds. *Fitzpatrick's Dermatology in General Medicine*. 7th Ed. New York, NY: McGraw-Hill; 2008:1007–1015.

Falagas ME, Angelousi AG, Peppas G. Imiquimod for the treatment of actinic keratosis: A meta-analysis of randomized controlled trials. *J Am Acad Dermatol*. 2006 Sep;55(3):537–538.

James WD, Berger TG, Elston DM. Epidermal nevi, neoplasms, and cysts. In: James WD, Berger TG, Elston DM, Odom RB, eds. *Andrews' Diseases of the Skin: Clinical Dermatology*. 10th Ed. Philadelphia, PA: Saunders Elsevier; 2006:641–643.

Lee PK, Harwell WB, Loven KH, et al. Long-term clinical outcomes following treatment of actinic keratosis with imiquimod 5% cream. *Dermatol Surg*. 2005 Jun;31(6):659–664.

Rigel DS, Cockerell CJ, Carucci J, et al. Actinic keratosis, basal cell carcinoma and squamous cell carcinoma. In: Bolognia JL, Jorizzo JL, Rapini RP, eds. *Dermatology*. 2nd Ed. St. Louis, MO: Mosby; 2008:1645–1651.

Szeimies RM, Gerritsen MJ, Gupta G, et al. Imiquimod 5% cream for the treatment of actinic keratosis: Results from a phase III, randomized, double-blind, vehicle-controlled, clinical trial with histology. *J Am Acad Dermatol*. 2004 Oct;51(4):547–555.

Thompson SC, Jolley D, Marks R. Reduction of solar keratoses by regular sunscreen use. *N Engl J Med*. 1993 Oct;329(16):1147–1151.

Confluent and Reticulated Papillomatosis

◼◼ Diagnosis Synopsis

Confluent and reticulated papillomatosis is a rare cutaneous disorder of as-yet undetermined etiology with clinical features resembling acanthosis nigricans. It has been speculated that the disorder may be due to an endocrine disturbance, abnormal keratinocyte differentiation and maturation, an abnormal host reaction to bacteria or fungi, or that it may be hereditary.

Recently, a case of confluent and reticulated papillomatosis from which a species of *Dietzia*, an actinomycete, was isolated was reported. The clinical response of the disease to antimicrobial treatment lends support to possible infectious etiology.

Confluent and reticulated papillomatosis is clinically characterized by hyperpigmented, hyperkeratotic, very thin papules, usually on the trunk. These papules coalesce into reticulated plaques. The lesions are usually asymptomatic but may be pruritic. The disorder typically affects young adults, and is more common in women and those with darker skin types. While responsive to treatment, the disease is usually chronic and marked by exacerbations and remissions.

Look For

Lesions begin as hyperkeratotic or very thin, slightly verrucous 1 to 2 mm papules that enlarge and coalesce to form reticulated papules (Figs. 4-285–4-286). Skin markings are often accentuated, and there may be slight overlying scale (Figs. 4-287–4-288). Early lesions may be erythematous, but they typically become gray-brown over time.

Lesions usually begin on the chest or abdomen and spread centrifugally. The face, neck, and proximal extremities may also be involved.

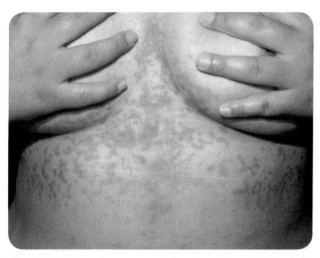

Figure 4-285 Confluent and reticulated papillomatosis on the neck with hyperpigmented papules surrounding islands of normal skin.

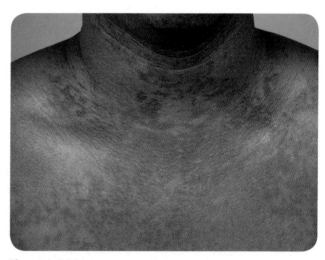

Figure 4-286 Confluent and reticulated papillomatosis on the neck with sharp borders between the affected and normal skin.

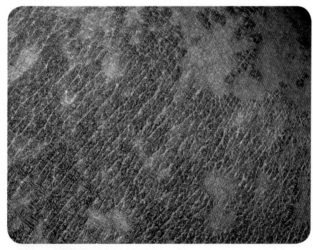

Figure 4-287 Confluent and reticulated papillomatosis on the chest with relatively flat papules.

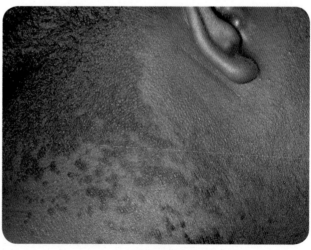

Figure 4-288 Confluent and reticulated papillomatosis on the neck and chest with varying degrees of hyperpigmentation.

Dark Skin Considerations

Early lesions may be difficult to appreciate in darker-skinned individuals.

Diagnostic Pearls

- Scraping the lesions may produce a fine scale. KOH preparations are negative.
- The mucous membranes are spared.

Differential Diagnosis and Pitfalls

- Acanthosis nigricans
- Macular amyloidosis
- Darier disease
- Pityriasis rubra pilaris
- Seborrheic keratoses
- Tinea versicolor
- Dermatopathia pigmentosa reticularis
- Epidermal nevus syndrome
- Erythema dyschromicum perstans
- Dowling-Degos disease (reticulated pigmented anomaly of the flexures)
- Dyskeratosis congenital
- Erythema ab igne
- Prurigo pigmentosa
- Incontinentia pigmenti

Best Tests

- Perform a KOH preparation and fungal culture of skin scraping to rule out a fungal infection. On occasion, concomitant *Pityrosporum* infections may be detected.
- Skin biopsy may be helpful.

Management Pearls

- Treatment is for cosmetic reasons.
- Overweight patients with confluent and reticulated papillomatosis have experienced the regression of lesions with weight loss.

Therapy

The most consistently helpful results in the treatment of confluent and reticulated papillomatosis have been achieved with oral minocycline (50–100 mg p.o. twice daily).

Other antibiotic regimens have had purported success:

- Azithromycin—250 to 500 mg p.o. three times weekly
- Clarithromycin—500 mg p.o. daily
- Erythromycin—1,000 mg p.o. daily
- Tetracycline—500 mg p.o. twice daily
- Cefdinir—300 mg p.o. twice daily

The following retinoids may also be tried:

- Topical—tretinoin cream (0.025%, 0.05%, 0.1%)—apply nightly; tazarotene—apply nightly
- Systemic—isotretinoin—0.5 to 1 mg/kg p.o. divided, twice daily; acitretin 25 to 50 mg p.o. daily

Other topical treatments that have shown mixed results include:

- Selenium sulfide—apply to affected area once daily for 10 min and then rinse
- Ketoconazole—apply to affected areas twice daily
- Calcipotriene 0.005% cream—apply to affected areas twice daily

Suggested Readings

Atasoy M, Ozdemir S, Akta? A, et al. Treatment of confluent and reticulated papillomatosis with azithromycin. *J Dermatol.* 2004 Aug;31(8):682–686.

Cockerell CJ, Larsen F. Benign epidermal tumors and proliferations. In: Bolognia JL, Jorizzo JL, Rapini RP, eds. *Dermatology.* 2nd Ed. St. Louis, MO: Mosby; 2008:1677–1678.

Jang HS, Oh CK, Cha JH, et al. Six cases of confluent and reticulated papillomatosis alleviated by various antibiotics. *J Am Acad Dermatol.* 2001 Apr;44(4):652–655.

Montemarano AD, Hengge M, Sau P, et al. Confluent and reticulated papillomatosis: Response to minocycline. *J Am Acad Dermatol.* 1996 Feb;34 (2 Pt 1):253–256.

Scheinfeld N. Confluent and reticulated papillomatosis: A review of the literature. *Am J Clin Dermatol.* 2006;7(5):305–313.

Darier Disease

Diagnosis Synopsis

Darier disease (keratosis follicularis) is an autosomal dominantly inherited disease that usually presents in early adolescence to mid-adult life with greasy, hyperkeratotic papules. The peak age of onset is in the second decade of life. The pathogenesis involves mutations in the *ATP2A2* gene, which encodes a sarco/endoplasmic reticulum calcium-ATPase pump (SERCA2). Although disease penetrance is high, expression is variable, and sporadic mutations may occur. There is no gender predilection.

After onset, the disease is lifelong. It may be accentuated or only prominent in the spring and summer, when exposures to heat, perspiration, and UV light are increased. Other exacerbating conditions/factors may include trauma, menstruation, and certain drugs (e.g., lithium and oral corticosteroids). The lesions of Darier disease may be pruritic, painful, or malodorous. Along with the appearance, these symptoms may lead to significant psychosocial distress. Patients are at an increased risk of bacterial or viral skin infections.

Linear, segmental, or unilateral presentations are uncommon variants of the disease caused by mutations in the same gene.

Look For

Small, symmetrical, skin-colored or yellow-brown papules, most frequently on the chest and face in a so-called seborrheic distribution, including the scalp and the retroauricular folds (**Figs. 4-289 and 4-290**). Intertriginous lesions are also seen. Pits may be seen on the palms and soles, and the hard palate may also be involve (**Fig. 4-291**). Hemorrhagic lesions can occur on the palms and soles as well. Papules (usually 0.5 to 1.0 cm in size) can be crusted, eroded, or verrucous in texture. Rarely, lesions have a unilateral or herpes zoster-like distribution. Lesions are frequently described as greasy.

Nail plates are thin, have chips and cracks along the nail margin, and often have parallel white or red bands in the nail bed. A V-shaped notch in the free edge of a nail is characteristic (**Fig. 4-292**).

Dark Skin Considerations

The lesions often have a dirty-gray coloration in darker-skinned individuals.

Diagnostic Pearls

- The lesions have a rough surface, which, upon gentle palpation, feels like the surface of very coarse sandpaper or a fine grater.

?? Differential Diagnosis and Pitfalls

- Follicular eczema has a similar distribution, as do follicular occlusion syndromes, perforating disorders, granuloma annulare, and some tumors of the appendages. They do not have the characteristic skin biopsy.
- Grover disease (transient acantholytic disease) has a similar biopsy but has a different age of onset (e.g., fourth or fifth decade).
- Hailey-Hailey disease is more erosive and is more common in intertriginous areas.
- Seborrheic dermatitis
- Pemphigus foliaceous

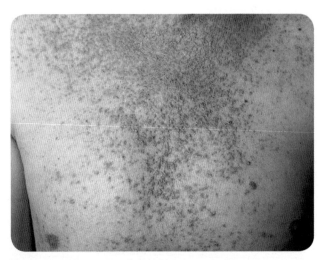

Figure 4-289 Discrete hyperkeratotic papules on the mid chest are characteristic in Darier disease.

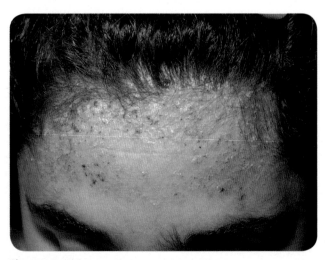

Figure 4-290 The forehead may be red with crusted erosions extending onto the scalp.

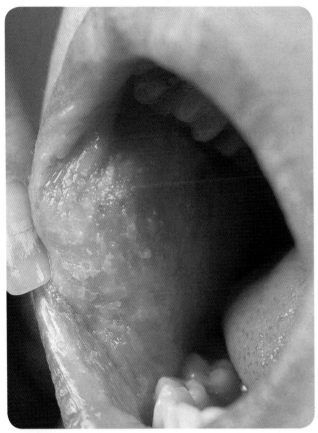

Figure 4-291 White intraoral papules and plaques are not rare in Darier disease.

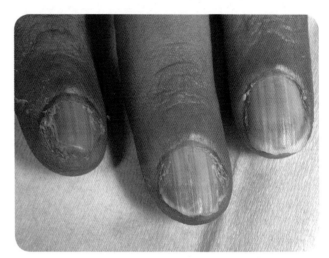

Figure 4-292 Nail plates may be thin with distal V-shaped nicking, and the nail beds may have longitudinal white and red bands.

- Treat any complicating infection aggressively, and adjust systemic retinoid dosages to find the optimum therapeutic window. Patients may be able to stop retinoids during the winter. With the newer retinoids, there is little rationale for using high doses of vitamin A to treat this disorder. Because therapy with retinoids is long term, the avoidance of pregnancy in females is essential. It is important to discuss with and follow-up patients for the long-term, bony side effects of retinoids.
- Superinfection with herpes simplex virus (HSV), a well-characterized complication termed Kaposi varicelliform eruption, is treated with appropriate antiviral agents. If suspicion is high, treatment is merited despite a negative viral culture.

- Acne
- Acanthosis nigricans
- Confluent reticulate papillomatosis
- Chronic vesiculobullous diseases such as bullous pemphigoid, pemphigus vulgaris, pemphigus foliaceous, and pemphigus vegetans

✓ Best Tests

- Skin biopsy is usually characteristic.
- Perform a skin swab for bacterial or viral culture if infection is suspected.

▲▲ Management Pearls

- Be certain of the diagnosis with family history or biopsy.
- Basic measures for all patients with Darier disease include sun protection and the use of cool cotton clothing, soap substitutes, emollients, and mild keratolytics (urea or lactic acid moisturizers).

Therapy

Topical retinoids (tretinoin 0.025% to 0.1%, adapalene 0.1%, or tazarotene 0.05% nightly) can be useful, although the dosage needs to be closely adjusted, as irritation is frequent and can lead to erosion. The concomitant use of low-potency topical corticosteroids may help control irritation.

Darier disease responds well to systemic retinoids such as isotretinoin (Accutane, starting dose 0.5 mg/kg/day) or acitretin (Soriatane, starting dose of 10 to 25 mg daily), both of which have teratogenetic potential. Women of childbearing potential should use two different birth control measures to avoid pregnancy. These drugs should be used by those familiar with them and their side effects.

(Continued)

Other therapies with purported success in case reports include topical 5-fluorouracil, topical tacrolimus, oral contraceptives, dermabrasion, laser treatment (carbon dioxide and Er:YAG), and photodynamic therapy. The treatment of hyperhidrosis with injections of botulinum toxin A may be useful in selected patients.

Impetiginized lesions can be treated locally with mupirocin or, if extensive, with the appropriate systemic antibiotics (i.e., dicloxacillin or cephalexin).

Oral acyclovir (or one of its congeners) is indicated in the case of HSV superinfection.

Suggested Readings

Burge S. Management of Darier's disease. *Clin Exp Dermatol.* 1999 Mar;24(2):53–56.

Cooper SM, Burge SM. Darier's disease: epidemiology, pathophysiology, and management. *Am J Clin Dermatol.* 2003;4(2):97–105.

Hovnanian A. Acantholytic disorders of the skin: Darier-White disease, acrokeratosis verruciformis, Grover disease, and Hailey-Hailey disease. In: Fitzpatrick TB, Wolff K, eds. *Fitzpatrick's Dermatology in General Medicine.* 7th Ed. New York, NY: McGraw-Hill; 2008:432–436.

Kontochristopoulos G, Katsavou AN, Kalogirou O, et al. Letter: Botulinum toxin type A: an alternative symptomatic management of Darier's disease. *Dermatol Surg.* 2007 Jul;33(7):882–883.

Rubegni P, Poggiali S, Sbano P, et al. A case of Darier's disease successfully treated with topical tacrolimus. *J Eur Acad Dermatol Venereol.* 2006 Jan;20(1):84–87.

Sehgal VN, Srivastava G. Darier's (Darier-White) disease/keratosis follicularis. *Int J Dermatol.* 2005 Mar;44(3):184–192.

Dermatitis, Atopic (Eczema)

▪▪ Diagnosis Synopsis

Atopic dermatitis, also known as atopic eczema, is a condition primarily affecting allergy-prone people (often with atopic triad of eczema, allergic rhinitis, and asthma). The exact cause of the condition is unknown; however, a defective function of the skin barrier due to mutations in the gene that encodes filaggrin is thought to play a major role. Most patients have marked xerosis and an inability to retain moisture in the skin. Atopy may include the presence of allergen-specific immunoglobulin E. The clinical presentation ranges from weeping and crusted areas of eczema to papules or lichenified plaques. Infants and children are most frequently affected, but the condition may persist into adulthood.

There is no known cure for atopic dermatitis. Environmental triggers such as heat, low (or high) humidity, detergents/soaps, abrasive clothing (e.g., wools), chemicals, smoke, and stress aggravate atopic dermatitis. The disorder is associated with intense itching that is aggravated by scratching. Scratching increases the chances of cutaneous infections because it produces breaks in the skin. Patients with atopic dermatitis are more prone to impetiginization with *Staphylococcus aureus* and infection with herpes simplex virus (eczema herpeticum).

Dark Skin Considerations

Atopic dermatitis has been found to be twice as common in blacks as in whites in some studies.

Immunocompromised Patient Considerations

HIV-infected individuals may be more predisposed to developing herpes simplex virus superinfection (eczema herpeticum).

◉ Look For

Thickened, scaly, erythematous papules and plaques involving the flexural surfaces. Lesions are most prominent on the face, neck, antecubital fossae, popliteal fossa, and extremities in general (Figs. 4-293–4-296). The nose is often spared. Impetiginized plaques can develop thick, oozing, yellow crusts.

Chronic papules and plaques can be deeply pigmented.

Allergy to eggs, cow's milk, and peanuts is common.

Nipples, in women, may be extensively involved bilaterally.

Dark Skin Considerations

Blacks frequently have extensive follicular accentuation and shininess without obvious lichenified plaques. They also have more post-inflammatory hyperpigmentation and hypopigmentation than those with lighter skin.

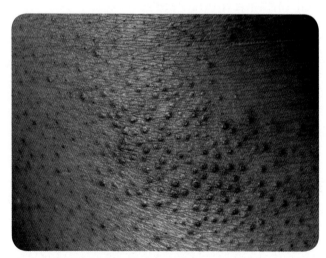

Figure 4-293 Patients with dark skin often have closely grouped papules in atopic dermatitis, called papular atopic dermatitis.

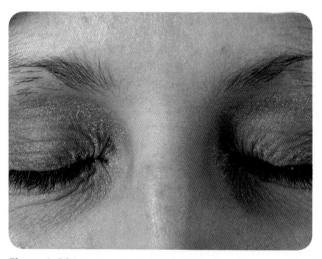

Figure 4-294 Erythema, periorbital thickening, and accentuation of skin markings (lichenification) in atopic dermatitis.

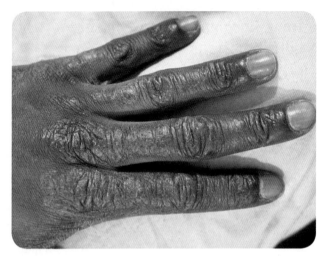

Figure 4-295 Marked lichenification of the dorsal hand and fingers with sharp borders in atopic dermatitis.

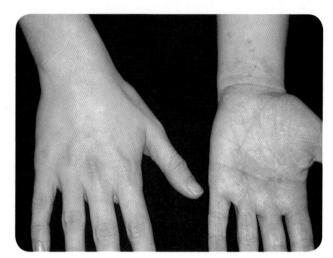

Figure 4-296 Lichenification of the wrist, pink papules, lichenification, erosions, and increased palmar markings (hyperlinear palms) in atopic dermatitis.

Diagnostic Pearls

- Make sure to obtain an adequate childhood and family history of allergies and skin disease.
- In the adult patient, persistent dry skin or persistent eyelid dermatitis may be a clue to atopic dermatitis.
- In general, it is rare for an adult without a personal or family history of atopy to develop atopic dermatitis. Such patients should be referred to dermatology to rule out another entity, specifically cutaneous T-cell lymphoma.

?? Differential Diagnosis and Pitfalls

- Seborrheic dermatitis—The distribution of lesions is often a helpful clue in distinguishing this entity from atopic dermatitis.
- Allergic contact dermatitis
- Irritant contact dermatitis
- Pityriasis rubra pilaris
- Glucagonoma syndrome
- Pellagra
- Lichen simplex chronicus
- Nummular eczema
- Scabies
- HIV-associated dermatitis
- Cutaneous T-cell lymphoma/mycosis fungoides—If an adult patient has persistent "eczema" that is not adequately responding to therapy, this entity should be ruled out with skin biopsies.
- Tinea corporis
- Psoriasis
- In children, in particular, consider Wiskott-Aldrich syndrome, selective IgA deficiency, Letterer-Siwe disease,

hyper IgE syndrome, and Netherton syndrome, as these conditions may display similar eruptions.

✓ Best Tests

- Take a careful history, as this is primarily a clinical diagnosis.
- In a few select cases, the following investigations may help rule out imitators:
  - Skin biopsy
  - Serum immunoglobulin levels (IgE, IgA, IgM, and IgG); serum IgE level is elevated in 80% of patients
  - Oral food challenges, RAST, or skin allergy testing
  - HIV test

▲▲ Management Pearls

- Secondary bacterial infection may exacerbate atopic dermatitis. Treat with a 10-day course of oral antibiotics to cover *S. aureus* infection.
- Counsel patients on the typical triggers, and encourage their avoidance. Factors that are known to exacerbate atopic dermatitis include stress, inappropriate bathing habits (e.g., prolonged, hot showers), infection, irritants (e.g., detergents), sweating, and environmental allergens.
- Emollients and moisturizing skin-care routines are essential. Recommend nonsoap cleansers or moisturizing soaps. Have the patient apply emollients such as petroleum jelly, ointments, or creams to damp skin after bathing and again 3 or more times during the day.
- Refer chronic, recalcitrant, or severe cases to a dermatologist.

Therapy

Use topical corticosteroids to treat active, inflamed plaques. Use class 6 and 7 topical steroids on the face and mid- to high-potency preparations on the trunk and extremities. Be careful of atrophy from use in skin folds and occluded areas. Patients frequently become sensitive to a component of topical medications. Ointments are recommended, as these usually contain fewer preservatives and stabilizers.

Patients should specifically be instructed to apply the topical steroids to the affected areas prior to application of an emollient.

Localized Disease

Mid-potency topical corticosteroids (class 3 and 4) need supervision with scheduled follow-up to observe for steroid atrophy.

- Triamcinolone cream, ointment—apply twice daily (15, 30, 60, 120, 240 g)
- Mometasone cream, ointment—apply twice daily (15, 45 g)
- Fluocinolone cream, ointment—apply twice daily (15, 30, 60 g)

Use low-potency topical steroids on areas of thinner skin on the face and intertriginous areas.

Desonide or Aclovate ointment or cream 30 g twice daily

Tacrolimus ointment 0.03%, 0.1% twice daily

Pimecrolimus 1% cream twice daily

Extensive Disease

UVB light therapy, PUVA (psoralen plus UVA), or UVA I may be used. Reserve low doses of cyclosporin A (100 mg/day), oral tacrolimus (1 to 3 mg/day), or azathioprine for resistant disease. Narrow-band UVB is an emerging therapy.

Antihistamine may be helpful. Consider one of the following antihistamines:

- Diphenhydramine hydrochloride (25 and 50 mg tablets or capsules): 25 to 50 mg nightly or every 6 h as needed
- Hydroxyzine (10 and 25 mg tablets): 12.5 to 25 mg, every 6 h as needed
- Cetirizine hydrochloride (5 and 10 mg tablets): 5 to 10 mg/day
- Loratadine (10 mg tablets): 10 mg tablet once daily
- Antibiotic therapy is beneficial when there is evidence of impetiginization. Direct coverage toward *S. aureus*.

Suggested Readings

Ashcroft DM, Dimmock P, Garside R, et al. Efficacy and tolerability of topical pimecrolimus and tacrolimus in the treatment of atopic dermatitis: Meta-analysis of randomised controlled trials. *BMJ*. 2005 Mar;330(7490):516.

Brenninkmeijer EE, Schram ME, Leeflang MM, et al. Diagnostic criteria for atopic dermatitis: a systematic review. *Br J Dermatol*. 2008 Apr;158(4):754–765.

Hanifin JM, Cooper KD, Ho VC, et al. Guidelines of care for atopic dermatitis, developed in accordance with the American Academy of Dermatology (AAD)/American Academy of Dermatology Association "Administrative Regulations for Evidence-Based Clinical Practice Guidelines". *J Am Acad Dermatol*. 2004 Mar;50(3):391–404.

Leung DY, Eichenfield LF, Boguniewicz M. Atopic dermatitis (atopic eczema). In: Fitzpatrick TB, Wolff K, eds. *Fitzpatrick's Dermatology in General Medicine*. 7th Ed. New York, NY: McGraw-Hill; 2008:146–158.

Palmer CN, Irvine AD, Terron-Kwiatkowski A, et al. Common loss-of-function variants of the epidermal barrier protein filaggrin are a major predisposing factor for atopic dermatitis. *Nat Genet*. 2006 Apr;38(4):441–446. Epub 2006 Mar 19.

Rodriguez-Serna M, Mercader P, Pardo J, et al. Kaposi's varicelliform eruption in an HIV-positive patient after laser resurfacing. *J Eur Acad Dermatol Venereol*. 2004 Nov;18(6):711–712.

Williams HC. Clinical practice. Atopic dermatitis. *N Engl J Med*. 2005 Jun;352(22):2314–2324.

Dermatitis, Contact

Diagnosis Synopsis

Allergic contact dermatitis is a delayed hypersensitivity reaction (type IV cell-mediated reaction). The most frequent sensitizers in the general population are fragrance, nickel, neomycin, formaldehyde, chromates, rubber chemicals, lanolin, other common environmental chemicals, and poison ivy and other plants.

Nickel is found in jewelry, belt buckles, green paints, and metal closures on clothing. Chromates are found in shoe and glove leathers. Rubber chemicals are found in gloves, respirators, balloons, and elastic in garments. Neomycin is common in triple antibiotic first aid ointments and other combination topical preparations. Eye preparations, eardrops, and some vaccines also cause allergic contact dermatitis. Other common allergen-containing products include cosmetics, soaps, and dyes. Allergic contact dermatitis can occur at any age. A detailed allergen exposure history should be elicited.

Dark Skin Considerations

It remains unclear if allergic contact dermatitis occurs with the same frequency in blacks as in whites. Blacks have a higher sensitivity to paraphenylenediamine (PPDA) and thiourea. The PPDA difference may be explained by the fact that hair dyes for dark hair have higher levels of PPDA or that blacks experience a cross reaction to systemic thiazide diuretics and oral antidiabetic drugs used to treat diseases more common in blacks (e.g., hypertension).

Immunocompromised Patient Considerations

Although sensitivity tends to persist, delayed-type sensitivity reactions may be lost with the progression of HIV infection.

Look For

In acute cases, lesions tend to be vesicular or bullous (Figs. 4-297 and 4-298). Subacute cases are papular, erythematous, and scaly (Fig. 4-299). Look for well-demarcated borders and geometric shapes with straight edges and right angles (Figs. 4-300–4-302). Eyelid edema is frequently seen when the allergen is innocently transferred from finger to lid (Fig. 4-303). Affected areas are typically severely pruritic. Contact dermatitis can be found at any body location.

Dark Skin Considerations

Scaling, red to deep brown-red plaques, vesicles, and bullae in acute cases. When the dermatitis is chronic, thickened plaques develop (Fig. 4-304) and secondary bacterial infection is possible.

Immunocompromised Patient Considerations

Secondary bacterial infection may be more common in immunosuppressed patients.

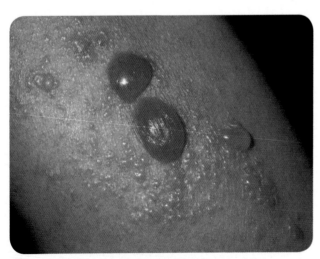

Figure 4-297 Rhus dermatitis often presents with both small vesicles and large bullae.

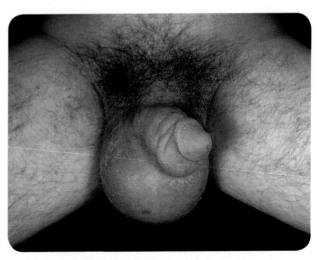

Figure 4-298 Rhus dermatitis with penile and scrotal edema. Vesicles may not be obvious in these locations.

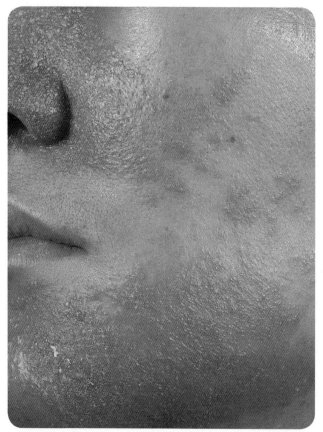

Figure 4-299 Pinpoint papules and vesicles on an erythematous base, with a sharp cutoff at the edges from contact dermatitis due to a theatrical mask.

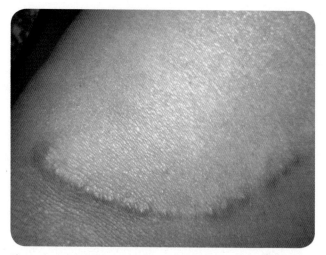

Figure 4-300 Linear vesicles are very suggestive of Rhus dermatitis.

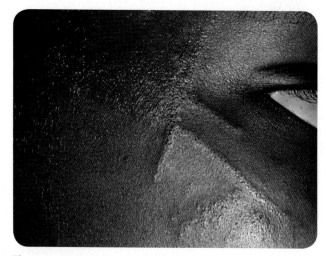

Figure 4-301 Multiple linear sets of vesicles in Rhus dermatitis.

●● Diagnostic Pearls

- Diagnosis and etiology is often based upon clinical exam and history.
- Individual lesions have well-demarcated borders, often with geometric shapes with straight edges and right angles.
- The distribution of the rash should drive the examiner's history to possible allergen exposures. Facial distributions often suggest a personal skin care product. Ear lobes suggest nickel allergy from earrings. Hand dermatitis should provoke questions regarding occupation, hobbies, and habits. There are photo-dependent allergic reactions as well.

?? Differential Diagnosis and Pitfalls

- Irritant contact dermatitis
- Tinea corporis
- Erysipelas
- Erythema multiforme
- Psoriasis
- Scabies
- Herpes simplex virus infection
- Insect bite reaction
- Seborrheic dermatitis
- Mycosis fungoides
- Dyshidrotic eczema
- Stasis dermatitis
- Nummular eczema
- Lichen simplex chronicus
- Cellulitis
- Atopic dermatitis
- Impetigo

✓ Best Tests

- The diagnosis can often be made with a careful history and physical examination. Conduct patch testing to verify the allergen in cases of allergic contact dermatitis.

235

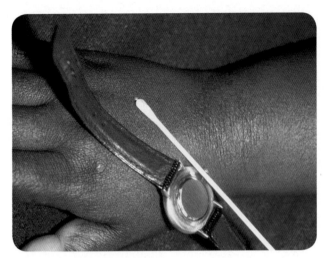

Figure 4-302 Contact dermatitis from nickel in a watch case.

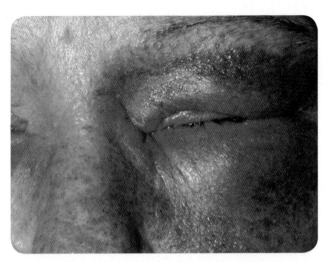

Figure 4-303 Edematous contact dermatitis from fragrance.

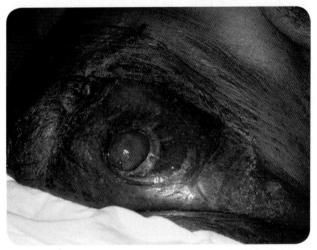

Figure 4-304 Chronic contact dermatitis from adhesive for ostomy appliance.

change ingredients or the patient may be newly sensitized. Preservatives in topical corticosteroids are common contactants, as can be the corticosteroid itself. Soap substitutes and emollients are often helpful to minimize irritation and soothe the affected skin.

- For patients needing systemic treatment, do not prescribe a 6-day course of quickly tapering steroids. The delayed hypersensitivity reaction is at least a 2-week process, and shorter courses of oral steroids will result in rebound of the dermatitis.

- Skin biopsy, which demonstrates dermatitis, helps confirm an "eczema," but it will not differentiate between different types (allergic contact, atopic, etc.) and does not identify the allergen.

▲▲ Management Pearls

- Identify the inciting allergen, if possible. Treatment is aimed at preventing contact with the allergen and control of symptoms, including antihistamines and topical and oral corticosteroids.
- Recommend the patient avoid common triggers (e.g., fragrance, lanolin, nickel) and buy recommended soaps, cleansers, and cotton gloves (as opposed to latex gloves). Do not disregard preparations that have been used for some time because over-the-counter preparations often

Therapy

High-potency topical corticosteroids on truncal and extremity skin.

High-potency topical corticosteroids (class 2)

- Fluocinonide cream, ointment—apply twice daily (15, 30, 60, 120 g)
- Desoximetasone cream, ointment—apply twice daily (15, 60, 120 g)
- Halcinonide cream, ointment—apply twice daily (15, 60, 240 g)
- Amcinonide ointment—apply twice daily (15, 30, 60 g)

Mid-potency topical corticosteroids (classes 3 and 4)

- Triamcinolone cream, ointment—apply twice daily (15, 30, 60, 120, 240 g)
- Mometasone cream, ointment—apply twice daily (15, 45 g)
- Fluocinolone ointment, cream—apply twice daily (15, 30, 60 g)

Use mild-potency topical steroids on thinner skin and class 6 and 7 steroids on the face and intertriginous areas (desonide cream, lotion, or ointment twice daily). Use steroid ointments that have fewer preservatives in them if there seems to be flaring with multiple topical medications.

Topical calcineurin inhibitors (pimecrolimus 1% cream and tacrolimus 0.1% ointment) applied twice daily may be an alternative to topical corticosteroids in the treatment of the inflammatory response, if the patient tolerates them.

If the patient's condition is exacerbated with the use of topical steroids, consider an allergy to this agent. This would be an indication for referral to dermatology for patch testing and further management.

Antihistamines

- Diphenhydramine hydrochloride—25 to 50 mg every 6 to 8 h, as needed
- Hydroxyzine—25 mg every 6 h, as needed
- Cetirizine hydrochloride—5 to 10 mg daily
- Loratadine—one 10 mg tablet daily

In severe cases involving large body areas, use a 14-day course of oral prednisone 0.5 mg/kg each morning and taper only slightly during the interval. For example, start at 40 mg/day and taper by 10 mg every 3 days to 0 mg.

Antibiotics may be indicated when there is evidence of impetiginization. Topical mupirocin or an oral cephalosporin (e.g., cephalexin) or penicillinase-resistant penicillin (e.g., dicloxacillin) will often suffice.

Treatment with PUVA/UVB or certain immune-modulating drugs (azathioprine, cyclosporine, and methotrexate) has also been tried.

Suggested Readings

American Academy of Allergy, Asthma and Immunology, American College of Allergy, Asthma and Immunology. Contact dermatitis: a practice parameter. *Ann Allergy Asthma Immunol.* 2006 Sep;97(3 Suppl. 2):-S1–S38.

Azurdia RM, King CM. Allergic contact dermatitis due to phenol-formaldehyde resin and benzoyl peroxide in swimming goggles. *Contact Dermatitis.* 1998 Apr;38(4):234–235.

Belsito DV. The diagnostic evaluation, treatment, and prevention of allergic contact dermatitis in the new millennium. *J Allergy Clin Immunol.* 2000 Mar;105(3):409–420.

Belsito DV. Occupational contact dermatitis: Etiology, prevalence, and resultant impairment/disability. *J Am Acad Dermatol.* 2005 Aug;53(2):-303–313.

Cohen DE, Heidary N. Treatment of irritant and allergic contact dermatitis. *Dermatol Ther.* 2004;17(4):334–340.

Cohen DE, Jacob SE. Allergic contact dermatitis. In: Fitzpatrick TB, Wolff K, eds. *Fitzpatrick's Dermatology in General Medicine.* 7th Ed. New York, NY: McGraw-Hill; 2008:135–146.

Corazza M, Virgili A. Allergic contact dermatitis due to nickel in a neoprene wetsuit. *Contact Dermatitis.* 1998 Nov;39(5):257.

Drake LA, Dorner W, Goltz RW, et al. Guidelines of care for contact dermatitis. Committee on Guidelines of Care. *J Am Acad Dermatol.* 1995 Jan;32(1):109–113.

Gudi VS, White MI, Ormerod AD. Allergic contact dermatitis from dibutylthiourea in a wet suit. *Dermatitis.* 2004 Mar;15(1):55–56.

James WD, Berger TG, Elston DM. Contact dermatitis and drug eruptions. In: James WD, Berger TG, Elston DM, Odom RB, eds. *Andrews' Diseases of the Skin: Clinical Dermatology.* 10th Ed. Philadelphia, PA: Saunders Elsevier; 2006:91–115.

Krob HA, Fleischer AB, D'Agostino R, et al. Prevalence and relevance of contact dermatitis allergens: A meta-analysis of 15 years of published T.R.U.E. test data. *J Am Acad Dermatol.* 2004 Sep;51(3):349–353.

Martellotta D, Di Costanzo L, Cafiero M, et al. Contact allergy to p-tert-butylphenol formaldehyde resin and zinc diethyldithiocarbamate in a wet suit. *Dermatitis.* 2008 Mar–Apr;19(2):E3–E4.

Vaswani SK, Collins DD, Pass CJ. Severe allergic contact eyelid dermatitis caused by swimming goggles. *Ann Allergy Asthma Immunol.* 2003 Jun;90(6):672–673.

■■ Diagnosis Synopsis

Dyshidrotic dermatitis (dyshidrotic eczema and pompholyx) is generally defined as a recurrent vesicular eruption limited to the hands (most often the sides of the digits) and sometimes the feet. The etiology is unknown. The lesions are extremely pruritic. Dyshidrotic dermatitis has been associated with contact irritants and allergens, atopic dermatitis, dermatophyte and bacterial infections, hyperhidrosis, hot weather, and emotional stress. Some cases spontaneously resolve. There is no gender predilection. Treatment is aimed at the symptomatic relief and control of vesiculation.

Look For

Small, tense, clear fluid-filled blisters at the lateral aspects of the digits (Fig. 4-305). The vesicles are deep seated in appearance (often referred to as "tapioca pudding" lesions) and may converge to form bullae. In severe cases, lesions can become large and extend to the palmar surfaces (Figs. 4-306 and 4-307). Interdigital maceration may be present. Once vesicles rupture, thin, scaly papules and plaques can form. The presence of scale can make it difficult to see the primary deep-seated vesicles that are the hallmark of dyshidrotic dermatitis (Fig. 4-308).

Patients with long-standing disease may have nail changes (transverse ridges, thickening, pitting).

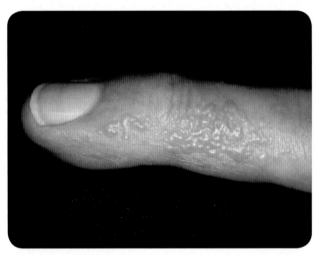

Figure 4-305 Clear vesicles on sides of fingers in dyshidrotic dermatitis (dyshidrotic eczema).

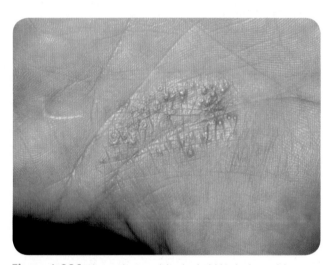

Figure 4-306 Clear palmar vesicles in dyshidrotic dermatitis.

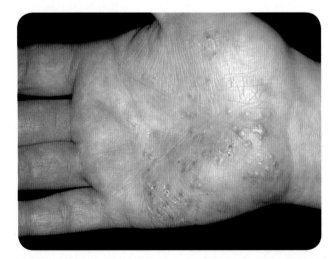

Figure 4-307 Vesicles and crusts on palmar surface in dyshidrotic dermatitis.

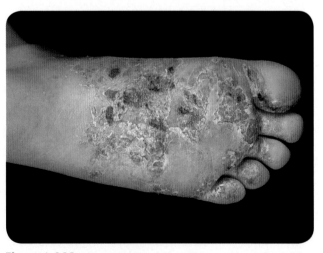

Figure 4-308 Severe crusting and erosions on volar surface of foot consistent with dyshidrotic dermatitis.

Diagnostic Pearls

- When limited to the feet, all efforts to exclude dermatophyte infection should be made.
- Scraping the undersurface of the roof of bullae can often lead to a positive fungal scraping and culture while studies of other portions of the lesions may be negative.

Differential Diagnosis and Pitfalls

- Distinguishing idiopathic dyshidrotic dermatitis from allergic contact dermatitis can be difficult, although contact dermatitis often involves the dorsum of the hand. An extensive history of environmental exposure should be gathered when a vesicular hand rash is present.
- Dermatophyte infection (e.g., tinea pedis and/or manuum)
- Herpes simplex virus
- Pustular psoriasis
- Pemphigus vulgaris
- Bullous pemphigoid
- Impetigo
- Scabies
- Infantile acropustulosis

✓ Best Tests

- This is usually a clinical diagnosis. Biopsy is confirmatory but does not help establish the etiology.
- Further testing may be done to rule out other conditions:
  - Patch testing (allergic contact dermatitis)
  - KOH preparation of scrapings (dermatophyte)
  - Bacterial culture (bacterial infection)
  - Biopsy for direct immunofluorescence (bullous pemphigoid)

Management Pearls

- To manage vesicles and bullae, use compresses (Burow solution). Drain large bullae, leaving the roof intact. A symptomatic relief of pruritus can be obtained with lotions or creams containing pramoxine, camphor, or menthol. Systemic antihistamines may also help. The removal of any irritating agents and class 2 and 3 steroids with or without occlusive vinyl gloves are the mainstays of treatment.
- A brief course of oral prednisone may be necessary, but patients often cannot tolerate being tapered off this therapy. Likewise, monthly Kenalog 40 IM injections are not recommended because of long-term side effects and possible aseptic necrosis of the hip.

Therapy

Conservative measures as above, plus a high-potency topical steroid initially (classes 2 and 3).

High-potency topical corticosteroids (class 2)

- Fluocinonide cream, ointment—apply twice daily (15, 30, 60, 120 g)
- Desoximetasone cream, ointment—apply twice daily (15, 60, 120 g)
- Halcinonide cream, ointment—apply twice daily (15, 60, 240 g)
- Amcinonide ointment—apply twice daily (15, 30, 60 g)

Mid-potency topical corticosteroids (classes 3 and 4)

- Triamcinolone cream, ointment—apply twice daily (15, 30, 60, 120, 240 g)
- Mometasone cream, ointment—apply twice daily (15, 45 g)
- Fluocinolone ointment, cream—apply twice daily (15, 30, 60 g)

Or if severe, use a superpotent topical steroid for a short 2-week course, and schedule close follow-up (class 1)

- Clobetasol 0.05% cream—apply twice daily (15, 30, 45 g)
- Betamethasone 0.05% cream—apply twice daily (15, 30, 45 g)
- Diflorasone 0.05% cream—apply twice daily (15, 30, 60 g)
- Halobetasol cream—apply twice daily (15, 50 g)

Beware of skin atrophy with potent and superpotent steroids!

Topical tacrolimus 0.1% ointment twice daily can be used alone or in combination with topical corticosteroids.

Severe cases can be treated with short courses of prednisone, beginning with 0.5 mg/kg each morning with gradual taper over 2 weeks, but beware of the difficulty tapering these patients.

Chronic, severe disease can be treated with topical PUVA (psoralen and UVA phototherapy administered by a dermatologist) or other systemic immunosuppressives (including azathioprine and methotrexate).

Botulinum toxin injections have also been used in refractory cases.

Suggested Readings

Doshi DN, Kimball AB. Vesicular palmoplantar eczema. In: Fitzpatrick TB, Wolff K, eds. *Fitzpatrick's Dermatology in General Medicine.* 7th Ed. New York, NY: McGraw-Hill; 2008:162–167.

Friedmann PS, Wilkinson M. Occupational dermatoses. In: Bolognia JL, Jorizzo JL, Rapini RP, eds. *Dermatology.* 2nd Ed. St. Louis, MO: Mosby; 2008:233.

Lofgren SM, Warshaw EM. Dyshidrosis: Epidemiology, clinical characteristics, and therapy. *Dermatitis.* 2006 Dec;17(4):165–181.

MacConnachie AA, Smith CC. Pompholyx eczema as a manifestation of HIV infection, response to antiretroviral therapy. *Acta Derm Venereol.* 2007;87(4):378–379.

Polderman MC, Govaert JC, le Cessie S, et al. A double-blind placebo-controlled trial of UVA-1 in the treatment of dyshidrotic eczema. *Clin Exp Dermatol.* 2003 Nov;28(6):584–587.

Swartling C, Naver H, Lindberg M, et al. Treatment of dyshidrotic hand dermatitis with intradermal botulinum toxin. *J Am Acad Dermatol.* 2002 Nov;47(5):667–671.

Warshaw EM. Therapeutic options for chronic hand dermatitis. *Dermatol Ther.* 2004;17(3):240–250.

■ Diagnosis Synopsis

Irritant contact dermatitis is a reaction caused by direct physical or chemical injury to the epidermis. The damage caused by an irritant leads to inflammation, manifested in the skin as erythema, edema, and scaling. Irritant contact dermatitis should be differentiated from true allergic contact dermatitis, which is a delayed type-IV hypersensitivity (immune) reaction. Patients typically present complaining of a burning or stinging sensation early in the course of irritant contact dermatitis. Symptoms and a rash usually follow the exposure by hours if the irritant is strong; this is in contrast to allergic contact dermatitis where symptoms are usually delayed by approximately 2 days following exposure. As the irritation becomes chronic and the skin continually inflamed, pruritus can become a predominant symptom.

The hands are the most common location for irritant contact dermatitis, though any body surface can be involved, including the genitals. Patients with a history of atopic dermatitis are particularly predisposed. Environmental factors include repeated exposure to water or frequent hand washing, soaps and solvents, fiberglass, mild acids, and alkalis. Dry air can also predispose to irritant contact dermatitis. Exposures are frequently occupational. High-risk jobs include cleaning, health care, food preparation, and hairdressing. Irritant contact dermatitis can occur at any age. It is more common in women.

◉ Look For

Look for erythematous macules, vesicles, bullae, erosions, or plaques. Plaques develop scale and fissuring in chronic areas of irritant contact dermatitis (Fig. 4-309). In acute cases, patches and plaques may have a sharp border corresponding to the areas of chemical exposure (Figs. 4-310 and 4-311). Fingertip irritant contact dermatitis can have desquamation, fissures, and scaling (Fig. 4-312). Irritant contact dermatitis can be found anywhere on the body but is most common on the hands.

Individuals with chronic irritant contact dermatitis may display signs of secondary lichenification of the skin due to repetitive rubbing of the area.

●● Diagnostic Pearls

- Look for a sharp border or "cutoff" of the involved areas and normal nearby skin.
- There may be certain telltale signs, such as drip marks and splatter patterns.
- Irritant contact dermatitis has less of a tendency to spread than does allergic contact dermatitis.

?? Differential Diagnosis and Pitfalls

- Allergic contact dermatitis
- Atopic dermatitis
- Tinea corporis, pedis, or manus—When a patient presents with scaling lesions (especially on the hands or feet), it is important to perform a potassium hydroxide (KOH) preparation to rule out a fungal etiology.
- Xerotic dermatitis/eczema craquelé
- Phytophotodermatitis
- Drug eruption
- Dyshidrotic dermatitis
- Intertrigo if present in skin fold
- Erythrasma
- Candidiasis
- Cellulitis

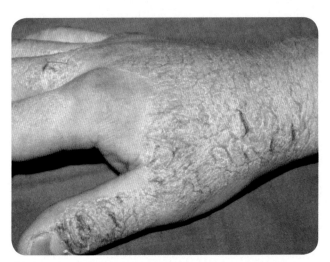

Figure 4-309 Red skin with multiple fissures suggests irritant contact dermatitis.

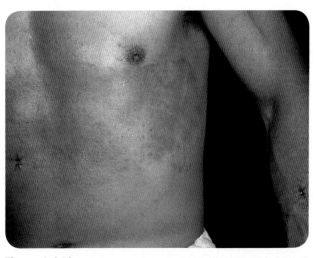

Figure 4-310 Irritant contact dermatitis from a "mustard plaster."

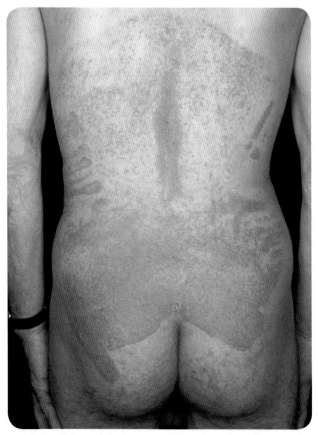

Figure 4-311 Irritant contact dermatitis from a prespinal anesthesia preparation. Note the geometric pattern and sharp cutoff.

- Erysipelas
- Nummular dermatitis
- Stasis dermatitis
- Cutaneous T-cell lymphoma

✓ Best Tests

- Irritant contact dermatitis is a clinical diagnosis and a diagnosis of exclusion; no laboratory studies exist to confirm that irritant dermatitis is the definitive diagnosis.
- Patch testing is used to rule out true allergic contact dermatitis.
- If scaling plaques are present, consider a KOH study to rule out a dermatophyte infection, such as tinea pedis, corporis, or manus.
- Take a detailed history of the patient's occupational, recreational, and home exposures. It may be valuable to instruct the patient to keep a diary of such exposures.

Management Pearls

- Prevention is of paramount importance. Remove the offending exposure, and protect the skin from reexposure.

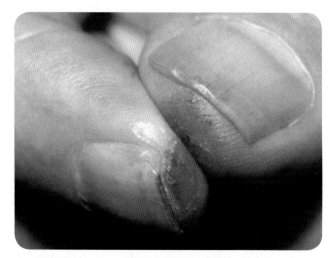

Figure 4-312 Irritant contact dermatitis from cigarettes.

Educate patients about common irritants; proper skin care, including the use of moisturizers; and protective clothing, such as gloves and aprons. The use of cotton gloves worn under occlusive gloves is superior to the use of occlusive gloves alone.
- For irritated skin in body folds, consider a barrier cream with zinc oxide paste.

Therapy

The patient should use petroleum jelly or a non-comedogenic moisturizing cream applied directly to wet skin after bathing or washing. These emollients should be applied frequently (at least twice daily) to moisturize and protect the skin. If a topical steroid is used, the steroid should be applied prior to the emollient.

Mild-to-moderate-strength topical steroids may have some benefit if inflammation is pronounced. High-potency topical steroids are infrequently used by dermatologists in the management of irritant contact dermatitis.

Mid-potency topical corticosteroids (classes 3 and 4)—until inflammation subsides (usually <1 week)

- Triamcinolone cream, ointment—apply twice daily (15, 30 g)
- Mometasone cream, ointment—apply twice daily (15 g)
- Fluocinolone ointment, cream—apply twice daily (15, 30 g)

Use a mild-potency topical steroid on thinner skin and a class 6 and 7 steroid on the face (desonide cream, lotion, or ointment applied twice daily [30 g]). Transition the patient to a lower-potency agent once inflammation begins to abate. Corticosteroid ointment preparations are preferable to creams and lotions, as these contain fewer preservatives and patients are, therefore, less likely to develop sensitization.

Topical calcineurin inhibitors (pimecrolimus 1% cream and tacrolimus 0.1% ointment) applied twice daily may be an alternative to topical corticosteroids in the treatment of the inflammatory response, if the patient tolerates them.

Other treatments include low-dose cyclosporine (3 mg/kg/day) and UVB or PUVA-bath phototherapy, but patients requiring this level of therapy require evaluation and treatment by a dermatologist.

Suggested Readings

Dong H, Kerl H, Cerroni L. EMLA cream-induced irritant contact dermatitis. *J Cutan Pathol.* 2002 Mar;29(3):190–192.

English JS. Current concepts of irritant contact dermatitis. *Occup Environ Med.* 2004 Aug;61(8):674, 722–726.

Friedmann PS, Wilkinson M. Occupational dermatoses. In: Bolognia JL, Jorizzo JL, Rapini RP, eds. *Dermatology.* 2nd Ed. St. Louis, MO: Mosby; 2008:233–234.

Kucenic MJ, Belsito DV. Occupational allergic contact dermatitis is more prevalent than irritant contact dermatitis: A 5-year study. *J Am Acad Dermatol.* 2002 May;46(5):695–699.

Ramsing DW, Agner T. Efficacy of topical corticosteroids on irritant skin reactions. *Contact Dermatitis.* 1995 May;32(5):293–297.

Slodownik D, Lee A, Nixon R. Irritant contact dermatitis: A review. *Australas J Dermatol.* 2008 Feb;49(1):1–9; quiz 10–11.

Diagnosis Synopsis

Nummular dermatitis (nummular eczema) is a particular form of dermatitis characterized by pruritic, coin-shaped, scaly plaques. It is of uncertain etiology, but the onset is associated with triggers such as frequent bathing, irritating and drying soaps, skin trauma, interferon therapy for hepatitis C, and exposure to irritating fabrics such as wool. Venous stasis may be a predisposing factor to developing lesions on the legs. Many authorities consider it to be a form of eczema, and some patients often have some of the signs and symptoms associated with classic atopic dermatitis.

Nummular dermatitis is pruritic but may be less pruritic than other common diagnoses with scaly plaques (e.g., tinea). Autoeczematization (widespread eczematous eruption secondary to triggers such as infection or severe localized eczema) and impetiginization (superinfection of impaired skin barrier) may take place. Nummular dermatitis is commonly encountered in young women with typical atopic dermatitis. It also frequently occurs in middle-aged to older men. There is no known ethnic predilection.

Look For

Round or coin-shaped, erythematous, scaly plaques, often with minute fissures, erosions, or crust located within (Figs. 4-313–4-316). They may begin as papules or vesicles, which then coalesce. Plaques may also develop a central clearing.

The plaques are found on the trunk and/or the extremities, often in a symmetric distribution. The lesions may also involve the hands and feet, but not the face and scalp.

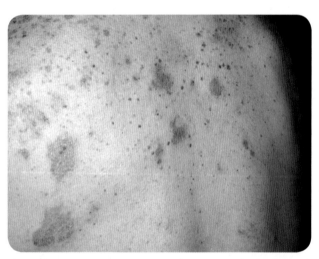

Figure 4-313 Nummular plaques usually have regular circular borders but at times may have irregular borders.

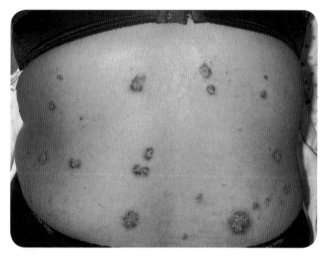

Figure 4-314 Multiple plaques with hyperkeratosis and crusting.

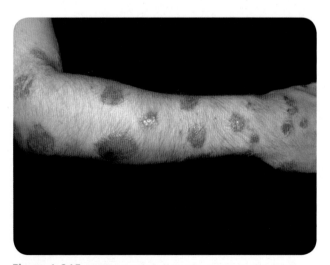

Figure 4-315 Multiple eroded plaques in nummular dermatitis.

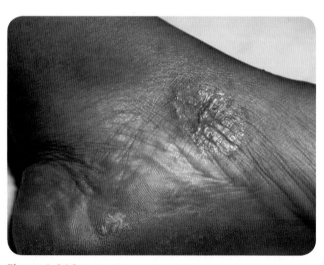

Figure 4-316 Nummular plaque on foot.

Dark Skin Considerations

Erythema may be less prominent in darker-skinned patients.

Diagnostic Pearls

- The scale of psoriasis is thicker and more silvery. Auspitz sign is present.
- Tinea corporis usually has leading scale (scale on the outside of the plaque).
- Atopic dermatitis may exhibit more lichenification.

?? Differential Diagnosis and Pitfalls

- Tinea corporis
- Psoriasis
- Atopic dermatitis
- Hailey-Hailey disease
- Lichen simplex chronicus
- Fixed drug eruption
- Mycosis fungoides (especially when lesions localize to the buttocks of adults)
- Eczema craquelé
- Contact dermatitis, irritant or allergic
- Small plaque parapsoriasis
- Pityriasis rosea
- Seborrheic dermatitis

✓ Best Tests

- Swab any crusted plaques for bacterial culture and sensitivity testing.
- Perform a skin scraping and KOH preparation to rule out a fungal infection.
- A skin biopsy will confirm the clinical diagnosis, although this is usually not necessary.

Management Pearls

- Look for signs of secondary bacterial infection, and treat with anti-staphylococcal antibiotics if necessary. The choice of antibiotic should be based on patterns of antimicrobial resistance within your community.
- Patients may benefit from using a humidifier, in the winter months in particular.
- Encourage patients to wear loose-fitting clothing and avoid irritating fabrics such as wool.

Therapy

Instruct the patient to apply thick emollients, such as petroleum jelly, at least twice daily. Patients should take short (5 min or less) lukewarm baths or showers, use mild soaps on axillary and groin areas, and apply emollients while the skin is still damp. Use a mid-to-high-potency (classes 2 to 5) topical corticosteroid applied directly to the lesions twice daily. The topical steroid should be applied prior to the emollient.

Class 2
- Fluocinonide cream, ointment—apply twice daily (15, 30, 60,120 g)
- Desoximetasone cream, ointment—apply twice daily (15, 60, 120 g)
- Halcinonide cream, ointment—apply twice daily (15, 60, 240 g)
- Amcinonide ointment—apply twice daily (15, 30, 60 g)

Classes 3 and 4
- Triamcinolone cream, ointment—apply twice daily (15, 30, 60, 120, 240 g)
- Mometasone cream, ointment—apply twice daily (15, 45 g)
- Fluocinolone ointment, cream—apply twice daily (15, 30, 60 g)

For extensive disease, consider UVB phototherapy plus emollients. Systemic corticosteroids and other immunosuppressants have also been used to treat extensive disease. Once these medications are under consideration, the patient requires evaluation and treatment by a dermatologist.

If pruritus is severe, systemic antihistamines may provide some relief, especially in the evening:

- Diphenhydramine hydrochloride—25 to 50 mg every 6 to 8 h, as needed
- Hydroxyzine—25 mg every 6 h, as needed
- Cetirizine hydrochloride—5 to 10 mg daily
- Loratadine—10 mg daily

Suggested Readings

Burgin S. Nummular eczema and lichen simplex chronicus/prurigo nodularis. In: Fitzpatrick TB, Wolff K, eds. *Fitzpatrick's Dermatology in General Medicine.* 7th Ed. New York, NY: McGraw-Hill; 2008:158–162.

Gutman AB, Kligman AM, Sciacca J, et al. Soak and smear: A standard technique revisited. *Arch Dermatol.* 2005 Dec;141(12):1556–1559.

James WD, Berger TG, Elston DM. Atopic dermatitis, eczema, and noninfectious immunodeficiency disorders. In: James WD, Berger TG, Elston DM, Odom RB, eds. *Andrews' Diseases of the Skin: Clinical Dermatology.* 10th Ed. Philadelphia, PA: Saunders Elsevier; 2006:82.

Diagnosis Synopsis

Perioral dermatitis (including steroid rosacea) is a localized inflammatory disorder of uncertain etiology. It manifests as an erythematous papular and pustular eruption with fine scaling involving the nasolabial folds, chin, and upper lip. It is seen almost exclusively in women aged between 18 and 40. A number of factors have been implicated in causing this condition, but medications such as topical glucocorticoids (including inhalers) and oral contraceptives are frequent etiologies.

Look For

Monomorphous, red papules, both grouped and individually on the chin, lips, and nasolabial folds (Figs. 4-317–4-320).

There may be pustules, and there may be associated scaling and erythema. On occasion, lesions are periocular.

Perioral dermatitis characteristically spares the skin immediately adjacent to the vermilion border.

Dark Skin Considerations

In blacks, pustules can predominate.

Diagnostic Pearls

- Perioral dermatitis is a relatively new disease since the 1950s, which suggests a new etiological agent.
- Differentiate from rosacea based on the absence of flushing and telangiectasias. Perioral dermatitis also tends to occur in a younger age group.

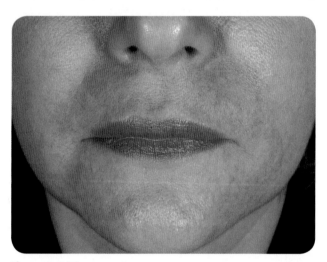

Figure 4-317 Groups of lesions often surround the mouth in perioral dermatitis.

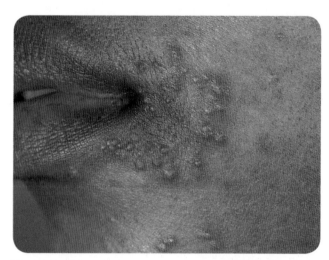

Figure 4-318 Individual lesions of perioral dermatitis are morphologically uniform.

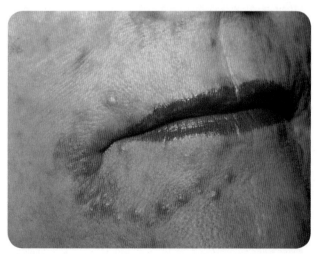

Figure 4-319 Lesions do not oppose the vermilion border in perioral dermatitis.

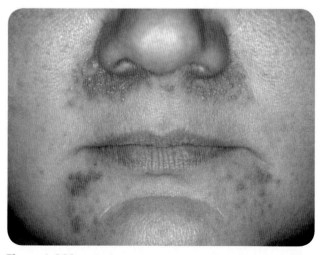

Figure 4-320 Symmetrical groups of lesions are common in perioral dermatitis.

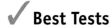

?? Differential Diagnosis and Pitfalls

- Rosacea
- Granulomatous periorificial dermatitis
- Lupus miliaris disseminata faciei
- Seborrheic dermatitis
- Atopic dermatitis
- Contact dermatitis
- Gram-negative folliculitis
- Acne

✓ Best Tests

- This is a clinical diagnosis. A skin biopsy could be suggestive of the diagnosis but is not diagnostic.

▲▲ Management Pearls

- If the perioral dermatitis was triggered by the use of mid- or high-potency topical steroids (as in steroid rosacea), then use low-potency class 6 or 7 steroids to taper because the disorder will flare if corticosteroids are discontinued abruptly. Patients must be warned that they will likely flare before they improve after the topical steroid is stopped.

Therapy

In patients with a history of steroid exposure, topical corticosteroids should be discontinued with tapering as necessary. Topical tacrolimus ointment 0.1% has been shown to be beneficial in these patients.

Topical and oral antibiotics may also be used. These are of particular value in patients with no history of topical steroid use.

Topical antibiotics
- Topical tetracycline solution applied to affected area twice daily
- Topical erythromycin solution applied to affected area twice daily
- Topical metronidazole (0.75% gel) applied to affected area twice daily
- Topical azelaic acid (20% cream) applied to affected area twice daily
- Topical clindamycin lotion applied to the affected area twice daily

Oral antibiotics
- Tetracycline 500 mg twice daily for 1 month, then taper to 1 p.o. daily for 2 weeks
- Doxycycline 100 mg twice daily for 1 month, then taper slowly over several weeks
- Erythromycin 333 mg every 8 h

Treatment is often required for several months.

Suggested Readings

Chamlin SL, Lawley LP. Perioral dermatitis. In: Fitzpatrick TB, Wolff K, eds. *Fitzpatrick's Dermatology in General Medicine*. 7th Ed. New York, NY: McGraw-Hill; 2008:709–712.

Hafeez ZH. Perioral dermatitis: An update. *Int J Dermatol*. 2003 Jul;42(7):514–517.

James WD, Berger TG, Elston DM. Granulomatous facial dermatitis. In: James WD, Berger TG, Elston DM, Odom RB, eds. *Andrews' Diseases of the Skin: Clinical Dermatology*. 10th Ed. Philadelphia, PA: Saunders Elsevier; 2006:249.

Schwarz T, Kreiselmaier I, Bieber T, et al. A randomized, double-blind, vehicle-controlled study of 1% pimecrolimus cream in adult patients with perioral dermatitis. *J Am Acad Dermatol*. 2008 Jul;59(1):34–40.

Siegel MA. Perioral dermatitis. *J Am Dent Assoc*. 2006 Aug;137(8):1121–1122.

Veien NK, Munkvad JM, Nielsen AO, et al. Topical metronidazole in the treatment of perioral dermatitis. *J Am Acad Dermatol*. 1991 Feb;24 (2 Pt 1):258–260.

Dermatitis, Seborrheic

Diagnosis Synopsis

Seborrheic dermatitis is a common inflammatory papulosquamous disease of uncertain etiology associated with the sebaceous follicle regions of the body, face, scalp, and chest. The pathogenesis may be related to an abnormal immune response to *Malassezia*, a genus of yeast that commonly colonizes the skin. There are two clinical presentations: infantile, which is in the first 3 months of life and self-limited; and adult, with an estimated prevalence of up to 5%. Men tend to be affected more than women. There is often dryness, pruritus, erythema, and fine, greasy scaling in characteristic sites: the scalp, face (especially the eyebrows and nasolabial folds), anterior chest, external ear canal, posterior ears, eyelid margins (blepharitis), groin (scrotum or labia minora), and perianal area. One or multiple sites may be involved. Certain medications may cause seborrheic dermatitis to flare, such as gold compounds, phenothiazines, lithium, methyldopa, griseofulvin, psoralens, stanozolol, and interferon alpha. Even with treatment, the disease tends to be chronic. Remissions and exacerbations should be expected.

Seborrheic dermatitis is often better in the summer and worse in the winter.

There is no apparent racial predilection. The condition may appear worse in men.

Immunocompromised Patient Considerations

Associated *Pityrosporum* folliculitis may be seen in immunocompromised patients. Seborrheic dermatitis is seen in up to 85% of HIV-infected patients at all stages of disease. It is also often seen in patients with Parkinson disease. The course is chronic and relapsing and may be difficult to treat.

Look For

Loose, bran-like or greasy scales within erythematous, fine patches or plaques involving the scalp, eyebrows, eyelids, lips, ears, and skin folds, especially the nasolabial folds (Figs. 4-321–4-323). It may also involve the anterior chest and umbilicus. Occasionally, crusted plaques are seen. The color may range from yellow-red to pink. Scale is less evident in intertriginous areas (Figs. 4-324 and 4-325).

What is classically referred to as "dandruff" represents a mild form of this dermatitis.

Dark Skin Considerations

In blacks, facial lesions may be arcuate or annular, have discrete papules, and have moderate hypopigmentation. Sometimes plaques are crusted, and in blacks, these plaques are usually grayish in color.

Immunocompromised Patient Considerations

Lesions may be more widespread and pronounced in immunocompromised patients.

Diagnostic Pearls

- If scales are difficult to remove, consider psoriasis and examine the patient in characteristic locations (especially extensor surfaces).
- Facial seborrheic dermatitis is often associated with rosacea.

Immunocompromised Patient Considerations

Lesions may be more widespread and pronounced in immunocompromised patients.

?? Differential Diagnosis and Pitfalls

- Tinea (corporis, capitis, or cruris)
- Psoriasis—The distinction between psoriasis and seborrheic dermatitis may be difficult at times, and there may be an overlap condition, sometimes referred to as "sebo-psoriasis."

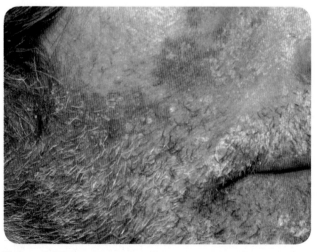

Figure 4-321 Scaling and erythema is common within the beard region in seborrheic dermatitis.

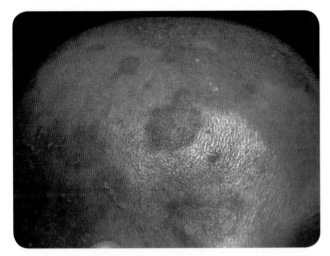

Figure 4-322 Annular erythematous plaques with overlying greasy, yellow scale on the scalp in seborrheic dermatitis.

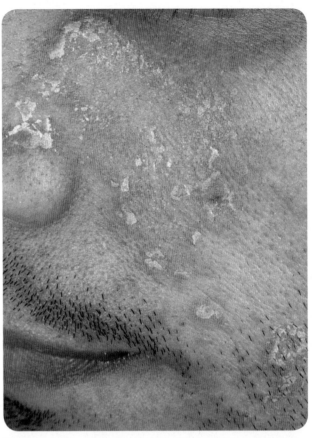

Figure 4-323 Scale and erythema on the face in seborrheic dermatitis.

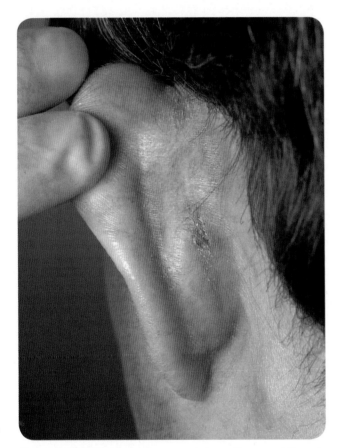

Figure 4-324 The intertriginous area between the ear and the scalp is a common location for seborrheic dermatitis.

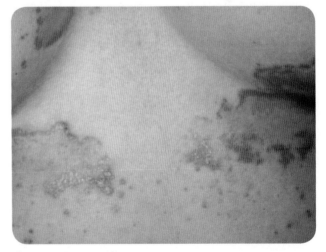

Figure 4-325 Intertriginous areas (e.g., below the breasts) are common sites for seborrheic dermatitis.

- Intertrigo
- Erythrasma
- Perioral dermatitis
- Contact dermatitis, irritant or allergic
- Rosacea
- Impetigo

- Pityriasis versicolor
- Nummular dermatitis
- Atopic dermatitis
- Pityriasis rosea
- Darier disease
- Eczema craquelé

- Candidiasis
- Dermatomyositis—The eyelid erythema seen in this condition has a more violaceous hue.

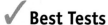 Best Tests

- This is usually a clinical diagnosis; a skin biopsy can be suggestive of but not diagnostic for this disease.
- Consider a skin scraping with a KOH preparation to rule out tinea.
- Consider HIV testing, especially in patients with risk factors/severe disease whose HIV status is unknown.
- Zinc deficiency may lead to a seborrhea-like eruption; consider obtaining a zinc level, especially in patients with poor nutritional status.

▲▲ Management Pearls

- After lesions are controlled, the patient may be weaned from therapy, but they should restart therapy at the smallest manifestation of the disease.
- Instruct the patient to avoid the use of harsh deodorant soaps. A soap substitute is probably best.

Immunocompromised Patient Considerations

Disease is typically more difficult to control in HIV-infected individuals. It may not improve with antiretroviral therapy.

Therapy

For the scalp

- Ketoconazole 2% shampoo—Apply to the wet scalp when first entering the shower. Use approximately twice weekly. The lather should also be used to cleanse the face and any other involved areas.
- 2% Pyrithione zinc shampoos
- 1% Ciclopirox shampoo twice weekly

- For dense scalp scale, consider fluocinolone acetonide 0.01% in peanut oil—Apply nightly and then shampoo out in the morning. An alternative is overnight applications of Bakers P&S solution; apply nightly and shampoo out in the morning (120 and 240 mL).

Alternative shampoos also include tar and salicylic acid–based preparations and 2.5% selenium sulfide shampoo.

Nonscalp disease

Ketoconazole is the first-line treatment.

- Ketoconazole cream twice daily (15 and 30 g) until clear

Although topical steroids may result in rapid clearing, they can induce rosacea. Thus, if necessary, only mild topical steroids should be used.

Use only mild topical steroids (class 6 or 7):

- Desonide cream, lotion—apply twice daily (15, 30, 60 g)
- Hydrocortisone cream 2.5%—apply twice daily (1, 2 oz)

Suggested Readings

Dreno B, Moyse D. Lithium gluconate in the treatment of seborrhoeic dermatitis: A multicenter, randomised, double-blind study versus placebo. *Eur J Dermatol.* 2002 Nov–Dec;12(6):549–552.

Gupta AK, Batra R, Bluhm R, et al. Skin diseases associated with Malassezia species. *J Am Acad Dermatol.* 2004 Nov;51(5):785–798.

Gupta AK, Bluhm R, Cooper EA, et al. Seborrheic dermatitis. *Dermatol Clin.* 2003 Jul;21(3):401–412.

Gupta AK, Kogan N. Seborrhoeic dermatitis: current treatment practices. *Expert Opin Pharmacother.* 2004 Aug;5(8):1755–1765.

James WD, Berger TG, Elston DM. Seborrheic dermatitis, psoriasis, recalcitrant palmoplantar eruptions, pustular dermatitis, and erythroderma. In: James WD, Berger TG, Elston DM, Odom RB, eds. *Andrews' Diseases of the Skin: Clinical Dermatology.* 10th Ed. Philadelphia, PA: Saunders Elsevier; 2006:191–193.

Plewig G, Jansen T. Seborrheic dermatitis. In: Fitzpatrick TB, Wolff K, eds. *Fitzpatrick's Dermatology in General Medicine.* 7th Ed. New York, NY: McGraw-Hill; 2008:219–225.

Swinyer LJ, Decroix J, Langner A, et al. Ketoconazole gel 2% in the treatment of moderate to severe seborrheic dermatitis. *Cutis.* 2007 Jun;79(6):475–482.

Dermatitis, Stasis

Diagnosis Synopsis

Stasis dermatitis is a cutaneous vascular disease of venous insufficiency and venous hypertension resulting in an acute or chronic dermatitis and pigmentary change of the lower legs. It usually begins on the medial malleolus but may become circumferential over time. Obesity, congestive heart failure, deep vein thrombosis (DVT), history of a leg fracture, venous hypertension secondary to prolonged standing, and congenital absence of venous valves are all associated conditions. Complications include infection and ulceration. Topical antibiotics such as neomycin are often applied to the dermatitis, which may act as a trigger in worsening the dermatitis. The incidence increases with advancing age.

Stasis dermatitis is often mistaken for cellulitis. Unlike cellulitis, the lesions of stasis dermatitis are often scaly and present bilaterally. While the patient may complain of severe pain and present with a red leg, signs of infection (fever, elevated white blood cell count, lymphadenopathy, and lymphatic streaking) will be absent. Frequently, other signs of venous insufficiency will also be apparent on physical examination.

Immunocompromised Patient Considerations

In immunocompromised patients, other entities, such as leukemia cutis, may mimic stasis dermatitis. If patient is unresponsive to therapy, early referral to dermatology is recommended.

Look For

Erythematous, scaly plaques involving the ankle and distal lower leg (Figs. 4-326–4-328). In chronic cases, red and yellow mottling and brown patches of pigmentation can be accompanied by an eczematous dermatitis as venous return shunts into the superficial vessels. Plaques may be exudative or lichenified. Other skin changes that are indicative of venous insufficiency include edema, varicosities, and atrophic patches (atrophie blanche). In some cases, patches may be distributed specifically over venous varicosities. Venous ulcers commonly occur in chronic stasis dermatitis (Fig. 4-329).

Advanced disease may have associated woody induration due to the chronic ischemia of the adipose tissue (lipodermatosclerosis).

Diagnostic Pearls

- Not every dermatitis on the lower legs should be called stasis dermatitis. Lichen simplex chronicus occurs in this location, and actual compromise of the venous circulation should be demonstrated before making this diagnosis. Stasis dermatitis can be unilateral but is often bilateral.
- Ask about a prior history of phlebitis or DVT, and look for varicosities (have patient stand while examining), signaling incompetent valves in the venous system.

?? Differential Diagnosis and Pitfalls

- Cellulitis—Patient is more likely to be febrile and ill-appearing. There is less associated scale in cellulitis.

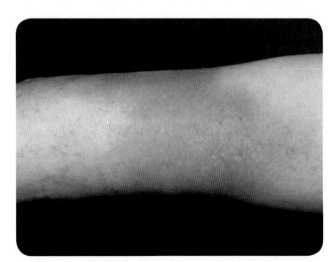

Figure 4-326 Edema and erythema characterize stasis dermatitis.

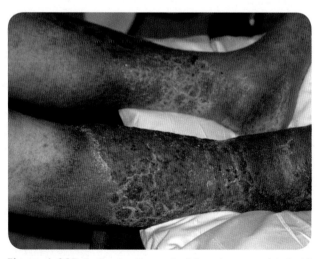

Figure 4-327 Scaling is often part of the edema associated with stasis dermatitis.

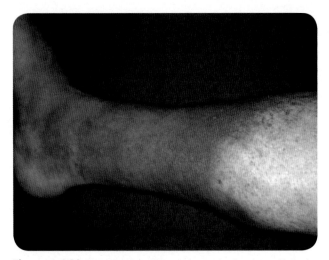

Figure 4-328 There is often fibrous change in the shape of the leg resembling an inverted champagne bottle.

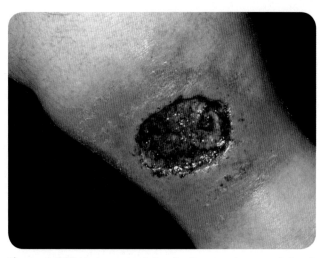

Figure 4-329 A clean-edged ulcer is often seen in areas of chronic stasis dermatitis.

- Xerosis
- Contact dermatitis—Concomitant contact dermatitis in patients with stasis dermatitis is common, often because these patients self-treat with many topical agents prior to seeking medical attention.
- Eczema craquelé
- Atopic dermatitis
- Cutaneous T-cell lymphoma
- Necrobiosis lipoidica
- Pretibial myxedema
- Nummular dermatitis
- Tinea corporis or pedis—A potassium hydroxide preparation should be performed to rule out this entity.
- Psoriasis
- Lichen simplex chronicus
- Schamberg disease and other pigmented purpuras
- Vasculitis
- Lymphedema

Immunocompromised Patient Differential Diagnosis

It is important to keep the differential broad in an immunocompromised patient.

✓ Best Tests

- Combined skin and vascular exam with specific attention to lower extremity pulses.
- Doppler ultrasound to evaluate the venous system is often a useful adjunct and should always be performed in suspected cases of DVT.
- Skin biopsy is rarely indicated.

▲▲ Management Pearls

- Doppler ultrasonography to assess arterial flow is prudent in patients with risk factors for peripheral vascular disease prior to the institution of compression therapy.
- If the patient has significant arterial disease, compression should be avoided until the patient is evaluated by a vascular surgeon.
- Consultation with a vascular surgeon may also be indicated in patients whose venous disease is amenable to surgical intervention (such as vein removal).
- Open excoriations or erosions may be treated with a topical antibiotic to prevent infection, but be aware that these agents may incite contact dermatitis (choose metronidazole).

Therapy

Compression stockings are a necessary long-term measure. They should be tailored to fit the patient and to the degree of venous insufficiency. Some suggested pressure gradients are the following:

- 15 to 20 mmHg—indicated for mild varicose veins and minor leg swelling
- 20 to 30 mmHg—indicated for moderate edema and moderate to severe varicosities
- 30 to 40 mmHg—indicated for chronic venous insufficiency, severe edema, DVT and post-thrombotic syndrome, venous ulceration, lymphedema, and orthostatic hypotension

Correct or maximize the treatment of other underlying factors, such as diabetes mellitus, peripheral vascular disease, anemia, obesity, or tobacco abuse. Exercise, as safely tolerated, should be encouraged. Minimize trauma to the area. Patients should be instructed to keep their legs elevated when at rest and to moisturize the skin with bland emollients in between flares.

Diuretics are rarely helpful in the management of stasis dermatitis.

Acute cases of stasis dermatitis require mid-to-high-potency topical corticosteroids applied twice daily.

High-potency topical corticosteroids (class 2)

Caution: Use only to reduce erythema and then decrease potency of corticosteroid to classes 4 to 6.

- Fluocinonide cream, ointment—apply twice daily (15, 30, 60, 120 g)
- Desoximetasone cream, ointment—apply twice daily (15, 60, 120 g)
- Halcinonide cream, ointment—apply twice daily (15, 60, 240 g)
- Amcinonide ointment—apply twice daily (15, 30, 60 g)

Mid-potency topical corticosteroids (classes 3 and 4)

- Triamcinolone cream, ointment—apply twice daily (15, 30, 60, 120, 240 g)
- Mometasone cream, ointment—apply twice daily (15, 45 g)
- Fluocinolone cream, ointment—apply twice daily (15, 30, 60 g)

Use steroid ointments (these have fewer preservatives) if there seems to be flaring with multiple topical medications. Allergic contact dermatitis may be a complication of treatment.

Wet-to-damp saline gauze dressings can be applied to weeping areas.

Treat impetiginized lesions with a topical (mupirocin) or systemic (dicloxacillin and cephalexin) antibiotic directed against *Staphylococcus* and *Streptococcus*.

Immunocompromised Patient Considerations

Early referral to dermatology is indicated if patient is not responding appropriately to initial therapeutic measures.

Suggested Readings

Dillon RS. Treatment of resistant venous stasis ulcers and dermatitis with the end-diastolic pneumatic compression boot. *Angiology*. 1986 Jan;37(1):47–56.

James WD, Berger TG, Elston DM, et al. Cutaneous vascular diseases. In: James WD, Berger TG, Elston DM, Odom RB, eds. *Andrews' Diseases of the Skin: Clinical Dermatology*. 10th Ed. Philadelphia, PA: Saunders Elsevier; 2006:845–846.

Papadavid E, Panayiotides I, Katoulis A, et al. Stasis dermatitis-like leukaemic infiltration in a patient with myelodysplastic syndrome. *Clin Exp Dermatol*. 2008 May;33(3):298–300.

Raju S, Hollis K, Neglen P. Use of compression stockings in chronic venous disease: patient compliance and efficacy. *Ann Vasc Surg*. 2007 Nov;21(6):790–795.

Yosipovitch G, DeVore A, Dawn A. Obesity and the skin: skin physiology and skin manifestations of obesity. *J Am Acad Dermatol*. 2007 Jun;56(6):901–916; quiz 917–920.

▪▪ Diagnosis Synopsis

Porokeratosis is a disorder of keratinization characterized by a distinct peripheral thin, ridge-like scale that corresponds histologically to a thin, angled column of epidermal parakeratotic cells that extends through the stratum corneum. Disseminated superficial actinic porokeratosis (DSAP) is a very common form of porokeratosis. DSAP is thought to have autosomal dominant inheritance with onset in the third or fourth decade of life. Women are affected three times more frequently than men. Risk factors for developing this disorder also include exposure to ultraviolet radiation and immunosuppression. Patients with DSAP may complain of exacerbations during the summer months with increased pruritus or burning sensation. Fair-skinned individuals are more prone to develop this disorder. The potential for transformation to squamous cell carcinoma exists but is rare. The lesions are minimally elevated keratotic papules symmetrically distributed on sun-exposed sites.

Immunocompromised Patient Considerations

DSAP is frequently associated with immunosuppressive conditions and conditions in which immunosuppressive medications are used, including HIV, organ transplants, Crohn disease, lymphomas, and cirrhosis.

◉ Look For

In DSAP, there are small annular-shaped, minimally elevated papules ranging from 2 to 5 mm in size (Figs. 4-330–4-332). They are numerous in number and may appear in the hundreds.

The papules are skin colored, brownish-red, or brown colored and have a scaly, distinct edge. Look carefully for the scaly ridge, which is often subtle (Fig. 4-333). The ridge on clinical exam corresponds to the cornoid lamellae seen histopathologically. The papule may attain a size of up to 10 mm. Papules may coalesce to form plaques.

These lesions are characteristically located on sun-exposed sites such as the extensor surface of the arms and the legs. The face is also affected in some patients, but certain regions are characteristically spared, such as the inguinal folds, palms and soles, and mucous membranes.

●● Diagnostic Pearls

- The papules of DSAP are quite distinct with a thin outer scaly ridge.
- DSAP typically occurs on the sun-exposed extremities.

?? Differential Diagnosis and Pitfalls

Although DSAP is distinct in its clinical appearance, it may still need to be differentiated from the following list of diseases:

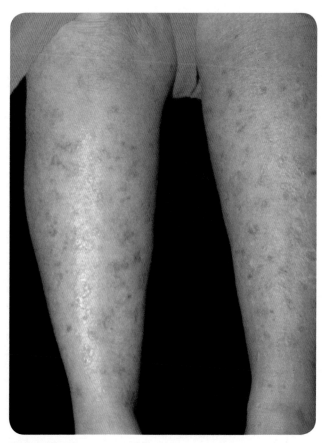

Figure 4-331 DSAP with shiny, slightly raised papules.

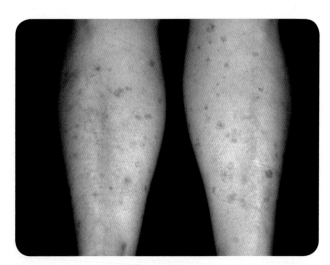

Figure 4-330 DSAP with multiple brownish, scaly papules.

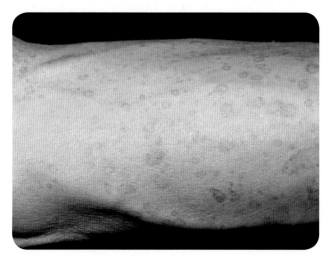

Figure 4-332 DSAP. A biopsy may be necessary to distinguish from flat seborrheic keratoses.

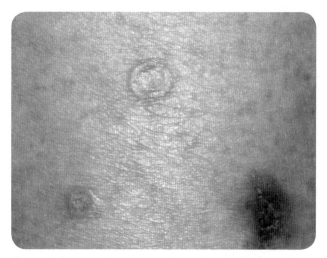

Figure 4-333 DSAP on atrophic skin with annular lesions.

- Actinic keratoses have scale throughout the lesion, where as in DSAP, scale forms a peripheral, thin ridge.
- Granuloma annulare
- Lichen planus
- Seborrheic keratoses have a more "stuck-on" appearance.
- Tinea corporis—A KOH preparation may be performed to rule out this entity.
- Flat warts

✓ Best Tests

- DSAP can often be a clinical diagnosis. If unsure of the diagnosis, a skin biopsy will show the near pathognomic cornoid lamella with its column of parakeratotic cells extending through the entire thickness of the stratum corneum. The specimen must include the raised hyperkeratotic ridge. While there are many forms of porokeratosis, DSAP is uniquely diagnosed when dozens to hundreds of scaling red-brown papules appear on the sun-exposed extremities.

▲▲ Management Pearls

- As treatment can be difficult, emphasis should be placed on avoiding exposure to strong sunlight and diligently using a broad-spectrum sunscreen with protection against both UVA and UVB, with an sun protection factor greater than 35.

Immunocompromised Patient Considerations

DSAP may improve or resolve as the patient's immune system is restored.

Therapy

The treatment of DSAP can be difficult. Because the risk of progression to skin cancer is quite low, the treatment side effects and risks must be taken into account prior to proceeding with treatment. Patients are often managed with diligent sun avoidance and emollients with no further interventions.

A few studies have investigated the use of topical 5-fluorouracil in DSAP suggesting benefit.

Other Topical Therapies
- Topical steroids of high potency such as fluocinonide cream and ointment—15, 30, 60 g twice daily may be applied.
- Keratolytics
- Topical retinoids
- Imiquimod 5%

Oral retinoids, such as isotretinoin and etretinate, have been used with some measure of success, but recurrence is high after discontinuation.

Oral isotretinoin—20 mg daily—combined with a topical cream, such as 5-fluorouracil, is effective.

Liquid nitrogen can be applied to individual macules. Scabs or blisters form 24 h after treatment.

Cryosurgery has also been used.

Photodynamic therapy is available for treatment and has the added advantage of treating precancerous spots before they become visible.

Immunocompromised Patient Considerations

Treatment of the immunosuppressive condition or discontinuation of immunosuppressive medications may lead to an improvement of DSAP.

Suggested Readings

Cavicchini S, Tourlaki A. Successful treatment of disseminated superficial actinic porokeratosis with methyl aminolevulinate-photodynamic therapy. *J Dermatolog Treat*. 2006;17(3):190–191.

James WD, Berger TG, Elston DM. Genodermatoses and congenital anomalies. In: James WD, Berger TG, Elston DM, Odom RB, eds. *Andrews' Diseases of the Skin: Clinical Dermatology*. 10th Ed. Philadelphia, PA: Saunders Elsevier; 2006:566–567.

Kang BD, Kye YC, Kim SN. Disseminated superficial actinic porokeratosis with both typical and prurigo nodularis-like lesions. *J Dermatol*. 2001 Feb;28(2):81–85.

Nayeemuddin FA, Wong M, Yell J, et al. Topical photodynamic therapy in disseminated superficial actinic porokeratosis. *Clin Exp Dermatol*. 2002 Nov;27(8):703–706.

O'Regan GM, Irvine AD. Porokeratosis. In: Fitzpatrick TB, Wolff K, eds. *Fitzpatrick's Dermatology in General Medicine*. 7th Ed. New York, NY: McGraw-Hill; 2008:443.

Panasiti V, Rossi M, Curzio M, et al. Disseminated superficial actinic porokeratosis diagnosed by dermoscopy. *Int J Dermatol*. 2008 Mar;47(3): 308–310.

Shumack SP, Commens CA. Disseminated superficial actinic porokeratosis: a clinical study. *J Am Acad Dermatol*. 1989 Jun;20(6):1015–1022.

Shumack S, Commens C, Kossard S. Disseminated superficial actinic porokeratosis. A histological review of 61 cases with particular reference to lymphocytic inflammation. *Am J Dermatopathol*. 1991 Feb;13(1): 26–31.

■■ Diagnosis Synopsis

Eczema craquelé is also known as winter itch, asteatotic eczema, xerotic eczema, and desiccation dermatitis. These entities represent the extreme end of the spectrum of xerosis (dry skin).

Xerosis is the predisposing factor to the development of eczema craquelé. It refers to a condition of rough, dry skin texture with fine scale and occasionally fine fissuring. It is often pruritic. The pathogenesis involves a decrease in the amount of lipids in the stratum corneum and a deficiency in the water-binding capacity of this layer. The most common cause of xerosis is aging; however, it can be associated with a number of environmental factors and/or disease states, such as low humidity, frequent bathing, harsh soaps, congenital and acquired ichthyoses, atopic dermatitis, hypothyroidism, Down syndrome, renal failure, malnutrition and malabsorptive states, HIV, lymphoma, liver disease, Sjögren syndrome, carcinomatosis, and certain drugs. Asteatotic dermatitis is a rare presentation of zinc deficiency.

Eczema craquelé begins as dry skin that progresses to superficially fissured, inflamed, and sometimes crusted dermatitis. A generalized dermatitis can develop. The condition is seen mostly in elderly individuals. This may be due to decreased sebaceous/sweat gland activity and keratin synthesis in elderly persons, as well as a host of other factors such as malnutrition, drugs, and underlying illnesses. The condition is exacerbated by low humidity and frequent bathing without moisturizing. Pruritus is frequent, and painful lesions can occur if the fissures are deep.

Immunocompromised Patient Considerations

Xerosis is a common early skin finding in patients with HIV, with the severity of progression of xerosis mirroring HIV progression.

◉ Look For

Xerosis usually has a slow and indolent course, progressing over years. It is characterized by dry, dull, rough skin with fine bran-like scales that flake off easily (Figs. 4-334–4-336). In contrast, eczema craquelé usually has a more acute or subacute onset. It is characterized by redness and tight-appearing, polygonally cracked skin with fine, interconnected horizontal and vertical fissures (Fig. 4-337). This forms an irregular network of fissures and cracks, similar to broken window glass. It is most severe on the distal legs and occasionally the arms and trunk. The face, scalp, groin, and axillae are usually spared from the fine, dry scales of the condition. Crusting, oozing, and bleeding fissures may be seen in advanced cases.

●● Diagnostic Pearls

- Patients will often have a history of heating using a wood stove, washing with harsh soaps, taking frequent or very hot showers, and/or a winter climate with low humidity.
- The appearance of this dermatitis has been described as "cracked porcelain," "crazy pavement," and like a "dried-up riverbed."

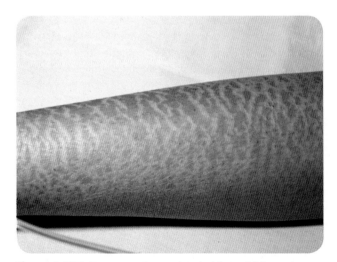

Figure 4-334 Severe xerosis associated with renal failure.

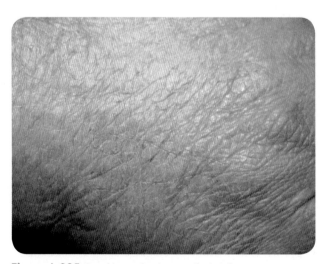

Figure 4-335 Dry skin on the dorsum of a hand.

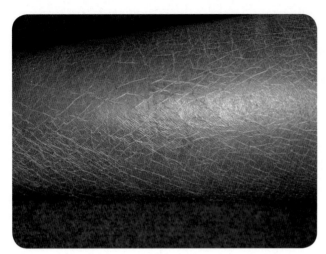

Figure 4-336 Xerosis with extensive shattered-glass pattern on the leg.

?? Differential Diagnosis and Pitfalls

- Ichthyosis vulgaris is also worse in the winter.
- Other ichthyoses
- Hypothyroidism causes very dry skin and may increase the tendency to get eczema craquelé.
- Eczema craquelé may be aggravated by topical agents or have superimposed irritant or contact dermatitis from these agents.
- Xerosis
- Stasis dermatitis
- Atopic dermatitis
- Tinea corporis
- Mycosis fungoides
- Chronic contact dermatitis
- Nummular eczema
- Scabies
- Seborrheic dermatitis

✓ Best Tests

- This is usually a clinical diagnosis. Further testing may reveal a systemic cause. Check for thyroid function, renal function, liver function, HIV, zinc level, malabsorption, cancer, or Sjögren syndrome if clinical suspicion warrants (lesions are widespread or fail to respond to therapy).

▲▲ Management Pearls

- Treat superficial crusts and signs of impetiginization with oral antibiotics for 7 to 10 days.
- Tell patients to avoid too frequent and too hot baths or showers.
- Encourage patients to use mild soaps and invest in a humidifier.

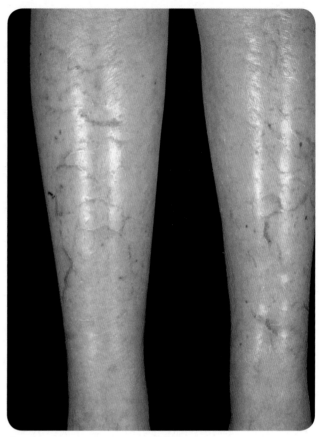

Figure 4-337 Cracking of the skin with red fissures (eczema craquelé) is often part of severe and prolonged xerosis.

Therapy

Instruct the patient to frequently apply a thick moisturizing cream or ointment such as petroleum jelly to wet skin. Eczema craquelé is best treated with heavy emollients after bathing. Immediate application of a moisturizing cream to the damp skin following bathing will "hold in" moisture.

Use a mild- to mid-potency topical steroid on inflamed areas. They may be used under occlusion for 24 to 48 h, if desired.

Mid-potency topical corticosteroids (classes 3 and 4)

- Triamcinolone cream, ointment—apply twice daily (15, 30, 60, 120, 240 g)
- Mometasone cream, ointment—apply twice daily (15, 45 g)
- Fluocinolone ointment, cream—apply twice daily (15, 30, 60 g)

Mid-potency topical corticosteroids for thinner skin (classes 6 and 7)

- Desonide cream, lotion, or ointment—apply twice daily (30 g)
- Use ointments (these have fewer preservatives in them) if the condition seems to be flaring with multiple topical medications. Avoid the use of neomycin.

Suggested Readings

Draelos ZD, Ertel K, Hartwig P, et al. The effect of two skin cleansing systems on moderate xerotic eczema. *J Am Acad Dermatol*. 2004 Jun;50(6): 883–888.

Fritsch PO, Reider N. Other eczematous eruptions. In: Bolognia JL, Jorizzo JL, Rapini RP, eds. *Dermatology*. 2nd Ed. St. Louis, MO: Mosby; 2008:200–201.

Ghali FE. Improved clinical outcomes with moisturization in dermatologic disease. *Cutis*. 2005 Dec;76(6 Suppl.):13–18.

Guillet MH, Schollhammer M, Sassolas B, et al. Eczema craquelé as a pointer of internal malignancy—a case report. *Clin Exp Dermatol*. 1996 Nov;21(6):431–433.

Johnson AW. Soap opera and winter itch: synthetic detergent bars (syndets) provide superior mildness compared with soaps. *Skinmed*. 2004 Sep–Oct;3(5):251; author reply 251–253.

Keenan WF. Comparative efficacy of two different formulations on xerosis. *J Am Acad Dermatol*. 1990 Oct;23(4 Pt 1):769–770.

Kumar B, Saraswat A, Kaur I. Mucocutaneous adverse effects of hydroxyurea: A prospective study of 30 psoriasis patients. *Clin Exp Dermatol*. 2002 Jan;27(1):8–13.

Li LF, Lan YZ. Bathing and generalized asteatotic eczema: a case-control study. *Br J Dermatol*. 2008 Jul;159(1):243–245.

Lodén M. Role of topical emollients and moisturizers in the treatment of dry skin barrier disorders. *Am J Clin Dermatol*. 2003;4(11):771–788.

Norman RA. Xerosis and pruritus in the elderly: Recognition and management. *Dermatol Ther*. 2003;16(3):254–259.

Proksch E. The role of emollients in the management of diseases with chronic dry skin. *Skin Pharmacol Physiol*. 2008;21(2):75–80.

Sparsa A, Boulinguez S, Liozon E, et al. Predictive clinical features of eczema craquelé associated with internal malignancy. *Dermatology*. 2007;215(1):28–35.

Wehr RF, Krochmal L. Considerations in selecting a moisturizer. *Cutis*. 1987 Jun;39(6):512–515.

Wilson D, Nix D. Evaluation of a once-daily moisturizer used to treat xerosis in long-term care patients. *Ostomy Wound Manage*. 2005 Nov;51(11):52–60.

Ichthyosis Vulgaris and Other Ichthyoses

Diagnosis Synopsis

The ichthyoses represent a heterogenous group of disorders characterized by a defective ability to properly form the outermost layers of the skin (ie, stratum corneum). Among other things, abnormal cornification in these diseases results in fine "fish-like" scale. The name ichthyosis gets its origin from the Greek word *ichthys*, meaning fish. The ichthyoses can be inherited or acquired. Here, we will discuss the most common of the inherited ichthyoses, ichthyosis vulgaris, and acquired ichthyosis (AI).

Ichthyosis vulgaris is an autosomal dominant disease (with variable penetrance) resulting from a loss-of-function mutation in the filaggrin gene. It is the most common disorder of cornification, affecting approximately 1 million people in the United States. Lack of functional filaggrin protein results in impaired keratinization leading to an increased adherence of the stratum corneum. Clinically, this is characterized by excessive fish skin-like scaling and desquamation beginning in the first few months of life (i.e., not present at birth). It is associated with extreme dryness secondary to epidermal water loss through abnormal skin barrier function. Coincident hair loss may occur, as may pruritus or a burning sensation. It is more prominent in winter and in climates with low relative humidity, with symptoms usually improving in warm, moist climates. Patients with the loss of a single filaggrin allele usually have a more favorable course with less severe symptoms, usually alleviating in intensity by adulthood. In contrast, mutations in both filaggrin alleles are thought to confer more severe and prolonged disease. There is no known ethnic or sex predilection. Hydration, lubrication, and keratolysis are the mainstays of therapy.

Ichthyosis vulgaris is often seen in association with atopic dermatitis and keratosis pilaris. As many as 50% of ichthyosis vulgaris patients also have atopic dermatitis. Furthermore, up to 50% of atopic dermatitis patients have a filaggrin mutation (compared to approx. 8% in the general population).

Rarely, the ichthyosis vulgaris-like disease that presents in adult patients, AI, is almost always associated with an underlying disease state such as malignancy, nonmalignant conditions, and medications. The most common associated malignancy is Hodgkin disease; however, it has also been reported with non-Hodgkin lymphomas; multiple myeloma; mycosis fungoides; carcinoma of the breast, lung, cervix, and liver; and sarcomas, including Kaposi sarcoma. The skin changes often occur simultaneously or after the diagnosis of malignancy. AI may be seen with chronic metabolic disturbances (malnutrition, malabsorption, renal failure, hyperparathyroidism, hypopituitarism, hypothyroidism, and diabetes). It also occurs on occasion with connective tissue disease (e.g., systemic lupus and dermatomyositis) as well as with sarcoidosis, leprosy (Hansen disease), and post-bone marrow transplant (graft-versus-host disease).

Drug-induced AI may be caused by cholesterol-lowering agents, butyrophenones, dixyrazine, maprotiline, cimetidine, allopurinol, hydroxyurea, and clofazimine. Disease severity depends upon the course of the associated disorder. AI often remits after the treatment of underlying malignancy.

Immunocompromised Patient Considerations

AI is often seen in HIV infection, usually with a low CD4 + count and not necessarily associated with malignancy. It may occur with higher frequency in HIV-infected Hispanics and blacks. It has been suggested that AI may be a harbinger for acute graft-versus-host disease in immunosuppressed patients postallogenic transplant.

Look For

Dry, fine-scaling skin forming a network of polygonal fish skin-like scale (Figs. 4-338–4-340). The condition is usually most apparent on the extensor extremities. It usually spares intertriginous areas secondary to increased moisture and humidity in these regions. Hyperkeratosis of the palms and soles with hyperlinearity (increased skin markings) can also be observed. In more severe cases, painful fissuring of the palms and soles can be observed (Fig. 4-341).

AI resembles ichthyosis vulgaris with symmetric, fine scale of trunk, limbs, and often the scalp, sparing the flexures and the face. Scales vary in size from 1 mm to 1 cm and are white, brown, or gray (Fig. 4-342). The lower extremities and back may have more pronounced changes.

Dark Skin Considerations

In those of African descent, extremely dry, brownish or gray, flaky or "ashy" skin may be a mild form of ichthyosis vulgaris.

Diagnostic Pearls

- Look for accentuated palmar creases and scaly palms.
- Symptoms are improved in the summer months.
- Adult onset of ichthyosis (i.e., AI) mandates investigation for underlying disease.

Differential Diagnosis and Pitfalls

- The main considerations in the differential diagnosis of ichthyosis vulgaris are other inherited ichthyoses, mainly X-linked ichthyosis, lamellar ichthyosis, and epidermolytic hyperkeratosis.

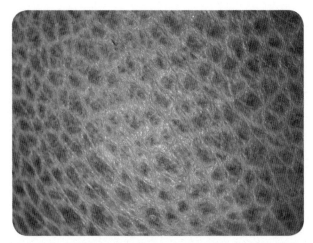

Figure 4-338 X-linked ichthyosis has well-demarcated brown scale.

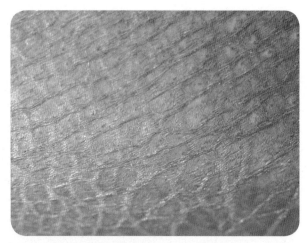

Figure 4-339 Woman with darkly pigmented skin with fine white scales consistent with ichthyosis vulgaris.

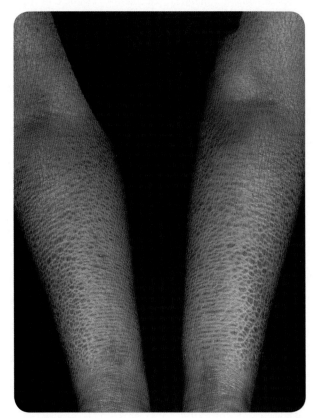

Figure 4-340 Antecubital fossae are often clear in ichthyosis vulgaris.

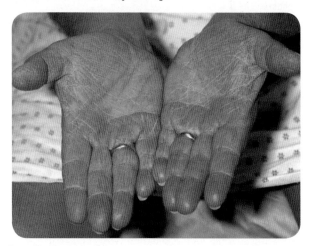

Figure 4-341 Ichthyosis vulgaris frequently has red and scaly palms with frequent fissures.

characterized by large thick, plate-like scale diffusely distributed over the entire body. Collodion membrane at birth, ectropion, eclabium, heat intolerance, and scarring alopecia are frequently associated findings.

- Epidermolytic hyperkeratosis (also called bullous congenital ichthyosiform erythroderma) is an autosomal dominant disorder caused by mutations in the genes encoding keratin 1 (KRT1) and keratin 10 (KRT10). Approximately 50% of the time, it arises from a spontaneous mutation (i.e., it is not inherited). It is characterized by erythroderma, bullae, and erosions from birth. As the patient ages, erythroderma is gradually replaced with severe hyperkeratosis with or without palmoplantar involvement. It is associated with frequent skin infections, malodor, defects in gait, and disfigurement.

Other considerations in the differential diagnosis include the following:

- Eczema craquelé
- Generalized xerosis
- Atopic dermatitis

- X-linked ichthyosis results from a mutation in the steroid sulfatase (STS) gene. It only occurs in males and is characterized by large dark, adherent scale on the extremities (including flexures), trunk, neck, and lateral face. It is associated with corneal opacities and cryptorchidism.
- Lamellar ichthyosis is an autosomal recessive disease caused by a mutation in either the transglutaminase-1 (TGM1) gene, the ABC tansporter-12 (ABCA12) gene, or the cytochrome P450 4F22 (CYP4F22) gene. It is

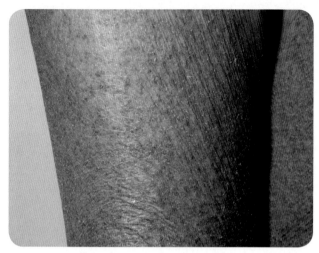

Figure 4-342 Ichthyosis vulgaris-like changes in a patient with lymphoma.

- Contact dermatitis (allergic or irritant)
- Drug reaction

✓ Best Tests

- This diagnosis can often be made clinically, but skin biopsy is characteristic.
- Specific investigations, such as mutational analysis and STS activity, may be illustrative if other hereditary forms of ichthyosis are being considered.
- Cases of AI warrant a search for an underlying systemic disease or malignancy. Skin biopsy is not diagnostic, showing changes identical to ichthyosis vulgaris.

▲▲ Management Pearls

- Emollients are the mainstay of therapy. Creams applied after bathing help the epidermis retain water. Moisturizing bath oils may be useful. Instruct the patient to use only nondrying soaps or nonsoap cleansers.
- Soaking the skin and mechanically exfoliating with a textured sponge or loofah will help to remove hyperkeratosis.
- The humidification of the environment, particularly during winter, is advisable.
- AI may improve with therapy of underlying disease.

Therapy

Patients should use a noncomedogenic moisturizing cream applied directly to wet skin after bathing and at least one other time each day. Hydration of skin and application of ointments is necessary to prevent water evaporation. Alpha hydroxy acids, such as lactic, glycolic, or pyruvic acids, twice daily may be more helpful than petrolatum.

For more scaling or hyperkeratotic areas, a keratolytic agent containing an alpha hydroxy acid, salicylic acid, or urea can be used (salicylic acid 4% to 12% lotion or cream and ammonium lactate 12% cream or lotion) applied twice daily. Urea or propylene glycol emollients act as humectants and are in many over-the-counter products. Keratolytics (salicylic acid) help to remove scale.

Salicylic acid, lactic acid, and calcipotriene preparations should not be used over the entire body due to risk of systemic absorption, but may be used to localized areas.

Topical retinoids (tretinoin 0.1% and tazarotene 0.05% gel) applied once daily for weeks to months have been used with success.

Topical vitamin D ointment (calcipotriol) can be tried.

In severe recalcitrant cases, systemic retinoids (isotretinoin, acitretin) have delivered acceptable results. However, systemic retinoids can lead to xerosis and, therefore, should be used with caution.

Mid-potency topical steroids on thin skin and class 6 and 7 steroids on the face (desonide cream, lotion, or ointment twice daily) can be prescribed when itching or dermatitis is coexistent. Use steroid ointments that have fewer preservatives in them if there seems to be flaring with multiple topical medications.

AI abates when the underlying condition is treated appropriately.

Suggested Readings

DiGiovanna JJ, Robinson-Bostom L. Ichthyosis: Etiology, diagnosis, and management. *Am J Clin Dermatol.* 2003;4(2):81–95.

Goldsmith LA, Baden HP. Management and treatment of ichthyosis. *N Engl J Med.* 1972 Apr;286(15):821–823.

Hernández-Martín A, González-Sarmiento R, De Unamuno P. X-linked ichthyosis: An update. *Br J Dermatol.* 1999 Oct;141(4):617–627.

Kaplan MH, Sadick NS, McNutt NS, et al. Acquired ichthyosis in concomitant HIV-1 and HTLV-II infection: a new association with intravenous drug abuse. *J Am Acad Dermatol.* 1993 Nov;29(5 Pt 1):701–708.

Moore RL, Devere TS. Epidermal manifestations of internal malignancy. *Dermatol Clin.* 2008 Jan;26(1):17–29, vii.

Oji V, Traupe H. Ichthyoses: Differential diagnosis and molecular genetics. *Eur J Dermatol.* 2006 Jul–Aug;16(4):349–359.

Okulicz JF, Schwartz RA. Hereditary and acquired ichthyosis vulgaris. *Int J Dermatol.* 2003 Feb;42(2):95–98.

Shwayder T. Disorders of keratinization: Diagnosis and management. *Am J Clin Dermatol.* 2004;5(1):17–29.

Diagnosis Synopsis

Non-bullous impetigo is a highly contagious superficial skin infection primarily caused by *Staphylococcus aureus* in industrialized countries. However, group A streptococcus (*Streptococcus pyogenes*) remains a common cause of non-bullous impetigo in developing countries. It has a predilection for children and is the most common cause of bacterial infection in this age group. Impetigo in adults usually results from extensive close contact with infected children or dermatologic conditions that predispose to superficial infection, such as minor trauma, atopic dermatitis, or infestation (e.g., scabies). Small epidemics can occur in crowded environments such as army barracks.

Clinically, impetigo presents as erythematous vesicles and/or pustules that quickly transition into superficial erosions with a characteristic "honey-colored" crust. Lesions are most commonly seen on the face (e.g., around the nose and mouth) and extremities. With the exception of mild lymphadenopathy, patients with impetigo generally have no associated systemic symptoms.

Although methicillin-resistant *S. aureus* (MRSA) infection of the skin usually presents as recurrent furunculosis or skin abscesses, MRSA has been shown to cause impetigo. Culture and sensitivities should always be performed in patients with lesions suspicious for cutaneous infection, and empiric coverage for MRSA should be instituted if clinical suspicion is high.

Immunocompromised Patient Considerations

Pyodermas including impetigo are quite common in HIV-infected patients. Additionally, pyodermas are found in immunosuppressed transplant patients, especially in the first months following transplant. Recurrent bouts of impetigo are more common in immunocompromised patients. This may be due to persistent nasal carriage of *Staphylococcus*, which has been reported to be as high as 50% in patients with HIV.

Look For

"Honey-" or golden-yellow crusted plaques, sometimes with small inflammatory halos (Figs. 4-343–4-346). The initial superficial vesicles are rarely seen, as they are fragile and transient.

The face is the most common location, particularly around the nose. However, any skin site can be involved if compromise to the epithelial barrier is present, such as that caused by minor skin trauma or lesions of atopic dermatitis.

Diagnostic Pearls

- Lesions may persist for weeks or months and can develop atrophy under a tightly adherent crust.
- Non-bullous impetigo is very infectious and may spread among school children, especially sports teams practicing contact sports (e.g., wrestling).

Immunocompromised Patient Considerations

Recurrent impetigo may be an indicator of an immunocompromised state.

?? Differential Diagnosis and Pitfalls

- A diagnosis of non-bullous impetigo is often mistakenly disregarded due to the lack of inflammation or induration.
- Superficial fungal infection
- Atopic dermatitis
- Contact dermatitis
- Erysipelas
- Cellulitis
- Burns
- Candidiasis
- Erythema multiforme
- Insect bite reaction
- Tinea
- Herpes simplex virus (HSV)
- Varicella
- Scabies
- Pemphigus foliaceus

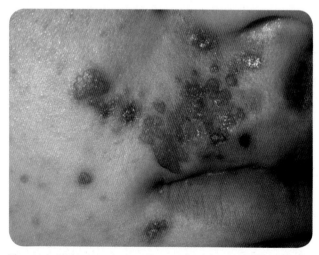

Figure 4-343 Multiple areas with superficial brown (honey-colored) crusting on the face. Impetigo can easily be mistaken for herpes simplex infection.

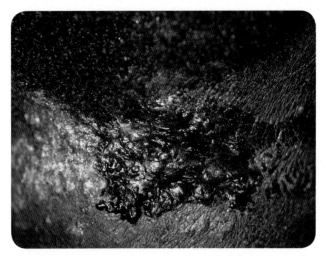

Figure 4-344 The posterior neck of this patient has multiple crusts, some of which are hemorrhagic.

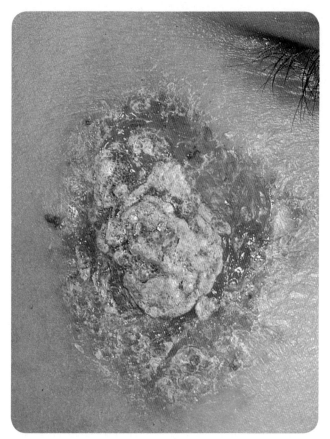

Figure 4-345 Heavily crusted superficial plaque of impetigo.

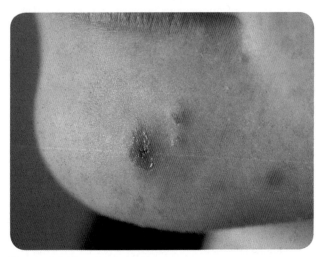

Figure 4-346 Very superficial crusted erosion of impetigo.

Immunocompromised Patient Differential Diagnosis

- HSV
- Varicella
- Herpes zoster
- Seborrheic dermatitis

✓ Best Tests

- Gram stain of exudate/lesional fluid will reveal Gram-positive cocci. Bacterial culture of a skin lesion with susceptibilities.

▲▲ Management Pearls

- To aid in keeping the lesions dry and promote healing, remove the crust by soaking in warm water, hydrogen peroxide, or aluminum acetate (Burow solution). If localized, the lesions can be treated with topical mupirocin; if widespread, the patient needs systemic antibiotics to clear the lesions.
- Given the prevalence of MRSA, maintain a high index of suspicion for this diagnosis, and make the initial choice of empiric antibiotic therapy accordingly. It is helpful to be aware of patterns of antimicrobial resistance within your community.
- Eradication of MRSA nasal carriage may be attempted with an application of 2% mupirocin cream to the nares. The combination of rifampin plus TMP-SMX has also been shown to temporarily eradicate MRSA colonization.
- Impetigo is very infectious, especially between household members. The infected individual should use separate towels and soap, and avoid sharing stuffed animals.

Precautions: Standard and Contact (Isolate patient, wear gloves and a gown, limit patient transport, and avoid sharing patient-care equipment.)

Therapy

Localized Disease

Local warm tap water soaks for 15 to 20 min three times daily followed by an application of mupirocin ointment. In patients who develop resistance to mupirocin, retapamulin may be used.

Widespread Disease

- Penicillin 250 mg p.o. three times daily for 7 to 10 days for streptococcal impetigo
- Cephalexin 250 to 500 mg p.o. four times daily for 7 to 10 days
- Erythromycin 250 mg p.o. four times daily for 7 to 10 days
- Dicloxacillin 250 mg p.o. four times daily for 7 to 10 days

Standard cephalosporins and penicillins are of no benefit in treating MRSA. In various studies, CA-MRSA has demonstrated a high degree of susceptibility to TMP-SMX and rifampin (100%), clindamycin (95%), and tetracycline (92%). Inducible resistance to clindamycin should be excluded by performing a D-zone disk-diffusion test.

Clindamycin 300 to 400 mg p.o. three times daily for 7 to 10 days.

Suggested Readings

Adachi J, Endo K, Fukuzumi T, et al. Increasing incidence of streptococcal impetigo in atopic dermatitis. *J Dermatol Sci*. 1998 May;17(1):45–53.

Anstead GM, Quinones-Nazario G, Lewis JS. Treatment of infections caused by resistant Staphylococcus aureus. *Methods Mol Biol*. 2007;391:227–258.

Donovan B, Rohrsheim R, Bassett I, et al. Bullous impetigo in homosexual men—a risk marker for HIV-1 infection? *Genitourin Med*. 1992 Jun;68(3):159–161.

Durupt F, Mayor L, Bes M, et al. Prevalence of Staphylococcus aureus toxins and nasal carriage in furuncles and impetigo. *Br J Dermatol*. 2007 Dec;157(6):1161–1167.

Feder HM, Abrahamian LM, Grant-Kels JM. Is penicillin still the drug of choice for non-bullous impetigo? *Lancet*. 1991 Sep;338(8770):803–805.

Hirschmann JV. Antimicrobial therapy for skin infections. *Cutis*. 2007 Jun;79(6 Suppl.):26–36.

Koning S, Verhagen AP, van Suijlekom-Smit LW, et al. Interventions for impetigo. *Cochrane Database Syst Rev*. 2004;(2):CD003261.

Moran GJ, Krishnadasan A, Gorwitz RJ, et al.; EMERGEncy ID Net Study Group. Methicillin-resistant S. aureus infections among patients in the emergency department. *N Engl J Med*. 2006 Aug;355(7):666–674.

Diagnosis Synopsis

There are many conditions that prompt patients to scratch when no primary visible dermatitis is evident. In the past, these entities have fallen under the umbrella term of "neurocutaneous dermatoses," or, more colloquially put, "pruritus without rash." Factors that cause the sensation of pruritus and thereby prompt patients to scratch include the following: underlying medical illnesses, an underlying nerve disorder, systemic drugs, and an underlying psychiatric illness.

Here we will discuss the following:

1. Generalized pruritus secondary to an underlying medical illness
2. Neuropathic pruritus—localized pruritus secondary to underlying lesion in the central or peripheral nervous system
3. Drug-induced pruritus
4. Neurotic excoriations and delusions of parasitosis

Generalized Pruritus Secondary to an Underlying Medical Illness

Generalized pruritus without primary skin lesions is, in many cases, caused by an underlying disease process that manifests in the skin as itch. Some of the most common causes are end-stage renal disease, chronic liver disease, cholestasis, thyroid disease, HIV, iron deficiency anemia, intestinal parasitosis, and malignancy. In these patients, treating the underlying cause effectively alleviates the itch.

Neuropathic Pruritus

Neuropathic pruritus is pruritus without dermatitis that is usually localized to a specific region of the body. Itch in this context is thought to result from a primary neurologic disorder manifesting in the skin as itch in a specific nerve distribution. Pruritus ani, pruritus scroti, pruritus vulvae, notalgia paresthetica, brachioradial pruritus, and scalp pruritus are examples of such conditions. Pruritus ani is characterized by intense bouts of violent itching centered on the anal area. Pruritus scroti and pruritus vulvae are similar to pruritus ani, but the itching is localized to the scrotum and vulva, respectively. Notalgia paresthetica is a localized pruritus of the back, presenting as an ill-defined area of hyperpigmentation. Brachioradial pruritus is itching or burning along the extensor arms, forearms, and upper back. Notalgia paresthetica and brachioradial pruritus have a strong association with disease of the cervical and/or thoracic spine. Scalp pruritus is itching localized to the scalp, primarily in the elderly. It is a diagnosis of exclusion, after common causes for scalp pruritus have been ruled out (i.e., seborrheic dermatitis, psoriasis, and lichen simplex chronicus). Collectively, these conditions can result from pathology anywhere along the nerve tract

(nerve root, cutaneous nerve ending, etc.). Thus, a thorough workup should include a detailed history to ascertain as to whether the patient is being locally exposed to exogenous pruritic substances (fiberglass, etc.) as well as imaging studies to determine if there is proximal nerve pathology (i.e., nerve impingement).

Drug-induced Pruritus

In some instances, generalized pruritus can occur as a side effect from a systemic drug. This may occur as a direct effect, primarily localized to the skin or indirectly as a result of the drug causing damage to internal viscera that manifests in the skin as itch (similar to pruritus of systemic disease). Drugs that commonly cause itch in a direct fashion are beta-blockers, retinoids, tamoxifen, busulfan, clofibrate, 8-methoxypsoralen, opioids, tramadol, methamphetamine, chloroquine, clonidine, gold salts, and lithium. Drugs that can indirectly cause pruritus by inducing cholestasis include estolate, estrogens, ACE-inhibitors, and sulfonamides. Hepatotoxic drugs that can indirectly induce pruritus include acetaminophen, anabolic steroids, phenytoin, isoniazid, sulfonamides, minocycline, and amoxicillin/clavulanic acid.

Neurotic Excoriations and Delusions of Parasitosis

Neurotic excoriations are a result of compulsively and habitually scratching and picking at the skin. Unlike patients with factitial dermatitis (discussed elsewhere), those with neurotic excoriations will usually admit their involvement in creating the lesion. There is a strong relationship between neurotic excoriations and underlying mental illness, most often obsessive compulsive disorder (OCD) and depression. The disorder is predominantly seen in middle-aged females but can be seen in almost any age. The continued scratching can lead to the itch-scratch-rash cycle, further perpetuating the condition. Individuals who take street drugs, especially cocaine and methamphetamines (crystal meth) are prone to neurotic excoriations. Pruritus-inducing drugs such as narcotics, especially heroin, may result in neurotic excoriations as well. Patients with neurotic excoriations will admit that they do not know what is causing the itch and are open to many possibilities. In contrast, patients with delusions of parasitosis have a false and fixed belief that they are infested by parasites. These patients have narrow and fixed delusions centered on their skin. Pruritus is often accompanied by the sensation of bugs biting and crawling on their skin.

Look For

In some cases of generalized pruritus, there are no skin lesions at all. More commonly, skin lesions are present, but there are no identifiable primary dermatologic lesions. Instead, linear erosions and (in chronic cases) lichenified papules or plaques are typically distributed on the extensor surfaces of the arms and forearms, in addition to the scalp, face, upper back, and buttocks (Figs. 4-347–4-350). Lesions can range from millimeters to centimeters and are often in different stages of development or healing. Broken hairs may be seen, and scarring alopecia may develop if the patient picks at his/her scalp. Lesions are typically seen in areas that the patient can scratch with his/her hands, usually sparing the mid-central back. Pruritus ani can present as anal bleeding from tears in the anal mucosa as a result of intense scratching. By definition, no erythema or scaling is observed in scalp pruritus.

Dark Skin Considerations

Like in the skin of whites, in patients with dark skin, neurotic excoriations can appear hypopigmented and/or hyperpigmented.

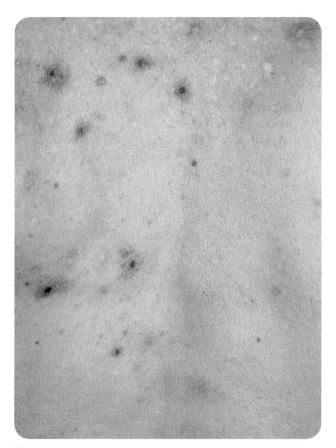

Figure 4-347 Multiple excoriations in an adult woman. Lesions can involve difficult-to-reach locations like the mid back.

 Diagnostic Pearls

- Lesions usually spare the mid-line upper back, where the skin is typically out of reach of the patient's hands.

?? Differential Diagnosis and Pitfalls

The differential diagnosis of pruritus without primary lesions can be broken down into primary medical, primary psychiatric, and primary drug-induced causes.

Primary Medical Cause

Hepatitis, HIV, lymphoma and other malignancies, pregnancy, uremia, polycythemia vera, hyperthyroidism and hypothyroidism, iron deficiency anemia, xerosis, intestinal parasitosis.

Primary Psychiatric Cause (Neurotic Excoriations)

Depression, trichotillomania, generalized anxiety disorder, tic disorder, OCD, body dysmorphic disorder, factitial dermatitis, somatization, hypochondriasis, borderline personality, delusions of parasitosis.

Primary Drug-Induced Cause

Although many drugs can cause pruritus (see above), some of the most common causes are antimalarials (e.g., chloroquine), narcotics, methamphetamines, and hydroxyethyl starch (frequently used blood plasma substitute).

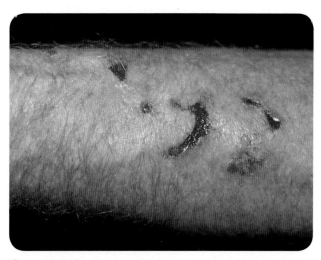

Figure 4-348 Self-induced lesions may have arcuate and other shapes suggesting external cause.

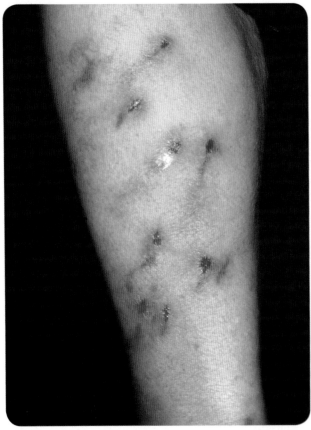

Figure 4-349 Linear erosions and ulcers suggest self-induced lesions.

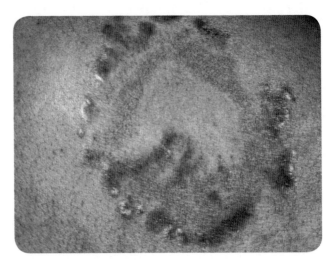

Figure 4-350 Interrupted annular lesion with hyperpigmentation suggests external etiology.

The differential diagnosis of pruritus ani includes allergic contact dermatitis (i.e., fragrance in toilet tissue), irritant contact dermatitis (i.e., leakage of rectal mucus), anal gonorrhea, anal mycosis, erythrasma, pinworm infestation, seborrheic dermatitis, lichen planus, and psoriasis.

The differential diagnosis of pruritus scroti includes lichen simplex chronicus, candidiasis (dermatophytes usually spare the scrotum), and allergic contact dermatitis (i.e., topical corticosteroids).

The differential diagnosis of pruritus vulvae includes lichen sclerosus, candidiasis, dysesthetic vulvodynia, and psoriasis.

The differential diagnosis of scalp psoriasis includes seborrheic dermatitis, psoriasis, dermatomyositis, and lichen simplex chronicus.

Immunocompromised Patient Differential Diagnosis

A case of generalized herpes simplex virus infection mimicking neurotic excoriations has been reported in a patient with AIDS.

✓ Best Tests

- The occlusion of the eroded lesions of neurotic excoriations can often establish the etiology, as they will gradually heal if protected from scratching or rubbing.
- For the localized pruritic disorders, skin biopsy is often necessary to rule out an underlying cutaneous cause.

▲▲ Management Pearls

- In generalized pruritus without rash, a thorough workup should be performed to rule out underlying disease states. A detailed medication history should be performed with special attention paid to the onset of pruritus and the initiation of various systemic medications known to cause pruritus.
- In the case of neurotic excoriations, reassure the patient that the problem is a common one and that manipulation may be contributing to continuance of the rash. Some patients scratch and excoriate during sleep; they should be questioned about sleep patterns. Have the patient keep their fingernails clipped very short. Refer patient to a mental health professional or a drug treatment center, if applicable. For the localized pruritic disorders, an underlying cause must be definitively ruled out.

Therapy

The pruritus of systemic disease is alleviated by treating the underlying disease state and/or discontinuing the offending medication. Palliative treatment can be attempted with emollients, topical corticosteroids, and oral antihistamines. Gabapentin has been shown to be efficacious in certain patients with uremic pruritus.

For neurotic excoriations, therapy should be targeted at the underlying psychiatric issues. SSRIs have shown favorable responses in decreasing OCD manifestations. To treat the lesions, occlusive dressings, topical antipruritics, and antihistamines may be effective. Steroid injections may help existing dermatitis but will not prevent the formation of new excoriated plaques. Systemic antibiotics are useful if the lesions are infected, although this is not typical.

For pruritus ani, stringent toilet care should be exercised with cleansing of the anal area (with soft cellulose tissue paper) after defecation. Topical corticosteroids and/or topical tacrolimus can be used to alleviate pruritus.

Low-potency topical corticosteroids can be used in pruritus scroti and pruritus vulvae.

Physical therapy and/or surgery can alleviate brachioradial pruritus.

Scalp pruritus can be treated with topical corticosteroid shampoos, oral antihistamines, and low doses of doxepin.

Suggested Readings

Binder A, Fölster-Holst R, Sahan G, et al. A case of neuropathic brachioradial pruritus caused by cervical disc herniation. *Nat Clin Pract Neurol.* 2008 Jun;4(6):338–342.

Cyr PR, Dreher GK. Neurotic excoriations. *Am Fam Physician.* 2001 Dec;64(12):1981–1984.

Don PC, Torakawa JT, Bitterman S. Herpetic infection mimicking chronic neurotic excoriations in AIDS. *Int J Dermatol.* 1991 Feb;30(2):136–138.

James WD, Berger TG, Elston DM. Pruritus and neurocutaneous dermatoses. In: James WD, Berger TG, Elston DM, Odom RB, eds. *Andrews' Diseases of the Skin: Clinical Dermatology.* 10th Ed. Philadelphia, PA: Saunders Elsevier; 2006:61.

Vila T, Gommer J, Scates AC. Role of gabapentin in the treatment of uremic pruritus. *Ann Pharmacother.* 2008 Jul;42(7):1080–1084.

Diagnosis Synopsis

Palmoplantar keratoderma (PPK) is thickening of the palms and/or soles that cannot be attributed to friction alone. Cases are either inherited or acquired. Heritable PPKs are identified by the presence of a family history and childhood onset; they may manifest in isolation, as the defining feature of a syndrome, or as a minor aspect of a syndrome (e.g., congenital ichthyoses, Darier disease).

Hereditary PPKs are approached and classified by the pattern of hyperkeratosis: diffuse, focal (often occurring over weight-bearing areas), or punctate.

- Diffuse Hereditary PPK
  - Vorner (epidermolytic) PPK and Unna-Thost (nonepidermolytic) PPK are the result of keratin mutations and show waxy or verrucous, white-yellow, symmetric hyperkeratosis.
  - Mal de Meleda is a rare diffuse hereditary PPK associated with *SLURP1* mutations and features stocking-glove distribution of hyperkeratosis with malodor and nail changes.
  - Vohwinkel syndrome (mutilating PPK) has two variants: the classic form associated with deafness and the connexin gene *GJB2*; and the loricrin variant associated with loricrin mutations and ichthyosis. The PPK shows a diffuse honeycomb pattern. Additional features include starfish-shaped keratotic plaques on dorsal hands, feet, elbows, and knees as well as constricting digital bands termed "pseudo-ainhum," which may progress to auto-amputation.
  - Papillon-Lefèvre syndrome is associated with mutations in the gene that encodes cathepsin C and demonstrates diffuse PPK, periodontal disease with the loss of teeth, and frequent cutaneous and systemic pyogenic infections.
  - Other diffuse hereditary PPKs include Greither syndrome, Bart-Pumphrey syndrome (PPK with knuckle pads, leukonychia, and deafness), Huriez syndrome (PPK with scleroatrophy), Clouston syndrome (hidrotic ectodermal dysplasia), Olmsted syndrome (mutilating PPK with periorificial plaques), diffuse nonepidermolytic PPK with sensorineural deafness, and Naxos disease (diffuse nonepidermolytic PPK with wooly hair and cardiomyopathy).
- Focal Hereditary PPK
  - Isolated focal PPKs (striate PPKs) are due to autosomal dominant mutations in genes encoding desmosomal proteins. Lesions favor pressure points on feet and may present as linear plaques on hands.
  - Howel-Evans syndrome is associated with mutations in the TOC gene, focal weight-bearing area plantar hyperkeratosis, milder palm involvement, and development of esophageal carcinoma.
  - Richner-Hanhart syndrome is associated with mutations in the gene that encodes tyrosine aminotransferase. The accumulation of tyrosine leads to focal (or diffuse) hyperkeratotic plaques on the hands, feet, elbows, and knees, corneal inflammation/ulceration, and mental retardation in some cases. Diets low in phenylalanine and tyrosine may prevent complications.
  - Focal PPK may also be seen in pachyonychia congenita type I and type II (syndromes with nail, skin, teeth, and eye anomalies) as well as Carvajal syndrome (striate focal epidermolytic PPK with wooly hair and dilated cardiomyopathy).
- Punctate Hereditary PPK or Keratosis Punctata (may not appear until adolescence or after)
  - Punctate PPKs are characterized by autosomal dominant inheritance and multiple firm 2 to 8 mm papules on the palms and soles. A pattern with lesions favoring palmar creases has been identified in patients of African descent.
  - Focal acral hyperkeratosis and acrokeratoelastoidosis present as 2 to 4 mm papules (some umbilicated) at the marginal borders of hands and feet.

Acquired PPKs occur later in life and have no associated family history.

They may be subdivided as follows:

- Keratoderma climactericum—Seen in menopausal women, often associated with obesity or hypertension; pressure points on the soles of the feet are affected first.
- Infectious PPK—Associated with dermatophytosis, leprosy, HIV, syphilis, crusted scabies, and human papillomavirus infections.
- Chemical/drug-induced PPK—Associated with exposure to arsenic, halogenated aromatic chemicals such as dioxin, venlafaxine, verapamil, hydroxyurea, etodolac, quinacrine, proguanil, methyldopa, practolol, doxorubicin, bleomycin, hydroxyurea, imatinib, capecitabine, tegafur, lithium, gold, and mexiletine.
- Dermatosis-related PPK—May be associated with atopic and contact dermatitis, psoriasis, reactive arthritis (keratoderma blennorrhagicum), lichen planus, lichen nitidus, lupus erythematosus, and pityriasis rubra pilaris.
- PPK as a feature of systemic disease—Hypothyroidism, myxedema, diabetes mellitus, and chronic lymphedema.
- Malnutrition-associated PPK
- Aquagenic keratoderma—Most often affects palms in patients in the second decade of life. Symptoms develop within 5 min of immersion in water.
- Paraneoplastic PPK—Acrokeratosis paraneoplastica of Bazex is associated with squamous cell carcinoma of the upper gastrointestinal (GI) tract, and "tripe palms" is associated with pulmonary or gastric malignancies. Other malignancies with associated paraneoplastic PPK include breast, bladder, skin, myeloma, mycosis fungoides, and Sézary syndrome.
- Idiopathic PPK—a diagnosis of exclusion.

Look For

Thickening of the palms and/or soles with variable areas affected (Figs. 4-351–4-354). Sometimes, there is plate-like scale or confluent, brown-to-yellow thickening. Patterns include diffuse, focal, and punctate. In the focal variants, the areas of hyperkeratosis can be very well defined.

Lesions that extend beyond the plantar or palmar skin may occur. These are referred to as "transgrediens."

Dark Skin Considerations

In keratosis punctata, look for 2 to 4 mm keratotic depressions on the palms and soles. A variant favoring the creases of the palms is commonly seen in black patients and can be somewhat painful.

Diagnostic Pearls

- Assessment begins by characterizing cases as inherited or acquired.
- Hereditary PPK cases are initially evaluated by pattern (diffuse, focal, or punctuate), by the presence or absence of transgrediens, accompanying symptoms, and of course by features of the family history. Refer inherited cases to a dermatologist or geneticist.
- Acquired cases should be evaluated with history and physical examination attuned to the list provided in the synopsis section. If no diagnosis is evident, limited diagnostic testing is indicated, including fungal scrapings, chest radiograph, TSH, CBC, ANA, RPR, HIV, and PPD. If the cause remains obscure after these tests, an age- and sex-appropriate search for malignancy is indicated,

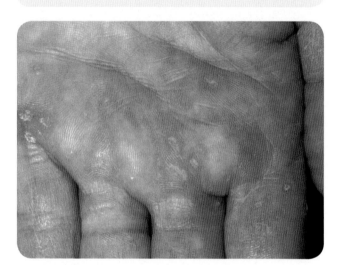

Figure 4-351 Punctate palmar-plantar lesions are often painful.

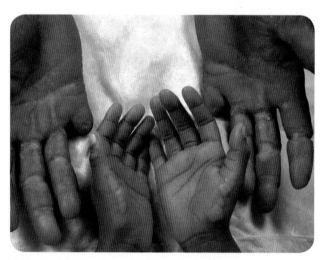

Figure 4-352 Keratoderma of Vohwinkel, with autoamputation and constricting digital bands in a father and palmar plaques on his son's palms laterally.

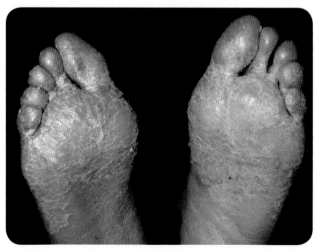

Figure 4-353 Diffuse palmar-plantar hyperkeratosis is frequently complicated by dermatophyte infection, as in this patient.

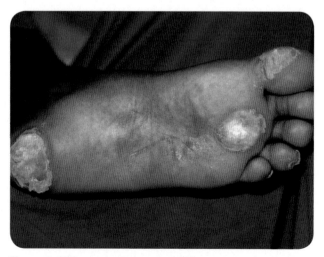

Figure 4-354 PPK is often accentuated over sites with pressure.

including CT scans of the chest/abdomen/pelvis, upper and lower GI tract endoscopy, and cystoscopy. Only if these are negative, should the designation of idiopathic PPK be assigned.

- Symmetry is usual, but asymmetric changes should prompt consideration of infectious or dermatosis-related PPK.

?? Differential Diagnosis and Pitfalls

Acquired Conditions that may have PPK as a Feature

- Psoriasis
- Atopic dermatitis
- Dyshidrotic eczema
- Contact dermatitis
- Pityriasis rubra pilaris
- Reactive arthritis (formerly Reiter syndrome)
- Acrodermatitis paraneoplastica of Bazex
- Tinea pedis/manuum
- Arsenical exposure
- Acanthosis nigricans (tripe palms are associated)
- Acquired ichthyosis associated with a malignancy
- Cutaneous T-cell lymphoma
- Lymphedema

Additional Inherited Conditions that may have PPK as a Feature (see Diagnosis Synopsis for Inherited Conditions in which PPK Predominates)

- Congenital ichthyoses
- Erythrokeratodermas
- Ectodermal dysplasias
- Dyskeratosis congenita
- Darier disease
- Basal cell nevus syndrome
- Incontinentia pigmenti
- Epidermolysis bullosa simplex
- Kindler syndrome
- Naegeli-Franceschetti-Jadassohn syndrome

PPK may occasionally be confused with corns and callosities or warts.

✓ Best Tests

- Biopsy can usually differentiate warts from PPK but is often not helpful in defining the underlying cause of an acquired keratoderma. In hereditary cases, the presence or absence of epidermolysis on histopathology may narrow the differential diagnosis.

- Scrape any scaly lesions and examine under the microscope with KOH to rule out a fungal infection. Dermatophytosis may be the cause of PPK or a treatable complication of a PPK.
- Consider thyroid function testing if the clinical scenario warrants, as cases of PPK associated with myxedema have been reported.
- Genetic testing in inherited cases.

▲▲▲ Management Pearls

Saline soaks and the paring down of hyperkeratotic areas are important adjunctive treatments.

Therapy

Treat any identifiable underlying condition (e.g., infection, malignancy, dermatosis, hypothyroidism) or stop any causative agents such as drugs.

Topical keratolytics are the mainstay of treatment. Examples include 5% to 10% salicylic acid, 10% lactic acid, 10% to 40% propylene glycol, or a 10% to 40% urea cream applied once or twice daily to thickened skin. Overnight occlusion may enhance the results.

Topical retinoids are also efficacious, but their use may be limited by irritation: tretinoin 0.1% gel or 0.1% cream nightly. Systemic retinoids (isotretinoin approx. 1 mg/kg daily, acitretin 25 to 50 mg daily) should be considered second-line and require careful monitoring for toxicities.

Alternative therapies that have demonstrated some efficacy include the following:

- Surgical excision and grafting
- Topical calcipotriol
- Topical corticosteroids
- Psoralen plus UVA (PUVA), sometimes combined with acitretin or isotretioin
- Dermabrasion
- Carbon dioxide laser

Suggested Readings

Itin PH, Fistarol SK. Palmoplantar keratodermas. *Clin Dermatol.* 2005 Jan–Feb;23(1):15–22.

James WD, Berger TG, Elston DM, et al. Pityriasis rosea, pityriasis rubra pilaris, and other papulosquamous and hyperkeratotic diseases. In: James WD, Berger TG, Elston DM, Odom RB, eds. *Andrews' Diseases of the Skin: Clinical Dermatology.* 10th Ed. Philadelphia, PA: Saunders Elsevier; 2006:211–215.

Krol AF. Keratodermas. In: Bolognia J, Jorizzo JL, Rapini RP, eds. *Dermatology*. 2nd Ed. St. Louis, MO: Mosby; 2008:777–789.

Milstone LM, Rizzo W, Richard G. Disorders of cornification. In: Spitz JL. *Genodermatoses: A Clinical Guide to Genetic Skin Disorders*. 2nd Ed. Philadelphia, PA: Lippincott Williams & Wilkins; 2005:30–31.

Patel S, Zirwas M, English JC. Acquired palmoplantar keratoderma. *Am J Clin Dermatol*. 2007;8(1):1–11.

Son SB, Song HJ, Son SW. Successful treatment of palmoplantar arsenical keratosis with a combination of keratolytics and low-dose acitretin. *Clin Exp Dermatol*. 2008 Mar;33(2):202–204.

Diagnosis Synopsis

In lichen planus (LP), autoreactive T lymphocytes attack keratinocytes in the skin, mucous membranes, hair follicles, or nail units. The etiology is unclear, but viruses, medications, or contact allergens have all been implicated. At the microscopic level, LP and its many variants show a stereotypical "lichenoid" pattern: a dense band of mononuclear cells obscures the dermo-epidermal junction, and basal keratinocytes demonstrate vacuolar degeneration indicative of immune-mediated apoptosis.

Clinically, the classic skin changes consist of itchy, small, flat-topped, red to purple papules that are most commonly seen on the volar wrists. Papules can be widespread and involve the trunk, inner thighs, shins, hands, oral mucosa, and genitalia (e.g., erosive or annular lesions on the glans penis or vulvovaginal LP). Oral LP often presents as lacy net-like, white plaques, though a variety of morphologies can be seen in the mouth. Oral lesions may accompany skin lesions or present in isolation, and oral LP may have a protracted or chronic course, less often seen with cutaneous LP. Lichen planopilaris, the hair follicle variant of LP, is typified by erythema and scale around hair follicles and scarring hair loss, most commonly on the scalp. Nail changes of LP—induced by lichenoid assault on the nail matrix—include fissuring, longitudinal ridging, and lateral thinning.

LP is most common in adults in the fourth to sixth decades of life, but it may occur at any age. There is no known predilection for either sex or for any ethnicity.

Certain medications cause an LP-like eruption. Prominent culprits include captopril, enalapril, labetalol, propranolol, methyldopa, propranolol, chloroquine, hydroxychloroquine, quinacrine, thiazide diuretics, penicillamine, quinidine, and gold salts. The longer list includes antimicrobials, other antihypertensives, psychotropic medications of diverse classes, anticonvulsants, oral hypoglycemic agents, diuretics, metals, nonsteroidal anti-inflammatory drugs (NSAIDs), and many others.

LP can spontaneously resolve, usually after a year, or follow a remitting or chronic course. It has been described in inconsistent association with hepatitis B and C, other chronic liver diseases, and diseases of altered immunity such as myasthenia gravis, ulcerative colitis, dermatomyositis, vitiligo, and alopecia areata. Oral LP may occur on mucosal surfaces apposed to amalgams and other dental restorative materials.

Look For

The classic description is given by the five Ps: purple, planar, polygonal, pruritic, papules most commonly seen on the volar wrists and flexural surfaces (Fig. 4-355). Papules can

also be widespread and involve the trunk, inner thighs, shins, hands, and genitalia. As the lesions become older, their surfaces develop adherent scales that form fine, grayish-white streaks called Wickham striae.

Useful as they are, the five Ps describe only the classic lesion; additional morphologies of LP are encountered on human skin:

- Hypertrophic
- Atrophic
- Erosive
- Follicular
- Annular
- Linear
- Guttate
- Actinic
- Bullous
- Ulcerative

Mucous membrane involvement may consist of lacy, net-like, white plaques with a violaceous base on the tongue or buccal mucosa (Fig. 4-356). Painful erosions and ulcers may also be seen, as well as atrophic, bullous, pigmented, and papular forms. Lesions may also be seen on the conjunctivae, the vulva, vagina, glans penis, anus, tonsils, larynx, and throughout the GI tract.

Lichen planopilaris presents as follicular-based scalp papules that progress to scarring alopecia. One variant of lichen planopilaris, the Graham-Little syndrome, is characterized by scarring alopecia of the scalp, nonscarring alopecia of the axilla and pubis, and typical mucocutaneous LP.

Nail changes such as thickening, splitting, ridges, and grooves can accompany the skin manifestations (Fig. 4-357). Pterygia may form on the proximal nail fold. Hypertrophic LP commonly involves the hands and feet.

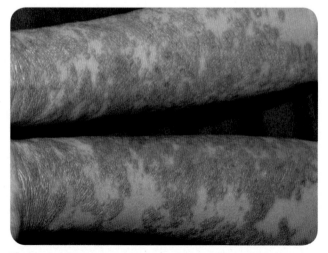

Figure 4-355 Lichen planus as purple polygonal papules on flexor forearms and wrist.

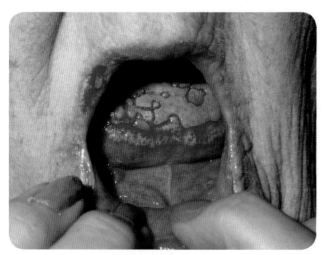

Figure 4-356 Oral ulcers and erosions are not uncommon in LP.

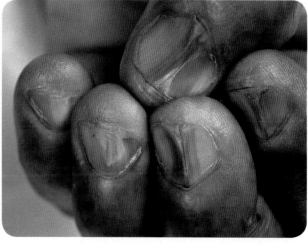

Figure 4-357 LP can cause partial or complete destruction of the nail matrix and can have pterygium with the posterior nail fold overgrowing and connecting with the nail bed.

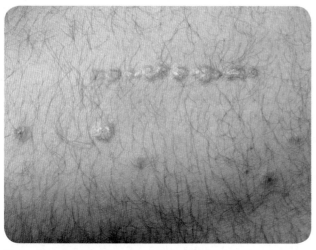

Figure 4-358 LP papules can sometime be linear from trauma (called the isomorphic response or Koebner phenomena).

Dark Skin Considerations

In darker-skinned patients, typical papules are of a gray or particularly deep purple to black color.

While LP shows no ethnic predilection, postinflammatory hyperpigmentation is typically prominent and lasting in blacks. Hypertrophic lesions, as well as the usually rare erosive and bullous palmoplantar LP, may occur more commonly in blacks. With the resolution of erosive LP, hyperpigmented scars remain in areas previously involved by persistent violaceous erythema. A silvery white or gray lace-like appearance of the surface of the oral mucosa is commonly encountered in black patients.

Diagnostic Pearls

- If you suspect LP on the glabrous (nonhair-bearing) skin, look closely within the mouth for the white or gray reticular plaques involving the buccal mucosa and/or tongue. Mucous membrane involvement may also occur in the absence of other lesions.
- Linear lesions may be present as a result of trauma (Koebner phenomenon) (Fig. 4-358).
- Nail changes are often more marked in those who are not white.

Differential Diagnosis and Pitfalls

In any location, consider drug-induced LP/lichenoid drug eruption; refer to the synopsis for a list of commonly implicated agents. Characteristics of lichenoid drug reaction, as opposed to nondrug-associated LP, include older mean age, more generalized distribution, paucity of Wickham striae, common and persistent hyperpigmentation, frequent photodistribution, sparing of mucous membranes, and distinct histologic characteristics.

Differential Diagnosis of Cutaneous LP

- Psoriasis
- Subacute cutaneous lupus erythematosus
- Chronic graft-versus-host disease
- Granuloma annulare
- Sarcoidosis
- Warts
- Pityriasis rosea

- Secondary syphilis (palm and sole lesions)
- Lichen simplex chronicus
- Prurigo nodularis
- Amyloidosis
- Kaposi sarcoma
- Tinea corporis
- Lichen nitidus
- Lichen spinulosus
- LP-like keratosis
- Erythema dyschromicum perstans
- Mycosis fungoides

Differential Diagnosis of Oral and Mucosal LP

- Oral candidiasis
- Leukoplakia
- Pemphigus vulgaris
- Seborrheic dermatitis (genital lesions)
- Lichen sclerosus (vulvar lesions)

Differential Diagnosis of Lichen Planopilaris

- Alopecia areata
- Seborrheic dermatitis
- Discoid lupus erythematosus
- Pseudopelade of Brocq
- Frontal fibrosing alopecia (regarded by some a variant of lichen planopilaris)
- Other scarring alopecias

Differential Diagnosis Nail Apparatus LP

- Alopecia areata, which has specific nail manifestations
- Onychomycosis
- Psoriasis

✓ Best Tests

- Skin biopsy will confirm the diagnosis, although it can often be made clinically.
- Practitioners in geographic locales in which LP is associated with hepatitis virus infections will consider obtaining serologic tests for hepatitis B and C as well as a liver function panel.

▲▲ Management Pearls

- Oral LP needs to be followed and managed carefully. Patients with persistent, severe oral LP are at higher risk for oral squamous cell carcinoma (SCC). In one large retrospective series, approximately 2% developed oral SCC, commonly on the lateral border of the tongue.
- Consultation with a dermatologist is recommended. Consider a dental consultation for severe oral LP.

Therapy

Withdraw any potential offending medication.

The control of pruritus may be achieved with the use of oral antihistamines or topical antipruritic agents such as lotions containing menthol, camphor, pramoxine, phenol, or doxepin hydrochloride.

Antihistamines

- Diphenhydramine: 25 to 50 mg nightly or every 6 h, as needed
- Hydroxyzine: 12.5 to 25 mg, every 6 h, as needed
- Cetirizine hydrochloride: 5 to 10 mg per day
- Loratadine: 10 mg daily

First-line therapy otherwise consists of topical or intralesional corticosteroids. Topical corticosteroids, in cream or ointment formulations, should be applied twice daily to only the lesions. Initially, use a high-potency topical steroid (class 2 or 3).

High-potency topical corticosteroids (*class* 2)

- Fluocinonide cream, ointment—apply twice daily
- Desoximetasone cream, ointment—apply twice daily
- Halcinonide cream, ointment—apply twice daily
- Amcinonide ointment—apply twice daily

Mid-potency topical corticosteroids (*classes* 3 *and* 4)

- Triamcinolone cream, ointment—apply twice daily
- Mometasone cream, ointment—apply twice daily
- Fluocinolone ointment, cream—apply twice daily

For severe disease, a superpotent topical steroid can be tried for a short 2-week course, but be sure to schedule a close follow-up.

Superpotent topical corticosteroids (*class* 1)

- Clobetasol 0.05% cream, ointment—apply twice daily
- Betamethasone 0.05% cream—apply twice daily
- Diflorasone 0.05% cream—apply twice daily
- Halobetasol—apply twice daily

Triamcinolone acetonide (3 to 10 mg/cc and in some cases up to 20 mg/cc) may be infiltrated into thicker papules and plaques at 1-month intervals. Be wary of skin atrophy.

Systemic corticosteroids can be used as a second-line treatment or in those with severe disease: prednisone 30 to 60 mg p.o. daily for 2 to 6 weeks, followed by a slow taper over several weeks. Oral metronidazole has also been used (500 mg p.o. twice daily), as have systemic retinoids (isotretinoin 0.5 mg/kg p.o. daily or acitretin 30 mg p.o. daily for 8 weeks). Severe cases have also been treated with narrow-band UVB or PUVA.

Alternative treatments with less evidence to support their use include topical 0.1% tacrolimus ointment twice daily, trimethoprim-sulfamethoxazole (two tabs p.o. twice daily for 5 days), cyclosporine (1 to 2 mg/kg p.o. daily), and photodynamic or UVA1 therapy. Anecdotal case reports and small series have also touted the efficacy of sulfasalazine, antimalarials, griseofulvin, itraconazole, tacrolimus, mycophenolate mofetil, azathioprine, levamisole, interferon, thalidomide, and enoxaparin. Many of these require careful patient screening and monitoring.

Oral LP
Treated with many of the same therapies, such as topical corticosteroids, topical tacrolimus, and intralesional corticosteroids. Fluocinolone gel applied with a cotton swab 4 times daily is a good choice. Oral disease is also treated with systemic corticosteroids and retinoids, topical retinoids, and hydroxychloroquine and immunosuppressive agents. Cyclosporine (compounded by a pharmacist in olive oil and applied using a cotton swab or swish and spit four times daily) may also be of benefit.

Palliative mouthwashes can be used for symptom control. Consider a cocktail of diphenhydramine elixir, aluminum/magnesium hydroxide antacid, and viscous lidocaine in a 1:1:1 ratio (sometimes called "magic mouthwash"). Swish and spit several times daily, as needed, for oral discomfort. Patients should avoid irritative or caustic foods and tobacco use.

Vulvovaginal LP
Most commonly treated with superpotent topical steroids or topical calcineurin inhibitors (e.g., tacrolimus ointment). Permanent scarring complications and malignancy have been identified as risks in vulvovaginal LP.

Lichen Planopilaris
First-line treatment for mild to moderate disease (involving <10% of the scalp) is intralesional injection of triamcinolone acetonide 10 mg/mL administered every 4 to 6 weeks. Rapidly progressive or severely symptomatic disease may be arrested with oral prednisone 1 mg/kg daily tapered over 2 to 4 months. Cases refractory to intralesional therapy may require treatment with oral immunomodulators that require careful patient screening and monitoring:

- Hydroxychloroquine 200 mg twice daily
- Cyclosporine 3 to 5 mg/kg daily
- Mycophenolate mofetil 500 to 1,000 mg twice daily

Other treatments reported for lichen planopilaris include oral retinoids, thalidomide, topical tacrolimus, and oral antimicrobials such as griseofulvin, dapsone, and tetracyclines. Topical minoxidil may have an adjunctive role.

Suggested Readings

Akdeniz S, Harman M, Atmaca S, et al. The management of lichen planus with low-molecular-weight heparin (enoxaparin). *Int J Clin Pract.* 2005 Nov;59(11):1268–1271.

Bauzá A, España A, Gil P, et al. Successful treatment of lichen planus with sulfasalazine in 20 patients. *Int J Dermatol.* 2005 Feb;44(2):158–162.

Boyd AS, Neldner KH. Lichen planus. *J Am Acad Dermatol.* 1991 Oct;25(4):593–619.

Cooper SM, Wojnarowska F. Influence of treatment of erosive lichen planus of the vulva on its prognosis. *Arch Dermatol.* 2006 Mar;142(3):289–294.

Goldblum OM. Lichen planus. *Skinmed.* 2002 Sep–Oct;1(1):52–53.

Goldstein AT, Metz A. Vulvar lichen planus. *Clin Obstet Gynecol.* 2005 Dec;48(4):818–823.

Güneş AT, Fetil E, Ilknur T, et al. Naproxen-induced lichen planus: report of 55 cases. *Int J Dermatol.* 2006 Jun;45(6):709–712.

Malhotra AK, Khaitan BK, Sethuraman G, et al. Betamethasone oral minipulse therapy compared with topical triamcinolone acetonide (0.1%) paste in oral lichen planus: A randomized comparative study. *J Am Acad Dermatol.* 2008 Apr;58(4):596–602.

Moyal-Barracco M, Edwards L. Diagnosis and therapy of anogenital lichen planus. *Dermatol Ther.* 2004;17(1):38–46.

Shiohara T, Kano Y. Lichen planus and lichenoid dermatoses. In: Bolognia J, Jorizzo JL, Rapini RP, eds. *Dermatology.* 2nd Ed. St. Louis, MO: Mosby; 2008:159–170.

Thompson DF, Skaehill PA. Drug-induced lichen planus. *Pharmacotherapy.* 1994 Sep–Oct;14(5):561–571.

Lichen Simplex Chronicus

Diagnosis Synopsis

Lichen simplex chronicus (LSC) is the cutaneous manifestation of chronic rubbing and/or scratching the skin from any source.

Clinically, lesions of LSC appear as well-defined plaques of lichenification and occasional scaling. Lichenification refers to thickened skin with enhanced skin markings as the result of friction from excessive scratching and rubbing. Individual papules may also be observed (prurigo nodularis), as may excoriations, which can become secondarily infected. As these lesions are self-induced, LSC is almost always distributed to areas of the body within hand's reach, most commonly on the back of the head and neck in women and in the genital (scrotum and perineum) area in men. LSC is more common in women and middle-aged-to-elderly patients.

The underlying precipitating factors inducing the patient to chronically scratch or rub their skin (causing lesions of LSC) are either known or unknown. LSC is commonly observed in uncontrolled atopic dermatitis and other dermatoses that have pruritus as a feature (e.g., insect bites, scabies). When LSC is observed on relatively normal skin with no obvious underlying cutaneous (or systemic) precipitants, psychological factors are thought to play a significant role. In either case, an itch-scratch cycle is initiated, and if allowed to continue unabated, plaques of LSC inevitably develop.

Immunocompromised Patient Considerations

Infection with HIV can cause generalized pruritus and, thus, may be an underlying precipitant of LSC.

Look For

Leathery plaques of thickened skin in which the normal texture is exaggerated (Figs. 4-359–4-362). Plaques may be slightly erythematous, and are often scaly and well demarcated. They may be hyperpigmented. Excoriations may be apparent as well.

Lesions are most common at the scalp, lateral and posterior neck, wrists and elbows, vulva or scrotum, and knees, lower legs, and ankles.

Dark Skin Considerations

Post-inflammatory hyperpigmentation is commonly seen in both the treated and untreated plaques of LSC in dark-skinned patients.

Diagnostic Pearls

- Even when the lesion has regressed temporarily, the fine skin markings are still accentuated. Postinflammatory hyperpigmentation is common.
- LSC is only found at locations that the patient can reach.

Differential Diagnosis and Pitfalls

- Psoriasis
- Mycosis fungoides
- Contact dermatitis
- Stasis dermatitis
- Hypertrophic lichen planus
- Hypertrophic discoid lupus

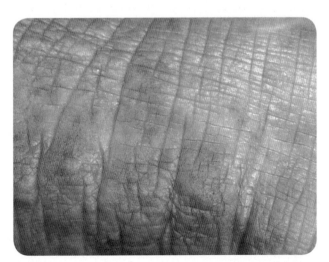

Figure 4-359 Marked accentuation of skin markings on the ankle is characteristic of LSC.

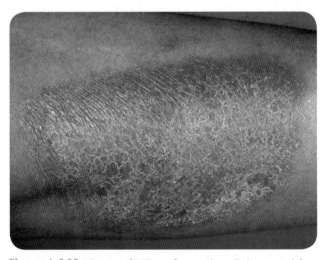

Figure 4-360 Plaques of LSC are frequently well demarcated from the surrounding skin.

278

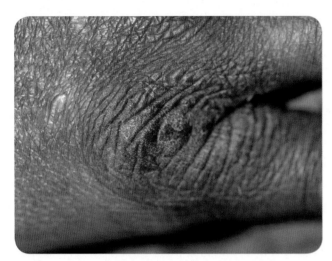

Figure 4-361 Accentuated skin markings characterize a plaque of LSC.

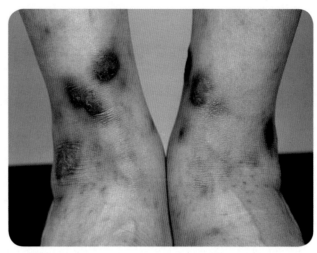

Figure 4-362 Very thick plaques of LSC merge with the diagnosis of prurigo nodularis.

- Multiple keratoacanthomas
- Dermatofibromas
- Verruca vulgaris
- Atopic dermatitis
- Acanthosis nigricans
- Extramammary Paget disease
- Acne keloidalis nuchae
- Notalgia paresthetica—localized pruritic area at one side of the mid-scapula area
- Bowen disease
- Pretibial myxedema
- Lichen amyloidosis

✓ Best Tests

- This diagnosis can often be made clinically.
- Skin biopsy may be performed to rule out other diagnoses (such as mycosis fungoides). Patch testing can be used to rule out allergic contact dermatitis.

▲▲ Management Pearls

- The goal of treatment is to eliminate environmental triggers and break the itch-scratch-rash-itch cycle. Stress upon patients the importance of not scratching lesions. Using barriers to cover plaques of LSC can eliminate scratching and lead to resolution.
- Maximize the treatment of any underlying skin disease. Use oral antihistamines to lessen pruritus. Keep skin well lubricated with a liberal use of emollients. If the itching is generalized, consider systemic causes of pruritus such as medications and renal, thyroid, hematologic, and hepatic abnormalities.

- Psychological evaluation and treatment, including psychoactive medications, behavioral therapy, and alternative treatments, such as hypnosis, have benefited some patients. In select cases, consider consultation with a mental health professional.

Therapy

High-potency or superpotent topical steroids (class 1 or 2) applied twice daily with or without occlusion is first-line therapy. Also consider flurandrenolide tape, a corticosteroid-impregnated tape (60 and 200 cm² rolls), that will serve as a reminder for the patient not to rub and deliver the topical steroid under occlusion. Change the tape once daily.

In general, start with a high-potency topical steroid (class 2 or 3) or a superpotent topical corticosteroid (class 1) if the condition is severe. Schedule close (i.e., 2 weeks) follow-up when using such agents. Decrease the potency and/or the frequency of application of the corticosteroid preparation as the lesions resolve to avoid inducing skin atrophy.

Superpotent topical corticosteroids (class 1)

- Clobetasol 0.05% cream—apply twice daily (15, 30, 45 g)
- Betamethasone 0.05% cream—apply twice daily (15, 30, 45 g)
- Diflorasone 0.05% cream—apply twice daily (15, 30, 60 g)
- Halobetasol cream—apply twice daily (15, 50 g)

(Continued)

High-potency topical corticosteroids (class 2)

- Fluocinonide cream, ointment—apply twice daily (15, 30, 60,120 g)
- Desoximetasone cream, ointment—apply twice daily (15, 60, 120 g)
- Halcinonide cream, ointment—apply twice daily (15, 60, 240 g)
- Amcinonide ointment—apply twice daily (15, 30, 60 g)

Mid-potency topical corticosteroids (classes 3 and 4)

- Triamcinolone cream, ointment—apply twice daily (15, 30, 60, 120, 240 g)
- Mometasone cream, ointment—apply twice daily (15, 45 g)
- Fluocinolone ointment, cream—apply twice daily (15, 30, 60 g)

Alternatively, intralesional injection with triamcinolone 3 to 5 mg/cc to the thickened plaque may be used.

For pruritus, the following antihistamines can be tried:

Diphenhydramine hydrochloride (25, 50 mg tablets or capsules)—25 to 50 mg nightly or every 6 h, as needed

- Hydroxyzine (10, 25 mg tablets)—12.5 to 25 mg every 6 h, as needed

- Cetirizine hydrochloride (5, 10 mg tablets)—5 to 10 mg per day
- Loratadine (10 mg tablets)—10 mg tablet once daily

Other treatments include 0.25% topical capsaicin cream (applied five times daily), cryosurgery, and 5% doxepin cream.

A topical antibiotic ointment (e.g., mupirocin) can be applied to impetiginized lesions.

Suggested Readings

Burgin S. Nummular eczema and lichen simplex chronicus/prurigo nodularis. In: Fitzpatrick TB, Wolff K, eds. *Fitzpatrick's Dermatology in General Medicine.* 7th Ed. New York, NY: McGraw-Hill; 2008:160–162.

Datz B, Yawalkar S. A double-blind, multicenter trial of 0.05% halobetasol propionate ointment and 0.05% clobetasol 17-propionate ointment in the treatment of patients with chronic, localized atopic dermatitis or lichen simplex chronicus. *J Am Acad Dermatol.* 1991 Dec;25(6 Pt 2):1157–1160.

Jones RO. Lichen simplex chronicus. *Clin Podiatr Med Surg.* 1996 Jan;13(1):47–54.

Lotti T, Buggiani G, Prignano F. Prurigo nodularis and lichen simplex chronicus. *Dermatol Ther.* 2008 Jan–Feb;21(1):42–46.

Lynch PJ. Lichen simplex chronicus (atopic/neurodermatitis) of the anogenital region. *Dermatol Ther.* 2004;17(1):8–19.

Virgili A, Bacilieri S, Corazza M. Managing vulvar lichen simplex chronicus. *J Reprod Med.* 2001 Apr;46(4):343–346.

Majocchi Granuloma

■ Diagnosis Synopsis

Majocchi granuloma (nodular granulomatous perifolliculitis) is a perifollicular and nodular process caused by the infection of the follicle with a dermatophyte fungal species. The disease process occurs when a dermatophyte invades the follicle, causing a granulomatous and/or suppurative reaction. Majocchi granuloma is most often caused by *Trichophyton rubrum* or, less commonly, *T. mentagrophytes* or *Epidermophyton floccosum*. These are the same fungal species typically responsible for the superficial dermatophyte infections tinea corporis or tinea pedis. Other dermatophyte species have been implicated as well.

Majocchi granuloma can occur from shaving and has been seen on the legs as well as the face. The involvement of the buttocks and genital skin has also been reported. The occlusion of the skin or simple trauma can also predispose to development of the lesion, as can the use of topical steroids on unsuspected tinea and immunosuppressed states. Depending on the cause, there may be differing clinical presentations.

Immunocompromised Patient Considerations

A deeper and more nodular form of Majocchi granuloma has also been reported in transplant patients and immunocompromised patients. HIV-infected individuals with tinea pedis may have a higher risk of progression to Majocchi granuloma on the feet and lower legs.

Look For

In the immunocompetent patient, look for pustules, papules, and nodules within erythematous, scaling plaques or occurring without the typical features of a dermatophyte infection (Figs. 4-363–4-366). Distended hair follicles with or without crusting may be observed. Affected areas may resemble a bacterial furuncle or carbuncle. Plaques typically occur on the extremities but can occur on any body surface except for the palms, soles, and mucous membranes.

Dark Skin Considerations

Black patients may have a greater predisposition to developing Majocchi granuloma from a superficial tinea, given the predisposition for pseudofolliculitis from ingrown hair shaft formation in this patient population.

Immunocompromised Patient Considerations

In the immunocompromised patient, look for deeper plaques and nodules, with or without pustules.

Diagnostic Pearls

- Look for a cluster or group of pustules within a plaque. Majocchi granuloma is within the differential of a patient

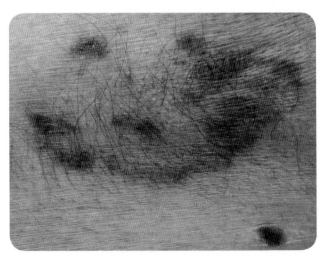

Figure 4-363 Papules in an annular configuration with purpura are suggestive of Majocchi granuloma.

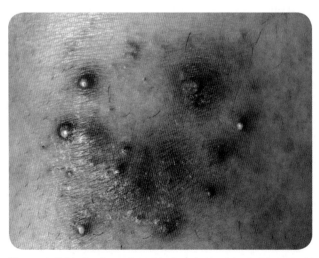

Figure 4-364 Papular and pustular lesions consistent with Majocchi granuloma. Lesions may also be purpuric.

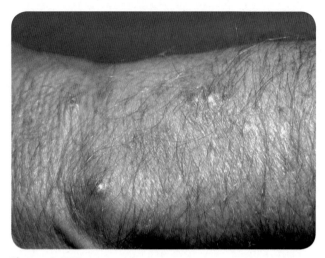

Figure 4-365 Papular and pustular papules on a hairy region are very suggestive of Majocchi granuloma.

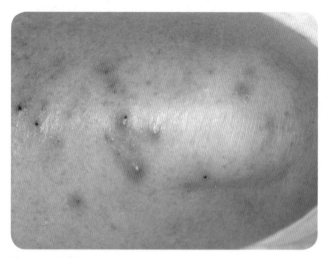

Figure 4-366 Papular and pustular lesions require mycology studies to rule out dermatophyte infection.

treated with a topical antifungal. Shaving (especially in women) and a history of occlusion with bandages or ointments are predisposing factors.
- Patients may have concomitant onychomycosis and/or tinea pedis.

?? Differential Diagnosis and Pitfalls

- Herpes simplex infection including herpetic folliculitis
- Furunculosis
- Bacterial folliculitis
- Pseudofolliculitis barbae
- Acne keloidalis nuchae
- Lymphocytoma cutis
- Kaposi sarcoma
- Abscess
- Nodular scabies
- Kerion

✓ Best Tests

- Preliminary testing should include a KOH and fungal culture.
- A skin biopsy with fungal stains and tissue culture is the best test because KOH examination is often negative, especially if a topical antifungal has been used recently.
- Bacterial and viral cultures will rule out bacterial folliculitis and herpes simplex.

▲▲ Management Pearls

- Advise patients to abstain from shaving or to shave less frequently, if possible.

- Topical corticosteroids and combination corticosteroid/antifungal preparations should not be used.

Immunocompromised Patient Considerations

Culture confirmation of the pathogenic organism is essential in immunocompromised patients, as atypical organisms may be causative. Majocchi granuloma due to *Aspergillus fumigatus* in a patient with AIDS has been reported.

Therapy

Systemic antifungal medications are the treatment of choice. Topical agents alone are not effective, as the organism is in follicles and the perifollicular dermis:

- Terbinafine—250 mg daily for 4 weeks in the immunocompetent. Consider 6 to 8 weeks of terbinafine therapy in the immunocompromised patient.
- Itraconazole pulse therapy—200 mg twice daily for 1 week, with 2 weeks off therapy; then, repeat the cycle for a total of three pulses. Itraconazole 200 mg twice daily for 2 to 3 months in the immunocompromised patient.

Suggested Readings

Chang SE, Lee DK, Choi JH, et al. Majocchi's granuloma of the vulva caused by Trichophyton mentagrophytes. *Mycoses*. 2005 Nov;48(6):382–384.

Cho HR, Lee MH, Haw CR. Majocchi's granuloma of the scrotum. *Mycoses*. 2007 Nov;50(6):520–522.

Elgart ML. Tinea incognito: An update on Majocchi granuloma. *Dermatol Clin.* 1996 Jan;14(1):51–55.

Elmets CA. Management of common superficial fungal infections in patients with AIDS. *J Am Acad Dermatol.* 1994 Sep;31(3 Pt 2):S60–S63.

Gupta AK, Groen K, Woestenborghs R, et al. Itraconazole pulse therapy is effective in the treatment of Majocchi's granuloma: A clinical and pharmacokinetic evaluation and implications for possible effectiveness in tinea capitis. *Clin Exp Dermatol.* 1998 May;23(3):103–108.

Gupta AK, Prussick R, Sibbald RG,et al. Terbinafine in the treatment of Majocchi's granuloma. *Int J Dermatol.* 1995 Jul;34(7):489.

James WD, Berger TG, Elston DM. Diseases resulting from fungi and yeasts. In: James WD, Berger TG, Elston DM, Odom RB, eds. *Andrews' Diseases of the Skin: Clinical Dermatology.* 10th Ed. Philadelphia, PA: Saunders Elsevier; 2006:302–303.

Saadat P, Kappel S, Young S, et al. Aspergillus fumigatus Majocchi's granuloma in a patient with acquired immunodeficiency syndrome. *Clin Exp Dermatol.* 2008 Jul;33(4):450–453.

Smith KJ, Neafie RC, Skelton HG, et al. Majocchi's granuloma. *J Cutan Pathol.* 1991 Feb;18(1):28–35.

Diagnosis Synopsis

Pityriasis lichenoides et varioliformis acuta (PLEVA), or Mucha-Habermann disease, is a T-cell lymphoproliferative disorder that is characterized by the acute onset of asymptomatic crops of erythematous papules. The papules spontaneously resolve within weeks and recur at a later time. Due to its recurrent nature, PLEVA lesions demonstrate varying stages of evolution and include small ulcers, crusted papules, vesicles, pustules, and varicella-like scarring. PLEVA eruptions are most commonly found in the male pediatric population but can occur in both genders, in all ages, and in all ethnicities.

While the etiology is not known, the histologic infiltrate is composed of monoclonal CD8+ T lymphocytes. This may help explain its association with lymphomas and cutaneous T-cell lymphoma (CTCL).

Pityriasis lichenoides chronica (PLC) is a related but more chronic form. In contrast to the crusts, vesicles, and pustules seen in PLEVA, PLC takes on a more indolent course and is characterized by crops of scaly erythematous papules that spontaneously regress over months (instead of weeks).

Variants of PLEVA include those with systemic manifestations such as fever, generalized lymphadenopathy, malaise, arthralgias, and arthritis. A severe variant, pityriasis lichenoides, ulceronecrotic, hyperacute (PLUH), is defined by more severe cutaneous and systemic findings. Large lesions with necrotic centers, ulcers, and diffuse purpuric papules can occur. Higher fevers, myalgias, arthralgias, CNS, and gastrointestinal symptoms have been described. PLUH carries a 25% mortality rate and is considered a dermatologic emergency.

PLEVA is generally viewed as a benign lymphoproliferative disorder that lasts from 1 to 3 years, depending on the distribution of lesions. However, there are case reports of progression to CTCL. No guidelines have been established for monitoring this possible progression.

Look For

Widely scattered, round, erythematous or purpuric lichenoid papules, small nodules, and macules in varying sizes and stages of evolution (Figs. 4-367–4-370). Lesions can have central vesiculation, hemorrhagic crusts, small eschars, or shallow ulcers. The lesions of the PLC variant tend to have smaller papules with some scale.

The lesions are most commonly scattered across the trunk, buttocks, and proximal extremities, but they may also occur on the face, palms, soles, and scalp.

The lesions of ulceronecrotic PLEVA are typically larger and covered by a black crust. They heal with scarring.

Dark Skin Considerations

PLEVA can result in significant residual macular hypopigmentation in darkly pigmented skin.

Diagnostic Pearls

- PLEVA is characterized by scattered lesions in multiple stages of evolution/healing.

Differential Diagnosis and Pitfalls

- Skin biopsy will aid in the diagnosis. The key entities to rule out in the differential diagnosis include lymphomatoid papulosis, drug reaction, small vessel vasculitis, varicella, and arthropod reactions.
- Lymphomatoid papulosis—Predominantly CD30 + cells in the infiltrate, in older patients, characterized by more

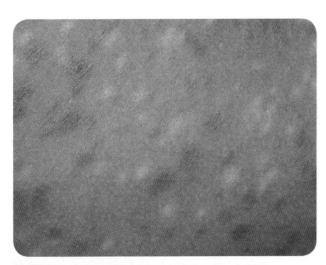

Figure 4-367 Atrophic and red papular lesions of PLEVA.

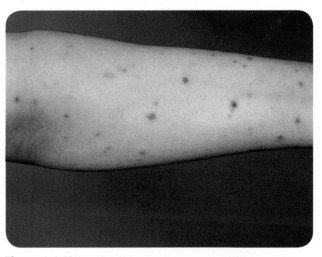

Figure 4-368 Papular and purpuric lesions in PLEVA.

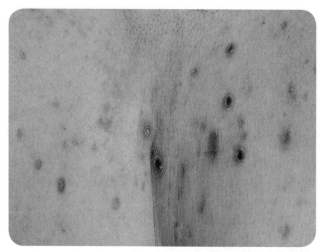

Figure 4-369 Papular, purpuric, and ulcerative lesions in PLEVA.

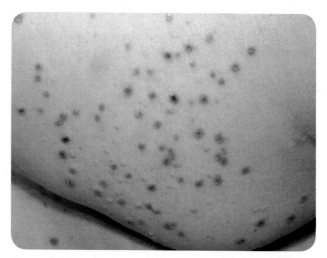

Figure 4-370 Papular, purpuric, and ulcerative lesions in PLEVA.

nodular lesions, and active lesions do not spontaneously resolve as quickly as PLEVA.

- Drug eruptions—Often present with urticarial, macular, or vesicular/bullous lesions. In addition, systemic symptoms are more pronounced than seen with classic PLEVA, including fever, lymphadenopathy, and facial edema. Eosinophilia on CBC and histology are often seen (but not an invariable finding). A medication history helps make this diagnosis.
- Vasculitis—Check serologies for RF, ANA, anti-ds DNA, ANCA, cryoglobulins. C3, C4 levels. Lesions are mostly purpuric and more monomorphous.
- Varicella—Prodrome of mild fever, malaise, and myalgia followed by pruritic erythematous papules. Lesions are pruritic. Recurrent eruptions are not a feature of varicella.
- Arthropod bites
- Dermatitis herpetiformis—Exquisitely pruritic. Ruled out by direct immunofluorescence on the skin biopsy.
- Pityriasis rosea—Herald patch, scaly papules/plaques. Crusts, vesicles, and bullae are not common findings.
- Lichen planus—Very pruritic, lesions are typically monomorphous and rarely crusted.
- Folliculitis
- Perforating dermatoses
- Toxoplasmosis
- Primary HIV infection
- Erythema multiforme
- Guttate psoriasis

Immunocompromised Patient Differential Diagnosis

- Disseminated herpes simplex virus—Mostly vesicular and bullous lesions. Patient will be more systemically ill.
- Secondary syphilis—Check RPR, history of chancre.

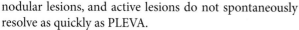 **Best Tests**

- Skin biopsy will usually confirm the diagnosis.
- Lab tests to look for underlying disease or rule out diagnoses in the differential diagnosis list include:
  - ASO
  - EBV IgM/IgG viral capsid antigen and nuclear antigen antibody
  - Hepatitis B, C, and HIV screens
  - Monospot or heterophil antibody test
  - RPR or VDRL
  - Throat culture
  - *Toxoplasma* Sabin-Feldman dye test, ELISA, and indirect immunofluorescence/hemagglutination

 Management Pearls

- Large ulcerations in the ulceronecrotic form of PLEVA require local wound care.
- There is evidence to support that the distribution of lesions can predict outcome. Patients with disseminated involvement of the skin have an average clinical course of 11 months, while those with lesions restricted to extremities have demonstrated an average clinical course of 33 months.
- There is an occasional association with non-Hodgkin lymphoma and T-cell lymphomas of the skin.

Therapy

The lesions tend to spontaneously resolve without treatment, and no randomized controlled trials have been performed. However, success has been reported with

(Continued)

antibiotics, UV light therapy, retinoids, immunosuppressants, and steroids.

Systemic antibiotics:

- Tetracycline 500 mg three to four times daily (adult)
- Erythromycin 250 mg four times daily (adult)
- Sulfonamides, dapsone, penicillin, streptomycin, and isoniazid

Sun, narrowband UVB, or PUVA have been reported helpful. Narrowband UVB has achieved complete response in patients with a mean cumulative dose of approximately 20 J/cm² over 40 exposures.

Retinoids:

- Acitretin 25 to 50 mg daily

Immunosuppressants:

- Methotrexate 0.3 mg/kg weekly; do not exceed 20 mg per week

Steroids:

- Topical steroids can be applied for mild to moderate disease
- Prednisone 40 to 60 mg daily for PLEVA with systemic manifestations

Combination therapy (antibiotics plus PUVA or methotrexate plus PUVA) may be superior for the rare ulceronecrotic form.

Pruritus can be treated with the following antihistamines:

- Diphenhydramine hydrochloride (25 and 50 mg tablets or capsules): 25 to 50 mg nightly or every 6 h as needed
- Hydroxyzine (10 to 25 mg tablets): 12.5 to 25 mg, every 6 h as needed
- Cetirizine hydrochloride (5 and 10 mg tablets): 5 and 10 mg per day
- Loratadine (10 mg tablets): 10 mg tablet once daily

Suggested Readings

Bowers S, Warshaw EM. Pityriasis lichenoides and its subtypes. *J Am Acad Dermatol.* 2006 Oct;55(4):557–572; quiz 573–576.

Fink-Puches R, Soyer HP, Kerl H. Febrile ulceronecrotic pityriasis lichenoides et varioliformis acuta. *J Am Acad Dermatol.* 1994 Feb;30(2 Pt 1):261–263.

Khachemoune A, Blyumin ML. Pityriasis lichenoides: Pathophysiology, classification, and treatment. *Am J Clin Dermatol.* 2007;8(1):29–36.

Pinton PC, Capezzera R, Zane C, et al. Medium-dose ultraviolet A1 therapy for pityriasis lichenoides et varioliformis acuta and pityriasis lichenoides chronica. *J Am Acad Dermatol.* 2002 Sep;47(3):410–414.

Tsuji T, Kasamatsu M, Yokota M, et al. Mucha-Habermann disease and its febrile ulceronecrotic variant. *Cutis.* 1996 Aug;58(2):123–131.

Wood GS, Hu CH, Garret AL. Parapsoriasis and pityriasis lichenoides. In: Fitzpatrick TB, Wolff K, eds. *Fitzpatrick's Dermatology in General Medicine.* 7th Ed. New York, NY: McGraw-Hill; 2008:240–243.

Pityriasis Rosea

Diagnosis Synopsis

Pityriasis rosea is a common cutaneous eruption that arises spontaneously, is asymptomatic or pruritic, and is self-limited in nature. Classically, a solitary pink or flesh-colored patch or scaly plaque appears first—the herald patch—in an otherwise healthy adolescent or young adult. Several days later, the ensuing eruption appears. The rash consists of multiple erythematous, scaly papules and plaques that favor the trunk and upper extremities. The face, palms, and soles are usually spared. While the exact cause remains unclear, several observations support a viral etiology. These include flu-like prodromal symptoms in some patients, the absence of recurrence (suggesting an immune response with specificity and cell memory to a pathogen), seasonal variation, and case clustering (suggesting possible "outbreaks").

Current investigational efforts have largely focused on human herpesvirus 6 and 7 (HHV-6 and HHV-7). There is usually a higher incidence in the spring and fall, but it can occur year-round. The condition is most common in patients between 15 and 40 years of age. Women are affected more than men, but there is no ethnic predilection. Clinical variations include eruptions lasting for 5 months or more and prodromal symptoms such as fever, malaise, and arthralgias. Up to a quarter of patients can experience mild to severe pruritus.

Immunocompromised Patient Considerations

Pityriasis rosea occurring during pregnancy may be associated with premature birth or fetal demise, especially if erupting during the first 15 weeks of pregnancy.

Look For

Salmon-colored oval or circular patches and plaques with an associated fine, central scaling (Figs. 4-371–4-373). The condition usually begins with one larger truncal plaque or patch, known as the herald patch. Then, after several days or weeks, new patches and plaques form in a "Christmas tree" distribution on the back (the long axis of oval lesions following skin fold lines) (Fig. 4-374). Pruritus may be lacking altogether or be very intense.

There are many variants, including a vesicular form, a pustular form, a papular form, and forms mimicking urticaria and erythema multiforme. Lesions may also appear purpuric or papular. Facial lesions are rare. Unusual variants of pityriasis rosea are where lesions are concentrated in the axillae and groin (the "inverse" form) or occur unilaterally.

Dark Skin Considerations

The typical "salmon-pink" color is not easily apparent in darkly pigmented skin; instead, pityriasis rosea lesions are more papular, scaly, and hyperpigmented than plaque- or patch-like. Postinflammatory hyperpigmentation is more commonly seen in darker-skinned individuals.

Diagnostic Pearls

- Lymphadenopathy is a rare finding.

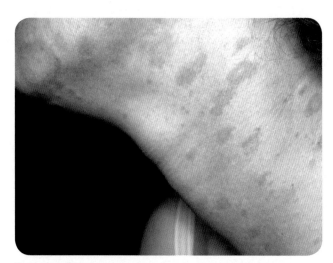

Figure 4-371 Pityriasis rosea with a herald patch on the chin and many plaques with their long axes parallel to lines of cleavage on the neck.

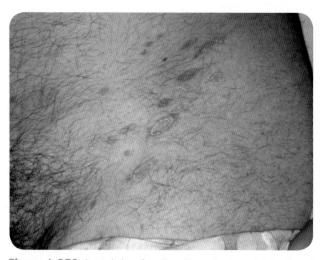

Figure 4-372 Central rim of scale and papules in a distribution of the lines of cleavage in pityriasis rosea.

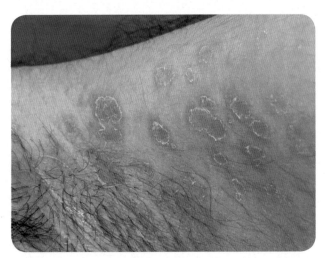

Figure 4-373 Multiple lesions of pityriasis rosea in the axilla with prominent annular scales.

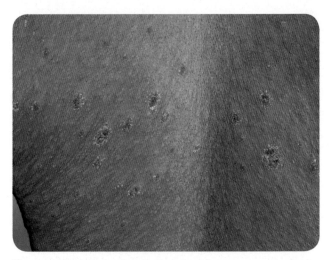

Figure 4-374 Oval, crusted lesions in a Christmas-tree distribution on the trunk in pityriasis rosea.

?? Differential Diagnosis and Pitfalls

- Secondary syphilis—systemic systems are more pronounced, including lymphadenopathy, fevers, history of primary chancre, condyloma lata; if remotely suspicious, check syphilis serologies
- Drug eruption
- Tinea corporis
- Tinea versicolor
- Nummular eczema—very pruritic; this is the most common complaint
- Guttate psoriasis—smaller size and thicker scale
- Parapsoriasis
- Erythema multiforme
- Urticaria
- Lichen planus
- Pityriasis lichenoides chronica

✓ Best Tests

- Diagnosis is usually made on clinical grounds.
- Skin biopsy is rarely indicated because histology is nonspecific and the clinical picture is characteristic.
- Syphilis serology with clinical suspicion (systemic symptoms, lymphadenopathy, history of primary chancre, condyloma lata, and HIV)
- KOH examination of skin scrapings when considering tinea infection.

▲▲ Management Pearls

- The acute onset and widespread involvement often causes significant concern for the patient or parents. Education and assurance of the benign nature may assist in management.

Therapy

Antipruritics (such as lotions containing camphor, menthol, or pramoxine), oatmeal baths, and antihistamines can provide symptomatic relief.

Antihistamines:

- Diphenhydramine hydrochloride (25 and 50 mg tablets or capsules): 25 to 50 mg nightly or every 6 h as needed
- Hydroxyzine (10 and 25 mg tablets): 12.5 to 25 mg every 6 h as needed
- Cetirizine hydrochloride (5 and 10 mg tablets): 5 to 10 mg per day
- Loratadine (10 mg tablets): 10 mg once daily

Topical corticosteroids may also help improve itch and appearance by decreasing inflammation.

Mid-potency topical corticosteroids (*classes 3 and 4*)

- Triamcinolone cream, ointment—apply twice daily (15, 30, 60, 120, 240 g)
- Mometasone cream, ointment—apply twice daily (15, 45 g)
- Fluocinolone ointment, cream—apply twice daily (15, 30, 60 g)

Although it requires referral to a phototherapy center, broadband ultraviolet B therapy (UVB) has been shown to be effective in shortening the course of pityriasis rosea and relieving symptoms; three to five treatments per week, at a dose strong enough to induce faint erythema.

Oral erythromycin has been used in the past, but current studies do not support its effectiveness for pityriasis rosea.

Suggested Readings

Allen RA, Janniger CK, Schwartz RA. Pityriasis rosea. *Cutis.* 1995 Oct;56(4):198–202.

Blauvelt A. Pityriasis rosea. In: Fitzpatrick TB, Wolff K, eds. *Fitzpatrick's Dermatology in General Medicine.* 7th Ed. New York, NY: McGraw-Hill; 2008:362–366.

Chuh A, Chan H, Zawar V. Pityriasis rosea—evidence for and against an infectious aetiology. *Epidemiol Infect.* 2004 Jun;132(3):381–390.

Chuh AA, Dofitas BL, Comisel GG, et al. Interventions for pityriasis rosea. *Cochrane Database Syst Rev.* 2007 Apr;(2):CD005068.

Chuh AA, Molinari N, Sciallis G, et al. Temporal case clustering in pityriasis rosea: A regression analysis on 1379 patients in Minnesota, Kuwait, and Diyarbakir, Turkey. *Arch Dermatol.* 2005 Jun;141(6):767–771.

Drago F, Broccolo F, Zaccaria E, et al. Pregnancy outcome in patients with pityriasis rosea. *J Am Acad Dermatol.* 2008 May;58(5 Suppl. 1):S78–S83.

Drago F, Ranieri E, Malaguti F, et al. Human herpesvirus 7 in pityriasis rosea. *Lancet.* 1997 May;349(9062):1367–1368.

González LM, Allen R, Janniger CK, et al. Pityriasis rosea: An important papulosquamous disorder. *Int J Dermatol.* 2005 Sep;44(9):757–764.

Pierson JC, Dijkstra JW, Elston DM. Purpuric pityriasis rosea. *J Am Acad Dermatol.* 1993 Jun;28(6):1021.

Sezer E, Saracoglu ZN, Urer SM, et al. Purpuric pityriasis rosea. *Int J Dermatol.* 2003 Feb;42(2):138–140.

Valkova S, Trashlieva M, Christova P. UVB phototherapy for Pityriasis rosea. *J Eur Acad Dermatol Venereol.* 2004 Jan;18(1):111–112.

Pityriasis Rubra Pilaris

Diagnosis Synopsis

Pityriasis rubra pilaris (PRP) is characterized by an acute cutaneous eruption that is often accompanied by pruritus and/or pain. Classic cutaneous lesions include follicular papules on an erythematous base coalescing to form large orange-red plaques but with characteristic islands of sparing. PRP commonly begins on the scalp and rapidly spreads in a craniocaudal direction, and has the potential to quickly progress to erythroderma over several weeks' time. Additional features include an orange-red palmoplantar keratoderma and sparing of the mucous membranes. PRP can be classified into five clinical types based on age of onset, cutaneous features, and clinical course. In classic adult PRP, more than 80% of patients will experience spontaneous remission within 3 years.

The etiology of PRP has not been clearly defined. The onset of disease has been associated with myositis, myasthenia gravis, hypothyroidism, HIV, infection, and malignancy. In addition, UV exposure and minor skin trauma prior to the onset of PRP have been reported. While there are reports of heritable forms, the large majority of PRP cases are acquired and without gender predilection. The incidence of the acquired form occurs in two peaks: during the first and second decades and the sixth decade.

Look For

Discrete, follicular, scaling papules coalescing in areas to confluent, orange-red plaques (Figs. 4-375–4-377). These often begin on the scalp and may expand to involve most of the body. There is orange hyperkeratosis of the palms and soles, sometimes with painful fissuring.

Nail changes include a thickened yellow-brown nail plate with subungual debris (Fig. 4-378).

Oral mucosal changes are very rare, but when present can include gray or whitish papules or plaques, erythema, or erosions.

Dark Skin Considerations

In darkly pigmented skin, the follicular prominence of lesions can be marked.
Also look for marked hyperkeratosis of the palms and soles.

Diagnostic Pearls

Several features facilitate the differentiation of PRP from psoriasis, and they include the following:

- Islands of normal skin within larger plaques are characteristically seen in PRP
- Orange-red, waxy-like keratoderma of the palms and soles are also features seen in PRP
- Nail oil-drop changes and nail pitting are characteristic of psoriasis
- A family history of psoriasis is often seen in psoriatic patients
- PRP and psoriasis are histologically different, and a biopsy will aid in the diagnosis

Immunocompromised Patient Considerations

- PRP has been described in HIV-infected patients who may or may not also have acne conglobata or hidradenitis-like lesions.

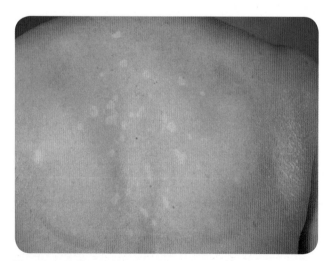

Figure 4-375 Islands of normal skin surrounded by red, scaling skin are characteristic of PRP.

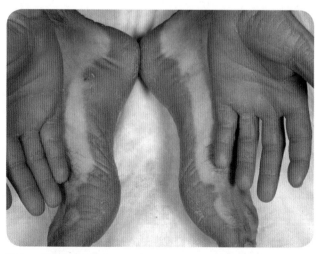

Figure 4-376 Prominent yellow palmar and plantar hyperkeratosis is characteristic of PRP.

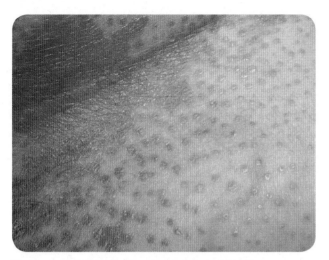

Figure 4-377 Follicular hyperkeratotic lesions in PRP.

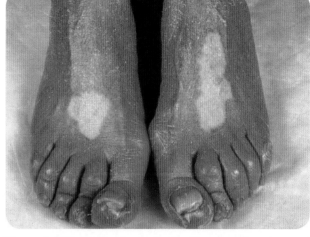

Figure 4-378 Islands of normal skin with surrounding plaques of PRP.

?? Differential Diagnosis and Pitfalls

Skin biopsy will greatly aid in the diagnosis.

- Psoriasis—See Diagnostic Pearls
- Seborrheic dermatitis—Much more responsive to standard therapies. PRP is often resistant to conventional therapies for seborrheic dermatitis. In addition, the progression of body surface involvement will distinguish PRP from seborrheic dermatitis.
- Mycosis fungoides/Sézary syndrome—Generalized lymphadenopathy, circulating malignant lymphocytes as determined by flow cytometry, leonine facies, a CD4/CD8 ratio more than 10 as determined by flow cytometry.
- Erythrokeratoderma variabilis—More than 90% of patients present within the first year of life.
- Drug eruption—Often present with urticarial, exanthematous, or vesicular/bullous lesions. In addition, systemic symptoms are more pronounced, including fever, lymphadenopathy, and facial edema. Eosinophilia on CBC and histology are often seen (but not an invariable finding). Medication history will help.
- Atopic dermatitis—Patients are often aware of their atopic history, and the condition commonly starts in childhood. Look for lichenified plaques on the flexural surfaces and neck.

✓ Best Tests

- Skin biopsy will usually aid in confirming the diagnosis and differentiating PRP from psoriasis.
- Other laboratory and radiologic investigations are not routinely necessary. Depending on the clinical situation, a search for HIV infection or underlying malignancy may be indicated.

- Patients who develop erythroderma should be evaluated for electrolyte abnormalities, hypoalbuminemia, and secondary infection.

▲▲ Management Pearls

- Some immediate relief can be gained from the application of potent topical steroids under occlusion, alternating with a solution of propylene glycol and lactic acid under occlusion. However, these modalities have little long-term therapeutic benefits. Heavy emollients, such as petroleum jelly or Aquaphor, may relieve fissuring and help erythrodermic skin retain moisture. Emollients such as 12% lactic acid cream or lotion (Lac-Hydrin 12%) may be helpful on areas of keratoderma.
- The morbidity of PRP is due to the erythroderma. Measures should be taken to prevent the progression of PRP to erythroderma. Complications of erythroderma include volume shifts (i.e., lower extremity edema) secondary to loss of fluids and proteins, tachycardia-induced high output cardiac failure, and thermoregulatory dysregulation (hypothermia and hyperthermia).

Therapy

No large controlled trials have been performed. Prednisone 40 to 60 mg per day is effective in controlling the disease and can be tapered while instituting one of the following:

- Retinoids are effective but must be used cautiously in women of child-bearing age due to their teratogenic effects. Physicians prescribing these medications must closely supervise the therapy, including monthly urine

(Continued)

HCG, CBC, triglyceride level, liver function tests, and two forms of contraception in women.

- Acitretin (10, 25 mg)—Begin at 25 mg daily, advance to 50 mg, and possibly 75 mg daily depending on weight.
- Isotretinoin (20, 40 mg) 0.5 to 1.5 mg/kg daily with food.
- Methotrexate (10 to 30 mg weekly)—Well-known side effects of methotrexate include hepatoxicity, myelosuppression, and conversion from latent to active tuberculosis or histoplasmosis. Take with folic acid 1 mg daily or leucovorin 5 mg weekly.
- Azathioprine 1 mg/kg daily for 6 to 8 weeks, and increase by 0.5 mg/kg every 2 to 4 weeks; do not exceed 2.5 mg/kg/day.
- Cyclosporin A 2.5 mg/kg daily (twice daily dosing) for 4 weeks. Increase by 0.5 mg/kg daily every 2 to 4 weeks. Do not exceed 5 mg/kg/day. Infliximab (Remicade) for refractory cases. Administer 5 mg/kg IV infusion followed by 5 mg/kg at 2 and 6 weeks after the first infusion, then subsequently every 2 months.
- Phototherapy can exacerbate PRP or induce remission. Success has been reported using treatment with narrow-band UVB (TL-01) in combination with acitretin. Extracorporeal photochemotherapy has also demonstrated success.

Suggested Readings

Bruch-Gerharz D, Ruzicka T. Pityriasis rubra pilaris. In: Fitzpatrick TB, Wolff K, eds. *Fitzpatrick's Dermatology in General Medicine.* 7th Ed. New York, NY: McGraw-Hill; 2008:232–236.

Caplan SE, Lowitt MH, Kao GF. Early presentation of pityriasis rubra pilaris. *Cutis.* 1997 Dec;60(6):291–296.

Clayton BD, Jorizzo JL, Hitchcock MG, et al. Adult pityriasis rubra pilaris: A 10-year case series. *J Am Acad Dermatol.* 1997 Jun;36(6 Pt 1):959–964.

De D, Dogra S, Narang T, Radotra BD, et al. Pityriasis rubra pilaris in a HIV-positive patient (Type 6 PRP). *Skinmed.* 2008 Jan–Feb;7(1):47–50.

Dicken CH. Treatment of classic pityriasis rubra pilaris. *J Am Acad Dermatol.* 1994 Dec;31(6):997–999.

Durairaj VD, Horsley MB. Resolution of pityriasis rubra pilaris-induced cicatricial ectropion with systemic low-dose methotrexate. *Am J Ophthalmol.* 2007 Apr;143(4):709–710.

Haenssle HA, Bertsch HP, Emmert S, et al. Extracorporeal photochemotherapy for the treatment of exanthematic pityriasis rubra pilaris. *Clin Exp Dermatol.* 2004 May;29(3):244–246.

Kaskel P, Peter RU, Kerscher M. Phototesting and phototherapy in pityriasis rubra pilaris. *Br J Dermatol.* 2001 Feb;144(2):430.

Liao WC, Mutasim DF. Infliximab for the treatment of adult-onset pityriasis rubra pilaris. *Arch Dermatol.* 2005 Apr;141(4):423–425.

Paranjothy B, Shunmugam M, MacKenzie J, et al. Peripheral ulcerative keratitis in pityriasis rubra pilaris. *Eye.* 2007 Jul;21(7):1001–1002.

Sehgal VN, Jain S, Kumar S, et al. Familial pityriasis rubra pilaris (adult classic-I): A report of three cases in a single family. *Skinmed.* 2002 Nov–Dec;1(2):161–164.

Prurigo Nodularis

Diagnosis Synopsis

Prurigo nodularis is a chronic condition of uncertain etiology. Patients present with multiple discrete, severely pruritic nodules that mostly appear on the dorsal extremities and anterior areas of the thighs and legs. The lesions are rarely seen on the face. The lesions are brought about by repetitive rubbing or scratching discrete areas of the skin, and patients often state that they are unable to stop doing so. Prurigo nodularis may be secondary to skin conditions associated with pruritus, such as atopic dermatitis and xerosis, as well as systemic conditions associated with generalized pruritus without a primary skin rash such as psychiatric conditions, HIV infection, renal or hepatic impairment, malignancies, and others.

Lesions are firm dome-shaped, smooth-topped or crusted 1 to 2 cm nodules that enlarge slowly over time. The lichenification of the lesions is often not present. It is most commonly seen in middle-aged to elderly patients and may be more common in women.

Dark Skin Considerations

Perforating folliculitis with superimposed prurigo nodularis has been reported in black patients on hemodialysis. In patients with HIV-AIDS, those with darker skin types are at higher risk of developing prurigo nodularis.

Immunocompromised Patient Considerations

Immunosuppressed patients, including those with HIV/AIDS, appear to have an increased incidence of prurigo nodularis. With HIV, occurrence is most common in patients with CD4 counts of less than 50/mL who are not taking antiretroviral therapy. Patients with chronic viral hepatitis may also develop prurigo nodularis. Coinfection with hepatitis C and HIV increases this risk.

Look For

Nodules and papules that range in size from 0.5 to 2 cm in diameter enlarge slowly over time. The nodules can be very firm and thick, and are usually limited to the extremities. They may have scaly or crusted centers and appear hyperpigmented or violaceous (Figs. 4-379 and 4-380). Often, central excoriations are present (Fig. 4-381). Bacterial superinfection is not uncommon. Persistent prurigo nodularis may evolve into anetoderma, a loss of skin elasticity with a resultant soft depression.

Dark Skin Considerations

Those with darker skin often have dark gray or hypopigmented centers.

Diagnostic Pearls

- Lesions are almost always in areas that can be scratched or rubbed, especially on the extremities. The "butterfly sign" refers to the area on the mid-upper back that is frequently spared (Fig. 4-382), as patients are unable to reach/scratch this zone.

Immunocompromised Patient Considerations

In patients with HIV or viral hepatitis, worsening of pruritus may mirror the progression of the viral infection (e.g., increased viral loads).

?? Differential Diagnosis and Pitfalls

Top considerations:

- Multiple keratoacanthomas
- Hypertrophic lichen planus
- Pemphigoid nodularis
- Nodular scabies

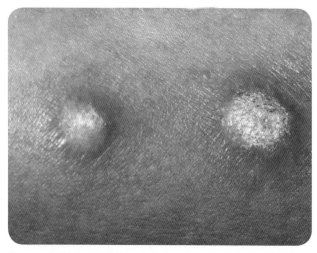

Figure 4-379 Irregular hyperkeratotic, pruritic papules with surrounding normal skin are characteristic of prurigo nodularis.

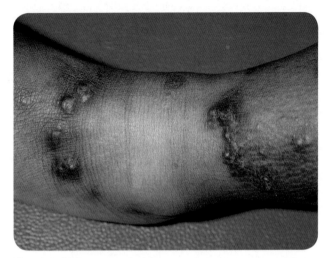

Figure 4-380 Hyperpigmentation is common in prurigo nodularis.

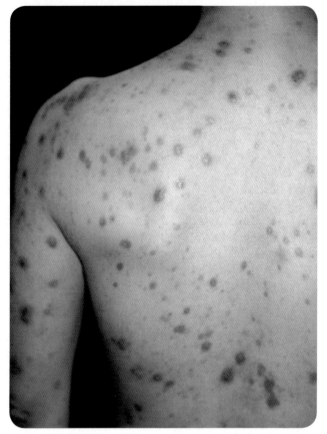

Figure 4-382 Relative sparing of a difficult-to-reach location—the mid back—in prurigo nodularis.

Figure 4-381 Excoriation of the papules is common in prurigo nodularis.

The following diagnoses can also mimic the lesions of prurigo nodularis:

- Keloids
- Acne keloidalis nuchae
- Hypertrophic actinic keratosis/cutaneous horn
- Hypertrophic scars
- Lymphoma
- Pseudolymphoma
- Lymphomatoid papulosis
- Warts
- Molluscum contagiosum
- Mastocytosis
- Cutaneous amyloidosis
- Dermatofibromas
- Pilomatrixomas
- Foreign body reactions
- Chondrodermatitis nodularis helicis

- Xanthomas
- Knuckle pads
- Multicentric reticulohistiocytosis
- Persistent insect bite reaction
- Mycosis fungoides
- Perforating skin disorders such as Kyrle disease

✓ Best Tests

- Skin biopsy will confirm the clinical impression.
- Culture for bacteria if there is any indication of pyoderma.
- Consider HIV testing if the patient's HIV status is unknown.
- Obtain a CBC, liver and thyroid function tests, and a chemistry panel to rule out hematologic malignancies and renal or hepatic disease as a cause of pruritus.
- An elevated serum IgE may indicate atopy.
- A thorough history and physical is often the most important evaluation for underlying causes of prurigo nodularis. If there is any suspicion of lymphoma based on a review of systems, a chest radiograph and/or abdominal CT scan may be obtained.

▲▲ Management Pearls

- The very indolent nature of these lesions should be communicated to the patient early in the course so that he or she can develop appropriate expectations. These lesions are very difficult to treat because they are chronically picked and scratched by the patient. Stopping the itch-scratch cycle is paramount for the patient to improve.

Therapy

This can be a difficult condition to treat. If an underlying disorder is discovered to be the cause of the intense pruritus, make every attempt to maximize the treatment of this disorder.

Control itch with the following soothing emollients (containing menthol, pramoxine, camphor), capsaicin cream (0.025% to 0.3%, applied four to six times daily) and antihistamines:

- Diphenhydramine hydrochloride (25, 50 mg tablets or capsules): 25 to 50 mg nightly or every 6 h as needed
- Hydroxyzine (10, 25 mg tablets): 12.5 to 25 mg every 6 h as needed
- Cetirizine hydrochloride (5 and 10 mg tablets): 5 to 10 mg per day
- Loratadine (10 mg tablets): 10 mg once daily

Have the patient apply Cordran tape or superpotent topical steroids (eg, clobetasol) to only the lesions. The tape has the added benefit of occluding the lesions and preventing further scratching.

Intralesional therapy with triamcinolone 5 to 10 mg/cc can also be helpful.

Cryosurgery should be attempted on only 1 or a few lesions to prove efficacy. Warn patients about the risk of hypopigmentation or hyperpigmentation and further scarring.

PUVA, UVB, and narrow-band UVB phototherapy have successfully been used for more diffuse lesions. Naltrexone may also be effective by acting on the central and peripheral itch pathways, which are in part mediated by opioid receptors. Severe refractory cases have been treated with thalidomide (100 to 300 mg daily) and cyclosporine (3 to 4.5 mg/kg daily). Refer the patient to a dermatologist if you are considering these therapies.

Psychiatric interventions also represent a major component of therapy in many patients. Antianxiety and antidepressant medications are beneficial for a significant number of patients. Biofeedback, journaling, and counseling are also helpful for many patients to help break the itch-scratch cycle.

Immunocompromised Patient Considerations

Antihistamines are frequently of little benefit in patients with HIV-associated prurigo nodularis. Starting antiretroviral medications is often the most effective therapy for this patient population. In viral hepatitis as well, antiviral therapy often leads to improvement.

Severe refractory cases in HIV patients have been treated with thalidomide, but refer the patient to a specialist if you are considering this therapy.

Suggested Readings

Burgin S. Nummular eczema and lichen simplex chronicus/prurigo nodularis. In: Fitzpatrick TB, Wolff K, eds. *Fitzpatrick's Dermatology in General Medicine.* 7th Ed. New York, NY: McGraw-Hill; 2008:158–162.

Lee MR, Shumack S. Prurigo nodularis: a review. *Australas J Dermatol.* 2005 Nov;46(4):211–218; quiz 219–220.

Lotti T, Buggiani G, Prignano F. Prurigo nodularis and lichen simplex chronicus. *Dermatol Ther.* 2008 Jan–Feb;21(1):42–46.

Maurer T, Poncelet A, Berger T. Thalidomide treatment for prurigo nodularis in human immunodeficiency virus-infected subjects: Efficacy and risk of neuropathy. *Arch Dermatol.* 2004 Jul;140(7):845–849.

Maurer TA. Dermatologic manifestations of HIV infection. *Top HIV Med.* 2005 Dec–2006 Jan;13(5):149–154.

Ständer S, Luger T, Metze D. Treatment of prurigo nodularis with topical capsaicin. *J Am Acad Dermatol.* 2001 Mar;44(3):471–478.

Wallengren J. Prurigo: diagnosis and management. *Am J Clin Dermatol.* 2004;5(2):85–95.

Diagnosis Synopsis

Psoriasis is a chronic, intermittently relapsing inflammatory disease that is classically characterized by sharply demarcated erythematous, silvery, scaly plaques most often seen on the scalp, elbows, and knees. Additional sites of involvement include the nails, hands, feet, and trunk. Approximately 2% of the world's population suffers from psoriasis. Psoriasis can develop at any age, in both genders, and in all ethnicities, but it occurs most frequently in whites.

Psoriasis is a polygenic disease where genetically susceptible individuals with certain HLA types (HLA-Cw6, HLA-B13, HLA-B17, HLA-B37, HLA-Bw16) mount aberrant immune responses after exposure to infection, drug ingestion, hypocalcemia, psychogenic stress, and/or external injury to the skin. Aberrant T-cell function and keratinocyte responses are believed to be major culprits in the pathogenesis of psoriasis.

Chronic plaque psoriasis is the most common variant, and disease burden can range from 1% to 2% (mild disease) to greater than 90% (erythrodermic psoriasis) of the total body surface area (BSA). Classic findings include well-demarcated; circular, oval, or polycyclic; erythematous; silvery; scaly plaques that are often symmetric in distribution. Lesions are often mildly pruritic and resolve with postinflammatory hyper- or hypopigmentation. Scarring is not a feature of resolution. During exacerbations, erythematous papules usually surround existing plaques, and a ring of intense erythema surrounds the plaques. During resolution, plaques will have a decreased amount of scale and central clearing, creating annular psoriatic lesions. Lesions can last from months to years in the same location.

The clinician should be aware of several key points in patients with psoriasis:

- Cardiovascular disease—The presence of psoriasis may have an impact on other organ systems. Psoriatic patients have an increased relative risk for cardiovascular disease including cerebrovascular accidents, pulmonary emboli, and myocardial infarctions. Additional risk factors for cardiac disease (diabetes, cholesterol, hypertension, obesity, smoking, etc.) should be appropriately screened for and addressed.
- While research-oriented severity scales exist (Psoriasis Area and Severity Index), the BSA is generally used clinically as a reference for evaluating response to treatment.
- Variants include guttate psoriasis, erythrodermic psoriasis, pustular psoriasis, psoriatic arthritis, inverse psoriasis, and acrodermatitis continua of Hallopeau. Some variants coexist.
- Psoriatic arthritis: Up to 30% of psoriatic patients may have erosive psoriatic arthritis requiring systemic therapies.
- Pregnancy: Approximately 50% of pregnant females with psoriasis report improvement of disease burden. However, there are many reports that show pustular psoriasis development in pregnant females who are hypocalcemic.
- Oral or IM steroids: Only in rare cases, such as erythroderma or severe pustular psoriasis, should oral steroids be considered. This is because the use of systemic steroids will lead to severe psoriasis rebound after steroid discontinuation.

Look For

- Sharply demarcated, erythematous, silver-scaled plaques of the scalp, elbows, and knees. Additional sites of involvement include the hands, feet, and trunk (Figs. 4-383–4-386).
- Nails: Fingernails are affected more often than toenails. Nail pitting, onycholysis ("oil spots"), splinter hemorrhages, subungual hyperkeratosis, leukonychia (Fig. 4-387).

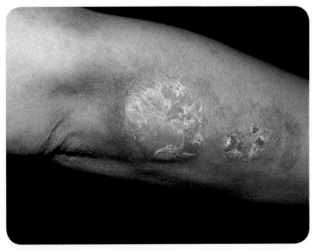

Figure 4-383 Well-delimited, red, scaly plaques of psoriasis in a typical location.

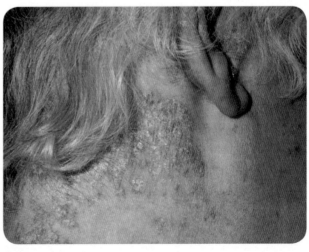

Figure 4-384 Psoriasis frequently affects the scalp and head or neck near the scalp.

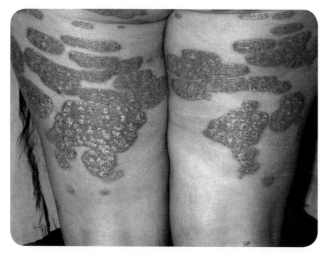

Figure 4-385 Psoriasis with multiple red plaques and prominent scale.

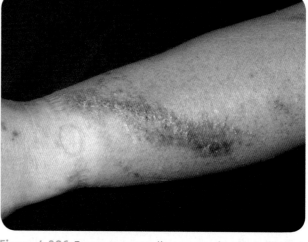

Figure 4-386 Trauma may cause linear areas of psoriasis (illustrating the Koebner phenomenon).

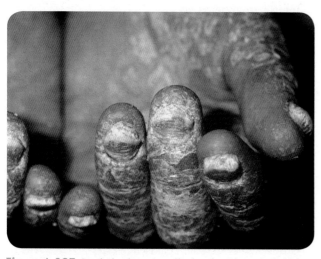

Figure 4-387 Psoriatic plaques on the hands with marked thickening and opacity of the nail plaques.

- Joints: In psoriatic arthritis, look for distal and proximal interphalangeal arthritis; "sausage digits" can be monoarticular or asymmetric oligoarthritis.
- Axilla, groin, intergluteal cleft: Locations for inverse psoriasis. Look for shiny erythematous, sharply demarcated plaques. Fissuring can be noted. Localized dermatophyte infections as well as *Candida* can trigger psoriasis in this area. Because of the moist environment and occlusion, heavy scale is not seen in these areas.

Diagnostic Pearls

- Very thick, silvery scale favors the diagnosis of psoriasis. The involvement of plaques in the navel and the gluteal cleft also favors a diagnosis of psoriasis. When in doubt, nail involvement favors psoriasis as well.

Immunocompromised Patient Considerations

- Psoriasis can occur even with very low CD4 counts. A flare of psoriasis or sudden onset of psoriasis may be an indicator of HIV infection.

?? Differential Diagnosis and Pitfalls

- Lichen planus—Very pruritic, associated with hepatitis C. Biopsy will differentiate psoriasis from lichen planus.
- Subacute cutaneous lupus erythematosus—Check ANA; will be positive in most lupus patients. SCLE is characterized by annular plaques with raised borders and central clearing or papulosquamous lesions that are restricted to sun-exposed skin.
- Pityriasis lichenoides chronica—Usually smaller papules. Biopsy will assist in differentiating from psoriasis, predominantly CD8+ T-cell infiltrate.
- Lymphomatoid papulosis—Crusted papules and smaller papules. Biopsy will assist in differentiating from psoriasis, predominantly CD30+ T-cell infiltrate.
- Pityriasis rubra pilaris—Look for orange-red, waxy-like keratoderma of the palms and soles. Islands of normal skin within larger plaques are characteristically seen in PRP. PRP and psoriasis are histologically different, and a biopsy will aid in the diagnosis. A family history of psoriasis is often noted in psoriatic patients.
- Mycosis fungoides—Generalized lymphadenopathy, circulating malignant lymphocytes as determined by flow cytometry, leonine facies, a CD4/CD8 ratio more than 10 as determined by flow cytometry.

- Secondary syphilis—Check RPR, and check for history of primary chancre and systemic symptoms.
- Chronic atopic dermatitis patients are often aware of their atopic history that commonly starts in childhood. Mild to moderate spongiosis is seen on histology. Look for lichenified plaques on the flexural surfaces and neck. More pruritic is seen than psoriasis.
- Contact dermatitis
- Nummular eczema—Intensely pruritic coin-shaped lesions, almost exclusively seen on the extremities.
- Lichen simplex chronicus—Common around the ankles.
- Seborrheic dermatitis—Sebaceous distribution
- Erythema annulare centrifugum
- Extramammary Paget disease
- Pityriasis rosea—Look for herald patch, collarette of scale, and orientation of lesions (fir-tree pattern in skin tension lines). Does not follow an intermittently relapsing course.
- Tinea corporis—Scale at leading edge of erythema with central clearing. Check KOH.
- Drug eruption—Drug eruptions often present with urticarial, exanthematous, or vesicular/bullous lesions. In addition, systemic symptoms are more pronounced than seen with classic psoriasis, including fever, lymphadenopathy, and facial edema. Eosinophilia on CBC and histology are often seen (but not an invariable finding). Look for nonsteroidal anti-inflammatory drugs (NSAIDs), sulfonamides, and penicillin.

Immunocompromised Patient Considerations

- Reactive arthritis (Reiter disease) with circinate lesions. Lesions on the glans penis and arthritis are difficult to differentiate from severe psoriasis flare.

✓ Best Tests

- This diagnosis is most often made clinically. If there is doubt, perform a skin biopsy.
- Consider plain films or bone scans in patients with joint complaints.

▲▲ Management Pearls

- Ultraviolet light is one of the best therapies to treat extensive or widespread disease. Consider narrow-band UVB three times weekly, or recommend natural sun exposure, if possible. Some cases of psoriasis are light induced, and this should be determined first by careful history.
- The National Psoriasis Foundation is an excellent resource for patients: http://www.psoriasis.org/home/

Immunocompromised Patient Considerations

- Therapy for HIV may improve psoriasis.

Therapy

Note that psoriasis is often too widespread to practically treat with topical agents or recalcitrant to topical therapy alone. However, this should be evaluated on a case-by-case basis because systemic treatments often require monitoring and carry a potential risk of systemic side effects. In addition, potent corticosteroids should not be used in the intertriginous areas due to skin thinning and striae formation.

Topical Treatments
High-potency topical corticosteroids (classes 1 and 2)

- Fluocinonide cream, ointment—apply twice daily (15, 30, 60, 120 g)
- Desoximetasone cream, ointment—apply twice daily (15, 60, 120 g)
- Halcinonide cream, ointment—apply twice daily (15, 60, 240 g)
- Amcinonide ointment—apply twice daily (15, 30, 60 g)
- Clobetasol cream, ointment—apply twice daily

Mid-potency topical corticosteroids (classes 3 and 4)

- Triamcinolone cream, ointment—apply twice daily (15, 30, 60, 120, 240 g)
- Mometasone cream, ointment—apply twice daily (15, 45 g)
- Fluocinolone cream, ointment—apply twice daily (15, 30, 60 g)

Vitamin D Analog
- Calcipotriene cream, ointment—Apply twice daily to affected areas (30, 60, 100 g tubes) (60 mL scalp solution). Therapy can be rotated with steroid treatment.

Tar-based Therapy
- 10% Liquor carbonis detergens in ointment—apply daily, compound 440 g jar
- Anthralin 0.1, 0.25, and 0.5 cream—begin with lowest strength, and apply short contact (e.g., 10 min); advance as tolerated
- Tar bath oils, 2.5% coal tar, (240, 180, 240 mL)

Scalp Therapy
Thick, scaly plaques within the scalp can be a difficult management problem. Consider loosening scale with an

oil-based treatment such as Baker P&S applied nightly (120 mL) or treating with fluocinolone peanut oil formulation applied nightly, supplied 120 mL. Have patient shampoo with tar-based shampoos.

Systemic Therapy

- Methotrexate 10 to 20 mg p.o. weekly
- Mycophenolate mofetil 1 g p.o. twice daily
- Cyclosporine 2 to 3 mg per kg p.o. daily
- Tacrolimus 1 to 3 mg p.o. daily
- Acitretin 25 to 50 mg p.o. daily
- TNF-alpha inhibitors (use as directed). Be sure to check PPD prior to use.
- Etanercept—50 mg SQ twice weekly for 3 months, then once weekly
- Alefacept—15 mg IM weekly for 12 weeks
- Infliximab
- Adalimumab

Ultraviolet Light

Can be used alone or in combination with acitretin systemically.

- Ultraviolet B (UVB) radiation (295 to 320 nm)—Perform three times weekly until remission is induced, followed by maintenance doses. Can be used alone or in conjunction with topical tar.
- Narrow-band UVB (311 nm)—Use three times weekly until remission is induced.
- Photochemotherapy (PUVA)—Increased risk of skin cancer over prolonged usage.
  - Patients ingest 8-methoxypsoralen with exposure to UVA within 2 h of ingestion; perform three times weekly in increasing doses until remission, then twice or once weekly as a maintenance dose.

- Bath PUVA involves dissolving the psoralen capsules in water, and affected skin is soaked for 15 to 30 min prior to UVA exposure.

Referral to dermatology is indicated for management with systemic medications.

Suggested Readings

Ashcroft DM, Li Wan Po A, Griffiths CE. Therapeutic strategies for psoriasis. *J Clin Pharm Ther.* 2000 Feb;25(1):1–10.

Boehncke WH, Elshorst-Schmidt T, Kaufmann R. Systemic photodynamic therapy is a safe and effective treatment for psoriasis. *Arch Dermatol.* 2000 Feb;136(2):271–272.

Gudjonsson JE, Elder JT. Psoriasis. In: Fitzpatrick TB, Wolff K, eds. *Fitzpatrick's Dermatology in General Medicine.* 7th Ed. New York, NY: McGraw-Hill; 2008:169–193.

Krueger G, Ellis CN. Psoriasis—recent advances in understanding its pathogenesis and treatment. *J Am Acad Dermatol.* 2005 Jul;53(1 Suppl. 1): S94–S100.

Menter A, Gottlieb A, Feldman SR, et al. Guidelines of care for the management of psoriasis and psoriatic arthritis: Section 1. Overview of psoriasis and guidelines of care for the treatment of psoriasis with biologics. *J Am Acad Dermatol.* 2008 May;58(5):826–850.

Menter A, Griffiths CE. Current and future management of psoriasis. *Lancet.* 2007 Jul;370(9583):272–284.

Schön MP, Boehncke WH. Psoriasis. *N Engl J Med.* 2005 May;352(18): 1899–1912.

Smith KE, Fenske NA. Cutaneous manifestations of alcohol abuse. *J Am Acad Dermatol.* 2000 Jul;43(1 Pt 1):1–16; quiz 16–18.

Stern RS. Psoralen and ultraviolet a light therapy for psoriasis. *N Engl J Med.* 2007 Aug;357(7):682–690.

Sterry W, Barker J, Boehncke WH, et al. Biological therapies in the systemic management of psoriasis: International Consensus Conference. *Br J Dermatol.* 2004 Aug;151(Suppl.) 69:3–17.

Yosipovitch G, DeVore A, Dawn A. Obesity and the skin: skin physiology and skin manifestations of obesity. *J Am Acad Dermatol.* 2007 Jun;56(6): 901–916; quiz 917–920.

Diagnosis Synopsis

Guttate psoriasis is a variant of psoriasis that is characterized by an acute, generalized eruption of small, discreet rain drop-like (hence the name, guttate) papules with fine scale that occurs 2 to 3 weeks after an upper respiratory infection. It most commonly occurs in children and is associated with an elevated anti-streptolysin O, anti-DNase B, or streptozyme titer. Guttate psoriasis can be pruritic, and postinflammatory pigmentary changes can follow. However, scarring and systemic symptoms such as fever, malaise, lymphadenopathy, myalgias, and arthralgias are usually absent.

Current evidence supports the theory that plaque psoriasis and guttate psoriasis are similar in that an environmental factor triggers an immune reaction in a genetically susceptible individual. The environment factor is often a streptococcal infection, and a T-cell driven immune reaction is elicited, leading to increased type 1 helper T-cells (Th1) activity and increased IFN-g and IL-2 cytokine levels. Regarding a genetically susceptible host, it has been demonstrated that HLA-Cw*0602–positive patients are more likely to develop guttate psoriasis.

Guttate psoriasis occurs in all races, both genders, and is most commonly seen in children and young adults aged younger than 30. The clinical course is unpredictable. In children, spontaneous remission over weeks to months is common, while in young adults, it may represent the first stage in the development of chronic plaque psoriasis.

In cases where a streptococcal infection cannot be identified, viruses such as rubella, roseola, and varicella have also been implicated as inciting factors. Medications have been cited as causative agents as well.

Look For

Hundreds of small, guttate (drop-like), scaly, erythematous papules concentrated on the scalp, face, neck, trunk, and extremities (Figs. 4-388–4-391). The palms and soles are usually spared, and the typical nail changes of psoriasis (e.g., oil-drop spots and pitting) may be absent.

Pharyngeal or perianal erythema may be present with concurrent streptococcal infection at these sites.

Dark Skin Considerations

In darkly pigmented skin, the lesions often appear gray in color, and sometimes the scales are silvery-white. Postinflammatory pigmentary changes can be quite prominent.

Diagnostic Pearls

- Sore throat is the most common associated factor in patients in the 20 to 30 year age group.

Differential Diagnosis and Pitfalls

- Pityriasis rosea—Look for a herald patch, collarette of scale, and orientation of lesions (fir-tree pattern in skin tension lines).
- Small plaque parapsoriasis—More common in middle aged and elderly; chronic asymptomatic patches.

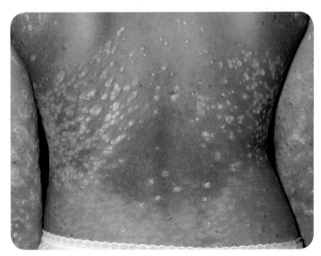

Figure 4-388 Small drop-like spots of guttate psoriasis may be seen during different stages of the disease, especially during an acute flare.

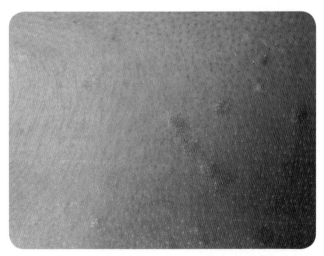

Figure 4-389 Small nonscaling guttate papules of psoriasis.

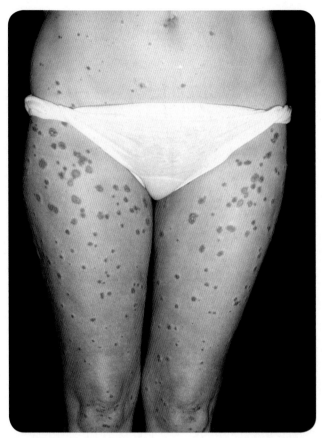

Figure 4-390 The papules are of various sizes with some very small guttate lesions on the abdomen. Scale is not obvious, and there is a perilesional ring of blanching that may be seen in psoriasis before treatment that is common in the late stages of treatment.

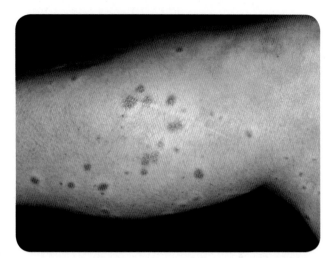

Figure 4-391 Guttate plaques of psoriasis; plaques may sometimes have surrounding blanching skin (Woronoff ring).

- Pityriasis lichenoides chronica—Biopsy will assist in differentiating from guttate psoriasis, predominantly CD8+ T-cell infiltrate.
- Secondary syphilis—Check RPR if strongly suspect; check for the history of primary chancre and systemic symptoms.
- Nummular dermatitis—Intensely pruritic, coin-shaped lesions almost exclusively seen on the extremities.
- Tinea corporis—Usually fewer isolated lesions. Check KOH.
- Tinea versicolor—Less scale and less inflammatory. KOH positive.
- Lymphomatoid papulosis—Biopsy will assist in differentiating from guttate psoriasis, predominantly CD30+ T-cell infiltrate.
- Psoriasiform drug eruption—Ask about medication history.
- Viral exanthem—Usually less scaly.

✓ Best Tests

- Often, this diagnosis can be made clinically based on history and its characteristic clinical appearance.

- Bacterial cultures of the throat or perianal area may help to isolate an organism in certain cases. The presence of antibodies to streptolysin O, anti-DNase B, or streptozyme can confirm previous infection.
- Perform a skin biopsy if the diagnosis is in doubt and a urinalysis if there is concern for post-streptococcal glomerulonephritis.

▲▲ Management Pearls

- Patients with guttate psoriasis need to be involved in a care plan of early treatment for bacterial pharyngitis, as recurrent episodes are common. The patient should have any symptoms of pharyngitis cultured and/or treated empirically for streptococcal pharyngitis. Early treatment can lessen the severity of each episode. In some cases, treatment of the underlying infection results in clearing of the psoriasis.
- Patients should refrain from scratching or rubbing lesions as skin trauma may lead to Koebnerization (spread of lesions within traumatized skin).

Therapy

Topical Therapies
Note that guttate psoriasis is often too widespread to practically treat with topical agents. However, this should be evaluated on a case-by-case basis because systemic treatments often require monitoring and carry a potential risk of systemic side effects.

Limited skin disease can be treated with topical (classes 2 to 4) corticosteroids.

(Continued)

High-potency Topical Corticosteroids (class 2)

- Fluocinonide cream, ointment—apply twice daily (15, 30, 60, 120 g)
- Desoximetasone cream, ointment—apply twice daily (15, 60, 120 g)
- Halcinonide cream, ointment—apply twice daily (15, 60, 240 g)
- Amcinonide ointment—apply twice daily (15, 30, 60 g)

Mid-potency Topical Corticosteroids (classes 3 and 4)

- Triamcinolone cream, ointment—apply twice daily (15, 30, 60, 120, 240 g)
- Mometasone cream, ointment—apply twice daily (15, 45 g)
- Fluocinolone ointment, cream—apply twice daily (15, 30, 60 g)

Calcipotriene—Can be used as an adjunct or replacement for steroids. Apply twice daily as a monotherapy, once daily as an adjunct.

Tazarotene—Apply 0.1% or 0.05% gel once daily.

Tacrolimus 0.1%—Apply to affected area twice daily. Use for facial and intertriginous areas.

Pimecrolimus 1%—Apply to affected area twice daily. Use for facial and intertriginous areas.

Ultraviolet Light
A suitable and popular modality for guttate psoriasis.

- Ultraviolet B (UVB) radiation (295 to 320 nm)—Perform three times weekly until remission is induced, followed by maintenance doses. Can be used alone or in conjunction with topical tar.
- Narrow-band UVB (311 nm)—Use three times weekly until remission is induced.
- Photochemotherapy (PUVA)—Clinicians should be aware of potential side effects and long-term risks:
  - Patients ingest 8-methoxypsoralen with exposure to UVA within 2 h of ingestion; perform three times weekly in increasing doses until remission, then twice or once weekly as a maintenance dose.
  - Bath PUVA involves dissolving the psoralen capsules in water, and affected skin is soaked for 15 to 30 min prior to UVA exposure.

Systemic Treatments
For severe or recalcitrant guttate psoriasis flares, systemic therapy can be considered.

- Methotrexate (10 to 15 mg p.o. weekly)
- Mycophenolate mofetil (1 g p.o. twice daily)
- Cyclosporine (2 to 3 mg/kg p.o. daily)
- Tacrolimus (1 to 3 mg p.o. daily)
- Acitretin (25 to 50 mg p.o. daily)

TNF-α inhibitors (as per package insert)—Note that no randomized trials have been performed with these agents, and there is no evidence that these should be employed as first-line agents.

- Etanercept
- Infliximab
- Adalimumab

Patients with recurrent episodes of streptococcal pharyngitis and guttate psoriasis may be helped by tonsillectomy; however, this has not been evaluated by a rigorous prospective trial.

Guttate psoriasis may be self-limiting or may respond to treatment of the underlying infection. There are controlled studies demonstrating *NO benefit* of systemic antibiotics in patients with guttate psoriasis and serologic evidence of a recent streptococcal infection. However, it is prudent to treat active streptococcal infection with a penicillin, cephalosporin, or erythromycin for 10 days:

- Amoxicillin 250 to 500 mg p.o. three times daily
- Penicillin VK 250 mg p.o. three to four times daily
- Cefuroxime 250 to 500 mg p.o. twice daily
- Erythromycin ethyl succinate 400 to 800 mg p.o. four times daily

Suggested Readings

Chalmers RJ, O'Sullivan T, Owen CM, et al. Interventions for guttate psoriasis. *Cochrane Database Syst Rev.* 2000;(2):CD001213.

Chalmers RJ, O'Sullivan T, Owen CM, et al. A systematic review of treatments for guttate psoriasis. *Br J Dermatol.* 2001 Dec;145(6):891–894.

Dogan B, Karabudak O, Harmanyeri Y. Antistreptococcal treatment of guttate psoriasis: A controlled study. *Int J Dermatol.* 2008 Sep;47(9): 950–952.

Menter A, Griffiths CE. Current and future management of psoriasis. *Lancet.* 2007 Jul;370(9583):272–284.

Owen CM, Chalmers RJ, O'Sullivan T, et al. Antistreptococcal interventions for guttate and chronic plaque psoriasis. *Cochrane Database Syst Rev.* 2000;(2):CD001976.

Stern RS. Psoralen and ultraviolet a light therapy for psoriasis. *N Engl J Med.* 2007 Aug;357(7):682–690.

Thappa DM, Laxmisha C. Suit PUVA as an effective and safe modality of treatment in guttate psoriasis. *J Eur Acad Dermatol Venereol.* 2006 Oct;20(9):1146–1147.

Psoriasis, Pustular

▪▪ Diagnosis Synopsis

Pustular psoriasis is an uncommon variant of psoriasis that is characterized by the presence of widespread, erythematous, sterile pustules on clinical examination and a predominantly neutrophilic infiltrate on a cellular level. Pustular psoriasis can be a severe inflammatory disease that requires hospitalization and aggressive therapy. Untreated disease can also progress to erythroderma. While many cases are idiopathic, risk factors that can trigger an episode include hypocalcemia, infection, a rapid withdrawal of corticosteroids (or weeks after an IM injection), pregnancy, medications (salicylates, lithium, iodine, trazodone, penicillin, interferon, hydroxychloroquine), and topical irritants such as tar and anthralin. Only a small number of patients have a preceding history of plaque-type psoriasis (Fig. 4-392).

There are 4 subtypes of pustular psoriasis. In the von Zumbusch type, there is an acute onset of generalized erythema and pustules with systemic manifestations including fever, skin tenderness, malaise, arthralgias, headache, and nausea. After several days, the pustules resolve to become confluent, scaling plaques. The exanthematic type is characterized by the acute onset of small pustules that are triggered by an infection or a drug. This subtype usually lacks systemic symptoms. The annular subtype is characterized by erythematous, annular lesions that have pustules at the advancing edge of a lesion and is associated with fever, malaise, and other systemic manifestations. The localized pattern occurs when pustules appear in existing psoriatic plaques. This can be seen in active plaques. Note that pustular psoriasis that occurs during pregnancy is termed impetigo herpetiformis.

Patients may experience relapses and remissions over a period of years. There is no racial predilection. Pustular psoriasis may occur in children but is more commonly seen in middle-aged adults.

Immunocompromised Patient Considerations

Fever and arthritis may be prominent features in the immunosuppressed patient. There may be an inflammatory polyarthritis with associated involvement of the plantar fascia and Achilles tendon. Relapses and remissions may occur over a period of years. It may be precipitated by use and withdrawal from systemic corticosteroids (e.g., weeks after an IM injection).

◉ Look For

Von Zumbusch Type

Clusters of sterile, 2 to 3 mm pustules on a background of erythema. Pustules may become confluent, forming large plaques of pus (Fig. 4-393). Flexures and the anogenital area are most commonly affected, but the palms, soles, and oral mucosa may also be involved. Pustules may form on the nail matrix, with subsequent loss of the nail plate. Fingertips can show atrophy with long-standing disease. Only rarely do other forms of psoriasis coexist with lesions of von Zumbusch type.

Annular Type

Pustules at the periphery of erythematous, annular lesions; located most commonly on the trunk (Fig. 4-394). The lesions expand peripherally, with healing occurring in the center.

Exanthematic Type

Acute onset of small, sterile pustules without significant systemic symptoms. Believed to have clinical and histological overlap with acute generalized exanthematous pustulosis (AGEP).

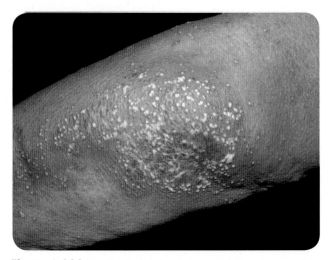

Figure 4-392 Small islands of pus in a slightly raised psoriatic plaque.

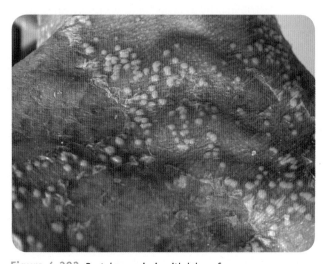

Figure 4-393 Pustular psoriasis with lakes of pus.

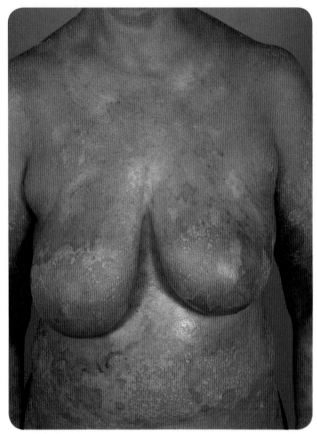

Figure 4-394 Psoriatic plaques with multiple pustules.

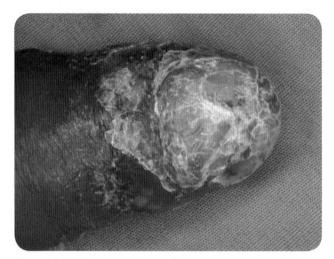

Figure 4-395 Pustular psoriasis on distal digit known as acrodermatitis continua.

Localized Types

- Pustulosis palmaris et plantaris—Palmar and/or plantar, 2 to 4 mm pustules, often located on the medial aspect of the foot and misdiagnosed as a bacterial or fungal infection.
- Acrodermatitis continua—Pustules on the fingertips and nail bed, often with subsequent nail dystrophy and loss (Fig. 4-395).

Dark Skin Considerations

Chronic subcorneal pustulosis with vasculitis is a rare variant of generalized pustular psoriasis described in black South Africans. Postinflammatory pigmentary changes can be quite prominent in darkly pigmented skin.

Diagnostic Pearls

- Spiking fevers and generalized discomfort may be suggestive of an alternative diagnosis, such as a systemic infectious disease. However, these patients often look ill and can be brought to the emergency room for evaluation.

- The annular type displays milder constitutional symptoms and is more common in infancy.

Immunocompromised Patient Considerations

- Associated plantar fasciitis and edema can lead to "AIDS gait," a type of limping gait where patients walk with feet inverted and extended to avoid pain.

?? Differential Diagnosis and Pitfalls

- AGEP—Clinically indistinguishable from pustular psoriasis. Time of onset and a drug history may help differentiate AGEP from pustular psoriasis. Antibiotics are the likely causative agents in AGEP. Histology can also help differentiate between the two. Also look for high fever, edema of the face, pustular eruption that occurs shortly after drug administration (<2 days), marked serum leukocytosis with neutrophilia, and associated petechiae, purpura, and vesicles in AGEP.
- Drug reaction with eosinophilia and systemic symptoms—Look for marked eosinophilia, visceral involvement (most commonly hepatitis), less acute onset, facial edema, and atypical lymphocytosis.
- Subcorneal pustular dermatosis (Sneddon-Wilkinson disease)—Associated with IgA paraproteinemia and is very responsive to dapsone. Pustular psoriasis is not responsive to dapsone and does not have an IgA paraproteinemia.
- Keratoderma blennorrhagicum seen in reactive arthritis disease—Look for characteristic associated findings including urethritis, arthritis, and ocular findings.

- Dyshidrotic eczema—Extremely pruritic, restricted to hands and feet, look for deep-seated vesicles that look like tapioca pudding.
- Erythema annulare centrifugum—To be considered when annular-type psoriasis is observed. No associated systemic findings. Individual lesions can last for months.
- Impetigo herpetiformis—Pustular psoriasis during pregnancy.
- Generalized herpes simplex

✓ Best Tests

- Skin punch biopsy for histology.
- Culture a pustule to rule out secondary bacterial super-infection.
- Some abnormalities that have been described include neutrophilia with WBC up to 30,000, absolute lymphopenia, elevated sedimentation rate, hypoalbuminemia, anemia, elevated transaminases, elevated alkaline phosphatase and bilirubin, and hypocalcemia. A decreased creatinine clearance has also been observed.

▲▲ Management Pearls

- Pustular psoriasis often responds dramatically and rapidly to systemic acitretin. Systemic corticosteroids (40 to 60 mg per day of prednisone of intravenous Solu-Medrol) *should be avoided* unless they are being used in the acute toxic phase to allow time for acitretin to take effect. In this case, a cautious, slow taper should be performed. Spontaneous resolution without therapy has also been described.
- Patients with severe, generalized disease (i.e., erythroderma) will often require hospital admission to ensure adequate hydration, nutrition, and temperature regulation.
- Consult a dermatologist. Other specialty consultations may be needed depending on the extent of systemic involvement or the occurrence of complications.

Therapy

Remove any precipitating causes and institute the proper supportive measures as dictated by disease severity (e.g., IV fluids, warming blankets for excessive heat loss, and bed rest). Bland emollients, compresses, and saline or colloidal oatmeal baths may be soothing. Monitor for and promptly treat any complicating infections.

Topical corticosteroids are often used, although the evidence to support their efficacy is poor.

First-line systemic medications include oral retinoids, methotrexate, cyclosporine, and certain biologics:

Retinoids
- Acitretin 25 to 50 mg p.o. daily; stop medication after resolution of pustules
- Isotretinoin 1 mg/kg p.o. daily

Antimetabolites
- Methotrexate 10 to 25 mg p.o. weekly
- Cyclosporine 2.5 to 5 mg/kg/day p.o. divided twice daily

Biologics
Biologic therapies such as infliximab, etanercept, and alefacept have shown promise in some patients. Currently, no guidelines exist for their use in pustular psoriasis, and infliximab has been reported to induce pustular psoriasis in case reports.

Phototherapy
Oral psoralen plus UVA (PUVA) is a viable treatment alternative if the patient can tolerate it, usually after first being stabilized with acitretin therapy. For example, acitretin is administered first at 25 to 50 mg for 1 week, then PUVA is performed three times per week. Once the resolution of the lesions has been accomplished, acitretin can be discontinued and maintenance phototherapy with PUVA or narrowband UVB can be continued as needed.

Additional treatment considerations include topical calcipotriol (be sure to monitor serum calcium), hydroxyurea, mycophenolate mofetil, 6-thioguanine, azathioprine, and colchicine.

Suggested Readings

Farber EM, Nall L. Pustular psoriasis. *Cutis.* 1993 Jan;51(1):29–32.

Gudjonsson JE, Elder JT. Psoriasis. In: Fitzpatrick TB, Wolff K, eds. *Fitzpatrick's Dermatology in General Medicine.* 7th Ed. New York, NY: McGraw-Hill; 2008:169–193.

Lee CS, Koo J. A review of acitretin, a systemic retinoid for the treatment of psoriasis. *Expert Opin Pharmacother.* 2005 Aug;6(10):1725–1734.

Martínez-Morán C, Sanz-Muñoz C, Morales-Callaghan AM, et al. Pustular psoriasis induced by infliximab. *J Eur Acad Dermatol Venereol.* 2007 Nov;21(10):1424–1426.

Mössner R, Thaci D, Mohr J, et al. Manifestation of palmoplantar pustulosis during or after infliximab therapy for plaque-type psoriasis: Report on five cases. *Arch Dermatol Res.* 2008 Mar;300(3):101–105.

Ozawa A, Ohkido M, Haruki Y, et al. Treatments of generalized pustular psoriasis: A multicenter study in Japan. *J Dermatol.* 1999 Mar;26(3):141–149.

Routhouska SB, Sheth PB, Korman NJ. Long-term management of generalized pustular psoriasis with infliximab: case series. *J Cutan Med Surg.* 2008 Jul–Aug;12(4):184–188.

Umezawa Y, Ozawa A, Kawasima T, et al. Therapeutic guidelines for the treatment of generalized pustular psoriasis (GPP) based on a proposed classification of disease severity. *Arch Dermatol Res.* 2003 Apr;295(Suppl. 1): S43–S54.

Diagnosis Synopsis

Palmoplantar pustulosis is a chronic eruption of the palms and soles composed of sterile vesicles and pustules. It is symmetric in distribution, often accompanied by painful fissuring, and is most commonly seen in women aged between 40 and 60. It often resolves spontaneously, and systemic symptoms are usually absent. The pathogenesis is not well understood. It is primarily a diagnosis of exclusion when the clinical exam does not suggest the diagnosis of dermatitis or psoriasis. Risk factors include focal infection, stress, and smoking. Only a minority of patients demonstrate classic plaque psoriasis elsewhere. Associated diseases include thyroid disease, sterile inflammatory bone lesions (part of the SAPHO syndrome: synovitis, acne, pustulosis, hyperostosis, and osteitis), psoriasis, and diabetes mellitus.

Look For

Deep-seated vesicles, pustules, and papules on the palms, often with surrounding erythema and scale (Figs. 4-396–4-399). There are often yellow-brown macules with the pustules.

Diagnostic Pearls

- Look for subtle signs of psoriasis, such as nail pitting or scale on the scalp, umbilicus, or gluteal cleft.
- Look for other manifestations of SAPHO syndrome (synovitis, acne, pustulosis, hyperostosis, and osteitis).

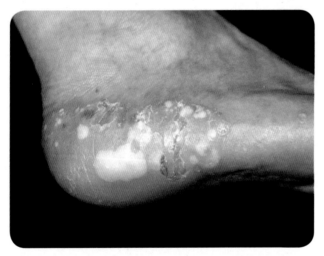

Figure 4-396 Large pustules in a red plaque.

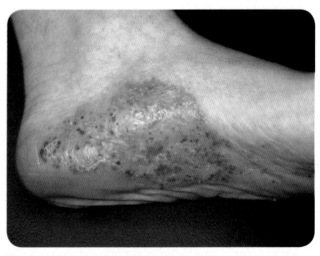

Figure 4-397 Red plantar plaque with vesicles.

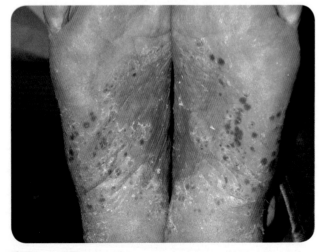

Figure 4-398 Symmetrical plantar plaques with crusts and deep pustules presenting as deep brown papules.

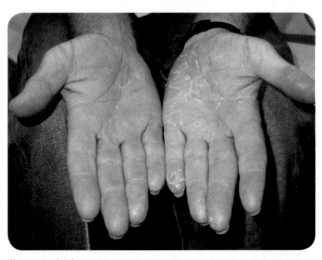

Figure 4-399 Annular scaling on the palmar surface in a late stage of palmoplantar pustulosis.

?? Differential Diagnosis and Pitfalls

- Pustular psoriasis—Widespread distribution, not restricted to palms and soles, acute eruption of sterile pustules resolving within days.
- Dyshidrotic eczema—Deep-seated vesicles of the palms, intensely pruritic.
- Tinea pedis or manus—Pruritic, erythematous, and scaly; KOH+.
- Infected atopic dermatitis—Perform culture when in doubt; atopic dermatitis will not be restricted to palms and soles; patient usually carries history of the diagnosis.
- Scabies—Look for burrows in the web spaces of the fingers; intensely pruritic; not restricted to palms and soles.

✓ Best Tests

- This is normally a clinical diagnosis of exclusion. KOH and fungal culture will exclude difficult-to-diagnose fungus. Consider thyroid function and glucose tolerance testing. Screen for arthropathy.

▲▲ Management Pearls

- Educate the patient about realistic expectations, and explain that this disease can be particularly difficult to treat.
- Advise smoking cessation in all patients who smoke.

Therapy

For mild cases, high-potency topical steroids under occlusion can be tried first.

High-potency Topical Corticosteroids (class 1 or 2)

- Fluocinonide cream, ointment—apply twice daily (15, 30, 60, 120 g)

- Desoximetasone cream, ointment—apply twice daily (15, 60, 120 g)
- Halcinonide cream, ointment—apply twice daily (15, 60, 240 g)
- Clobetasol cream, ointment—apply twice daily

For severe or recalcitrant cases, systemic retinoids, tetracycline, and PUVA are the treatments of choice:

- Acitretin—0.5 mg/kg p.o. daily or 25 mg p.o. daily
- Isotretinoin—40 to 80 mg p.o. daily
- Methotrexate—2.5 to 20 mg p.o. weekly
- Tetracycline—250 mg p.o. twice daily
- Topical hand and foot PUVA (Oxsoralen 10 to 40 mg p.o. daily)—two to three times a week

Cyclosporine (2.5 to 5 mg/kg/day) is considered second-line therapy due to its significant side effect profile.

Suggested Readings

Eriksson MO, Hagforsen E, Lundin IP, et al. Palmoplantar pustulosis: A clinical and immunohistological study. *Br J Dermatol*. 1998 Mar;138(3): 390–398.

Erkko P, Granlund H, Remitz A, et al. Double-blind placebo-controlled study of long-term low-dose cyclosporin in the treatment of palmoplantar pustulosis. *Br J Dermatol*. 1998 Dec;139(6):997–1004.

Ettler K, Richards B. Acitretin therapy for palmoplantar pustulosis combined with UVA and topical 8-MOP. *Int J Dermatol*. 2001 Aug;40(8):541–542.

Giménez-García R, Sánchez-Ramón S, Cuellar-Olmedo LA. Palmoplantar pustulosis: A clinicoepidemiological study. The relationship between tobacco use and thyroid function. *J Eur Acad Dermatol Venereol*. 2003 May;17(3):276–279.

Marsland AM, Chalmers RJ, Hollis S, et al. Interventions for chronic palmoplantar pustulosis. *Cochrane Database Syst Rev*. 2006 Jan;(1): CD001433.

Michaëlsson G, Gustafsson K, Hagforsen E. The psoriasis variant palmoplantar pustulosis can be improved after cessation of smoking. *J Am Acad Dermatol*. 2006 Apr;54(4):737–738.

Whittam LR, Wakelin SH, Barker JN. Generalized pustular psoriasis or drug-induced toxic pustuloderma? The use of patch testing. *Clin Exp Dermatol*. 2000 Mar;25(2):122–124.

Scabies

◼◼ Diagnosis Synopsis

Scabies is a parasitic infestation resulting when the mite, *Sarcoptes scabiei var. hominis*, burrows into and just below the stratum corneum in the epidermis (Fig. 4-400). It is transmitted most often via direct person-to-person contact and less frequently by fomites. Human scabies is extremely contagious, spreading between individuals who share close contact or living spaces. Prevalence rates are higher in children, residents of long-term care facilities, and sexually active persons, although scabies can appear in individuals of all ages, ethnicities, and socioeconomic groups. Factors that contribute to the persistence and spread of scabies are overcrowding, delays in diagnosis, and poor public health awareness. Outbreaks in health care facilities, such as nursing homes, can result in dozens of patients and staff becoming infected.

A typical infestation has 10 to 20 mites, but most patients mount an intense hypersensitivity reaction resulting in a widespread and intensely pruritic skin eruption. The hypersensitivity reaction usually develops 2 to 6 weeks after becoming colonized. The condition persists without medical treatment because the mite lays eggs that cause continued infestation. Canine scabies can be spread from dogs to humans but not between humans. Scabies can cause a generalized eruption resembling erythroderma in the elderly, the institutionalized, and patients with immunosuppression or neurologic dysfunction (so-called Norwegian scabies or, more appropriately, crusted scabies). In these patients, the mite burden is much higher, with thousands to millions of mites present on affected skin.

Immunocompromised Patient Considerations

Infestations in the immunocompromised patient are more common and more pronounced.

Scabies can cause a generalized eruption mimicking erythroderma in the elderly and the immunosuppressed. Crusted scabies is seen more frequently in patients with HIV and AIDS, with risk increasing as CD4 count decreases. Crusted scabies may be the presenting sign of HTLV infection. Patients with sensory nerve dysfunction, such as paraplegics and those with leprosy, are also at higher risk. Crusted scabies frequently presents with thick, scaly plaques and little pruritus despite high mite burden.

◉ Look For

The telltale diagnostic sign is the burrow. The burrow of the female scabies mite is a fine, thread-like, serpiginous line with a terminal tiny (smaller than a pin head), black speck representing the mite itself (Fig. 4-401). The burrow, along with small erythematous papules and vesicles, is seen mostly on the flexor wrists, elbows, and areolae, in the interdigital web spaces, axillae, and umbilicus, along the lower abdomen, and in the genital and buttocks regions. Scabies classically spares the head and neck areas. Note, however, that in many infested patients, obvious burrows may not be identified.

Secondary lesions are due to scratching and include excoriations, impetiginized lesions with crusts, and prurigo-like nodules.

Crusted scabies, as the name implies, consists of scaling and crusting of the skin, with ill-defined, widespread areas of erythema. Any site can be involved, but the most common are the arms and hands. Patients may present with generalized erythema and scaling. Nail dystrophy may be present, and the head and neck may be involved.

In adults, pruritic lesions on the areola in women and the penis and scrotum in men are highly suggestive of scabies (Fig. 4-402).

Immunocompromised Patient Considerations

Immunocompromised patients are much more likely to develop crusted scabies with diffuse redness and scaling. Individual burrows may not be visible in these patients, but the scales and crusts are typically teeming with mites (Fig. 4-403).

◉◉ Diagnostic Pearls

- Look closely for the burrow; mites are almost never found by scraping papules or excoriated lesions. The tiny black dot present at the edge of an intact linear papule represents a mite. Look for and/or inquire about lesions and symptoms in family members and caretakers.

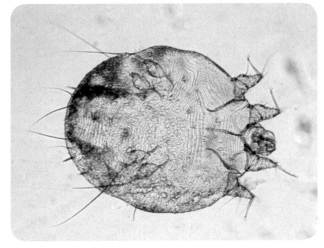

Figure 4-400 Adult scabies mite.

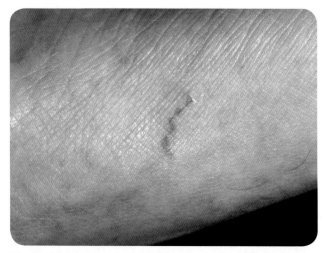

Figure 4-401 When seen, scabetic burrows can be scraped to reveal organisms and establish the diagnosis.

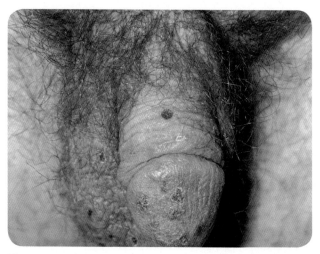

Figure 4-402 Penile crusts and erosions are very suggestive of scabies.

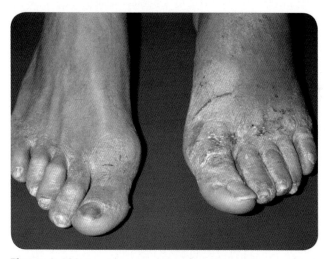

Figure 4-403 Immunosuppressed patients of any cause may have hyperkeratotic scabetic lesions teaming with organisms.

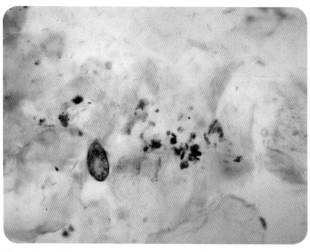

Figure 4-404 A scraping with scabies eggs and feces establishes the diagnosis.

- Pruritus tends to be more intense at night and when the patient is warm.
- A negative scabies prep does not rule out this diagnosis; mites can be infrequent and difficult to isolate in patients with normal immune function.

Immunocompromised Patient Considerations

- The diagnosis of scabies is often elusive in immunocompromised patients, and a high index of suspicion should be present for patients with immune suppression and pruritus without an obvious cause. Patients may present having seen multiple other physicians and many prior failed therapies if scabies has not been suspected.

?? Differential Diagnosis and Pitfalls

- Insect bites
- Papular urticaria
- Canine scabies—This mite can transiently infect humans but does not have the classical distribution of human scabies and cannot subsequently be passed from person to person.
- Atopic dermatitis
- Nummular eczema
- Folliculitis
- Impetigo
- Bedbug bites
- Varicella
- Contact dermatitis
- Dermatitis herpetiformis

- Seabather's eruption
- Dyshidrotic dermatitis
- Lichen planus
- Id reaction
- Neurotic excoriations
- Prurigo nodularis
- Acropustulosis of infancy
- Bullous pemphigoid—urticarial phase

Immunocompromised Patient Differential Diagnosis

- Condyloma acuminatum
- Molluscum contagiosum
- Bowenoid papulosis
- Allergic contact dermatitis
- Psoriasis
- Seborrheic dermatitis
- Exfoliative erythroderma due to another cause
- Secondary syphilis must be ruled out if a genital scabetic nodule is found

✓ Best Tests

- Perform a scabies prep. Put a small amount of mineral oil on the skin area to be tested, and take a no. 15 blade and gently remove the terminal end of the burrow where you see the tiny black speck. Apply this scraping to a glass slide, cover with oil and a cover slip, and examine under the microscope for the presence of the mite or its ova or fecal pellets, known as scybala (Fig. 4-404).
- Burrows may be more easily identified by covering a suspected burrow with the ink from a fountain or marking pen, then wipe away with an alcohol pad after a minute or two. The ink will penetrate the burrow, making it more visible.
- In cases of crusted scabies, add a few drops of 10% potassium hydroxide (KOH) solution to the skin scraping to break down the excess keratin. Scales will typically contain many mites.

▲▲ Management Pearls

- Treat the entire family and all close contacts. Close contacts may be infected but not yet symptomatic and will, therefore, be unaware of the infection. If untreated, such individuals will pass the mite back to others.
- Patients should be instructed to launder bed linens, towels, and clothing used in the last 72 h prior to treatment in hot water and dry on high heat. Items that cannot be laundered can be sealed in airtight plastic bags for 10 to

14 days. All carpets and upholstered furniture should be thoroughly vacuumed and the vacuum bags or canisters disposed of. It is important that such control measures coincide with the pharmacologic treatment of household members.
- Make sure to tell the patient that lesions can take a week or more to clear as the immune reaction will continue despite killing the mite with the treatment. Itching may persist for up to 4 weeks despite the complete eradication of live mites.
- Lesions may become secondarily infected with *Staphylococcus aureus*.
- Scabies is very difficult to eradicate from hospital settings once an outbreak has occurred. A prompt identification of affected patients and appropriate isolation is essential. Hospital infection control teams should be involved at the outset of case identification to help control spread.

Precautions: Standard and Contact (Isolate patient, wear gloves and a gown, limit patient transport, and avoid sharing patient-care equipment.)

Immunocompromised Patient Considerations

- Patients who have uncomplicated scabies and also are infected with HIV should receive the same treatment regimens as those who are HIV negative. HIV-infected patients and others who are immunosuppressed are at increased risk for crusted scabies. Ivermectin has been reported to be useful in small, noncontrolled studies and may be used in conjunction with topical therapy. Such patients should be managed in consultation with a specialist.

Therapy

CDC-Recommended Regimens
Permethrin cream (5%) applied to all areas of the body from the neck down and washed off after 8 to 14 h. The treatment is repeated again a week later.

OR

Ivermectin 200 µg/kg p.o. once. Repeat in 1 to 2 weeks.

Note that resistance to topical permethrin appears to be on the rise.

CDC-Recommended Alternative Regimen

Lindane (1%)—1 oz of lotion or 30 g of cream applied in a thin layer to all areas of the body from the neck down and thoroughly washed off after 8 h. Lindane is not recommended as first-line therapy because of toxicity. It should only be used as an alternative if the patient cannot tolerate other therapies or if other therapies have failed.

Lindane should not be used immediately after a bath or shower, and it should not be used by persons who have extensive dermatitis, women who are pregnant or lactating, or children aged younger than 2 years. Lindane resistance has been reported in some areas of the world, including parts of the United States. Seizures have occurred when lindane was applied after a bath or used by patients who had extensive dermatitis. Aplastic anemia after lindane use has also been reported.

Permethrin is effective and safe, and it is less expensive than ivermectin. One study demonstrated increased mortality among elderly, debilitated persons who received ivermectin, but this observation has not been confirmed in subsequent reports.

For patients with crusted scabies, an attempt should be made to remove as much of the crusted scale as possible prior to initiating therapy with a topical agent. Mechanical debridement can be facilitated with warm soaks followed by the application of a keratolytic agent (e.g., Lac-Hydrin cream). Such patients may require repeated applications of a topical antiscabietic.

Antihistamines for pruritus is an important adjunctive treatment:

- Diphenhydramine hydrochloride (25 and 50 mg tablets or capsules): 25 to 50 mg nightly or every 6 h as needed
- Hydroxyzine (10, 25 mg tablets): 10 to 25 mg every 6 h as needed
- Cetirizine hydrochloride (5 and 10 mg tablets): 5 to 10 mg per day
- Loratadine (10 mg tablets): 10 mg tablet once daily

Consider a short course of topical corticosteroids for patients in whom the reaction is severe. Intralesional corticosteroids have been used in the treatment of scabetic nodules.

Immunocompromised Patient Considerations
CDC-Recommended Regimen

- Permethrin cream (5%) applied to all areas of the body from the neck down and washed off after 8 to 14 h

And/or

- Ivermectin 200 µg/kg orally, repeated in 2 weeks

In infants and the elderly, topical permethrin should be applied from head to toe as the head and neck may be involved.

Suggested Readings

Centers for Disease Control and Prevention, Workowski KA, Berman SM. Sexually transmitted diseases treatment guidelines, 2006. *MMWR Recomm Rep.* 2006 Aug;55(RR-11):1–94.

Chosidow O. Clinical practices. Scabies. *N Engl J Med.* 2006 Apr; 354(16):1718–1727.

Chouela E, Abeldaño A, Pellerano G, et al. Diagnosis and treatment of scabies: a practical guide. *Am J Clin Dermatol.* 2002;3(1):9–18.

Hengge UR, Currie BJ, Jäger G, et al. Scabies: A ubiquitous neglected skin disease. *Lancet Infect Dis.* 2006 Dec;6(12):769–779.

Johnston G, Sladden M. Scabies: Diagnosis and treatment. *BMJ.* 2005 Sep;331(7517):619–622.

Meinking DL, Burkhart CN, Burkhart CG, et al. Infestations. In: Bolognia J, Jorizzo JL, Rapini RP, eds. *Dermatology.* 2nd Ed. St. Louis, MO: Mosby; 2008:1291–1295.

Scheinfeld N. Controlling scabies in institutional settings: A review of medications, treatment models, and implementation. *Am J Clin Dermatol.* 2004;5(1):31–37.

Stone SP, Goldfarb JN, Bacelieri RE. Scabies, other mites, and pediculosis. In: Fitzpatrick TB, Wolff K, eds. *Fitzpatrick's Dermatology in General Medicine.* 7th Ed. New York, NY: McGraw-Hill; 2008:2029–2037.

Usha V, Gopalakrishnan Nair TV. A comparative study of oral ivermectin and topical permethrin cream in the treatment of scabies. *J Am Acad Dermatol.* 2000 Feb;42(2 Pt 1):236–240.

Seabather's Eruption

Diagnosis Synopsis

Seabather's eruption is caused by envenomation and subsequent hypersensitivity to the larval form of marine coelenterates encountered in seawater. Larva of the thimble jellyfish, *Linuche unguiculata,* is the cause of eruptions in the Atlantic Ocean off the coastline of Florida, Mexico, and the Caribbean. The adult size is 5 to 20 mm (up to 3/4 in.), and the larval form is only 0.5 mm. Most cases occur between March and August. Off the coast of Long Island, NY, sea anemone larvae of *Edwardsiella lineata* have also been identified as causal.

Envenomation occurs when the larvae get caught beneath swimwear and stinging cells (nematocysts) discharge into the skin. The mechanical pressure of swimwear is hypothesized to, in part, trigger the firing of these cysts. Within a few hours, bathers develop a burning, itchy, papular eruption predominately in the area beneath the swimwear. The rash may blister and desquamate, and it can last up to 10 days. The itching can last 1 to 2 weeks. With ocular exposure, conjunctivitis may develop.

Systemic symptoms, more commonly seen in children and adolescents, include fever, malaise, headache, nausea, vomiting, diarrhea, and abdominal pain. No deaths have been reported.

Systemic hypersensitivity reactions, including anaphylaxis, are rare in jellyfish envenomations.

Look For

Look for a pruritic, papular rash found predominantly underneath swimwear (Figs. 4-405–4-408). This is in contrast to swimmer's itch, which typically appears at exposed skin sites after bathing in fresh water. Wheals or vesicles may also be present in seabather's eruption.

Diagnostic Pearls

- If jellyfish identification is necessary, nematocysts imbedded in the skin can be removed with sticky tape (or by scraping the skin), preserved, and sent for identification.

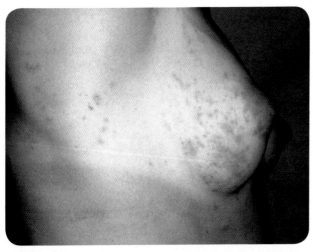

Figure 4-405 Typically, seabather's eruption papules and vesicles occur in locations covered by a bathing suit.

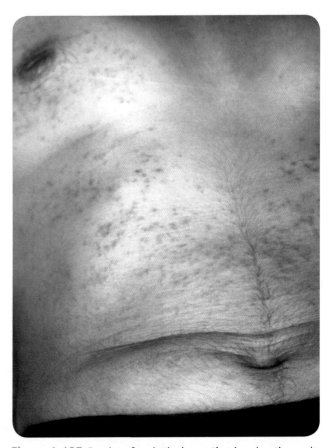

Figure 4-407 Papules of seabather's eruption in a location under a bathing suit.

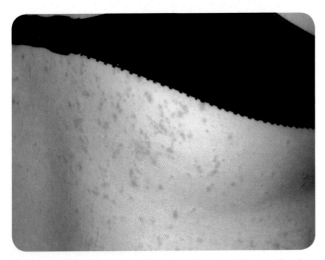

Figure 4-406 Scattered red papules of seabather's eruption in a location covered by a bathing suit.

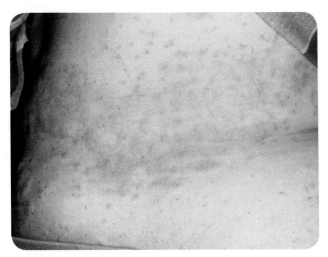

Figure 4-408 Seabather's eruption papules.

?? Differential Diagnosis and Pitfalls

- Contact dermatitis
- Folliculitis, especially *Pseudomonas*
- Insect bites
- Urticaria
- Swimmer's itch

✓ Best Tests

No specific tests are necessary as seabather's eruption is self-limited and treatment is tailored toward symptoms.

▲▲ Management Pearls

- Tell the victim to wash swimwear because remaining nematocysts can cause a recurrence next time it is worn. The bathing suit should be washed with soap and water and then dried with heat rather than air-dried.
- Patients with previous eruptions should shower—without swimwear—immediately after swimming in seawater to prevent recurrent outbreaks.

Therapy

Treatment for seabather's eruption is symptomatic. Options include soothing emollients such as calamine or camphor-menthol lotions and colloidal baths (oatmeal, etc.). Topical steroids (hydrocortisone or triamcinolone) as well as antihistamines are also effective. In cases of severe eruptions, with or without systemic symptoms, short courses of systemic corticosteroids have also been used.

Suggested Readings

Daly AS, Scharf MJ. Bites and stings of terrestrial and aquatic life. In: Fitzpatrick TB, Wolff K, eds. *Fitzpatrick's Dermatology in General Medicine*. 7th Ed. New York, NY: McGraw-Hill; 2008:2049.

Elston DM. Bites and stings. In: Bolognia J, Jorizzo JL, Rapini RP, eds. *Dermatology*. 2nd Ed. St. Louis, MO: Mosby; 2008:1316–1318.

Freudenthal AR, Joseph PR. Seabather's eruption. *N Engl J Med*. 1993 Aug;329(8):542–544.

Khachemoune A, Yalamanchili R, Rodriguez C. What is your diagnosis? Diagnosis: Seabather's eruption. *Cutis*. 2006 Mar;77(3):148, 151–152.

MacSween RM, Williams HC. Seabather's eruption—a case of Caribbean itch. *BMJ*. 1996 Apr;312(7036):957–958.

Tomchik RS, Russell MT, Szmant AM, et al. Clinical perspectives on seabather's eruption, also known as 'sea lice'. *JAMA*. 1993 Apr;269(13):1669–1672.

Wong DE, Meinking TL, Rosen LB, et al. Seabather's eruption. Clinical, histologic, and immunologic features. *J Am Acad Dermatol*. 1994 Mar;30(3):399–406.

Seborrheic Keratosis

◼◼ Diagnosis Synopsis

Seborrheic keratoses (SKs) are exceedingly common benign thickenings of the epidermis that typically appear on the chest and the back. There can be few or hundreds of these raised, "stuck-on"-appearing papules and plaques with well-defined borders. The etiology is unknown, although there is a familial trait for the development of multiple SKs with an autosomal dominant mode of inheritance. SKs are noninflammatory (unless traumatized) and typically arise slowly over time. They may be pruritic. In these cases, the patient may scratch or rub the lesions, causing redness, bleeding, or secondary infection to develop. The lesions tend to increase in incidence and number with increasing age.

Relatively rapid onset of numerous SKs can be a cutaneous sign of internal malignancy. Multiple eruptive SKs in association with a visceral cancer are referred to as the sign of Leser-Trélat. The most common associated malignancy is adenocarcinoma of the gastrointestinal tract.

◉ Look For

Pink, skin-colored, yellow-brown to brownish-black; waxy; "stuck-on"-appearing papules (Figs. 4-409–4-411). Pigmentation may be variable within a single lesion. Scratching the surface usually shows a scaling, rough appearance. The surface may appear verrucous (Fig. 4-412). Lesions are usually well circumscribed. They may occur on any body site, save for the palms, soles, and mucous membranes.

A clinical variant of the typical SK is a type of "skin tag." Distinct from a smooth skin tag, or acrochordon, these pedunculated 1 to 2 mm, furrowed, rough-surfaced polyps appear most commonly around the neck or in the axillae and show a surface morphology similar to that of the classic SK.

Dark Skin Considerations

Dermatosis papulosa nigra are often considered a variant and are most often seen as dark brown, 1 to 3 mm, hyperkeratotic papules on the faces of blacks. The lesions do not appear until puberty and initially look like freckles. They become more numerous and larger with age.

⬤⬤ Diagnostic Pearls

- The growths have a coarse, waxy scale that can be removed to show a raw, moist base.
- Individual lesions grow rapidly and reach a static size without further next growth.
- Close examination with a magnifying device, such as a magnifying lens or an episcope, can show the plug-like structure that is the gross manifestation of the microscopic horn cyst.

?? Differential Diagnosis and Pitfalls

- Melanoma is always in the differential of pigmented solitary lesions.
- Lentigo maligna
- Warts
- Epidermodysplasia verruciformis

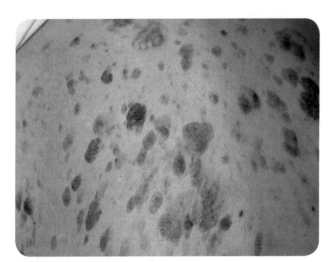

Figure 4-409 Multiple SKs are common, and may vary in size and in their degree of hyperpigmentation.

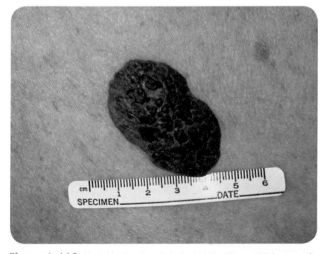

Figure 4-410 Very black seborrheic keratosis. The multiple smooth-surfaced papules (horn cysts) in the lesion are strong indications of the lesion being benign.

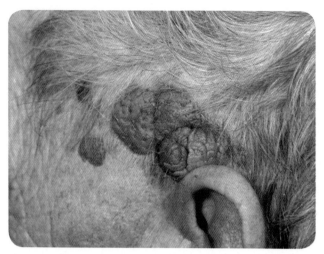

Figure 4-411 The even brown color and the uniform elevation make SKs more likely than lentigo maligna.

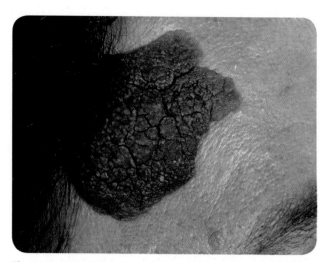

Figure 4-412 Very verrucous seborrheic keratosis sharply delimited from the surrounding skin. If present since childhood, epidermal nevus would be the likelier diagnosis.

- Epidermal nevus
- Pigmented basal cell carcinoma
- Melanocytic nevus
- Bowen disease
- Bowenoid papulosis
- Stucco keratosis
- Fibroepithelioma of Pinkus
- Acrokeratosis verruciformis of Hopf
- Cutaneous horn
- Arsenical keratosis
- Acrochordon
- Lentigo
- Nevus sebaceus

✓ Best Tests

- This diagnosis can usually be made clinically. If there is any concern for malignancy, however, the lesion must be excised and sent for histopathology.

▲▲▲ Management Pearls

- SKs are generally removed only for cosmetic reasons as the lesions have no malignant potential. Patient reassurance regarding the chronic and benign nature of these lesions is key.
- In patients with multiple SKs, a suspicious pigmented lesion may be overlooked. Also, multiple eruptive SKs should prompt a search for underlying internal malignancy, especially if the patient history or review of systems is suspicious for cancer.

Therapy

- Cryosurgery is the most common treatment method; however, this may leave an area of dyspigmentation.
- Curettage and cautery is another option.
- Chemical peels (i.e., trichloroacetic acid) have been used for small and superficial SKs.
- Laser therapy (pulsed CO_2 and ER:YAG) have demonstrated some efficacy.
- Shave excision can be used for larger lesions.

Suggested Readings

Braun RP, Rabinovitz H, Oliviero M, et al. Dermoscopic diagnosis of seborrheic keratosis. *Clin Dermatol.* 2002 May–Jun;20(3):270–272.

Herron MD, Bowen AR, Krueger GG. Seborrheic keratoses: A study comparing the standard cryosurgery with topical calcipotriene, topical tazarotene, and topical imiquimod. *Int J Dermatol.* 2004 Apr;43(4):300–302.

Pariser RJ. Benign neoplasms of the skin. *Med Clin North Am.* 1998 Nov;82(6):1285–1307, v–vi.

Sahin MT, Oztürkcan S, Ermertcan AT, et al. A comparison of dermoscopic features among lentigo senilis/initial seborrheic keratosis, seborrheic keratosis, lentigo maligna and lentigo maligna melanoma on the face. *J Dermatol.* 2004 Nov;31(11):884–889.

Schwartz RA. Sign of Leser-Trélat. *J Am Acad Dermatol.* 1996 Jul;35(1): 88–95.

Thomas I, Kihiczak NI, Rothenberg J, et al. Melanoma within the seborrheic keratosis. *Dermatol Surg.* 2004 Apr;30(4 Pt 1):559–561.

Thomas VD, Swanson NA, Lee KK. Benign epithelial tumors, hamartomas, and hyperplasias. In: Fitzpatrick TB, Wolff K, eds. *Fitzpatrick's Dermatology in General Medicine.* 7th Ed. New York, NY: McGraw-Hill; 2008: 1054–1056.

Syphilis, Secondary

▪▪ Diagnosis Synopsis

Syphilis is a sexually transmitted infection (STI) caused by the bacterium *Treponema pallidum* and is characterized by a chronic, intermittent, clinical course. It is transmitted from person to person via direct contact with a syphilis ulcer during vaginal, anal, or oral sex. Hence, the locations for syphilitic ulcers include the vagina, cervix, penis, anus, rectum, lips, and inside of the mouth. According to the Centers for Disease Control and Prevention (CDC), over 36,000 cases of syphilis were reported in the United States in 2006. Between 2005 and 2006, the number of primary and secondary syphilis cases increased by 11.8%. Sixty-four percent of syphilis cases were among men who have sex with men. An increased incidence of syphilis in the United States has been observed in black and Hispanic individuals, sex workers, individuals who sexually expose themselves to sex workers, and individuals with a history of other STIs and/or HIV.

The Natural History of Syphilis is as Follows

Primary Stage

- Primary lesion develops in 10 to 90 days (average of 3 weeks) after direct inoculation.
- Primary lesion is a painless, asymptomatic papule, followed by ulceration (chancre) and regional lymphadenopathy.
- Chancre lasts 3 to 6 weeks and heals spontaneously.
- All patients with primary syphilis will go on to develop secondary syphilis if left untreated.

Secondary Stage

- Characterized by hematogenous and lymphatic dissemination.
- Wide range of clinical manifestations but dominated by mucocutaneous and prodromal symptoms 3 to 10 weeks after the appearance of primary chancre.
- Cutaneous manifestations—Generalized nonpruritic papulosquamous eruption including the palms and soles, with pink to violaceous, scaly papules. Patchy alopecia of the scalp is also observed in secondary syphilis.
- Mucosal lesions—Ulcers, gray-colored plaques, and condyloma lata.
- Prodromal symptoms—Fever, weight loss, malaise, lymphadenopathy, myalgias, and sore throat.
- Mucocutaneous manifestations and prodromal symptoms last 3 to 12 weeks and resolve spontaneously.
- If left untreated, up to 25% of patients will relapse within the first 2 years.

Tertiary syphilis may appear months to years after secondary syphilis resolves and can involve the CNS, heart, bones, and skin.

Immunocompromised Patient Considerations

Genital ulcers caused by syphilis increase the risk of HIV transmission due to epithelial barrier compromise and increased numbers of macrophages and T-lymphocytes with HIV-specific receptors.

Note that HIV infection can alter the clinical presentation of syphilis. HIV-associated manifestations include multiple chancres, atypical cutaneous eruptions, increased severity of organ involvement (such as hepatitis and glomerulonephritis), and rapidly developing arteritis and neurosyphilis. Neurosyphilis can occur at any stage of syphilis.

◉ Look For

Wide range of clinical manifestations but dominated by mucocutaneous and prodromal symptoms 3 to 10 weeks after the appearance of primary chancre.

Cutaneous manifestations—Diffuse and generalized nonpruritic papulosquamous eruption including the palms and soles, with pink to violaceous, scaly papules. These can be followed by hyperpigmented, scaly macules on the palmar and plantar surfaces (Figs. 4-413–4-417).

Patchy alopecia with a "moth-eaten" appearance can be observed on the scalp.

Mucosal manifestations—Ulcers, gray-colored papules and plaques, and condyloma lata (wet-appearing, exophytic mucous-covered papules and plaques). Erythematous papules at the angles of the mouth with a central fissure.

Prodromal symptoms—Fever, weight loss, malaise, lymphadenopathy, myalgias, and sore throat.

Dark Skin Considerations

The most common presentation is hundreds of small superficial macules and papules (generalized). Macules typically occur in a symmetrical pattern on the face, shoulders, flanks, palms, soles, and genital regions.

While macules are more common in whites, blacks have a higher frequency of annular, follicular, papular, and pustular lesions. Annular plaques of secondary syphilis are more common in black patients and tend to be periorificial in distribution. Follicular lesions are also much more prevalent in black patients. Papular lesions in black patients tend to be hyperpigmented. Both papular and plaque lesions in black patients may have a pink or red color.

Palmoplantar lesions in blacks may be hyperkeratotic and may resolve with residual hyperpigmentation. They are often copper colored, especially in black patients. Truncal lesions may also leave hyperpigmented macules or, infrequently, lead to keloid formation.

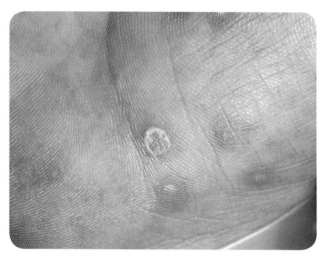

Figure 4-413 Secondary syphilis has nonvesicular, brown palmar papules that may have annular scaling.

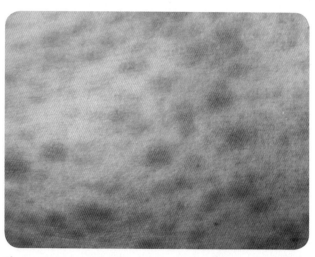

Figure 4-414 Papular, brown lesions of secondary syphilis on the trunk.

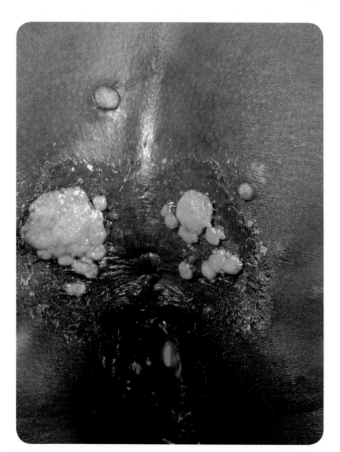

Figure 4-415 Genital lesions of secondary syphilis (condyloma lata).

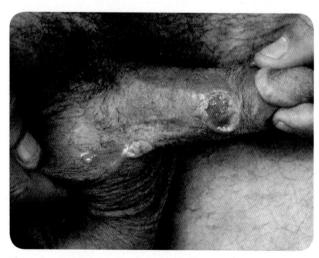

Figure 4-416 The lesions in chancroid are painful and more irregular than in syphilis.

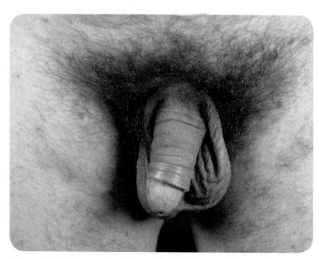

Figure 4-417 Red-brown papules on the penis, including the glans, and in the groin in secondary syphilis.

Diagnostic Pearls

Syphilis is considered "the great mimicker" and has evaded diagnosis on many occasions by many esteemed clinicians. The involvement of the palms and/or soles with macules and scaly papules should certainly raise suspicion for secondary syphilis. The presence of any one of the many signs of secondary syphilis should prompt serological testing in sexually active adults. Sir William Osler is quoted as saying, "The physician who knows syphilis knows medicine," and, "Syphilis is no respecter of age, sex, or station in life."

Immunocompromised Patient Considerations

In the immunocompromised patient, "the great mimicker" can present as more florid disease but can also be disguised as almost imperceptible disease. Multiple stages of disease can be present in the same patient (i.e., persistent primary chancre and the papulosquamous eruption of secondary syphilis).

?? Differential Diagnosis and Pitfalls

The following differential will be focused on the mucocutaneous findings of secondary syphilis.

Skin

- Lichen planus—Very pruritic, associated with hepatitis C, violaceous, scaly papules; consider tissue biopsy.
- Lichen amyloidosis—monomorphous papules
- Pityriasis rosea—Look for herald patch, collarette of scale, and orientation of lesions (fir-tree pattern in skin tension lines).
- Pityriasis rubra pilaris—Look for orange-red, waxy-like keratoderma of the palms and soles; consider tissue biopsy.
- Guttate psoriasis—Systemic signs absent, palms and soles are spared; biopsy will aid in diagnosis.
- Drug eruption—Cutaneous lesions of drug eruption tend to be different than those seen in syphilis. Drug eruptions often present with urticarial, exanthematous, or vesicular/bullous lesions. Eosinophilia on CBC and histology are often seen (but not an invariable finding). Look for nonsteroidal anti-inflammatory drugs (NSAIDs), sulfonamides, and penicillin medication history.
- Erythema multiforme—Characteristic target lesions (three concentric colors that are round and well demarcated) and occur more often on the extremities than on the trunk. Precipitating factors are infectious (herpes simplex virus, mycoplasma, etc.) and usually not medication related.
- Reactive arthritis (Reiter syndrome)

- Tinea—Check KOH.
- Scabies—Check for scabies mite in mineral oil.
- Sarcoidosis

Mucous Membrane

- Herpes simplex
- Aphthous ulcers
- Erythroplakia
- Erosions due to oral candidiasis
- Condyloma acuminata

Patchy Alopecia

- Alopecia areata
- Traction alopecia

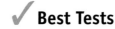 Best Tests

The diagnosis of syphilis includes the following strategies:

- Direct visualization of the bacteria via dark field microscopy
- Direct detection of the bacterial DNA via PCR
- Serologic antibody tests (nonspecific and treponemal specific)

Nontreponemal Tests (Detection of Antibodies to Cardiolipin)

- Venereal Disease Research Laboratory
- Rapid plasma reagin (RPR or STS)
- Titers correlate with disease activity, and, therefore, it is useful in screening and monitoring treatment
- False positives due to pregnancy, lupus erythematosus, lymphoma, antiphospholipid syndrome, cirrhosis, vaccinations, drug abuse, HIV, and other infectious diseases
- False negatives in HIV coinfected patients due to the "prozone effect," where an extremely high antibody titer must be diluted for the test to be positive. If clinical suspicion is high, dilute serum and retest.

Treponemal Specific Tests (To be Performed when Non-treponemal Test is Reactive)

- Microhemagglutination assay for *T. pallidum*
- Fluorescent treponemal antibody absorption test
- Not reactive in early primary syphilis
- Will remain positive forever, so not useful for monitoring response to treatment
- False positives in HIV infection, autoimmune diseases, and additional bacteria from treponeme and spirochete families

Note that an early primary lesion (<1 to 2 weeks) must be evaluated by dark-field examination or direct immunofluorescent microscopy of the spirochete (recall that primary lesion occurs *prior* to hematogenous dissemination, so serology will be negative early on).

Do not perform a dark-field examination on oral lesions because nonpathogenic spirochetes are present in normal oral flora.

▲▲ Management Pearls

- All patients diagnosed with syphilis should be screened for HIV infection and retested 3 months later if the first HIV test is negative.
- Patients with neurologic or ophthalmic symptoms should have CSF analysis and ocular slit lamp examination performed.
- It is not necessary to perform CSF analysis if the patient does not demonstrate neurologic symptoms.
- Pregnancy: Note that no alternative exists for penicillin. If the patient has a history of penicillin allergy, she should undergo desensitization.
- Management of sex partners: Persons exposed to an infected sexual partner within 90 days preceding the diagnosis of primary, secondary, or early latent syphilis may also be infected, irrespective of serologic results; such persons should be treated presumptively.

Therapy

Current CDC Guidelines
- Penicillin G, IM, or IV, for all stages of syphilis, remains the gold standard
- Type of preparation, dosage, and length of treatment depends on the stage and clinical manifestations

Primary and Secondary Syphilis
- Adults: Benzathine penicillin G 2.4 million units IM, single dose

Pregnancy
- Treatment during pregnancy is dictated by the penicillin schedule that is appropriate for the given stage of syphilis.
- Note that no alternative exists for penicillin. If the patient has a history of penicillin allergy, she should undergo desensitization.

Immunocompromised Patient Considerations

HIV-positive patients who contract early syphilis may be at an increased risk for neurologic complications and may have higher rates of treatment failure with currently recommended regimens. No treatment regimens for syphilis have been demonstrated to be more effective in preventing neurosyphilis in HIV-infected patients than the syphilis regimens recommended for HIV-negative patients. Careful follow-up post-therapy intervention is essential.

Suggested Readings

Angus J, Langan SM, Stanway A, et al. The many faces of secondary syphilis: A re-emergence of an old disease. *Clin Exp Dermatol.* 2006 Sep;31(5): 741–745.

Baughn RE, Musher DM. Secondary syphilitic lesions. *Clin Microbiol Rev.* 2005 Jan;18(1):205–216.

Bean WB. *Sir William Osler: Aphorisms from His Bedside Teachings and Writings.* Springfield, IL: Charles C. Thomas; 1968:133.

Centers for Disease Control and Prevention, Workowski KA, Berman SM. Sexually transmitted diseases treatment guidelines, 2006. *MMWR Recomm Rep.* 2006 Aug;55(RR-11):1–94.

David G, Perpoint T, Boibieux A, et al. Secondary pulmonary syphilis: Report of a likely case and literature review. *Clin Infect Dis.* 2006 Feb;42(3): e11–e15.

Domantay-Apostol GP, Handog EB, Gabriel MT. Syphilis: The international challenge of the great imitator. *Dermatol Clin.* 2008 Apr;26(2):191–202, v.

Dylewski J, Duong M. The rash of secondary syphilis. *CMAJ.* 2007 Jan; 176(1):33–35.

Lautenschlager S. Cutaneous manifestations of syphilis: Recognition and management. *Am J Clin Dermatol.* 2006;7(5):291–304.

Lee V, Kinghorn G. Syphilis: An update. *Clin Med.* 2008 Jun;8(3):330–333.

Osler W. *The Principles and Practice of Medicine.*7th Ed. New York, NY: D. Appleton; 1909:278.

Peterman TA, Furness BW. The resurgence of syphilis among men who have sex with men. *Curr Opin Infect Dis.* 2007 Feb;20(1):54–59.

Sanchez MR. Syphilis. In: Fitzpatrick TB, Wolff K, eds. *Fitzpatrick's Dermatology in General Medicine.* 7th Ed. New York, NY: McGraw-Hill; 2008:1955–1977.

Diagnosis Synopsis

Tinea Corporis

Tinea corporis, commonly known by the misnomer "ringworm," is an inflammatory or noninflammatory reaction to infection with dermatophyte fungi. The lesions usually take the form of annular, erythematous, scaly plaques. Fungal organisms of various causative species of the genera *Trichophyton, Microsporum,* or *Epidermophyton* are transmitted to humans by direct skin-to-skin contact with those infected (animals or humans, as in tinea corporis gladiatorum, common in wrestlers) or through fomites. Tinea corporis is more prevalent in warm, humid climates and may also occur as a result of the spread of infection from other body locations. See separate descriptions for discussions of tinea pedis (foot) and tinea cruris (groin). Majocchi granuloma, a variant deeper infection, is also discussed separately.

Tinea imbricata is a distinct form of tinea corporis caused by *Trichophyton concentricum*. It is more prevalent in tropical locales such as Central and South America, the South Pacific, and Southeast Asia.

Tinea incognito refers to an atypical presentation of tinea corporis or other tinea after a period of inadvertent treatment with topical corticosteroids.

Tinea Faciale

Tinea faciale, also known as tinea faciei, is a localized dermatophyte infection limited to the skin of the face. It may be called tinea barbae in males who shave. Common causative species include *T. tonsurans, M. canis, T. mentagrophytes,* and *T. rubrum*. The most common manifestation is that of pruritic, erythematous, annular, scaling plaques, most often on the cheeks, but the range of appearance is large, and the disease is often misdiagnosed for the lack of consideration. Tropical or humid climates are associated with more frequent and severe cases. Occasionally, tinea faciale may occur as the result of spread of a dermatophyte infection from another body location (e.g., the scalp).

Immunocompromised Patient Considerations

Tinea Corporis

In the immunocompromised patient, infection can be superficial or affect the dermis and perifollicular structures. When dermatophytes infect the follicle, deeper lesions appear, sometimes as nodules. Follicular infection is known as Majocchi granuloma. In the immunocompromised patient, infection can be quite similar to that in immunocompetent patients with superficial scaly plaques, pruritus, and lesions displaying the classic annular advancing, scaling border. However, infections without pruritus or "classic" features are also seen. Lesions can be quite extensive, covering multiple body zones in the immunocompromised patient. Sometimes they appear as noninflamed hyperkeratotic plaques that are microscopically loaded with fungi. Dermatophyte infections are frequently seen in untreated AIDS and solid organ transplant patients. Renal transplant patients are at even higher risk for tinea corporis. Some authors report the prevalence of dermatophytosis as similar in patients with HIV and healthy patients but that HIV patients may manifest more atypical, severe, and deep disease. Rare cases of death from dermatophytosis are reported in AIDS patients.

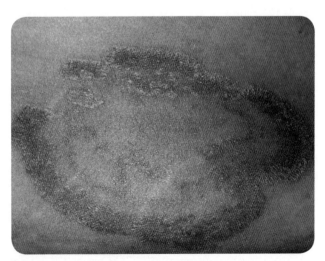

Figure 4-418 Complex polycyclic and arcuate papules and pustules are common in tinea corporis.

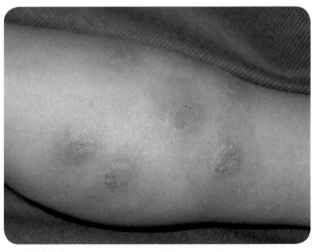

Figure 4-419 Tinea corporis lesions containing small vesicles; these frequently evolve into lesions with multiple annular scales.

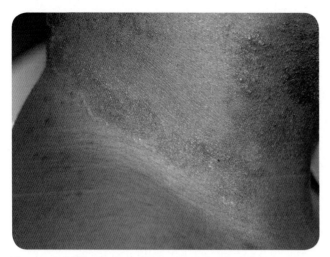

Figure 4-420 Hyperpigmentation is common in tinea corporis lesions in patients with darkly pigmented skin.

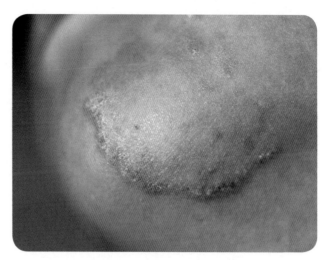

Figure 4-421 Polycyclic border characteristic of a dermatophyte infection on the face (tinea faciale).

Look For

Tinea Corporis

Annular, red, scaly plaques anywhere on the body. Plaques often have an active border, meaning that the advancing edge of the plaque has prominent scale with associated fungal hyphae. The central clearing of the elevated lesions leads to the appearance of the annular shape, and, thus, the description "ringworm." Papules, vesicles, and crusting may develop in the active border (Figs. 4-418–4-420).

Tinea imbricata consists of scaly plaques distinctly arranged in concentric rings, like the crosscut of a tree trunk.

Tinea incognito (lesions of tinea corporis inadvertently treated with topical corticosteroids) may present as patches or papules and plaques with less erythema and move subtle scale. Scattered pustules and hyperpigmentation may be present.

Tinea Faciale

On the face, tinea is most commonly seen on the cheeks but may also be located on the nose, the periocular region, the chin (Fig. 4-421), and the forehead. Lesions may look similar to those of tinea corporis but are prone to atypical appearances that frequently result in misdiagnosis. There may be single or multiple patches. Lesions may start as scaly papules that then develop a raised, advancing border with or without crusts, pustules, and vesicles. The central area may show pigmentary changes and less scale than the border.

Dark Skin Considerations

Tinea Corporis and Tinea Faciale
In blacks, erythema may be less conspicuous, but abundant scale may be more evident.

Immunocompromised Patient Considerations

Tinea Corporis
Plaques can cover large areas in the immunocompromised and can become deep within plaques. Dermal nodules; fluctuant, red nodules; and erosive lesions can be seen.

Diagnostic Pearls

Tinea Corporis

Dermatophytosis that has been treated with topical steroids can demonstrate the absence of redness and minimal scaling despite the lesion being loaded with fungi. If the skin scraping is negative in a lesion that has not been treated, the lesion is probably *not* fungal in etiology.

Tinea Faciale

Tinea faciale is most often misdiagnosed as seborrheic dermatitis or sebopsoriasis. Tinea barbae, a variant of tinea faciale that affects the beard area in men, is distinguished from bacterial folliculitis by the ease with which beard hairs are plucked (i.e., beard hair is plucked more easily in tinea barbae).

?? Differential Diagnosis and Pitfalls

Tinea Corporis

- Seborrheic dermatitis
- Psoriasis
- Parapsoriasis

- Candidiasis
- Erythrasma
- Impetigo
- Subacute cutaneous lupus erythematosus
- Tinea versicolor
- Granuloma annulare—typically no scale
- Mycosis fungoides
- Nummular dermatitis
- Secondary syphilis
- Pityriasis rosea
- Lyme disease
- Erythema annulare centrifugum
- Annular lichen planus
- Drug eruptions

Tinea Faciale

- Seborrheic dermatitis
- Atopic dermatitis
- Contact dermatitis
- Candidiasis
- Lupus erythematosus, discoid and subacute cutaneous
- Psoriasis
- Polymorphous light eruption and other photodermatoses
- Granuloma annulare
- Acne vulgaris
- Perioral dermatitis
- Rosacea
- Pityriasis alba
- Sarcoidosis
- Nummular dermatitis
- Secondary syphilis
- Pityriasis rosea
- Demodex folliculitis
- Pseudofolliculitis barbae
- Impetigo and other bacterial infections

 ## Best Tests

Tinea Corporis and Tinea Faciale

- Scrape the scaly, active border with a scalpel blade or the edge of a glass slide. Collect scale on a slide and cover with a cover slip. Direct a drop of 10% KOH (potassium hydroxide) solution to the edge of the coverslip. Under the microscope, observe for branching or curving fungal hyphae crossing cell borders.
- A fungal culture will allow species determination but takes several weeks.
- Certain species of dermatophyte (e.g., *M. canis*) will fluoresce under a Wood lamp.

▲▲ Management Pearls

Tinea Corporis

- Small, localized lesions can be treated topically. Extensive disease may require weeks of oral antifungal therapy.
- Topical agents should be applied at least 2 cm outside the border of the lesions and treatment continued for 1 week beyond the time of observed clinical resolution.

Tinea Faciale

- Small, localized lesions can be treated topically. Extensive disease or disease with concomitant tinea capitis will require treatment with oral antifungal agents.
- Infection in pets should be identified and treated, or reinfection is likely.

Therapy

Tinea Corporis and Tinea Faciale

Limited, localized disease should be treated topically. Allylamines (e.g., terbinafine and naftifine) and imidazoles (e.g., clotrimazole) are the mainstays of therapy. Allylamines may require shorter courses, but imidazoles are less expensive.

Use topical antifungals for 1 to 6 weeks, based on clinical response:

- Terbinafine 1% cream—apply once to twice daily
- Clotrimazole 1% cream—apply twice daily
- Econazole 1% cream—apply once to twice daily
- Oxiconazole 1% cream—apply twice daily
- Ciclopirox 0.77% cream, gel, or lotion—apply twice daily
- Ketoconazole 2% cream—apply once to twice daily
- Miconazole 2% cream—apply twice daily
- Naftifine 1% cream—apply once to twice daily
- Butenafine 1% cream—apply once to twice daily

Topical corticosteroids by themselves or in combination with antifungals are generally not indicated and are absolutely contraindicated in immunosuppressed patients. Combination steroid-antifungal therapy should not be used for tinea faciale. Use of corticosteroid-antifungal combinations in cases of diagnostic uncertainty may lead to persistent fungal infections and is not recommended.

Extensive disease, particularly when other body parts are involved, may require weeks of oral antifungal agents:

- Terbinafine 250 mg once a day for 2 to 4 weeks
- Itraconazole 100 to 200 mg twice a day for 1 week
- Fluconazole 150 to 300 mg once a week for 2 to 4 weeks
- Griseofulvin ultramicrosize 5 mg/kg/day for 4 to 8 weeks (generally reserved for severe cases)

Systemic antifungals are contraindicated in patients with liver disease; monitoring of liver enzymes is generally recommended. Drug interactions are frequent with systemic antifungals.

Mention is made here of tinea capitis, which affects hair and is much more common in children than in adults. Treatment is classically with griseofulvin or terbinafine.

Immunocompromised Patient Considerations

Localized disease may still be treated topically in immunocompromised patients.

Extensive disease may require longer courses of systemic antifungals than are used in immunocompetent patients. Drug interactions with antiretrovirals are rare in practice and nearly absent with oral terbinafine, which some regard as the drug of choice in patients with HIV/AIDS and extensive dermatophytoses.

Avoid topical corticosteroids in immunocompromised patients.

Suggested Readings

Adams BB. Tinea corporis gladiatorum. *J Am Acad Dermatol.* 2002 Aug;47(2):286–290.

Burkhart CN, Chang H, Gottwald L. Tinea corporis in human immunodeficiency virus-positive patients: case report and assessment of oral therapy. *Int J Dermatol.* 2003 Oct;42(10):839–843.

Cirillo-Hyland V, Humphreys T, Elenitsas R. Tinea faciei. *J Am Acad Dermatol.* 1993 Jul;29(1):119–120.

Drake LA, Dinehart SM, Farmer ER, et al. Guidelines of care for superficial mycotic infections of the skin: tinea corporis, tinea cruris, tinea faciei, tinea manuum, and tinea pedis. Guidelines/Outcomes Committee. American Academy of Dermatology. *J Am Acad Dermatol.* 1996 Feb;34(2 Pt 1):282–286.

Gupta AK, Chaudhry M, Elewski B. Tinea corporis, tinea cruris, tinea nigra, and piedra. *Dermatol Clin.* 2003 Jul;21(3):395–400, v.

Gupta AK, Cooper EA. Update in antifungal therapy of dermatophytosis. *Mycopathologia.* 2008 Nov–Dec;166(5–6):353–367.

Lebwohl M, Elewski B, Eisen D, et al. Efficacy and safety of terbinafine 1% solution in the treatment of interdigital tinea pedis and tinea corporis or tinea cruris. *Cutis.* 2001 Mar;67(3):261–266.

Lin RL, Szepietowski JC, Schwartz RA. Tinea faciei, an often deceptive facial eruption. *Int J Dermatol.* 2004 Jun;43(6):437–440.

Verma S, Heffernan MP. Superficial fungal infection: Dermatophytosis, onychomycosis, tinea nigra, piedra. In: Fitzpatrick TB, Wolff K, eds. *Fitzpatrick's Dermatology in General Medicine.* 7th Ed. New York, NY: McGraw-Hill; 2008:1814–1815.

Zinberg M, Werbitt RL, Lynfield YL. Recurrent fungal infection of the face: Diagnostic pitfalls. *Cutis.* 1984 Feb;33(2):180–182.

Diagnosis Synopsis

Tinea pedis (athlete's foot) is a localized inflammatory reaction to a fungal infection of the foot. The most common species of dermatophyte responsible are *Trichophyton rubrum*, *T. mentagrophytes*, and *Epidermophyton floccosum*. The condition causes dry scale on the feet, maceration between the toes and, in some cases, leads to the destruction of the nail plate (onychomycosis). Factors leading to this infection include high levels of humidity, occlusive footwear, and the use of communal pools or baths. Athletes are at increased risk. Tinea pedis may lead to a secondary (Gram-negative) bacterial infection, especially in diabetic patients. Tinea pedis is more common in men. There is no ethnic predilection, and prevalence of the condition increases with age.

Three patterns of foot involvement predominate: interdigital, moccasin, and vesiculobullous. More than one pattern may be present in a single patient.

Look For

Plaques on the dorsum of the foot may have an active border, meaning that the advancing edge of the plaque has prominent erythema and scale with associated fungal hyphae (Figs. 4-422–4-424). Plantar surfaces tend to have a powdery, white scale, sometimes in a "moccasin" distribution (i.e., the entire plantar foot and 2 to 3 cm surrounding the bottom). Web space involvement (the fourth web space is the most common) usually consists of white and macerated skin, and may represent a mixed infection with bacteria (Fig. 4-425). Fissuring may occur.

Bullous or vesiculobullous tinea pedis is an uncommon variant; in this form, tense vesicles appear on the soles due to the thick stratum corneum there. They may be gray, white, or brown in color.

Concomitant onychomycosis and/or tinea manuum (as in the two-foot-one-hand syndrome—named for two infected feet plus the dominant hand) may be present.

Diagnostic Pearls

- Dermatophytosis that has been treated with topical steroids can demonstrate the absence of redness and minimal scaling despite impressive fungal infection. If the skin scraping is negative in a lesion that has been treated with steroids, the lesion is probably *not* fungal in etiology.
- Use a Wood light to rule out toe web erythrasma by looking for a pink to red fluorescence.
- A dermatophytid reaction (also called the "id reaction") on the palms may occur in cases of bullous tinea pedis. This condition mimics dyshidrotic dermatitis in that both can demonstrate papules, vesicles, and, occasionally, pustules on the palms and lateral aspects of the fingers. The lesions on the hands do not contain fungi. The exact pathogenesis of this reaction is unknown, but it will clear with adequate treatment of the dermatophyte infection.

Differential Diagnosis and Pitfalls

- Web space erythrasma is typically hyperkeratotic but can be erosive.
- Bullous tinea pedis may be confused with friction blisters or autoimmune blistering disorders.
- Maceration with mixed bacteria
- Candidiasis
- Contact dermatitis

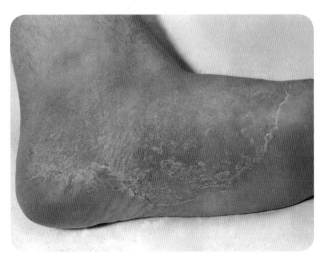

Figure 4-422 Red lesion with serpiginous scaling characteristic of tinea pedis.

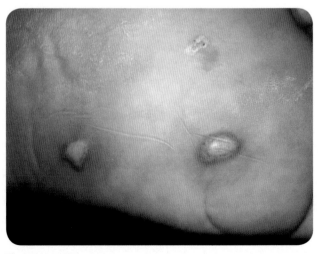

Figure 4-423 Dermatophyte infection may have vesicles or bullae with peripheral redness; the undersurface of the blister roof is loaded with fungi.

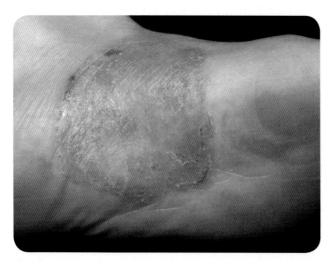

Figure 4-424 One presentation of tinea pedis includes inflammatory scaling plaques.

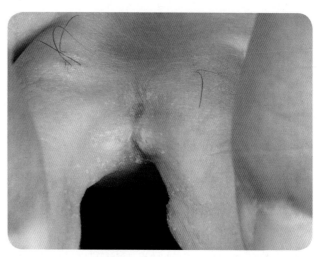

Figure 4-425 Interdigital scaling, redness, and painful fissures are common in tinea pedis.

- Psoriasis—Sometimes psoriasis may be limited to soles or may present in a palmoplantar distribution.
- Erythema multiforme
- Dyshidrotic dermatitis (also called dyshidrotic eczema or pompholyx)
- Pityriasis rubra pilaris
- Secondary syphilis
- Pitted keratolysis—A frequently overlooked condition that causes plantar pits and malodorous feet. Its cause is bacterial, and it responds to topical antibacterials such as clindamycin solution and aluminum chloride 20% solution for drying.

✓ Best Tests

- Scrape the scaly active border with a scalpel blade or the edge of a glass slide. If there are vesicles or bullae present, scrape the underside of the vesicle roof. Collect scale on a slide and cover with a coverslip. Direct a drop of 10% to 20% KOH (potassium hydroxide) solution to the edge of the coverslip. Under the microscope, observe for branching or curving fungal hyphae crossing cell borders.
- A fungal culture will allow species determination, but it will take several weeks.

▲▲ Management Pearls

- Small, localized lesions can be treated topically. Extensive disease may require oral antifungal agents.
- Encourage patients to wear protective footwear in communal bathing/swimming areas and to limit the use of highly occlusive footwear. Cotton socks are preferred, and these should be changed frequently when there is

excessive perspiration. Dry the feet and interdigital spaces completely before putting on clean socks.
- Old footwear can be a source of reinfection. It is advisable to treat potentially contaminated shoes with an antifungal powder (such as miconazole).
- Patients with severe interdigital maceration (also known as erosio interdigitalis blastomycetica) may benefit from the use of a topical astringent, such as aluminum acetate soaks, combined with topical antifungals and topical gentamicin cream to cover Gram-negative bacterial superinfections.

Therapy

Tinea pedis can often be treated with a topical antifungal cream. More extensive or complicated infections (bullous tinea pedis, tinea pedis with onychomycosis, infections in immunocompromised patients) may require systemic treatment.

Use Topical Antifungals for 1 to 6 weeks, Based on Clinical Response
- Terbinafine 1% cream—apply twice daily
- Clotrimazole 1% cream—apply twice daily
- Econazole 1% cream—apply twice daily
- Oxiconazole 1% cream—apply twice daily
- Ciclopirox 0.77% cream, gel, or lotion—apply twice daily
- Ketoconazole 2% cream—apply twice daily
- Miconazole 2% cream—apply twice daily
- Naftifine 1% cream—apply twice daily
- Butenafine 1% cream—apply twice daily

(Continued)

Note that treatments listed above are effective in the treatment of tinea pedis. Allylamines, such as terbinafine, naftifine, and butenafine, are more expensive than azoles, such as clotrimazole or miconazole, but they are less likely to result in treatment failure. Ciclopirox, miconazole, econazole, and naftifine have additional antibacterial activity and may be useful when bacterial superinfection is suspected. Topical corticosteroids are generally not indicated, though certain authors have suggested their concomitant use with antifungals when pruritus is intense. Patients with hyperkeratotic tinea pedis may benefit from a keratolytic agent such as salicylic acid or urea creams and lotions.

Regardless of the location of symptoms, topical antifungals should be applied in the web spaces and to the soles. To avoid recurrence, treatment should be continued for at least a week past the point of clinical clearing.

Extensive Disease or Disease Unresponsive to Topicals

- Terbinafine—250 mg daily for 2 weeks
- Itraconazole—100 to 200 mg daily for 2 to 4 weeks or 200 mg twice daily for 1 week
- Griseofulvin ultra-microsize 330 to 750 mg daily for 4 to 8 weeks
- Fluconazole—150 mg weekly for 2 to 4 weeks

Systemic antifungals are contraindicated in patients with liver disease and can cause liver failure and death, even in healthy patients. Monitoring of liver enzymes is recommended. Drug interactions are very common with systemic antifungals. If simultaneous treatment of onychomycosis is a goal, longer treatment courses than those listed here are required, but pulsed dosing of 1 week per month should be considered.

Suggested Readings

Crawford F. Athlete's foot. *Clin Evid.* 2005 Dec;(14):2000–2005.

Crawford F, Hollis S. Topical treatments for fungal infections of the skin and nails of the foot. *Cochrane Database Syst Rev.* 2007 Jul;(3):CD001434.

Drake LA, Dinehart SM, Farmer ER, et al. Guidelines of care for superficial mycotic infections of the skin: Tinea corporis, tinea cruris, tinea faciei, tinea manuum, and tinea pedis. Guidelines/Outcomes Committee. American Academy of Dermatology. *J Am Acad Dermatol.* 1996 Feb;34(2 Pt 1):282–286.

Field LA, Adams BB. Tinea pedis in athletes. *Int J Dermatol.* 2008 May;47(5):485–492.

Gupta AK, Cooper EA. Update in antifungal therapy of dermatophytosis. *Mycopathologia.* 2008 Nov–Dec;166(5–6):353–367.

Korting HC, Kiencke P, Nelles S, et al. Comparable efficacy and safety of various topical formulations of terbinafine in tinea pedis irrespective of the treatment regimen: Results of a meta-analysis. *Am J Clin Dermatol.* 2007;8(6):357–364.

Leyden JL. Tinea pedis pathophysiology and treatment. *J Am Acad Dermatol.* 1994 Sep;31(3 Pt 2):S31–S33.

Verma S, Heffernan MP. Superficial fungal infection: Dermatophytosis, onychomycosis, tinea nigra, piedra. In: Fitzpatrick TB, Wolff K, eds. *Fitzpatrick's Dermatology in General Medicine.* 7th Ed. New York, NY: McGraw-Hill; 2008:1815–1817.

Tinea Versicolor

▪▪ Diagnosis Synopsis

Tinea versicolor is also known as pityriasis versicolor. It is a superficial skin condition resulting from infection with yeast from the *Malassezia* genus—*M. globosa*, *M. sympodialis*, *M. furfur*, and possibly others. Clinically, the infection manifests as macules, papules, patches, and plaques with fine scale of varying pigmentation, primarily on the trunk. The distribution is worldwide, but the condition is most commonly found in tropical areas with high humidity and temperatures. Young adults and teenagers appear to be affected more frequently than older adults and young children in more temperate climates.

Risk factors other than high heat and humidity include oily skin, excessive sweating, pregnancy, poor nutrition, corticosteroid use, and some immunodeficiency states. Immunosuppression due to medications (as seen in transplant patients) is a known risk factor for tinea versicolor. Cyclosporine and azathioprine use have frequent associations with the condition. Patients with Cushing syndrome may have a higher incidence of tinea versicolor as well. This infection may be encountered in military personnel deployed in warm or tropical regions. Some patients may have a genetic predisposition to tinea versicolor and experience recurrent infections.

Because yeast normally dwells on the skin in minute amounts, the incubation period is unknown. The timeframe can range from weeks to months, and the disease typically begins during or just after the warmest months of the year. There are no associated systemic signs. Because this condition is so ubiquitous worldwide, it should be in the differential of any hypopigmented or hyperpigmented macules or patches on the body.

Immunocompromised Patient Considerations

Immunosuppression due to medications, as seen in transplant patients, is a risk factor for tinea versicolor. Patients with HIV/AIDS seem to be at equal risk as HIV-seronegative patients but may experience more extensive disease.

◉ Look For

Hyperpigmented or hypopigmented macules and patches or barely elevated papules/plaques, usually on the chest, back, and upper arms (Figs. 4-426–4-428). The macules may coalesce to form irregular patches. Most cases have a fine, dusty-appearing scale, but, in some cases, the scale may be so fine that it is imperceptible (Fig. 4-429).

Distinctly follicular forms may also occur. In *Pityrosporum* (prior genus name for *Malassezia*) folliculitis, lesions typically appear on the back, chest, and sometimes the extremities. Pruritus is more common with *Pityrosporum* folliculitis than with typical tinea versicolor. The primary lesion is a 2 to 3 mm perifollicular, erythematous papule or pustule. Only by appropriate culture and KOH examination can it be distinguished from a bacterial folliculitis.

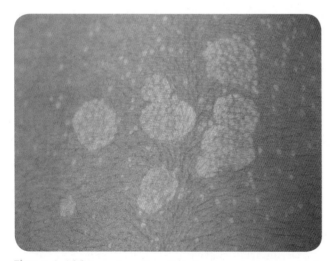

Figure 4-426 Large hypopigmented plaques and small papules in tinea versicolor.

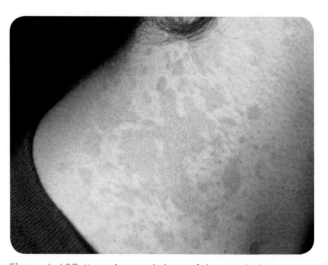

Figure 4-427 Hyperpigmented plaque of tinea versicolor.

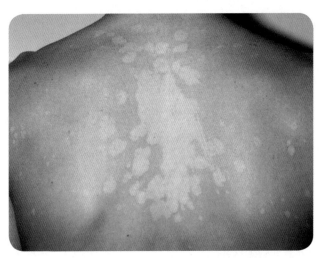

Figure 4-428 Typical location of a hypopigmented plaque of tinea versicolor.

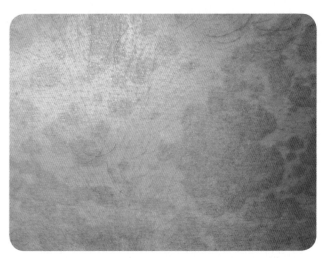

Figure 4-429 Red and slightly scaling plaques of tinea versicolor.

Dark Skin Considerations

Whereas tinea versicolor often presents as tan lesions in light-skinned patients, these are infrequent in black patients. Typical macules and patches in black patients are either hypopigmented or markedly hyperpigmented. Hypopigmented lesions are more prominent in the summer because sun exposure causes the patient's noninvolved skin to get darker while the tinea versicolor skin does not darken. Although these forms can also appear in fair-skinned patients, the findings are usually more prominent in black patients. Hyperpigmented lesions vary from gray to dark brown. The involvement of the face may be more common in black patients, especially in children.

Immunocompromised Patient Considerations

An inverse form with a different distribution (face, flexures, and extremities) is most often seen in immunocompromised patients.

Diagnostic Pearls

- Examination with a Wood lamp accentuates the pigmentary findings. This is especially important in those with very light skin pigmentation.
- Hyperpigmented or hypopigmented macules combined with a distribution of the upper trunk and neck is suggestive of tinea versicolor.

?? Differential Diagnosis and Pitfalls

- Confluent and reticulated papillomatosis of Gougerot and Carteaud presents with lesions in similar locations on the upper chest but has a negative skin scraping.
- Epidermodysplasia verruciformis may also mimic tinea versicolor but will not respond to antifungal therapies.
- Seborrheic dermatitis may mimic tinea versicolor, especially if there is involvement of the face.
- Erythema dyschromicum perstans
- Atopic dermatitis
- Pityriasis rosea
- Pityriasis alba
- Guttate psoriasis
- Nummular eczema
- Vitiligo
- Erythrasma
- Tinea corporis
- Patch stage mycosis fungoides
- Leprosy—only in patients living in endemic areas, not a consideration in travelers

✓ Best Tests

- Lightly scrape the scale within the skin lesions onto a glass slide and cover with a coverslip. Add a small drop of 10% KOH (potassium hydroxide) to the edge of the coverslip. The capillary action will be enough to wet the specimen. Examine under the microscope. Look for small hyphae and spores. Grape-like clusters of spores are often described as "meatballs," and the hyphae are described as having a "spaghetti" appearance.

▲ ▲ Management Pearls

- Tinea versicolor acquired in travel to tropical locales (or for those living in such places) can be difficult to treat. In these cases, oral therapy in combination with topical therapy may prove useful.
- Inform patients that skin color changes will typically resolve within 1 to 2 months of treatment (and sometimes much longer).
- The recurrence of tinea versicolor is very common, and most patients prone to it will require a preventive regimen in addition to a primary treatment regimen.
- Tinea versicolor is not contagious and is not due to poor hygiene.

Therapy

Systemic Treatment
- Ketoconazole 200 mg p.o. daily for 10 days or a single 400 mg dose
- Fluconazole 150 to 300 mg p.o. once weekly for 2 to 4 weeks or 300 mg p.o. repeated after 2 weeks
- Itraconazole 200 mg p.o. daily for 5 to 7 days

Oral ketoconazole and fluconazole have similar efficacy.

Topically, for Large Skin Areas
- Selenium sulfide 2.5% lotion—apply for 10 min daily for 7 days, repeat the same regimen in 1 month
- Pyrithione zinc 2% shampoo—apply for 10 min daily for 7 days, repeat the same regimen in 1 month
- Propylene glycol 50% in water—apply twice daily for 2 weeks
- Bifonazole 1% shampoo—apply daily for 3 weeks
- Ketoconazole 2% shampoo—apply daily to scalp and body for 5 to 10 min for 1 to 14 days

Topically, More Limited Areas
- Clotrimazole 1% cream—apply twice daily for 2 to 6 weeks
- Sulconazole 1% cream—apply daily for 2 weeks
- Econazole 1% cream—apply once to twice daily for 2 weeks
- Ketoconazole 2% cream—apply once to twice daily for 2 to 4 weeks
- Ciclopirox 0.77% cream or lotion—apply once or twice daily for 4 weeks

- Terbinafine 1% cream or solution—apply once or twice daily for 1 to 2 weeks

Prevention of Recurrence
- Selenium sulfide 2.5% lotion—apply first and third day of the month
- Ketoconazole 2% shampoo used lathered on scalp and body for 5 to 10 min once a week
- Ketoconazole 400 mg p.o. once a month
- Fluconazole 300 mg p.o. once a month
- Itraconazole 400 mg p.o. once a month

Note that the use of systemic antifungals carries a small risk of liver toxicity.

Suggested Readings

Borelli D, Jacobs PH, Nall L. Tinea versicolor: Epidemiologic, clinical, and therapeutic aspects. *J Am Acad Dermatol*. 1991 Aug;25(2 Pt 1):300–305.

Drake LA, Dinehart SM, Farmer ER, et al. Guidelines of care for superficial mycotic infections of the skin: Pityriasis (tinea) versicolor. Guidelines/Outcomes Committee. American Academy of Dermatology. *J Am Acad Dermatol*. 1996 Feb;34(2 Pt 1):287–289.

Farschian M, Yaghoobi R, Samadi K. Fluconazole versus ketoconazole in the treatment of tinea versicolor. *J Dermatolog Treat*. 2002 Jun;13(2):73–76.

Gupta AK, Ryder JE, Nicol K, et al. Superficial fungal infections: an update on pityriasis versicolor, seborrheic dermatitis, tinea capitis, and onychomycosis. *Clin Dermatol*. 2003 Sep–Oct;21(5):417–425.

Köse O, Bülent Taştan H, Riza Gür A, et al. Comparison of a single 400 mg dose versus a 7-day 200 mg daily dose of itraconazole in the treatment of tinea versicolor. *J Dermatolog Treat*. 2002 Jun;13(2):77–79.

Lange DS, Richards HM, Guarnieri J, et al. Ketoconazole 2% shampoo in the treatment of tinea versicolor: A multicenter, randomized, double-blind, placebo-controlled trial. *J Am Acad Dermatol*. 1998 Dec;39(6):944–950.

Rigopoulos D, Gregoriou S, Kontochristopoulos G, et al. Flutrimazole shampoo 1% versus ketoconazole shampoo 2% in the treatment of pityriasis versicolor. A randomised double-blind comparative trial. *Mycoses*. 2007 May;50(3):193–195.

Schwartz RA. Superficial fungal infections. *Lancet*. 2004 Sep–Oct;364(9440):1173–1182.

Sobera JO, Elewski BE. Fungal diseases. In: Bolognia J, Jorizzo JL, Rapini RP, eds. *Dermatology*. 2nd Ed. St. Louis, MO: Mosby; 2008:1135–1138.

Verma S, Heffernan MP. Superficial fungal infection: Dermatophytosis, onychomycosis, tinea nigra, piedra. In: Fitzpatrick TB, Wolff K, eds. *Fitzpatrick's Dermatology in General Medicine*. 7th Ed. New York, NY: McGraw-Hill; 2008:1828–1830.

Yazdanpanah MJ, Azizi H, Suizi B. Comparison between fluconazole and ketoconazole effectivity in the treatment of pityriasis versicolor. *Mycoses*. 2007 Jul;50(4):311–313.

Transient Acantholytic Dermatosis (Grover Disease)

■■ Diagnosis Synopsis

Transient acantholytic dermatosis (TAD), also known as Grover disease, is an intensely pruritic inflammatory skin disorder of uncertain etiology. It manifests most commonly as 1 to 4 mm red, scaly papules over the trunk. Histologically, there is focal acantholysis (separation of keratinocytes in the epidermis) and dyskeratosis (abnormal keratinocyte maturation). The disease favors middle-aged to elderly white men; case series show a male-to-female ratio of from 1.8 to 3:1. Although the cause has not been established, the condition has been linked to heat, sweating, excessive UV exposure, and ionizing radiation. One large retrospective study of outpatients found the disease diagnosed four times more commonly in the winter than in the summer, and it attributed this to dry skin as the cause. A study of inpatients found prolonged bed rest as a risk factor. Atopic patients may also be at higher risk. Treatment is symptomatic, as the condition is benign and often—but not always—self-limited.

◉ Look For

Small (1 to 4 mm) red papules or papulovesicles scattered on the trunk. The lesions may be widespread on the back (Figs. 4-430–4-433).

Less commonly, individual lesions may appear as pustules or even bullae. They can be seen on the extremities, neck, and shoulders as well, but they almost never occur on the palms, soles, or scalp.

●● Diagnostic Pearls

- Lesions frequently come in a single crop after sun exposure or heavy sweating. They may also appear after some cytokine therapies.
- Lesions may be crusted due to excoriation.

?? Differential Diagnosis and Pitfalls

- Papular urticaria
- Folliculitis (bacterial or *Pityrosporum*)—more pustules
- Acne—more pustules in younger patients
- Pemphigus foliaceus—larger erosions
- Miliaria rubra—occurs after prolonged occlusion
- Dermatitis herpetiformis—extensor surfaces, similarly pruritic
- Seborrheic dermatitis—sebaceous distribution, scaly plaques
- Drug eruption—more macular
- Herpes simplex—more painful
- Herpes zoster—dermatomal distribution
- Viral exanthem—macular
- Milia—white central papule
- Pityriasis rosea—herald patch, larger scaly papules and plaques
- Scabies—look for burrows on the web spaces
- Arthropod assault—larger erythematous papules
- Multiple lichen planus-like keratoses—larger papules
- Multiple actinic keratoses—more keratotic
- Darier disease—sebaceous distribution, lifelong history
- Irritant contact dermatitis—confluent plaques
- Pityriasis lichenoides—chronic scaling papules
- Secondary syphilis—scaling papules and plaques, history of chancre

✓ Best Tests

- Skin biopsy is often helpful, but TAD has several histopathologic features that resemble other conditions (e.g., other acantholytic diseases such as Darier disease, Hailey-Hailey disease, and pemphigus). Clinical correlation is necessary.

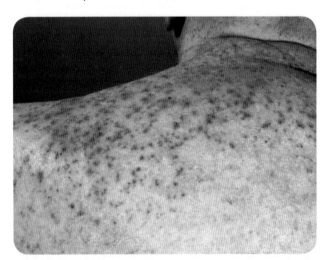

Figure 4-430 Multiple eroded hyperkeratotic papules are characteristic of TAD.

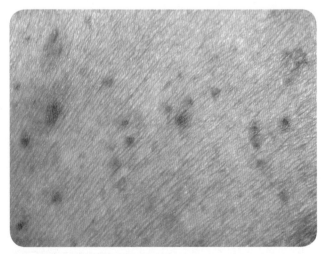

Figure 4-431 The lesions of TAD are often subtle and mimic folliculitis.

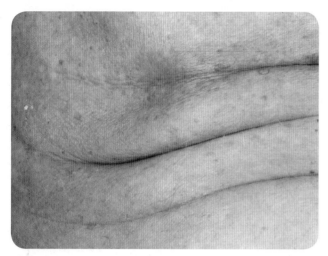

Figure 4-432 TAD in an 86 year old with a 2-year history of itching lesions.

▲▲ Management Pearls

- This can be a very difficult disease to manage due to the intense pruritus and only modestly effective therapeutic options. Patients should be instructed to avoid excessive heat and sweating, and to take measures to prevent xerosis (e.g., avoid excessive bathing and practice daily emollient use).
- Pramoxine or menthol-containing lotions or emollients may be soothing.

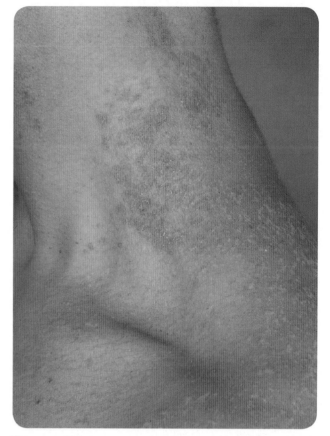

Figure 4-433 Individual small lesions of TAD with a plaque-like grouping of lesions.

Therapy

High-potency Topical Corticosteroids (class 2)

- Fluocinonide cream, ointment—apply twice daily
- Desoximetasone cream, ointment—apply twice daily
- Halcinonide cream, ointment—apply twice daily
- Amcinonide ointment—apply twice daily

Antihistamines
- Hydroxyzine: 10 to 50 mg p.o. every 6 h as needed
- Diphenhydramine hydrochloride: 25 to 50 mg p.o. every 6 h as needed
- Cetirizine: 10 to 20 mg twice daily

For more severe or recalcitrant disease, consider isotretinoin (0.5 to 1 mg/kg/day for 2 to 12 weeks), acitretin (0.5 mg/kg/day), systemic corticosteroids (prednisone approx. 10 to 60 mg daily with a taper over several weeks), psoralen plus UVA (PUVA), and vitamin A (50,000 U three times daily for 2 weeks), and even the simple application of triple antibiotic ointment have all been reported to be efficacious in case reports or small case series.

Suggested Readings

Davis MD, Dinneen AM, Landa N, et al. Grover's disease: Clinicopathologic review of 72 cases. *Mayo Clin Proc.* 1999 Mar;74(3):229–234.

French LE, Piletta PA, Etienne A, et al. Incidence of transient acantholytic dermatosis (Grover's disease) in a hospital setting. *Dermatology.* 1999;198(4):410–411.

Helfman RJ. Grover's disease treated with isotretinoin. Report of four cases. *J Am Acad Dermatol.* 1985 Jun;12(6):981–984.

Hovnanian A. Acantholytic disorders of the skin: Darier-White disease, acrokeratosis verruciformis, Grover disease, and Hailey-Hailey disease. In: Fitzpatrick TB, Wolff K, eds. *Fitzpatrick's Dermatology in General Medicine.* 7th Ed. New York, NY: McGraw-Hill; 2008:437–438.

Julliard KN, Milburn PB. Antibiotic ointment in the treatment of Grover disease. *Cutis.* 2007 Jul;80(1):72–74.

Parsons JM. Transient acantholytic dermatosis (Grover's disease): A global perspective. *J Am Acad Dermatol.* 1996 Nov;35(5 Pt 1):653–666; quiz 667–670.

Quirk CJ, Heenan PJ. Grover's disease: 34 years on. *Australas J Dermatol.* 2004 May;45(2):83–86; quiz 87–88.

Scheinfeld N, Mones J. Seasonal variation of transient acantholytic dyskeratosis (Grover's disease). *J Am Acad Dermatol.* 2006 Aug;55(2):263–268.

Yoo JH, Cho KH, Youn JI. A case of bullous transient acantholytic dermatosis. *J Dermatol.* 1994 Mar;21(3):194–196.

Diagnosis Synopsis

Common warts (verruca vulgaris) are benign skin proliferations caused by the human papillomavirus (HPV) types 2 and 4. They may be transmitted by direct or indirect contact. Autoinoculation is common. They can occur on virtually any epidermal surface, including mucosal surfaces, but common warts are most often seen on the hands, feet, and knees, and they present as flesh-colored, hyperkeratotic papules. Warts are more common in the immunocompromised and school-aged children. They also occur more frequently in whites.

Immunocompromised Patient Considerations

Widespread or extensive warts are often a presenting sign of an immunocompromised state. Warts, in general, tend to be more numerous in immunosuppressed patients and have a higher potential for malignant transformation.

Look For

Hyperkeratotic, skin-colored papules with a rough and irregular (verrucous) surface. They may vary in size (1 mm to >1 cm). There are usually several lesions scattered on the digits or extremities (Figs. 4-434–4-436).

Immunocompromised Patient Considerations

Extensive periungual warts or extensive facial warts can be seen with immunosuppression, in which case HIV testing would be warranted (Fig. 4-437).

Diagnostic Pearls

- Tiny black or red dots within the lesion are characteristic of common warts and represent thrombosed capillaries. These are best visualized by removing the surface of the wart with a no. 15 surgical blade.
- Common warts also cause an interruption in the normal skin lines (dermatoglyphics).

Differential Diagnosis and Pitfalls

- Keratoacanthomas have a central keratin crater.
- Squamous cell carcinoma can arise in preexisting warts and may be recalcitrant to therapy.
- Prurigo nodularis is characterized by pruritic papules and nodules.
- Perforating disorders tend to be follicularly based with a central core.
- Seborrheic keratoses have a characteristic "stuck-on," waxy appearance.
- Lichen planus lesions are typically more planar, violaceous, and pruritic.
- Cutaneous horns can arise from warts, hypertrophic actinic keratoses, seborrheic keratoses, and squamous cell carcinomas.
- Actinic keratoses tend to be scaly erythematous papules in sun-exposed areas of elderly individuals.
- Lichen nitidus is characterized by discrete, dome-shaped papules.
- A clavus, or corn, is a painful hyperkeratotic lesion with a central core that lacks the pinpoint thrombosed capillaries and retains normal skin dermatoglyphics. Clavi occur in sites of pressure and repeated friction.

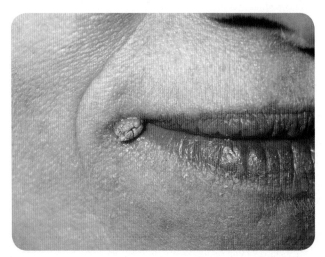

Figure 4-434 Warts are frequent at mucocutaneous junctions.

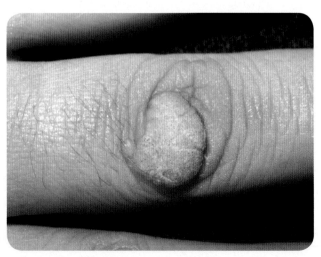

Figure 4-435 Hyperkeratotic plaque from a wart in a common location.

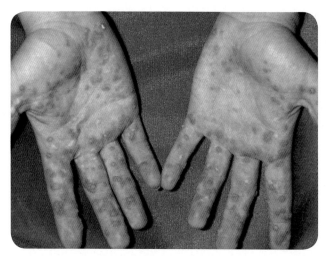

Figure 4-436 Extensive verrucae warrant careful immunological history and, at times, testing of immune function.

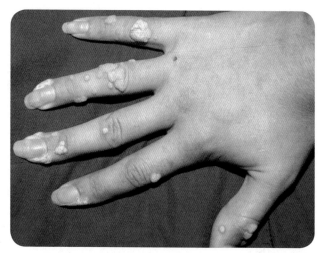

Figure 4-437 Common warts on the hand and periungually in a patient with acute lymphocytic leukemia.

- Foreign body reactions may have a history of trauma or inoculation.
- Molluscum contagiosum lesions are smooth, dome-shaped papules with a central umbilication.

Immunocompromised Patient Differential Diagnosis

Common warts can progress to squamous cell carcinoma in immunosuppressed patients.

✓ Best Tests

- This is usually a clinical diagnosis; however, biopsy is confirmatory if the diagnosis is in doubt.
- Lesions that are atypical or resistant to therapy should be biopsied to rule out squamous cell carcinoma.

▲▲ Management Pearls

- Warts typically remit spontaneously. Therefore, medical intervention is usually instituted for cosmetic reasons when the warts are located on the face or hands, or in immunosuppressed patients to decrease the spread of new lesions.
- Aggressive home therapy with 40% salicylic acid plaster available over the counter (OTC) applied daily or twice daily and taped on with strong adhesive tape (e.g., duct tape). Have the patient pare the wart down with a file or pumice stone between applications of each patch.

- Given the risk of scarring, surgical removal should be limited to only special cases.

Immunocompromised Patient Considerations

Warts in immunosuppressed patients can be more resistant to traditional therapy.

Dark Skin Considerations

Use caution with liquid nitrogen treatment in darkly pigmented individuals, as there is a greater risk of hyper- and hypopigmentation.

Therapy

Be sure to pare the wart down before cryosurgery or application of any topical therapy to improve the chance of treatment success.

Warts are benign and usually self-limited. Therefore, it is reasonable to not treat. Patients often request treatment, however, in which case therapeutic options include the following:

- Destructive therapy: 40% salicylic acid plasters/ointments (OTC) with strong adhesive tape as described above. Can leave on for 2 to 4 days, followed by paring or pumice stone. Alternatives include silver nitrate and glutaraldehyde solution.

(Continued)

- Cryotherapy using liquid nitrogen applied for 5 s with 1 to 3 freeze/thaw cycles. Trichloroacetic acid or monochloroacetic acid under occlusion for 48 to 72 h. Electrodesiccation and CO_2 laser therapy should be used with caution to avoid scarring.
- Topical medications: 5-fluorouracil (1% or 5% cream) applied daily or twice daily; or Imiquimod 5% cream can be applied three to five times per week for 6 weeks or longer until lesions disappear. An irritation of the lesions is expected. Tretinoin 0.1% cream or gel daily or twice daily as tolerated. Tretinoin can be combined with imiquimod as well.
- Intralesional immunotherapy: Topical diphenylcyclopropenone, topical squaric acid, intralesional *Candida* antigen, mumps antigen, and trichophyton antigens can sensitize patients to HPV. Intralesional interferon α-2b 1 mL of 1 million IU three times a week for 3 weeks.
- Intralesional chemotherapy: Intralesional bleomycin 0.5 U/mL with no more than 3 mL injected at one time. (Use with caution as scarring and neuropathy can result.)

Immunocompromised Patient Considerations

All therapies for warts can be used in immunosuppressed patients.

Suggested Readings

Ahmed I, Agarwal S, Ilchyshyn A, et al. Liquid nitrogen cryotherapy of common warts: cryo-spray vs. cotton wool bud. *Br J Dermatol.* 2001 May;144(5):1006–1009.

Androphy EJ, Lowy DR. Warts. In: Fitzpatrick TB, Wolff K, eds. *Fitzpatrick's Dermatology in General Medicine.* 7th Ed. New York, NY: McGraw-Hill; 2008:1914–1923.

Gibbs S, Harvey I. Topical treatments for cutaneous warts. *Cochrane Database Syst Rev.* 2006 Jul;(3):CD001781.

Gibbs S, Harvey I, Sterling J, et al. Local treatments for cutaneous warts: Systematic review. *BMJ.* 2002 Aug;325(7362):461.

Kirnbauer R, Lenz P, Okun MM. Human papillomavirus. In: Bolognia J, Jorizzo JL, Rapini RP, eds. *Dermatology.* 2nd Ed. St. Louis, MO: Mosby; 2008:1183–1198.

Lipke MM. An armamentarium of wart treatments. *Clin Med Res.* 2006 Dec;4(4):273–293.

Micali G, Dall'Oglio F, Nasca MR, et al. Management of cutaneous warts: An evidence-based approach. *Am J Clin Dermatol.* 2004;5(5):311–317.

Sterling JC, Handfield-Jones S, Hudson PM; British Association of Dermatologists. Guidelines for the management of cutaneous warts. *Br J Dermatol.* 2001 Jan;144(1):4–11.

■■ Diagnosis Synopsis

Plantar warts are common superficial skin growths caused by the human papillomavirus (HPV) types 1, 2, and 4. Plantar warts are hyperkeratotic papules that often form on pressure points such as the ball of the foot and the heel, but they may occur anywhere else on the sole. Lesions are often asymptomatic, but a callus overlying the wart on pressure points may lead to pain with pressure or walking. They are frequently transmitted person to person through exposure to the virus on locker room floors, public showers, and pool areas. They are slightly more common in females, young children, and immunocompromised patients.

Immunocompromised Patient Considerations

Widespread or extensive warts are often a presenting sign of an immunocompromised state.

Warts, in general, tend to be more numerous in immunosuppressed patients and have a higher potential for malignant transformation.

◉ Look For

Flat, hyperkeratotic, skin-colored papules often associated with overlying callus on the plantar surface of the foot (Figs. 4-438–4-441). Occasionally, several lesions can merge and form one large mosaic wart. Some plantar warts are inverted secondary to pressure.

●● Diagnostic Pearls

- Tiny black or red dots within the lesion are characteristic of warts and represent thrombosed capillaries. These are best visualized by removing the surface of the wart with a no. 15 surgical blade.
- Plantar warts also cause an interruption in the normal skin lines (dermatoglyphics).

?? Differential Diagnosis and Pitfalls

- A clavus, or corn, is a painful hyperkeratotic lesion with a central core that lacks the pinpoint thrombosed capillaries and retains normal skin dermatoglyphics. Clavi occur in sites of pressure and repeated friction.
- Foreign body reaction may have a history of trauma or inoculation.
- Acquired digital fibrokeratoma tends to have a smoother and more pedunculated appearance with a collarette of normal skin.
- Squamous cell carcinoma can arise in preexisting warts and may be recalcitrant to therapy.
- If the patient has recently traveled to a tropical area, consider tungiasis (infestation with a burrowing flea into the sole of the foot). Look for a firm, white papule with a central black dot.

Immunocompromised Patient Differential Diagnosis

Common warts and plantar warts can progress to squamous cell carcinoma in immunosuppressed patients.

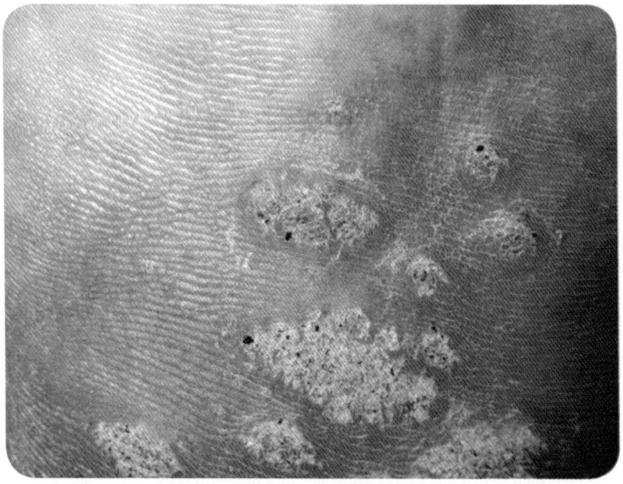

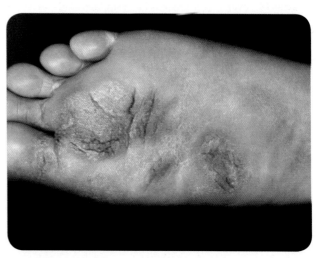

Figure 4-438 Small and large hyperkeratotic plaques, some with thrombosed capillaries characteristic of plantar warts.

Figure 4-439 Plantar warts often have massive hyperkeratosis and deep fissures.

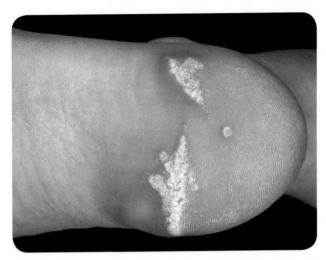

Figure 4-440 Recurrent linear plantar wart recurring after attempted surgical removal.

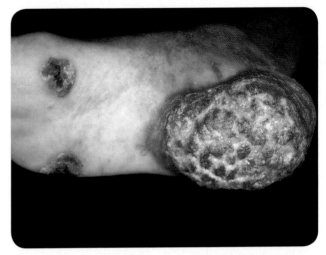

Figure 4-441 The large, thick plaque on the heel requires biopsy to exclude a squamous cell carcinoma arising in a wart.

✓ Best Tests

- This is usually a clinical diagnosis; however, biopsy is confirmatory if the diagnosis is in doubt.
- Lesions that are resistant to therapy should be biopsied to rule out squamous cell carcinoma.

▲▲ Management Pearls

- Plantar warts can remit spontaneously. Therefore, medical intervention is usually instituted for cosmetic reasons, if the wart is painful, or in immunosuppressed patients to decrease the spread of new lesions.
- Aggressive home therapy with 40% salicylic acid plaster available over the counter (OTC) applied daily or twice daily and taped on with strong adhesive tape (e.g., duct tape). Have the patient pare the wart down with a file or a pumice stone between applications of each patch.
- Given the risk of scarring, surgical removal should be limited to only special cases.
- Remind patients they will need multiple treatments and that plantar warts tend to recur. Advise the use of shower shoes or sandals in public locker rooms and showers.

Immunocompromised Patient Considerations

Warts in immunosuppressed patients can be more resistant to traditional therapy.

Dark Skin Considerations

Use caution with liquid nitrogen treatment in darkly pigmented individuals, as there is a risk of hyper- and hypopigmentation.

Therapy

Be sure to pare the wart down before cryosurgery or application of any topical therapy to improve the chance of treatment success.

Warts are benign and usually self-limited. Therefore, it is reasonable to not treat them. Patients often request treatment, however, in which case therapeutic options include the following:

- Destructive therapy: 40% Salicylic acid plasters/ointments (OTC) with strong adhesive tape as described above. Can leave on for 2 to 4 days, followed by paring or pumice stone. Alternatives include silver nitrate and glutaraldehyde solution.
- Cryotherapy using liquid nitrogen applied for 5 s with 1 to 3 freeze/thaw cycles. Trichloroacetic acid or monochloroacetic acid under occlusion for 48 to 72 h. Electrodesiccation and CO_2 laser therapy should be used with caution to avoid scarring.
- Topical medications: 5-fluorouracil (1% or 5% cream) applied once or twice daily; or imiquimod 5% cream can be applied three to five times per week for 6 weeks or longer until lesions disappear. An irritation of the lesions is expected. Tretinoin 0.1% cream or gel once or twice daily as tolerated. Tretinoin can be combined

with imiquimod as well. The occlusion of any topical therapy for plantar warts should improve efficacy.

- Intralesional immunotherapy: Topical diphenylcyclopropenone, topical squaric acid, intralesional *Candida* antigen, mumps antigen, and trichophyton antigens can sensitize patients to HPV. Intralesional interferon α-2b 1 mL of 1 million IU three times a week for 3 weeks.
- Intralesional chemotherapy: Intralesional bleomycin 0.5 U/mL with no more than 3 mL injected at one time. (Use with caution because scarring and neuropathy can result.)

Be careful when treating to not induce a scar on the bottom of the foot because this may be uncomfortable with ambulation.

Immunocompromised Patient Considerations

All therapies for warts can be used in immunosuppressed patients.

Suggested Readings

Androphy EJ, Lowy DR. Warts. In: Fitzpatrick TB, Wolff K, eds. *Fitzpatrick's Dermatology in General Medicine*. 7th Ed. New York, NY: McGraw-Hill; 2008:1914–1923.

Esterowitz D, Greer KE, Cooper PH, et al. Plantar warts in the athlete. *Am J Emerg Med*. 1995 Jul;13(4):441–443.

Gibbs S, Harvey I. Topical treatments for cutaneous warts. *Cochrane Database Syst Rev*. 2006 Jul;(3):CD001781.

Glover MG. Plantar warts. *Foot Ankle*. 1990 Dec;11(3):172–178.

Kirnbauer R, Lenz P, Okun MM. Human papillomavirus. In: Bolognia J, Jorizzo JL, Rapini RP, eds. *Dermatology*. 2nd Ed. St. Louis, MO: Mosby; 2008:1183–1198.

Landsman MJ, Mancuso JE, Abramow SP. Diagnosis, pathophysiology, and treatment of plantar verruca. *Clin Podiatr Med Surg*. 1996 Jan;13(1): 55–71.

Lipke MM. An armamentarium of wart treatments. *Clin Med Res*. 2006 Dec;4(4):273–293.

Sparling JD, Checketts SR, Chapman MS. Imiquimod for plantar and periungual warts. *Cutis*. 2001 Dec;68(6):397–399.

Bullous Pemphigoid and Pemphigus Vulgaris

◼◼ Diagnosis Synopsis

Bullous pemphigoid (BP) is a chronic autoimmune subepidermal blistering disease most frequently seen in the elderly. IgG autoantibodies bind to antigens that comprise the hemidesmosome adhesion complex in the basement membrane of the skin (BP180 or BP230). This triggers complement activation and the release of inflammatory mediators. The result is the formation of local or generalized, tense bullae. The disease can occur on any body surface, but mucous membrane involvement is rarely seen.

BP has been associated with other autoimmune diseases such as diabetes mellitus, thyroiditis, dermatomyositis, lupus erythematosus, rheumatoid arthritis, ulcerative colitis, myasthenia gravis, and multiple sclerosis. Therapeutic radiation or drugs (furosemide, nonsteroidal anti-inflammatory drugs (NSAIDs), captopril, penicillamine, and some antibiotics) have also been associated with BP. It may also follow certain nonbullous inflammatory skin diseases, such as psoriasis and lichen planus, or vaccination (most often in children). In whites, there has been a significant association with the DQB1*0301 allele, whereas Japanese patients have a higher frequency of alleles DRB1*04, DRB1*1101, and DQB1*0302.

The condition is often self-limiting, but it can become chronic over months to years. There is a wide spectrum of clinical severity. The disease can be generalized and severe, or patients may have only a few asymptomatic, localized bullae. There is no race or gender predilection. In some instances, early BP lesions will appear as pruritic urticarial papules and plaques (known as urticarial BP).

Pemphigus vulgaris (PV) is a chronic autoimmune intraepidermal blistering disease that can cause significant morbidity and serious complications. IgG autoantibodies are formed to the keratinocyte cell surface molecules desmoglein 1 and 3, creating problems with cell-cell adhesion (acantholysis). Bullae and erosions develop on skin and mucous membranes. Severe cases can be life threatening. Complications are related to the use of high dose steroids, secondary infection, loss of the skin barrier, and poor oral intake. It is also associated with other autoimmune diseases, especially myasthenia gravis. In **pemphigus foliaceus (PF)**, the autoantibody in question is directed against desmoglein 1 specifically. PF is generally a more benign form of pemphigus with no oral lesions and not resulting in severe illness. Recent sun exposure can exacerbate the condition. Pemphigus occurs in all ethnicities and equally in both sexes. PF usually occurs in middle age and PV in the fifth or sixth decade of life.

◉ Look For

Bullae of BP are tense compared to the flaccid bullae of PV or erosions of PF. In BP, bullae are most often seen on the lower abdomen, thighs, and forearms (Fig. 4-442). They can be extensive or localized, and there is a flexural predilection (Fig. 4-443). They may appear on normal-looking skin or have an erythematous base. Vesicles or bullae can be filled with either serous or blood-tinged fluid (Fig. 4-444). The lesions typically heal without scarring or milia formation.

In PV, the vesicles and erosions can affect mucosal surfaces, including conjunctiva and oral mucosa (Fig. 4-445). Large areas of epidermis can denude (Fig. 4-446), creating risk for bacterial infection and sepsis. Look for active vesicles at the margins of plaques. In PF, superficial blisters, crusted erosions, and scale are seen on the scalp, face, and trunk, often in a seborrheic distribution (Figs. 4-447 and 4-448). Lesions usually start on the trunk. Because the vesicles are superficial, patients often appear to have an infected eczema of the face and upper trunk.

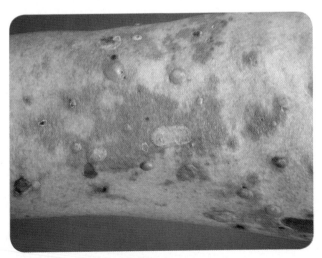

Figure 4-442 Urticarial plaques may accompany lesions in BP.

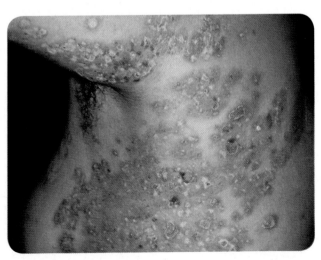

Figure 4-443 BP with active blisters and hyperpigmentation from previous episodes.

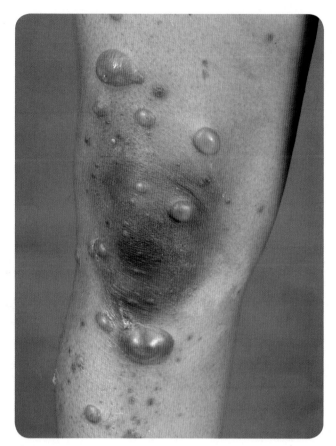

Figure 4-444 Tense, clear bullae on normal skin are characteristic of BP.

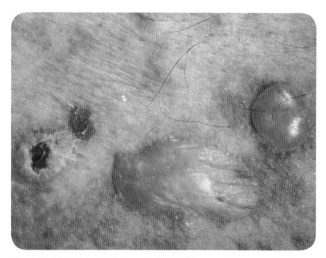

Figure 4-446 PV with bullae and erosions.

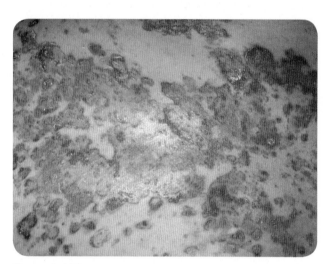

Figure 4-447 PF with bullae, erosions, and scaling.

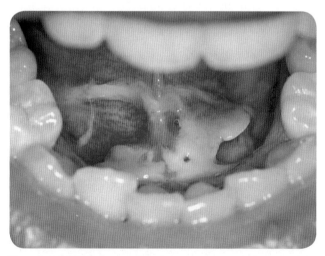

Figure 4-445 PV with oral ulcers.

Dark Skin Considerations

In BP, there can be fixed urticarial plaques that may be heavily pigmented in dark-skinned individuals.

●● Diagnostic Pearls

- Pruritus is prominent and may actually precede the appearance of skin lesions.
- BP should always be highly considered when tense bullae are present in patients aged older than 60.
- BP rarely has mucosal lesions, as compared with PV, which frequently begins with oral erosions.
- Early lesions in BP may be urticarial, but individual lesions of BP last longer than 24 h, as compared with true urticaria, where lesions last less than 24 h.
- Nikolsky sign, where slight friction induces an erosion or vesicle, is often absent in BP but present in pemphigus.
- The Asboe-Hansen sign ("bulla-spread phenomenon"), in which gentle pressure on an intact bulla forces the fluid to spread under the skin, away from the site of the pressure, may also be present in PV.

- Diabetic bullae, which often erode and are large in size, may be confused with BP, but they are commonly solitary.
- Older patients can get erythema multiforme (EM) from drugs or herpes infections; however, EM does not commonly present with frank bullae.
- Urticarial lesions are transient, lasting less than 24 h.
- Epidermolysis bullosa acquisita can be difficult to distinguish but may have the additional findings of milia; biopsy with direct immunofluorescence is helpful.
- Cicatricial pemphigoid is a scarring, blistering disease that involves the mucosal surfaces.
- Pemphigoid gestationis is a variant of BP that presents in pregnant or postpartum females.
- Linear IgA dermatosis often presents with a cluster of vesicles on an erythematous base.
- Dermatitis herpetiformis rarely has intact bullae secondary to excoriation.
- Bullous fixed drug eruption has a history of inciting drug and usually presents with a solitary lesion.
- Bullous impetigo will have associated honey-colored crust.
- Porphyria cutanea tarda or pseudoporphyria presents with bullae, milia, and hypertrichosis in sun-exposed areas.
- Sneddon-Wilkinson syndrome (subcorneal pustular dermatosis)
- Hailey-Hailey disease
- Drug-induced pemphigus (penicillamine, captopril, thiol-containing compounds)
- Paraneoplastic pemphigus (lymphoproliferative malignancy) usually involves the vermillion border of the lips.
- Toxic epidermal necrolysis
- Erosive lichen planus can involve the mucosa.

- Atopic dermatitis, contact dermatitis, and seborrheic dermatitis can mimic PF.
- Impetigo and bullous impetigo
- Mycosis fungoides
- Subacute cutaneous lupus erythematosus

✓ Best Tests

- Take a complete medication history.
- Skin biopsy of the edge of a bulla for H&E staining will reveal a bulla with associated eosinophilic infiltrate and characteristic patterns of blister location and acantholysis. Diagnosis is confirmed with direct immunofluorescence on a perilesional biopsy (Fig. 4-449). Eosinophilia is common.
- Serum ELISA for antibodies against desmogleins can be useful in PV and PF.

▲▲ Management Pearls

- Secondary infection of lesions should be treated aggressively with appropriate systemic antibiotics.
- There is usually no relationship to an underlying neoplasm, as compared to some other blistering disorders. A thorough history and general physical exam is usually sufficient. However, systemic symptoms or an atypical presentation should warrant further workup of underlying malignancy.
- Patients with pemphigus should be instructed to minimize trauma to the skin. Patients with PV may need dietary modifications (e.g., avoidance of caustic or hard foods). Sun avoidance and sun-protection measures (e.g., sunscreens and barrier clothing) should be instituted for patients with PF.

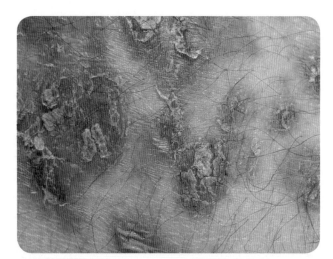

Figure 4-448 PF with erosions, crusts, and a few flaccid bullae.

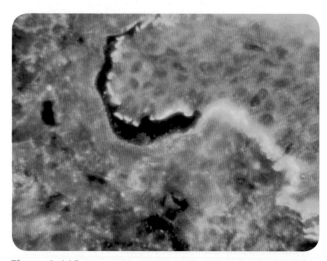

Figure 4-449 Immunofluorescent study showing IgG staining of the basement membrane zone and then the epidermal roof of the blister.

- Involve a dermatologist in the patient's care. Depending on the extent and severity of disease, consultations with dentistry, ophthalmology, or otolaryngology may be indicated.

Therapy

Avoid mechanical skin trauma.

Patients with oral disease may require a modified diet (e.g., soft foods).

BP
Localized Disease
- High-potency topical corticosteroids (clobetasol propionate) or intralesional steroids (triamcinolone acetonide).

Extensive Disease
- Prednisone at 0.5 to 1 mg/kg/day and taper slowly with clearing. Patients taking long-term systemic corticosteroids should receive calcium (at least 1 g daily) and vitamin D supplementation ± other method(s) of osteoporosis prevention.
- Recently, tetracycline (500 mg four times daily) in combination with nicotinamide (500 mg three times daily) or minocycline (100 mg twice daily) have been used for their anti-inflammatory effects and as steroid-sparing agents, though controlled studies have not yet been done to prove efficacy.
- Dapsone (50 to 100 mg per day), azathioprine (75 to 150 mg per day), mycophenolate mofetil (1.0 to 1.5 g twice daily), cyclophosphamide (1 to 3 mg/kg/day), cyclosporine (1 to 5 mg/kg/day), and methotrexate (5 to 10 mg weekly) also serve as important steroid-sparing agents. Their use should be considered if the patient requires several months of systemic corticosteroids in the range of 40 to 60 mg.
- For resistant cases, plasma exchange, IVIg, or rituximab (anti-CD20) can be attempted.

PV and PF
Initial therapy should be with prednisone with at least a dose of 1 mg/kg. If there is not a response within a few days, increasing the dose to 1.5 or 2 mg/kg is reasonable. Patients may be on steroids for months to years, and all of the side effects of corticosteroids must be considered and managed as preventively as possible.

Nicotinamide (1.5 g per day) with tetracycline (2 g per day) has been reported effective in a few patients with PF.

Other therapies for their steroid-sparing effects include the following:

- Mycophenolate mofetil (1.5 m twice daily)
- Azathioprine (100 to 300 mg per day)
- Dapsone (100 to 200 mg per day)
- Cyclophosphamide (50 to 200 mg per day)
- Cyclosporine (5 mg/kg/day)
- High-dose IVIg

Suggested Readings

Borradori L, Bernard P. Pemphigoid group. In: Bolognia JL, Jorizzo JL, Rapini RP, eds. *Dermatology*. 2nd Ed. St. Louis, MO: Mosby; 2008:431–438.

Di Zenzo G, Marazza G, Borradori L. Bullous pemphigoid: Physiopathology, clinical features and management. *Adv Dermatol*. 2007;23:257–288.

Joly P, Roujeau JC, Benichou J, et al; Bullous Diseases French Study Group. A comparison of oral and topical corticosteroids in patients with bullous pemphigoid. *N Engl J Med*. 2002 Jan;346(5):321–327.

Khumalo NP, Murrell DF, Wojnarowska F, et al. A systematic review of treatments for bullous pemphigoid. *Arch Dermatol*. 2002 Mar;138(3):385–389.

Nousari HC, Anhalt GJ. Pemphigus and bullous pemphigoid. *Lancet*. 1999 Aug;354(9179):667–672.

Saouli Z, Papadopoulos A, Kaiafa G, et al. A new approach on bullous pemphigoid therapy. *Ann Oncol*. 2008 Apr;19(4):825–826.

Stanley JR. Bullous pemphigoid. In: Fitzpatrick TB, Wolff K, eds. *Fitzpatrick's Dermatology in General Medicine*. 7th Ed. New York, NY: McGraw-Hill; 2008:475–480.

Vassileva S. Drug-induced pemphigoid: Bullous and cicatricial. *Clin Dermatol*. 1998 May–Jun;16(3):379–387.

Dermatitis Herpetiformis

Diagnosis Synopsis

Dermatitis herpetiformis is a chronic pruritic autoimmune blistering disorder associated with gluten-sensitive enteropathy. Over 90% of patients have associated gluten-sensitive enteropathy, although only 20% will show evidence of clinical disease. The pathogenesis involves the deposition of IgA immune complexes in the papillary dermis. The associated autoantigen is an epidermal transglutaminase. There is a genetic predisposition to the disease, as certain human leukocyte antigen (HLA) haplotypes, HLA class II DQ2, demonstrate an increased expression.

The disease manifests as an intermittent pruritic papulovesicular eruption over the extensor surfaces of the extremities. Many patients experience complete remission of their disease on a strict gluten-free diet. Patients are at an increased risk of developing Hashimoto thyroiditis, non-Hodgkin lymphoma, and GI lymphomas. Dermatitis herpetiformis is more common in men and individuals of Northern European descent.

Look For

Small, fragile, clustered vesicles located symmetrically over the elbows, knees, shoulders, and buttocks (Figs. 4-450–4-453). The face may also be involved. Cutaneous findings are usually limited to pinpoint erosions and excoriations; however, erythematous papules and urticarial plaques may also be seen. Due to the severe pruritus and secondary excoriation, intact vesicles are rare.

Diagnostic Pearls

- Symmetrically grouped, extremely pruritic lesions over extensor arms, legs, and buttocks.
- History of bloating and diarrhea associated with gluten-containing foods.
- Lesions may be worsened by iodides and certain non-steroidal anti-inflammatory drugs (NSAIDs).

Differential Diagnosis and Pitfalls

- Bullous pemphigoid presents with erythematous plaques and intact, tense bullae in older patients.
- Linear IgA bullous dermatosis presents with annular erythema and clustered vesicles.
- Eczematous dermatitis is also pruritic, with ill-defined, weeping erythematous plaques.
- Herpes simplex virus (HSV) has nonsymmetric, localized, clustered vesicles with more pain and less pruritus.
- Epidermolysis bullosa acquisita may have associated milia.
- Transient acantholytic dermatosis (Grover disease) is a pruritic papular eruption in the seborrheic regions of older men.
- Neurotic excoriations are distributed in areas within reach for the patient to scratch.
- Scabies manifests with interdigital burrows and involvement of the hands, wrists, and genital region, sparing the head.
- Papular urticaria may be associated with arthropod bites and is distributed over exposed areas.

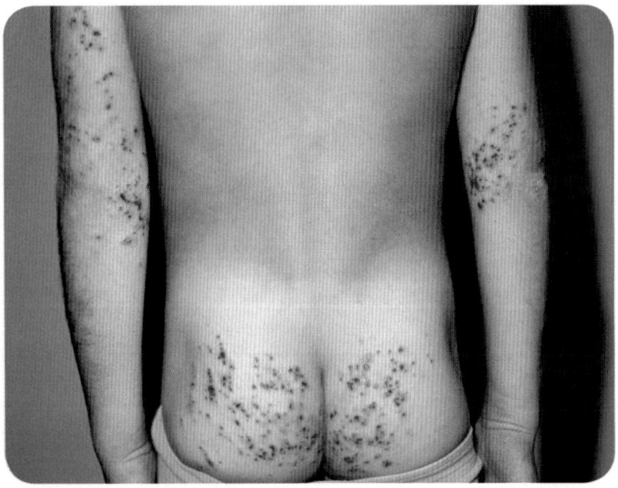

Figure 4-450 Closely grouped papulovesicular lesions characterize dermatitis herpetiformis.

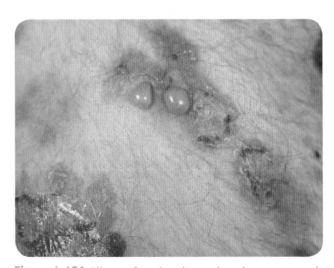

Figure 4-451 Blisters of varying sizes and erosions may occur in dermatitis herpetiformis.

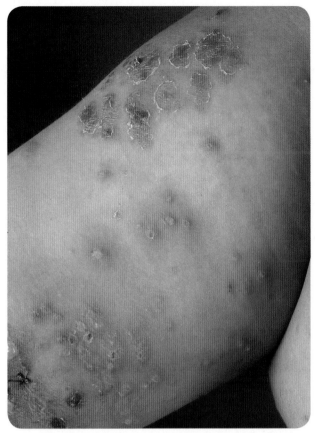

Figure 4-452 Small erosions, erythematous plaques, and annular scale in dermatitis herpetiformis.

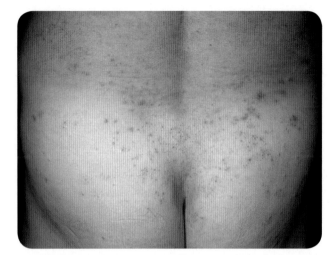

Figure 4-453 Characteristic location for dermatitis herpetiformis.

- Pemphigoid gestationis is characterized by tense bullae over the abdomen in pregnant women.
- Chronic prurigo consists of lichenified excoriated papules.

✓ Best Tests

- Skin biopsy of the edge of a lesion for histology and perilesional skin for direct immunofluorescence is diagnostic.
- Anti-gliadin, anti-endomysial, or anti-reticulin IgA antibodies can be detected by indirect immunofluorescence and are an index of gluten-sensitive enteropathy disease severity.

▲▲ Management Pearls

- A strict gluten-free diet alone can greatly ameliorate symptoms. Consider consultation with a dietician and/or a gastroenterologist.

Therapy

A gluten-free diet and dapsone are considered first-line therapy.

- Dapsone can be started at 25 to 50 mg p.o. daily with gradual increase to a maintenance dose of 100 mg p.o. daily. Dapsone will improve cutaneous disease but has no effect on intestinal involvement.
  Caution: Dapsone may produce hemolysis, methemoglobinemia, hypersensitivity, and a motor neuropathy. Obtain the following baseline studies: CBC, LFTs, and G-6-PD levels. After the initiation of therapy, monitor patients with a CBC every week for the first month, and then follow the CBC monthly for 5 months and LFTs every 6 months.
- Sulfapyridine 1 to 1.5 g p.o. daily may be substituted in cases of dapsone intolerance.
- Other therapies that have demonstrated some benefit in case reports and series include cyclosporine, colchicine, heparin, systemic corticosteroids, and tetracycline in combination with nicotinamide.

Suggested Readings

Fry L. Dermatitis herpetiformis: Problems, progress and prospects. *Eur J Dermatol.* 2002 Nov–Dec;12(6):523–531.

Hall RP III, Katz SI. Dermatitis herpetiformis. In: Fitzpatrick TB, Wolff K, eds. *Fitzpatrick's Dermatology in General Medicine.* 7th Ed. New York, NY: McGraw-Hill; 2008:500–505.

Hull CM, Zone JJ. Dermatitis herpetiformis and linear IgA bullous dermatosis. In: Bolognia JL, Jorizzo JL, Rapini RP, eds. *Dermatology.* 2nd Ed. St. Louis, MO: Mosby; 2008:447–452.

Leonard JN, Fry L. Treatment and management of dermatitis herpetiformis. *Clin Dermatol.* 1991 Jul–Sep;9(3):403–408.

Nicolas ME, Krause PK, Gibson LE, et al. Dermatitis herpetiformis. *Int J Dermatol.* 2003 Aug;42(8):588–600.

Diagnosis Synopsis

Infection with herpes simplex virus type 1 or type 2 (HSV-1 or HSV-2) usually presents as discrete groups of painful vesicles on orolabial or genital skin. However, in some instances, HSV infection may be diffuse, involving multiple sites of the body. When multiple regions of skin and/or internal viscera are concomitantly infected, the disease is termed disseminated HSV.

Clinically, disseminated HSV presents as a widespread eruption of vesicles, pustules, and/or erosions. Constitutional symptoms often occur and commonly consist of fever and regional lymphadenopathy. Most patients recover without adverse event, but progression to fatal disease can occur.

Two general groups of patients are at risk to develop disseminated HSV: patients with underlying skin disease and immunocompromised patients (see below).

Acute generalized infection of previously damaged skin with HSV is known as eczema herpeticum or Kaposi varicelliform eruption. This clinical picture may be seen in all age groups, but it most commonly occurs in the second and third decades. Most cases are due to HSV-1, but HSV-2 is also reported. Atopic dermatitis is the most common preceding condition, but the condition may also be seen in patients with various other underlying skin conditions such as Darier disease, pemphigus foliaceus, pityriasis rubra pilaris, Hailey-Hailey disease, congenital ichthyosiform erythroderma, mycosis fungoides, and patients with burns.

Immunocompromised Patient Considerations

Immunocompromised and pregnant patients have a higher risk of developing disseminated HSV. Diffuse cutaneous involvement can be associated with esophagitis meningitis, encephalitis, and fulminant hepatitis. Multiorgan failure and death can result. Prompt diagnosis and aggressive systemic antiviral therapy are keys to avoiding morbidity and mortality. In immunocompromised hosts, orofacial or genital lesions are not requisite in active disseminated HSV.

Look For

Look for monomorphic umbilicated vesicles; small, punched-out ulcers; or even hemorrhagic vesicles (Figs. 4-454–4-456). The typical grouping of vesicles and umbilication of vesicles may not be obvious. Vesicles, pustules, or erosions (Fig. 4-457) may be widespread.

Instead of small, discrete vesicles, lesions may present as erosions or ulcers, particularly in the perianal/perineal

location. These lesions may have scalloped borders suggesting their origins in groups of vesicles.

Lesions are frequently seen on the head, neck, and upper trunk. HSV infection can occur anywhere on the body, but it tends to spare the feet and lower legs.

Immunocompromised Patient Considerations

In the immunocompromised, severe disseminated HSV infections can present as large erosions, ulcers, or even hyperkeratotic, verrucous-appearing plaques that are similar in appearance to condylomatous plaques (Fig. 4-458).

Diagnostic Pearls

- Monomorphous diffuse, discrete, 2 to 3 mm hemorrhagic crusts or polycyclic, punched-out ulcers are common.

Immunocompromised Patient Considerations

In immunocompromised patients, orofacial or genital lesions are not requisite in active disseminated HSV.

Differential Diagnosis and Pitfalls

- Differentiate from zoster, which can also disseminate and present with vesicular and hyperkeratotic papules in immunocompromised patients.
- Impetigo (individual lesions may be super-infected with *Staphylococcus*)

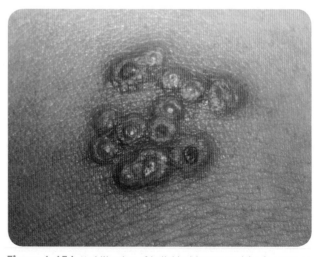

Figure 4-454 Umbilication of individual herpes vesicles is common.

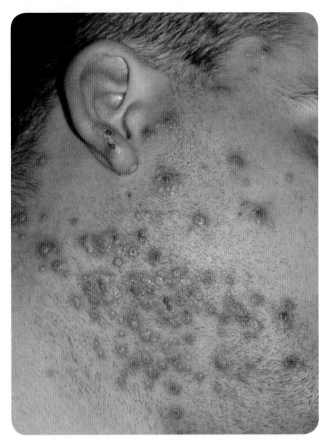

Figure 4-455 Extensive herpes in a herpes related to physical contact (herpes gladiatorum).

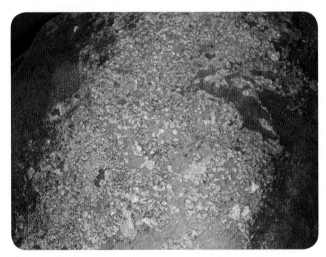

Figure 4-456 Disseminated herpes with large ulcerations.

- Varicella
- Vaccinia
- Coxsackie A16 infection
- Erythema multiforme
- Disseminated cytomegalovirus infection
- Autoimmune blistering disease

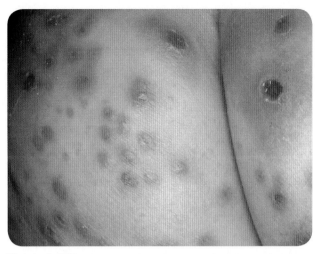

Figure 4-457 Disseminated herpes with erosions and ulcerations.

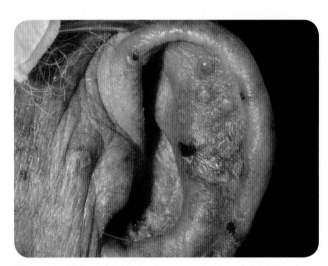

Figure 4-458 Disseminated herpes simplex secondary to prednisone used for immunosuppression.

✓ Best Tests

- Tzanck preparation for multinucleated giant cells (Fig. 4-459).
- Direct fluorescence antigen (DFA) testing is a rapid (<24 h) and sensitive test for HSV-1, HSV-2, and varicella-zoster virus. This test is performed by vigorously scraping the base of a vesicle with a sterile cotton-tipped swab or no. 15 blade and smearing the cells onto a glass slide from a DFA kit. The slide is then fixed (usually contained in a kit) and sent for immunofluorescence analysis. Individual slides must be sent for each virus suspected. Slides can be stored at room temperature for 24 h after fixation, if needed.
- PCR-based clinical assays are rapid, highly sensitive tests for both HSV-1 and HSV-2 detection.

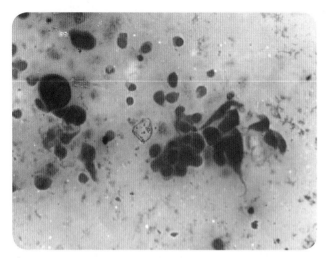

Figure 4-459 Large multinucleated and binucleated cells (upper left) and larger nuclei (in other portions of the figure) characteristic of a herpes virus infection.

- Viral culture of skin lesions.
- Bacterial culture with evidence of impetiginization.
- If there are neurologic signs or symptoms, perform a lumbar puncture with analysis of the cerebrospinal fluid (CSF). PCR can also be used to detect viral DNA in samples of CSF. Neuroimaging (i.e., MRI) is also employed.

▲▲ Management Pearls

- Some patients are best handled as outpatients if not acutely ill, to minimize contagion; however, many patients will require hospitalization and, often, weeks of antiviral therapy (depending on the degree of their immunodeficiency and extent of systemic involvement). Long-term antiviral suppression is often required after the initial infection is treated, as patients are now identified as predisposed to develop disseminated HSV.
- Consultations with infectious disease specialists and critical care physicians are often needed.

Precautions: Standard and Contact. (Isolate patient, wear gloves and a gown, limit patient transport, and avoid sharing patient-care equipment.)

Immunocompromised Patient Considerations

In HIV and AIDS, some patients have been refractory to intravenous acyclovir and have responded to IV foscarnet.

Therapy

Because the lesions are contagious, infection control measures should be followed to prevent both direct contact and dissemination to others and to other sites.

Maximize supportive care; many patients will require treatment and monitoring in an intensive care setting. Provide proper wound care, nutrition, hydration, and pain control.

Patients with disseminated HSV typically require treatment with intravenous antiviral agents. Very mild disease can be treated with oral acyclovir, although this is the exception. Systemic or topical antibiotics are often administered prophylactically or at the first signs of infection in open wounds. Dosing must be tailored to the clinical scenario.

Uncomplicated infection in an immunocompetent host:

- Acyclovir 5 to 10 mg/kg IV every 8 h, transitioning to oral acyclovir when clinically improves and lesions begin to crust over

Herpes simplex encephalitis:

- Acyclovir 10 to 15 mg/kg IV every 8 h for 2 to 3 weeks

Maintenance suppression:

- Acyclovir (400 mg p.o. twice daily) or valacyclovir (500 mg p.o. daily)

Immunocompromised Patient Considerations

Severe infection in an immunocompromised host:

- Acyclovir 5 to 10 mg/kg IV every 8 h for 1 to 2 weeks. Continuing treatment until all lesions are healing (i.e., crusted over) is recommended.
- Acyclovir-resistant HSV in an immunocompromised host:
  Foscarnet: 40 mg/kg IV every 8 to 12 h for 2 to 3 weeks. Continuing treatment until all lesions are healing (i.e., crusted over) is recommended.

Suggested Readings

Basse G, Mengelle C, Kamar N, et al. Disseminated herpes simplex type-2 (HSV-2) infection after solid-organ transplantation. *Infection.* 2008 Feb;36(1):62–64.

Chazotte C, Andersen HF, Cohen WR. Disseminated herpes simplex infection in an immunocompromised pregnancy: Treatment with intravenous acyclovir. *Am J Perinatol.* 1987 Oct;4(4):363–364.

Gelven PL, Gruber KK, Swiger FK, et al. Fatal disseminated herpes simplex in pregnancy with maternal and neonatal death. *South Med J.* 1996 Jul;89(7):732–734.

Herget GW, Riede UN, Schmitt-Gräff A, et al. Generalized herpes simplex virus infection in an immunocompromised patient—report of a case and review of the literature. *Pathol Res Pract.* 2005;201(2):123–129.

Kramer SC, Thomas CJ, Tyler WB, et al. Kaposi's varicelliform eruption: A case report and review of the literature. *Cutis.* 2004 Feb;73(2):115–122.

Lagrew DC, Furlow TG, Hager WD, et al. Disseminated herpes simplex virus infection in pregnancy. Successful treatment with acyclovir. *JAMA.* 1984 Oct;252(15):2058–2059.

Shenoy MM, Suchitra U. Kaposi's varicelliform eruption. *Indian J Dermatol Venereol Leprol.* 2007 Jan–Feb;73(1):65.

Whitley RJ. Herpes simplex virus infections of the central nervous system. A review. *Am J Med.* 1988 Aug;85(2A):61–67.

Whitley R, Barton N, Collins E, et al. Mucocutaneous herpes simplex virus infections in immunocompromised patients. A model for evaluation of topical antiviral agents. *Am J Med.* 1982 Jul;73(1A):236–240.

■■ Diagnosis Synopsis

Orofacial herpes simplex infections (also known as cold sores, fever blisters, or herpetic gingivostomatitis) are very common viral infections causing pain, vesicles, ulceration, and crusting of the perioral skin and oral mucosa. They should be considered within the differential diagnosis of a patient presenting with facial vesicles or crusts. Although the primary causative agent of orofacial disease is herpes simplex virus type 1 (HSV-1), involvement in this area can also be caused by herpes simplex virus type 2 (HSV-2), which is more commonly the cause of genital HSV.

HSV is highly contagious. It is spread by direct contact with virus-containing lesions. The majority of primary infections are asymptomatic, occurring without any signs of cutaneous disease. Symptomatic eruptions may be highly localized to a small area or involve the entire oropharynx and lips. Severe oral ulcerations can develop and be associated with fever, pharyngitis, lymphadenopathy, malaise, headache, foul breath, and difficulty eating. The primary episode usually resolves within 14 days. However, viral shedding from intraoral lesions can persist for several weeks after clinical lesions have resolved. Primary infections are more common in childhood.

Mucocutaneous HSV infection is characterized by initial outbreaks (primary infection), periods of latency (regional sensory ganglia), and recurrent flares localized to the area of the initial outbreak (recurrent infection). Stress, ultraviolet light, fever, tissue damage, and immunosuppression have all been associated with triggering recurrent flares. Recurrent flares are associated with a prodrome of burning, itching, and a tingling sensation before the actual lesions appear. Mucocutaneous eruptions are less severe than that of the primary infection and with less pain and a shorter duration.

The majority of patients have fewer than three outbreaks per year; however, a small percentage of patients have a minimum of six eruptions per year.

Immunocompromised Patient Considerations

Orofacial HSV infections are common and should be considered within the differential diagnosis of any immunocompromised patient presenting with facial vesicles, crusts, erosions, or ulcers. In the immunocompromised patient, eruptions tend to be more severe with larger areas involved, more pain, and longer duration. HSV infection should be considered in immunocompromised hosts with chronic mucosal erosions or ulcers. Oral infection with HSV-2 is more frequent in patients with HIV.

◉ Look For

Groups of umbilicated yellow or grayish vesicles, pinpoint ulcers, or erosions (Figs. 4-460–4-462). If the acute infection is severe, the vesicles will coalesce to form large grayish, membranous plaques. Vesicles at the vermilion border may show umbilication before they are denuded or crusted.

In the oral cavity, look for painful yellow ulcers on the mucosa involving any site but in particular the gingiva, dorsum of tongue, and buccal and labial mucosa. Ulcers are usually 2 to 4 mm in diameter but may coalesce to form larger, irregularly shaped ulcers with scalloped borders. It is rare to see intact blisters in the oral cavity. HSV infections are associated with the development of erythema multiforme.

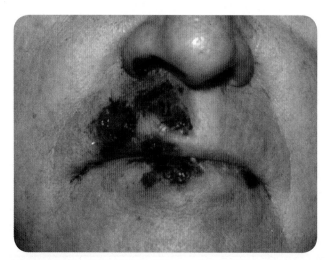

Figure 4-460 Grouped hemorrhagic crusts and ulcers characterize herpes infection.

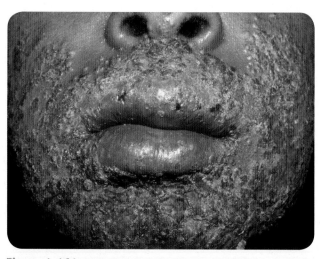

Figure 4-461 Crusted herpetic lesions may be difficult to distinguish from pyogenic infection.

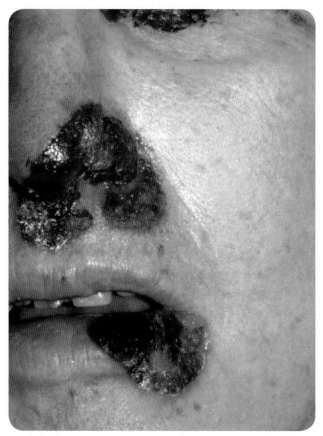

Figure 4-462 Herpetic lesions at skin-mucosal junctions of mouth, eye, and nares.

Immunocompromised Patient Considerations

In the immunocompromised patient, typical lesions may not be seen. Vesicles or erosions may be present, or, alternatively, thick hemorrhagic crusts or eschars may be the only morphologies apparent (Fig. 4-463).

Diagnostic Pearls

- Recurrent episodes do not have the same extent of involvement as the primary infection, unless the host is immunosuppressed.
- Recurrent HSV outbreaks tend to favor keratinized surfaces.

Immunocompromised Patient Considerations

Recurrent episodes can have the extensive involvement of the primary infection in the immunosuppressed host.

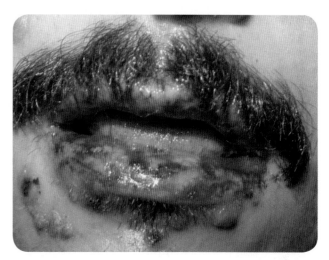

Figure 4-463 Extensive herpes simplex in a patient with AIDS.

?? Differential Diagnosis and Pitfalls

- With primary infection, fever and systemic complaints are more extensive than in immunobullous diseases such as pemphigus.
- Herpangina
- Hand-foot-and-mouth disease
- *Candida*
- Erosive lichen planus
- Stomatitis associated with chemotherapy
- Aphthous ulcers
- Impetigo
- Zoster
- Behçet disease
- Stevens-Johnson syndrome
- Erythema multiforme
- Pemphigus vulgaris
- Acute necrotizing ulcerative gingivitis

✓ Best Tests

- This diagnosis is frequently made on clinical grounds.
- An immediate confirmation of an acute herpetic infection (which includes infection with the varicella-zoster virus [VZV]) can be made by demonstrating multinucleated giant cells on Tzanck preparation.
- Direct fluorescence antigen testing (DFA) is a rapid (<24 h) and sensitive test for HSV-1, HSV-2, and VZV. This test is performed by vigorously scraping the base of a vesicle with a sterile cotton-tipped swab or no. 15 blade and smearing the cells onto a glass slide from a DFA kit. The slide is then fixed (usually contained in a kit) and sent for immunofluorescence analysis. Individual slides must be sent for each virus suspected. Slides can be stored at room temperature for 24 h after fixation, if needed.

- PCR-based clinical assays are rapid, highly sensitive tests for both HSV-1 and HSV-2 detection.
- Diagnosis can also be confirmed within a few days by viral culture.
- Particularly severe presentations of herpetic gingivostomatitis should prompt an investigation into the patient's immune status.

▲▲ Management Pearls

- In severe cases, the patient may be unable to take oral fluids and may need intravenous fluids and pain relief with narcotics.
- If episodes are frequent (six or more per year) and severe, consider suppressive therapy with oral acyclovir. Episodic oral therapy can be used in the patient who experiences tingling before the onset of vesicles. These patients should carry with them at least one oral dose and initiate therapy with the onset of symptoms.
- Advise patients about the risk of autoinoculation (e.g., of the eye), and encourage proper handwashing techniques.

Precautions: Standard and Contact. (Isolate patient, wear gloves and a gown, limit patient transport, and avoid sharing patient-care equipment.)

Therapy

In the past, patients were not prescribed antiviral agents, and the disease was allowed to run its natural, painful course. However, current thinking favors treatment to reduce the period of infectivity and to reduce pain and morbidity.

Pain control is important:

- 2% Viscous lidocaine—Swish and spit out 5 mL four to five times daily, as needed. This can also be mixed with equal volumes of Kaopectate (or Maalox) and Benadryl used in a similar manner.
- 1.0% Dyclonine HCl in aqueous solution—Swish and spit out 5 mL four to five times daily.
- Ice chips and popsicles are helpful for relieving mouth pain and providing some hydration.
- Nonsteroidal anti-inflammatory agents or acetaminophen is often sufficient for pain and fever.

Treatment with acyclovir or its prodrugs (valacyclovir or famciclovir) works best to target the virus. Topical antiviral agents may be useful during the primary episode to decrease viral shedding and patient discomfort, but they are generally less helpful in the management of recurrent outbreaks of HSV. Some topical agents include the following:

- Acyclovir 5% cream applied six times daily for 7 days
- Penciclovir 1% cream applied every 2 h while awake for 4 to 5 days

- Docosanol 10% cream applied five times daily for 5 to 10 days
- Cidofovir cream or gel applied once daily in cases of localized HSV that are resistant to acyclovir

Systemic (Oral) Antiviral Regimens
Acute
- Acyclovir 400 mg p.o. three times daily for 10 days
- Valacyclovir 500 mg p.o. twice daily for 5 days
- Famciclovir 500 mg p.o. three times daily for 5 days

Prophylactic-suppressive
- Acyclovir 400 mg p.o. twice daily
- Famciclovir 250 mg p.o. twice daily
- Valacyclovir 500 to 1,000 mg p.o. daily

Episodic
- Acyclovir 400 mg p.o. three times daily for 5 days
- Valacyclovir 2 g p.o. every 12 h for two doses, must be taken at the first sign of symptoms; or 500 mg p.o. twice daily for 5 days
- Famciclovir 500 mg p.o. three times daily for 5 days

Antistaphylococcal antibiotics (e.g., topical mupirocin) may be used in the prevention or treatment of superficial impetiginization.

Some patients find that outbreaks are triggered by sunlight or sunburn. In these patients, encourage the use of sun-protective clothing (e.g., hats), sunscreens, and sun avoidance.

Suggested Readings

Arduino PG, Porter SR. Oral and perioral herpes simplex virus type 1 (HSV-1) infection: Review of its management. *Oral Dis.* 2006 May;12(3):254–270.

Centers for Disease Control and Prevention, Workowski KA, Berman SM. Sexually transmitted diseases treatment guidelines, 2006. *MMWR Recomm Rep.* 2006 Aug;55(RR-11):1–94.

Fatahzadeh M, Schwartz RA. Human herpes simplex virus infections: Epidemiology, pathogenesis, symptomatology, diagnosis, and management. *J Am Acad Dermatol.* 2007 Nov;57(5):737–763; quiz 764–766.

Gilbert S, Corey L, Cunningham A, et al. An update on short-course intermittent and prevention therapies for herpes labialis. *Herpes.* 2007 Jun;14(Suppl. 1):13A–18A.

Gilbert S, McBurney E. Use of valacyclovir for herpes simplex virus-1 (HSV-1) prophylaxis after facial resurfacing: A randomized clinical trial of dosing regimens. *Dermatol Surg.* 2000 Jan;26(1):50–54.

Miller CS, Cunningham LL, Lindroth JE, Avdiushko SA. The efficacy of valacyclovir in preventing recurrent herpes simplex virus infections associated with dental procedures. *J Am Dent Assoc.* 2004 Sep;135(9):1311–1318.

Miller CS, Redding SW. Diagnosis and management of orofacial herpes simplex virus infections. *Dent Clin North Am.* 1992 Oct;36(4):879–895.

Whitley RJ, Roizman B. Herpes simplex virus infections. *Lancet.* 2001 May;357(9267):1513–1518.

Herpes Zoster (Shingles)

▪▪ Diagnosis Synopsis

Herpes zoster, or shingles, is a reactivation of a latent infection with the varicella-zoster virus, a member of the *Herpesviridae* family. After a primary infection (chickenpox), the virus lays dormant in dorsal root ganglia for life. Reactivation may be triggered by immunosuppression, certain medications, other infections, or different forms of physical or emotional stress. The onset of cutaneous herpes zoster typically involves a 1 to 3 day prodrome of pain or paresthesias in the affected dermatome followed by the eruption of erythematous papules and vesicles in the same distribution. The individual lifetime risk of developing herpes zoster is one in three.

Herpes zoster is usually confined to a distinct dermatome but can also be found in multiple contiguous or noncontiguous dermatomes (zoster multiplex). There may be small islands of lesions at a distant location. Disseminated zoster rarely occurs 5 to 10 days after the onset of dermatomal disease. It is defined as more than 20 lesions outside the initial dermatome of involvement. Associated symptoms can include pain, malaise, and headache. Thoracic dermatomal pain can simulate an acute myocardial infarction. Among herpes zoster patients, 10% to 25% will have eye involvement, termed herpes zoster ophthalmicus.

The most common complication is postherpetic neuralgia, defined as pain and neuropathic symptoms that persist beyond the resolution of the rash. Risk factors include older age, severity of herpes zoster prodromal pain, and severity of pain in the initial clinical presentation of acute herpes zoster. The pain of postherpetic neuralgia can be intractable and debilitating, and one of the goals of treatment is to prevent its development. Neuropathies may occur and include peripheral motor neuropathies, neurogenic bladder, and diaphragmatic paralysis. They are usually transient. Herpes zoster

encephalitis usually appears in the first 2 weeks after the onset of lesions and has a 10% to 20% mortality rate. Lesions are also at risk for bacterial superinfection. In extreme cases, necrotizing fasciitis may occur.

Immunocompromised Patient Considerations

There is an increased incidence of herpes zoster in immunocompromised persons, such as AIDS and cancer patients, transplant recipients, and patients on oral corticosteroids. Episodes of herpes zoster tend to be more extensive and longer lasting in these populations. Additionally, dermatomal herpes zoster is one of the most common immune restoration diseases occurring during the initial months of HAART therapy.

In underlying immunodeficiency, disseminated or generalized herpes zoster, multiple recurrences, systemic infection with visceral dissemination, and CNS involvement such as encephalitis, meningitis, myelitis, and polyneuritis have been reported.

◉ Look For

Grouped vesicles or small bullae on an erythematous base, usually (but not always) confined to a distinct dermatome and not crossing the midline (Figs. 4-464–4-466). The face in the trigeminal, and especially ophthalmic distribution (Fig. 4-467 and 4-468), and the trunk from T3 to L2 are most frequently affected.

Early lesions may be urticarial, grouped papules (Fig. 4-469). Vesicles may be confluent, sparse, or discrete. Commonly, vesicles become hemorrhagic, umbilicated, or

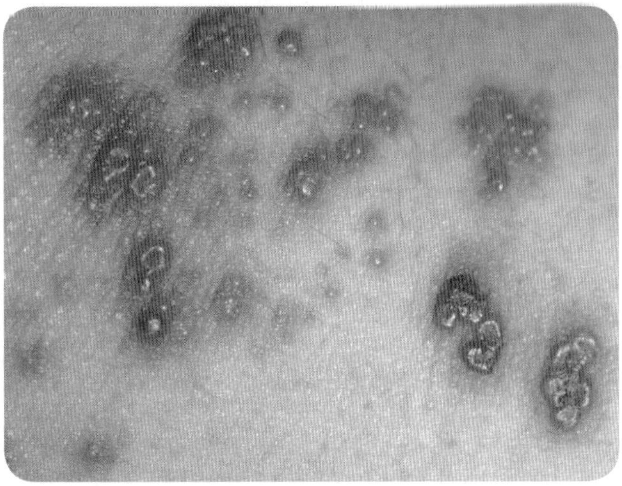

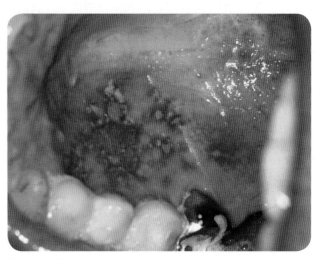

Figure 4-464 Prominent umbilication and some hemorrhagic lesions in herpes zoster.

Figure 4-465 Herpes zoster can involve the oral mucosa, the hard palate in this patient.

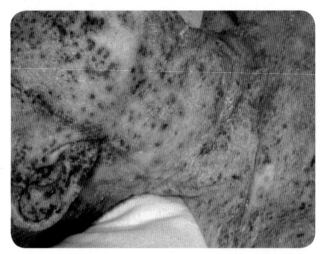

Figure 4-466 Disseminated zoster may be associated with malignancy or immunosuppression.

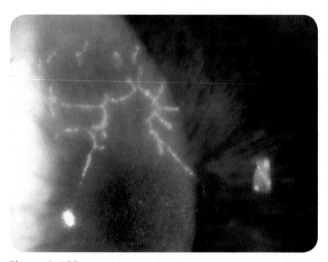

Figure 4-468 Dendritic corneal ulcer with ophthalmic zoster.

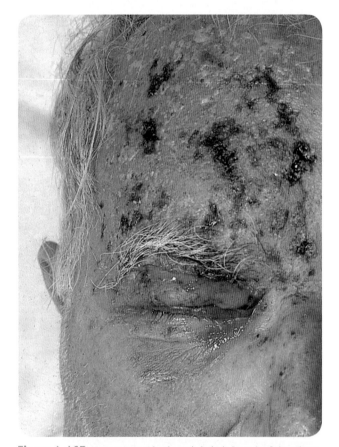

Figure 4-467 Herpes zoster in the ophthalmic branch of the trigeminal nerve often has corneal involvement.

pustular after several days. The lesions typically crust over and resolve after a 7 to 14 day course. Scarring is common.

Regional adenopathy may be seen. Some patients may suffer acute segmental neuralgia, known as zoster sine herpete, without ever developing a skin eruption.

Diagnostic Pearls

- Postherpetic neuralgia is more common in individuals aged older than 70.
- The Ramsey-Hunt syndrome consists of vertigo, ipsilateral facial weakness, and deafness from involvement of the geniculate ganglion.
- The involvement of the nasociliary branch of the ophthalmic nerve increases the risk of ocular complications such as conjunctivitis, lid ulcerations, keratitis, glaucoma, optic neuritis, optic atrophy, and panophthalmitis.

Differential Diagnosis and Pitfalls

- Herpes simplex virus infection
- Cellulitis
- Allergic contact or irritant contact dermatides
- Folliculitis
- Herpangina
- Insect bites
- Molluscum contagiosum
- Poxviruses (cowpox and monkeypox)
- Pyoderma gangrenosum
- Primary varicella infection
- During the prodromal phase, herpes zoster pain may mimic acute myocardial infarction or biliary colic.

Best Tests

- The Tzanck smear is the most rapid and least expensive test. A smear is made of cells scraped from the base of a vesicle or bulla, stained with Wright-Giemsa, and examined under the microscope for multinucleate giant cells.

352

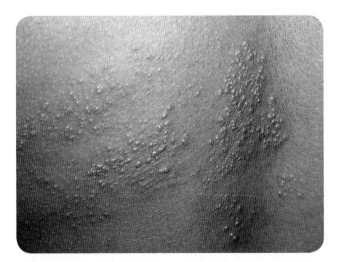

Figure 4-469 Early dermatomal zoster with a few umbilicated vesicles.

- Direct fluorescent antigen (DFA) and viral culture swab are less rapid but are the standard tests used when there is doubt about the diagnosis.
- PCR can be useful for detecting viral DNA in difficult or complicated cases (encephalitis, zoster sine herpete), although most disease is diagnosed clinically by typical appearance and distribution of lesions.
- Electron microscopy is rarely used.
- Consider the following additional tests based on the clinical scenario:
  - HIV testing
  - Lumbar puncture with CSF analysis
  - MRI of brain and/or spinal cord

▲▲ Management Pearls

- Patients with active vesicular lesions can spread the infection to immunocompromised hosts and, if the patient is a health care provider, he/she should take a leave of absence from work.
- The following consultations may be needed: dermatology, neurology, infectious disease, and/or ophthalmology (herpes zoster ophthalmicus).
- The CDC Advisory Committee on Immunization Practices recommends a single dose of the live attenuated zoster vaccine (similar to varicella vaccine but 14 times more potent) for adults aged 60 or older, whether or not they have had a previous episode of herpes zoster. The vaccine is contraindicated in the immunocompromised, those with an allergy to gelatin or neomycin, or those with active untreated tuberculosis. The vaccination decreases risk for both herpes zoster and postherpetic neuralgia.

Therapy

Antiviral therapy (acyclovir and pro-drug forms), if administered in the first 72 h after symptom onset (and possibly beyond that time), can shorten the length and severity of the acute episode and may help to decrease the likelihood of developing postherpetic neuralgia. A single published study supports the use of amitriptyline (25 mg daily) as an adjunct to an antiviral agent in acute herpes zoster to decrease the incidence of and pain associated with subsequent postherpetic neuralgia. Take into account the risk factors for developing postherpetic neuralgia: old age, severe pain in the acute episode of herpes zoster, and presence and severity of prodromal pain. Corticosteroids do not appear to prevent postherpetic neuralgia.

Aluminum acetate or Burow soaks can help to alleviate cutaneous symptoms. Patients routinely require oral analgesia. Consider nonsteroidal anti-inflammatory drugs (NSAIDs) and opioids, including controlled release of oxycodone in patients not rapidly responding to the initial regimen. The simultaneous prescription of stool softeners can prevent opioid-induced constipation. Observe for and promptly treat any secondary bacterial infection.

Antivirals
- Acyclovir 800 mg p.o. every 4 h for 7 to 10 days (frequently given five times daily)
- Famciclovir 500 mg p.o. every 8 h for 7 days
- Valacyclovir 1,000 mg p.o. every 8 h for 7 days

Note: Valacyclovir should not be used in immunosuppressed patients.

Foscarnet 40 mg/kg IV every 8 h for 10 days. Given as a 1-h infusion. This drug is reserved for cases resistant to acyclovir.

Therapies for Postherpetic Neuralgia
- Topical lidocaine 5% patch
- Tricyclic antidepressants (e.g., nortriptyline, start at 10 to 20 mg daily)
- Gabapentin 300 mg p.o. three times daily
- Pregabalin start at 75 mg at bedtime and then advance to up to 300 daily to twice daily
- Weak opioid agonist analgesics (e.g., tramadol 50 to 200 mg daily)
- Strong opioid agonist analgesics (e.g., controlled-release oxycodone)
- Topical capsaicin 0.075% cream

Immunocompromised Patient Considerations

- Acyclovir 10 mg/kg (or 500 mg/m²) IV every 8 h for 7 to 10 days

Suggested Readings

Bowsher D. The effects of pre-emptive treatment of postherpetic neuralgia with amitriptyline: A randomized, double-blind, placebo-controlled trial. *J Pain Symptom Manage*. 1997 Jun;13(6):327–331.

Decroix J, Partsch H, Gonzalez R, et al. Factors influencing pain outcome in herpes zoster: An observational study with valaciclovir. Valaciclovir International Zoster Assessment Group (VIZA). *J Eur Acad Dermatol Venereol*. 2000 Jan;14(1):23–33.

Dworkin RH, Johnson RW, Breuer J, et al. Recommendations for the management of herpes zoster. *Clin Infect Dis*. 2007 Jan;44(Suppl. 1):S1–S26.

Feller L, Wood NH, Lemmer J. Herpes zoster infection as an immune reconstitution inflammatory syndrome in HIV-seropositive subjects: A review. *Oral Surg Oral Med Oral Pathol Oral Radiol Endod*. 2007 Oct;104(4):455–460.

Gilden DH, Kleinschmidt-DeMasters BK, LaGuardia JJ, et al. Neurologic complications of the reactivation of varicella-zoster virus. *N Engl J Med*. 2000 Mar;342(9):635–645.

Harpaz R, Ortega-Sanchez IR, Seward JF; Advisory Committee on Immunization Practices (ACIP) Centers for Disease Control and Prevention (CDC). Prevention of herpes zoster: Recommendations of the Advisory Committee on Immunization Practices (ACIP). *MMWR Recomm Rep*. 2008 Jun;57(RR-5):1–30; quiz CE2–4.

Katz J, Cooper EM, Walther RR, et al. Acute pain in herpes zoster and its impact on health-related quality of life. *Clin Infect Dis*. 2004 Aug;39(3):342–348.

Madkan V, Sra K, Brantley J, et al. Human herpesviruses. In: Bolognia J, Jorizzo JL, Rapini RP, eds. *Dermatology*. 2nd Ed. St. Louis, MO: Mosby; 2008:1204–1208.

Plaghki L, Adriaensen H, Morlion B, et al. Systematic overview of the pharmacological management of postherpetic neuralgia. An evaluation of the clinical value of critically selected drug treatments based on efficacy and safety outcomes from randomized controlled studies. *Dermatology*. 2004;208(3):206–216.

Straus SE, Oxman ME, Schmader KE. Varicella and herpes zoster. In: Fitzpatrick TB, Wolff K, eds. *Fitzpatrick's Dermatology in General Medicine*. 7th Ed. New York, NY: McGraw-Hill; 2008:1885–1898.

Tyler KL, Beckham JD. Management of acute shingles (herpes zoster). *Rev Neurol Dis*. 2007;4(4):203–208.

Tyring SK. Management of herpes zoster and postherpetic neuralgia. *J Am Acad Dermatol*. 2007 Dec;57(6 Suppl.):S136–S142.

Diagnosis Synopsis

Cutaneous larva migrans (also known as creeping eruption, creeping verminous dermatitis, sandworm eruption, plumber's itch, and duck hunter's itch) is a parasitic infestation of the epidermis. It is caused by larvae of hookworms that infect domestic dogs and cats or humans (*Ancylostoma braziliense*, *A. caninum*, *A. duodenale*, and *Necator americanus*). It is usually acquired by walking barefoot on soil or sand contaminated with dog or cat feces that contains the larvae. After contact with the skin, larvae penetrate the epidermis and undergo a prolonged migration through the epidermis in a serpiginous, or "snake-like," fashion. The infection is almost always confined to the outer most layers of the skin (i.e., the epidermis) and very rarely penetrates to subcutaneous tissues and disseminates hematogenously.

Clinically, the cutaneous findings are characterized by intensely pruritic serpiginous tracts localized primarily to the ankles and feet; however, other areas of the body that have contacted infected soil may be involved. Lesions are often edematous, erythematous, and may have associated vesicles and bullae. The majority of patients present with more than one lesion. The migration of larvae begins approximately 4 days after entry and then progresses horizontally about 1 to 2 cm daily. Since the human is a "dead-end" host, the larvae typically spontaneously resolve, although lesions may persist for up to a month. Treatment is often undertaken for relief of intense pruritus and the possibility of bacterial superinfection. The disease is most commonly found in warm climates, with high incidence observed in southeastern United States, Central and South American, Africa, and the Caribbean.

Although rare, larvae can migrate beyond the skin, causing systemic disease characterized by pulmonary infiltrates and peripheral eosinophilia, termed Loeffler syndrome.

Immunocompromised Patient Considerations

Fever may be a presenting sign of cutaneous larva migrans in HIV-infected patients.

Look For

- Pruritic, raised, red, serpiginous, curvilinear trails with or without papules and/or vesicles (Figs. 4-470–4-473).
- The lesions are most commonly found on the ankles and feet but can be found on the buttocks, genitals, hands, or any area with direct contact with sand or soil.

Diagnostic Pearls

The patient almost always has a history of skin exposure to the ground or sand in warm climates. However, it may be weeks or months before the lesions appear, especially if the weather is cold. (The lesions may erupt during the change of seasons when the temperature rises.)

Differential Diagnosis and Pitfalls

- Cercarial forms of nonhuman schistosomes
- Swimmer's itch (cercarial dermatitis)

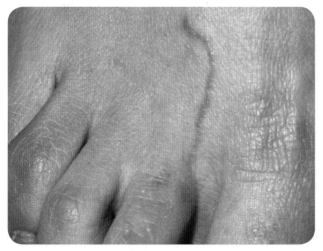

Figure 4-470 A red, serpiginous plaque on a dorsum of the foot is characteristic of cutaneous larva migrans.

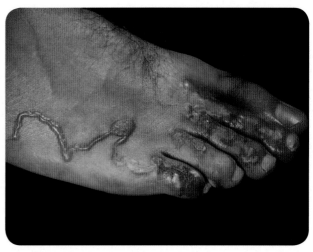

Figure 4-471 Long very, serpiginous plaque of cutaneous larva migrans.

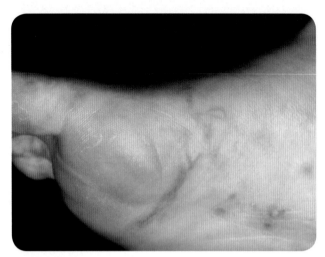

Figure 4-472 Plantar surface with multiple lesions of cutaneous larva migrans.

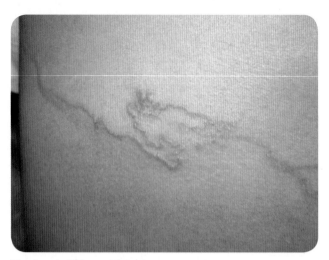

Figure 4-473 Complex serpiginous lesion of cutaneous larva migrans.

- Larval forms of marine coelenterates
- Portuguese man-of-war and jellyfish stings
- Strongyloides infestation
- Erythema annulare centrifugum
- Erythema chronicum migrans
- Figurate erythemas
- Phytophotodermatitis
- Contact dermatitis
- Tinea pedis
- Myiasis
- Loiasis
- Impetigo
- Dracunculiasis
- Gnathostomiasis
- Hookworm
- Foreign body

✓ Best Tests

- The diagnosis of cutaneous larva migrans is made clinically.
- Biopsy is not recommended, as the serpiginous tract lags behind the movement of the worm leading to usually negative or nonspecific biopsy histopathology. Rarely, peripheral eosinophilia may be present.

▲▲ Management Pearls

- Attempts at surgical extraction or treatment with liquid nitrogen should be avoided because the skin findings are a delayed reaction to the parasite (i.e., the worm is not directly under the lesion in most cases).
- This infection is self-limited and will eventually resolve without therapy; however, due to the intense pruritus and risk of superinfection, treatment is recommended.

Therapy

- Albendazole 200 mg p.o. twice daily for 5 days
- Ivermectin 200 µg/kg p.o. once
- Failure with one course of either ivermectin or albendazole is not unusual; simply repeat the course a second time.

Topical 10% to 15% thiabendazole is an option, but it often must be made to order by the pharmacy. Apply four times daily for 1 week. Include the area about 2 cm beyond the leading edge of the serpiginous trail.

Oral thiabendazole is also effective but frequently causes nausea, vomiting, and diarrhea. Dose at 10 mg/lb in patients less than 150 lb, and, at 150 lb or greater, dose with 1.5 g. Dose twice daily for 2 days, and repeat in a week if the lesions are still active.

Suggested Readings

Albanese G, Venturi C, Galbiati G. Treatment of larva migrans cutanea (creeping eruption): A comparison between albendazole and traditional therapy. *Int J Dermatol.* 2001 Jan;40(1):67–71.

Caumes E. Treatment of cutaneous larva migrans. *Clin Infect Dis.* 2000 May;30(5):811–814.

Caumes E, Carriere J, Datry A, et al. A randomized trial of ivermectin versus albendazole for the treatment of cutaneous larva migrans. *Am J Trop Med Hyg.* 1993 Nov;49(5):641–644.

Caumes E, Ly F, Bricaire F. Cutaneous larva migrans with folliculitis: Report of seven cases and review of the literature. *Br J Dermatol.* 2002 Feb;146(2):314–316.

Cayce KA, Scott CM, Phillips CM, et al. What is your diagnosis? Cutaneous larva migrans. *Cutis.* 2007 Jun;79(6):429, 435–436.

Hochedez P, Caumes E. Hookworm-related cutaneous larva migrans. *J Travel Med.* 2007 Sep–Oct;14(5):326–333.

Lederman ER, Weld LH, Elyazar IR, et al. GeoSentinel Surveillance Network. Dermatologic conditions of the ill returned traveler: An analysis from the GeoSentinel Surveillance Network. *Int J Infect Dis*. 2008 Nov;12(6): 593–602.

Nash TE. Visceral Larva Migrans and other unusual Helminth infections. In: Mandell GL, Bennett JE, Dolin R, eds. *Principles and Practice of Infectious Diseases*. 6th Ed. Philadelphia, PA: Elsevier; 2005:3295–3296.

Richey TK, Gentry RH, Fitzpatrick JE, et al. Persistent cutaneous larva migrans due to *Ancylostoma* species. *South Med J*. 1996 Jun;89(6): 609–611.

Roest MA, Ratnavel R. Cutaneous larva migrans contracted in England: A reminder. *Clin Exp Dermatol*. 2001 Jul;26(5):389–390.

Thomé Capuano AC, Catanhede Orsini Machado de Sousa S, Aburad de Carvalhosa A, et al. Larva migrans in the oral mucosa: Report of a case. *Quintessence Int*. 2006 Oct;37(9):721–723.

Veraldi S, Persico MC. HIV, cutaneous larva migrans and fever. *Int J STD AIDS*. 2007 Jun;18(6):433–434.

Miliaria Crystallina

■■ Diagnosis Synopsis

Miliaria is caused by the occlusion of the eccrine sweat ducts. There are various clinical patterns of miliaria depending on the level of occlusion.

Miliaria crystallina results from the blockage of the eccrine sweat duct in the stratum corneum, corresponding to the formation of asymptomatic pinpoint, fragile vesicles. Miliaria crystallina is most common in neonates, but is also seen in adults in the setting of bedridden patients with high fever and excessive sweating. The use of occlusive products prior to exercise may induce this as well. It is also more common in tropical climates.

When the occlusion of the sweat duct is deeper in the epidermis, miliaria rubra (prickly heat), miliaria pustulosa, or miliaria profunda may result.

◉ Look For

Presents with tiny, clear, superficial, noninflammatory vesicles that are 1 to 2 mm in diameter (occasionally larger) (Figs. 4-474–4-476). The vesicles are fragile and do not persist. They may become confluent (Fig. 4-477), and they most commonly involve areas occluded by clothing or bedding. After the vesicles rupture, they may leave behind areas of fine desquamation.

●● Diagnostic Pearls

- Vesicles are very fragile and rupture easily. Lesions are most prominent in areas occluded by bedding or clothing (e.g., the back in bedridden patients).

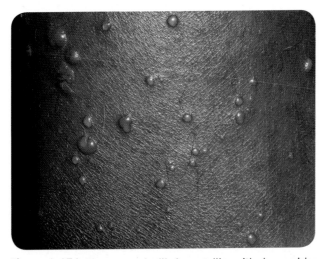

Figure 4-474 Biopsy-proved miliaria crystallina with clear vesicles of varying sizes.

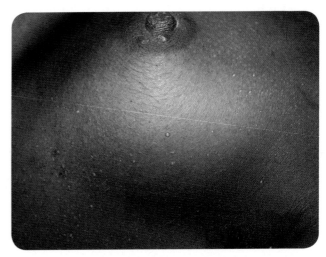

Figure 4-475 Scattered, clear miliarial vesicles on a breast.

Figure 4-476 Scattered, clear vesicles in miliaria crystallina.

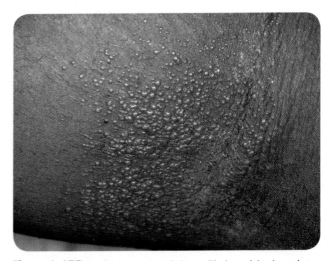

Figure 4-477 Confluent plaque of clear miliaria vesicles in an intertriginous location.

- Patients will often have a history of a recent high fever or a visit/move to a tropical climate.

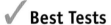 **Differential Diagnosis and Pitfalls**

- Lesions may resemble toxic epidermal necrolysis with the presence of desquamation. However, miliaria crystallina does not have the intense erythema, mucosal involvement, or systemic illness associated with toxic epidermal necrolysis.
- Vesicular drug eruption
- Varicella presents with vesicles on an erythematous base (e.g., "dewdrops on a rose petal") and with lesions in different stages.
- Folliculitis has follicular-based pustules.
- Herpes simplex presents with painful crops of vesicles that often occur near a mucosal surface.

✓ **Best Tests**

- A skin biopsy will confirm the diagnosis but is usually not necessary based on the clinical scenario and exam.
- If there is concern for infection, a culture may be performed.

▲▲▲ **Management Pearls**

- Treat any underlying causes of fever, and avoid occlusive clothing or products.
- Keep the patient in a cool environment; provide air conditioning, if possible.

Therapy

Miliaria crystallina is usually asymptomatic and self-limited; treatment is usually not required.

Cool baths or showers may enhance patient comfort. Encourage patients to wear loose-fitting clothing and expose the involved skin to the air, if possible. Antipyretics can help control fever and prevent subsequent miliaria formation. Patients should avoid heavy emollients, as they may exacerbate the problem.

Suggested Readings

Godkar D, Razaq M, Fernandez G. Rare skin disorder complicating doxorubicin therapy: Miliaria crystallina. *Am J Ther.* 2005 May–Jun;12(3): 275–276.

Haas N, Henz BM, Weigel H. Congenital miliaria crystallina. *J Am Acad Dermatol.* 2002 Nov;47(5 Suppl.):S270–S272.

Haas N, Martens F, Henz BM. Miliaria crystallina in an intensive care setting. *Clin Exp Dermatol.* 2004 Jan;29(1):32–34.

La Shell MS, Tankersley MS, Guerra A. Pruritus, papules, and perspiration. *Ann Allergy Asthma Immunol.* 2007 Mar;98(3):299–302.

▪▪ Diagnosis Synopsis

Porphyrias are the result of an accumulation of metabolites in the heme biosynthetic pathway; enzyme deficiencies are the cause.

Porphyria cutanea tarda (PCT) is the most common porphyria and is caused by an acquired (type I) or inherited autosomal dominant (type II) deficiency of uroporphyrinogen decarboxylase, the fifth of eight enzymes in the pathway. In most cases of PCT, even inherited cases, liver toxicity (e.g., from alcoholism, exogenous estrogens from contraceptives or hormone replacement, hepatitis C virus infection, iron overload, and liver tumors) causes or exacerbates the effects of the enzymatic deficiency. Photoexcitable uroporphyrins accumulate in the skin and damage it, clinically manifesting as skin fragility, blistering, hypertrichosis, scarring, and sclerodermoid features. Patients may also notice urine discoloration. Though historically associated with male alcoholics, an awareness of PCT in women with liver disease or who take exogenous estrogen has increased. The disease usually begins in middle age, sooner in alcoholics. There is no apparent predisposition in any ethnicity. Sun exposure—specifically violet light (wavelength 400 to 410 nm)—plays a major role in lesion development as photoexcited porphyrins generate the reactive oxygen species that damage the skin. Therefore, patients with PCT experience more symptoms in spring and summer months.

Immunocompromised Patient Considerations

PCT has also been reported with an increased frequency in HIV-infected patients; however, the increased incidence may be related to concomitant hepatitis C virus infection, drug-induced hepatotoxicity, or comorbid alcohol abuse.

◉ Look For

Tense vesicles, bullae, and erosions on sun-exposed areas, especially the hands and forearms. Erosions may be crusted and may heal with milia (small, superficial cysts) formation, hyperpigmentation, and hypopigmented atrophic scars (Figs. 4-478–4-480).

The hypertrichosis of the temples or the lateral cheeks is another important finding in PCT.

An erythematous or violaceous discoloration of the face, neck, and/or upper chest may be present.

Severe or advanced disease may exhibit sclerodermoid features, scarring alopecia, and onycholysis.

●● Diagnostic Pearls

- To establish a tentative diagnosis of PCT, immediately examine the patient's urine with a Wood lamp after acidifying it with 10% HCl or acetic acid. Look for an orange-red fluorescence (Fig. 4-481). This test is not particularly sensitive, however, and many tests are falsely negative.
- In the absence of intact bullae, heavily crusted erosions are very suggestive of PCT.

?? Differential Diagnosis and Pitfalls

- Rarely, patients may have an increased dermal fibrosis, resulting in skin that resembles the skin of patients with scleroderma, but they do not have associated GI or renal abnormalities.
- Pseudoporphyria secondary to certain drugs (nonsteroidal anti-inflammatory drugs, vitamin A derivatives, immunosuppressants, and chemotherapeutic agents)—patients have normal porphyrin levels.

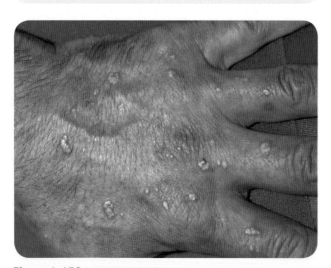

Figure 4-478 Multiple milia on the dorsum of the hands are suggestive of the precursor blisters of PCT.

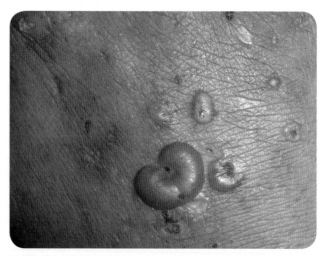

Figure 4-479 Tense blisters and milia in PCT.

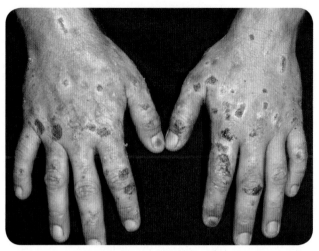

Figure 4-480 Erosions in this location may be the predominant lesion and suggest the need for porphyria testing.

- Variegate porphyria (VP)—may present with skin findings identical to PCT, but patients are also at risk for acute porphyric neurologic crises (not seen in PCT). VP is more common in whites of South African decent and may be differentiated from PCT by the pattern of porphyrins in urine, plasma, and fecal specimens (ratio of urine uroporphyrin to coproporphyrin is approximately 1:1 in VP but up to 8:1 in PCT).
- Hepatoerythropoietic porphyria—childhood onset with rare autosomal recessive uroporphyrin decarboxylase deficiency
- Hereditary coproporphyria
- Hydroa vacciniforme
- Bullous lupus erythematosus
- Photodrug eruption
- Epidermolysis bullosa
- Epidermolysis bullosa acquisita
- Acute dermatomyositis
- Polymorphous light eruption
- Morphea
- Contact dermatitis
- Bullous pemphigoid
- Bullous fixed drug eruption
- Bullous arthropod bites

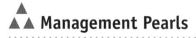 Best Tests

- Serum porphyrins should be analyzed. Uroporphyrins and coproporphyrins can also be measured from a quantitative 24-h urine collection or fecal specimens.
- Skin biopsy may be suggestive but is not diagnostic.

▲▲ Management Pearls

- Stress the importance of sun avoidance until remission can be induced.

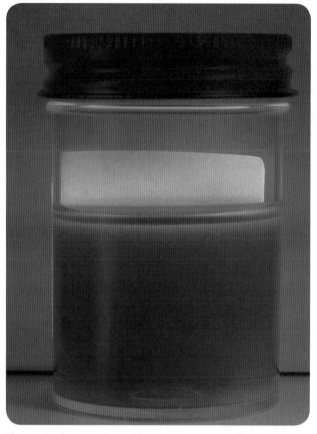

Figure 4-481 Red fluorescence of urine with Wood light in PCT.

- Work with the patient to reduce or eliminate alcohol use. Optimize the management of any hepatitis, if present. Encourage a decrease in consumption of iron-containing foods. Eliminate the use of estrogen, if possible. Ensure an adequate vitamin C intake.
- Depending on the extent of disease and underlying factors, consultations with specialists in hematology, gastroenterology (hepatology), and dermatology may be needed.
- Other tests to consider include the following:
  - Hematologic and iron studies, including serum ferritin and liver function tests
  - Hepatitis serology
  - HIV testing
  - Hemochromatosis gene analysis
  - Liver imaging or biopsy to identify underlying causative liver pathology
  - Fasting blood glucose and antinuclear antibodies (sometimes elevated in PCT)
  - α-fetoprotein may be useful as a screen for hepatocellular carcinoma
- Use urine porphyrin levels to monitor response to therapy.

361

Therapy

Emphasize sun avoidance and the use of broad-spectrum sunscreens such as zinc oxide or titanium dioxide. Sunscreens must cover the lower wavelength visible spectrum (i.e., violet light between 400 and 410 nm) to be helpful in PCT.

First-line specific treatment consists of phlebotomy and antimalarial drugs.

Serial Phlebotomy

Approximately 500 mL of blood should be removed weekly or biweekly (as the patient tolerates) until the hemoglobin reaches a value of 10 to 11 g/dL or until serum iron has reached 60 mg/dL. Many patients demonstrate serum or liver iron overload.

Antimalarials

Chloroquine (low dose)—125 mg twice weekly or hydroxychloroquine 200 mg twice weekly; usually more than a year of therapy is required. The patient must have their visual fields monitored by ophthalmology every 6 months.

Other therapies to consider include chelation with desferrioxamine and subcutaneous erythropoietin (50 to 100 units/kg three times weekly) for those who are anemic, in order to facilitate intermittent phlebotomy.

Suggested Readings

Badminton MN, Elder GH. Management of acute and cutaneous porphyrias. *Int J Clin Pract*. 2002 May;56(4):272–278.

Bickers DR, Frank J. The porphyrias. In: Fitzpatrick TB, Wolff K, eds. *Fitzpatrick's Dermatology in General Medicine*. 7th Ed. New York, NY: McGraw-Hill; 2008:1235–1242.

DeLeo V. Disorders of porphyrin metabolism. In: Spitz JL, ed. *Genodermatoses: A Clinical Guide to Genetic Skin Disorders*. 2nd Ed. Philadelphia, PA: Lippincott Williams & Wilkins; 2005:216–217.

Drobacheff C, Derancourt C, Van Landuyt H, et al. Porphyria cutanea tarda associated with human immunodeficiency virus infection. *Eur J Dermatol*. 1998 Oct–Nov;8(7):492–496.

Drobacheff C, Derancourt C, Van Landuyt H, et al. Porphyria cutanea tarda associated with human immunodeficiency virus infection. *Eur J Dermatol*. 1998 Oct-Nov;8(7):492–496.

Frank J, Poblete-Gutierrez P. Porphyria. In: Bolognia J, Jorizzo JL, Rapini RP, eds. *Dermatology*. 2nd Ed. St. Louis, MO: Mosby; 2008:641–651.

Köstler E, Wollina U. Therapy of porphyria cutanea tarda. *Expert Opin Pharmacother*. 2005 Mar;6(3):377–383.

Norman RA. Past and future: Porphyria and porphyrins. *Skinmed*. 2005 Sep–Oct;4(5):287–292.

Peters TJ, Sarkany R. Porphyria for the general physician. *Clin Med*. 2005 May–Jun;5(3):275–281.

Sarkany RP. The management of porphyria cutanea tarda. *Clin Exp Dermatol*. 2001 May;26(3):225–232.

Sassa S. Modern diagnosis and management of the porphyrias. *Br J Haematol*. 2006 Nov;135(3):281–292.

Smith KE, Fenske NA. Cutaneous manifestations of alcohol abuse. *J Am Acad Dermatol*. 2000 Jul;43(1 Pt 1):1–16; quiz 16–18.

Diabetic Dermopathy

▪▪ Diagnosis Synopsis

Diabetic dermopathy, commonly known as shin spots, is found in 50% of diabetics and is the most common cutaneous finding in patients with diabetes mellitus. The etiology of diabetic dermopathy is unclear. Previously, ischemia had been thought to be a causative factor, but studies found that blood flow to the skin was actually increased when compared to other surrounding areas. Trauma is also thought to be a causative factor. The incidence of diabetic dermopathy ranges from 9% to 55% in patients with diabetes mellitus. There is no clear variation of incidence between diabetic dermopathy in patients with noninsulin-dependant diabetes mellitus versus those with insulin-dependant diabetes mellitus.

There is, however, a correlation between the presence of skin lesions and the number of microangiopathic complications (retinal, neuropathic, and/or nephrogenic) present. As the number of complications present increases from 1 to 3, so does the number of lesions. Thus, the incidence of diabetic dermopathy in patients with all three complications is much higher than in patients with just one complication.

The incidence of diabetic dermopathy increases with age. It is typically seen in patients older than 50 years of age. Men show an increased incidence compared to women. Although located bilaterally, their distribution is asymmetric. Lesions do not itch or cause pain. The control of blood sugar levels does not affect the outcome of the lesions. There is no correlation between diabetic dermopathy and obesity or hypertension.

◉ Look For

Diabetic dermopathy presents as few or many macules, patches, and papular lesions that are dark brown to reddish-brown in color at the anterior lower legs (Figs. 4-482–4-484). They are usually oval, round, or linear in shape and smooth and well demarcated, though some papules can have scale or hemorrhagic crusts. They vary in size from 0.5 cm in diameter up to large patches covering most of the shin. Older lesions are covered with a thin scale, and appear atrophic and hyperpigmented.

Dark Skin Considerations

Diabetic dermopathy is diagnosed less frequently in darker-skinned individuals, perhaps because the macules are more difficult to discern.

●● Diagnostic Pearls

The presence of well-demarcated, hyperpigmented, atrophic scars on the shins of a diabetic patient strongly point to a diagnosis of diabetic dermopathy.

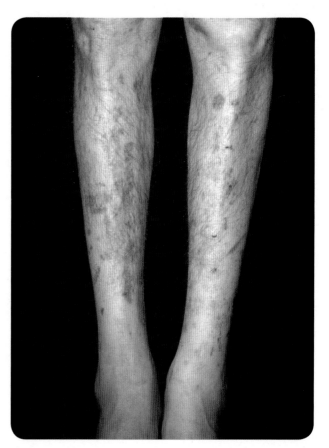

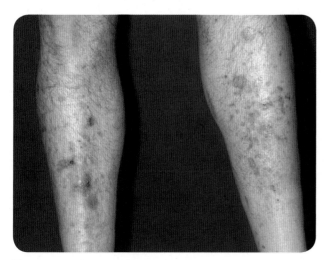

Figure 4-482 Multiple flat or atrophic hyperpigmented lesions characterize diabetic dermopathy.

Figure 4-483 The atrophic pigmented lesions are more prominent on the anterior shins, suggesting a role for trauma.

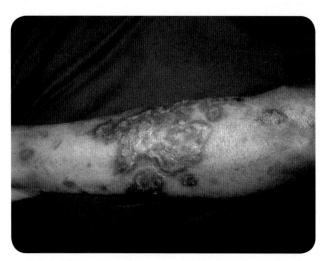

Figure 4-484 Lesions of diabetic dermopathy may occasionally be very hyperpigmented.

?? Differential Diagnosis and Pitfalls

- Stasis dermatitis
- Necrobiosis lipoidica diabeticorum—This entity also occurs on the shins but has a more yellow color and a firm, waxy consistency.
- Granuloma annulare
- Lichen planus
- Postinflammatory hyperpigmentation
- Psoriasis
- Neurotic excoriations
- Capillaritis (Schamberg disease)
- Lichen amyloidosis

✓ Best Tests

Diabetic dermopathy is a clinical diagnosis based on the appearance and location of the typically macular (occasionally papular) lesions.

Management Pearls

Because lesions are asymptomatic, the management of diabetes is the main concern.

Therapy

The treatment of diabetic dermopathy is nonspecific because lesions are asymptomatic. Blood sugar control is of paramount importance.

Suggested Readings

Ahmed I, Goldstein B. Diabetes mellitus. *Clin Dermatol.* 2006 Jul–Aug; 24(4):237–246.

James WD, Berger TG, Elston DM. Errors in metabolism. In: James WD, Berger TG, Elston DM, Odom RB, eds. *Andrews' Diseases of the Skin: Clinical Dermatology.* 10th Ed. Philadelphia, PA: Saunders Elsevier; 2006:540.

Köstler E, Porst H, Wollina U. Cutaneous manifestations of metabolic diseases: uncommon presentations. *Clin Dermatol.* 2005 Sep–Oct;23(5):457–464.

Morgan AJ, Schwartz RA. Diabetic dermopathy: A subtle sign with grave implications. *J Am Acad Dermatol.* 2008 Mar;58(3):447–451.

Romano G, Moretti G, Di Benedetto A, et al. Skin lesions in diabetes mellitus: prevalence and clinical correlations. *Diabetes Res Clin Pract.* 1998 Feb;39(2):101–106.

Wigington G, Ngo B, Rendell M. Skin blood flow in diabetic dermopathy. *Arch Dermatol.* 2004 Oct;140(10):1248–1250.

Necrobiosis Lipoidica

■■ Diagnosis Synopsis

Necrobiosis lipoidica (NL) is a disorder of collagen degeneration with granuloma formation and fat deposition. The exact cause is not known, but many theories have focused on the role of diabetic microangiopathy due to NL's strong association with diabetes mellitus, more commonly type I diabetes. Multiple studies have estimated the percentage of patients with diabetes at the time of presentation to range from 11% to 65%. Many more patients will have impaired glucose tolerance tests, develop diabetes at a later date, or have a positive family histories of diabetes. However, this disorder may occur in patients who are not diabetic.

NL typically presents with asymptomatic shiny, red-brown patches on the shins that are brought to a clinician's attention for cosmetic reasons. Occasionally, ulcerations and pain will occur after trauma to the areas. These lesions slowly enlarge over the course of months to years. NL may occur at any age, and there is no racial predilection. Women are affected three times as often as men.

Treatment for NL remains largely unsatisfactory, and the disease process is chronic and, for the most part, progressive.

◉ Look For

The presenting lesions of NL are often red-brown papules or nodules that enlarge over time. NL may also present as similarly colored patches or plaques.

Over time, these lesions coalesce into plaques and become yellow-brown, waxy, and atrophic centrally (Figs. 4-485 and 4-486). Telangiectasias are characteristic of NL.

Ulcers can occur at the sites of trauma and may be painful (Figs. 4-487 and 4-488).

NL most commonly affects the pretibial area, but other common locations are the ankles, calves, thighs, and feet. They are usually bilateral. Lesions have also been reported on the face, scalp, trunk, and arms.

Dark Skin Considerations

The characteristic yellow-brown color of chronic atrophic lesions may be difficult to appreciate in dark-skinned patients.

Lesions of cutaneous sarcoidosis may closely mimic NL.

●● Diagnostic Pearls

- NL tends to develop at an earlier age in patients with pre-existing diabetes.
- Koebnerization (lesions developing at trauma sites) may take place in NL.
- Upper extremity lesions tend to be more papulonodular in appearance.

?? Differential Diagnosis and Pitfalls

- Granuloma annulare
- Sarcoidosis
- Xanthomas
- Diabetic dermopathy
- Stasis dermatitis
- Epithelioid sarcoma
- Rheumatoid nodule(s)

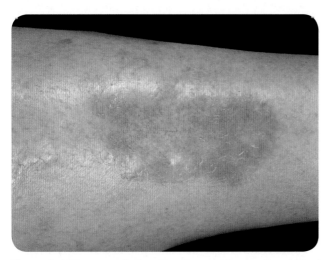

Figure 4-485 NL as a single yellow plaque with some dilated blood vessels on the shin, a characteristic location.

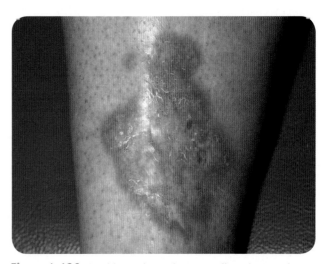

Figure 4-486 NL with scarring and orange-yellow pigmentation.

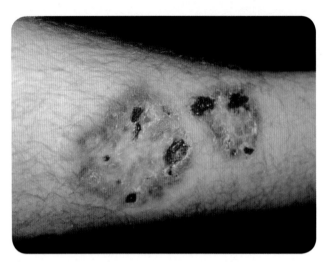

Figure 4-487 NL with severe atrophy and ulceration.

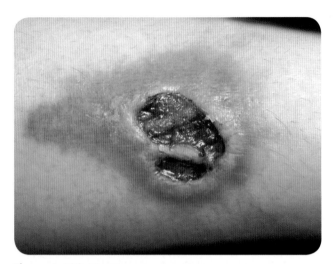

Figure 4-488 NL with severe ulceration.

- Necrobiotic xanthogranuloma
- Panniculitis, including erythema nodosum
- Morphea
- Lichen sclerosus
- Leprosy
- Deep fungal infections

Immunocompromised Patient Differential Diagnosis

It is important to rule out granulomatous infections including deep fungal, leprosy, and tertiary syphilis in this population.

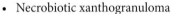

✓ Best Tests

Biopsy is characteristic.

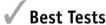

▲▲ Management Pearls

- In diabetics, the severity (or frequency) of the disease does not correlate with the degree of glycemic control. Nevertheless, it remains in the patient's best interest to optimize glucose control and to cease smoking, if applicable, to prevent further and future vascular compromise. Diabetics with NL have higher rates of retinopathy and neuropathy.
- Some clinicians advocate checking a glucose tolerance test to rule out occult diabetes in patients presenting with NL.
- Squamous cell cancers have been rarely reported in lesions of NL, related to trauma and chronic ulceration.

Therapy

Numerous therapies have been tried, but a substantial body of evidence to recommend some definitively over others is lacking.

Intralesional triamcinolone and 0.1% betamethasone under occlusion have demonstrated some success, as have the antiplatelet agents aspirin and dipyridamole. Systemic corticosteroids tapered over 5 weeks were effective in a small case series, though hyperglycemia was a reported side effect. There are single case reports and small series reporting the efficacy of pentoxifylline, topical tacrolimus, infliximab, psoralen plus UVA (PUVA), tretinoin, ticlopidine, mycophenolate mofetil, nicotinamide, clofazimine, and perilesional heparin injections.

Pulsed dye laser has been used to successfully treat prominent telangiectases.

In diabetics, ulcer prevention with leg rest, support stockings, and glucose control is important. If ulcers should develop, the same basic principles of meticulous wound care as for all diabetics apply.

Cyclosporine 2.5 mg/kg/day has healed ulcerated NL in a few cases, as has GM-CSF.

Surgical excision with split-thickness skin grafting should be kept as a last resort for recalcitrant ulcers.

A theoretical basis for the use of inhibitors of the gli-1 oncogene (including tacrolimus and sirolimus), which is upregulated in NL, has been described and may guide future therapeutic investigations.

Suggested Readings

Howard A, White CR Jr. Non-infectious granulomas. In: Bolognia J, Jorizzo JL, Rapini RP, eds. *Dermatology.* 2nd Ed. St. Louis, MO: Mosby; 2008:1429–1431.

Körber A, Dissemond J. Necrobiosis lipoidica diabeticorum. *CMAJ.* 2007 Dec 4;177(12):1498.

Köstler E, Porst H, Wollina U. Cutaneous manifestations of metabolic diseases: Uncommon presentations. *Clin Dermatol.* 2005 Sep–Oct; 23(5):457–464.

Macaron NC, Cohen C, Chen SC, et al. gli-1 Oncogene is highly expressed in granulomatous skin disorders, including sarcoidosis, granuloma annulare, and necrobiosis lipoidica diabeticorum. *Arch Dermatol.* 2005 Feb;141(2):259–262.

Marinella MA. Necrobiosis lipoidica diabeticorum. *Lancet.* 2002 Oct 12; 360(9340):1143.

McDonald L, Zanolli MD, Boyd AS. Perforating elastosis in necrobiosis lipoidica diabeticorum. *Cutis.* 1996 May;57(5):336–338.

Mendoza V, Vahid B, Kozic H, Weibel S. Clinical and pathologic manifestations of necrobiosis lipoidica-like skin involvement in sarcoidosis. *Joint Bone Spine.* 2007 Dec;74(6):647–649.

Moreno-Arias GA, Camps-Fresneda A. Necrobiosis lipoidica diabeticorum treated with the pulsed dye laser. *J Cosmet Laser Ther.* 2001 Sep;3(3): 143–146.

Yorav S, Feinstein A, Ziv R, Kaplan B, Schewach-Millet M. Diffuse necrobiosis lipoidica diabeticorum. *Cutis.* 1992 Jul;50(1):68–69.

Poikiloderma of Civatte

Diagnosis Synopsis

Poikiloderma of Civatte is a chronic benign skin condition caused by long-term sun exposure in fair-skinned adults. Poikiloderma of Civatte refers to a specific pattern of mottled erythema involving the lateral neck and the superior medial chest. Poikiloderma involves the clinical triad of telangiectasia, hyperpigmentation and/or hypopigmentation, and superficial (epidermal or superficial dermal) atrophy. This condition is typically brought to the attention of the clinician as a new rash even though it develops slowly over months to years. As many as half of all patients may complain of mild itching, burning, or flushing in affected areas. Poikiloderma of Civatte is a cosmetic problem typically affecting women more frequently than men and typically appears in and after the fifth decade of life. Contact sensitization to chemicals present in fragrances and cosmetics has been proposed as a cofactor in the development of this disorder.

Look For

Lateral and anterior neck with mottled pigmentation and erythema (Figs. 4-489–4-491). Fine telangiectasias are frequently seen. The lateral aspects of the midface (parotid and preauricular areas) are also commonly involved.

Dark Skin Considerations

Given its likely relationship to accumulated photodamage, poikiloderma of Civatte is rarely seen in patients of Fitzpatrick skin type IV and higher.

Diagnostic Pearls

Mottled erythema at the neck and superior chest with sparing of the naturally shaded area below the chin is the distribution of this condition (Fig. 4-492). Perifollicular skin is typically spared.

Differential Diagnosis and Pitfalls

- Contact dermatitis
- Photodermatitis
- Dermatomyositis
- Systemic lupus erythematosus
- Cutaneous T-cell lymphoma
- Parapsoriasis
- Bloom syndrome
- Rothmund-Thomson syndrome
- Melasma
- Erythromelanosis follicularis faciei
- Mastocytosis

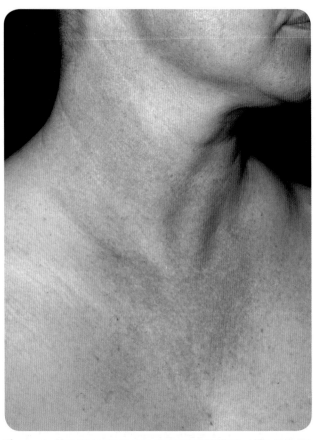

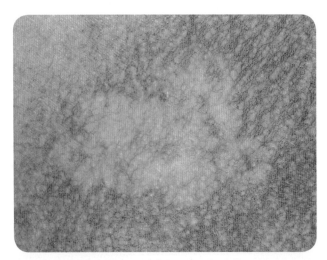

Figure 4-489 Prominent red follicular papules characterize poikiloderma of Civatte.

Figure 4-490 Wide band of sparing beneath the mandible in poikiloderma of Civatte.

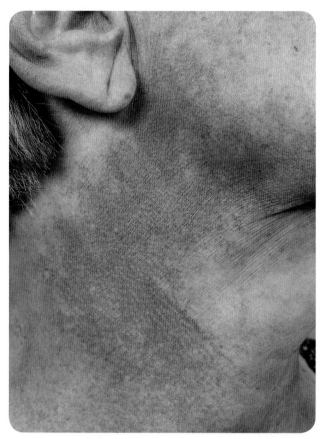

Figure 4-491 Facial involvement with the poikiloderma of Civatte is not unusual.

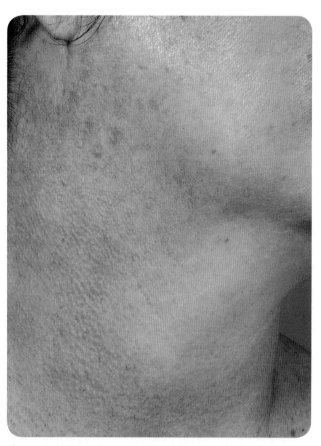

Figure 4-492 Poikiloderma of Civatte typically has patches of normal skin under the neck, where the skin has been protected from sunlight.

✓ Best Tests

This is a clinical diagnosis, although a skin biopsy will be confirmatory. Skin biopsy will reveal irregular basilar pigmentation, solar elastosis, telangiectasias, and mild epidermal atrophy.

▲▲ Management Pearls

Poikiloderma of Civatte is a benign condition for which treatment is optional and for cosmetic purposes only.

Therapy

If the patient is desirous of treatment, skin appearance can often be improved with pulsed-dye (685 to 695 nm) or KTP (potassium-titanyl-phosphate, 532 nm) laser treatments. Intense pulsed light systems have also produced beneficial results.

Sun avoidance and sun-protection measures (e.g., sunscreens and hats) will help to prevent worsening.

Suggested Readings

Batta K, Hindson C, Cotterill JA, Foulds IS. Treatment of poikiloderma of Civatte with the potassium titanyl phosphate (KTP) laser. *Br J Dermatol.* 1999 Jun;140(6):1191–1192.

Katoulis AC, Stavrianeas NG, Georgala S, et al. Poikiloderma of Civatte: A clinical and epidemiological study. *J Eur Acad Dermatol Venereol.* 2005 Jul;19(4):444–448.

Katoulis AC, Stavrianeas NG, Katsarou A, et al. Evaluation of the role of contact sensitization and photosensitivity in the pathogenesis of poikiloderma of Civatte. *Br J Dermatol.* 2002 Sep;147(3):493–497.

Katoulis AC, Stavrianeas NG, Panayiotides JG, et al. Poikiloderma of Civatte: A histopathological and ultrastructural study. *Dermatology.* 2007;214(2):177–182.

Langeland J. Treatment of poikiloderma of Civatte with the pulsed dye laser: A series of seven cases. *J Cutan Laser Ther.* 1999 Apr;1(2):127.

Lim HW, Hawk JL. Photodermatoses. In: Bolognia J, Jorizzo JL, Rapini RP, eds. *Dermatology.* 2nd Ed. St. Louis, MO: Mosby; 2008:1349.

Pérez-Bernal A, Muñoz-Pérez MA, Camacho F. Management of facial hyperpigmentation. *Am J Clin Dermatol.* 2000 Sep–Oct;1(5):261–268.

Ross BS, Levine VJ, Ashinoff R. Laser treatment of acquired vascular lesions. *Dermatol Clin.* 1997 Jul;15(3):385–396.

Rusciani A, Motta A, Fino P, et al. Treatment of poikiloderma of Civatte using intense pulsed light source: 7 years of experience. *Dermatol Surg.* 2008 Mar;34(3):314–349; discussion 319.

Radiation Dermatitis

Diagnosis Synopsis

Radiation-induced dermatitis is typically caused by radiotherapy for underlying malignancies. It may also result from exposure to radiation during interventional procedures such as coronary angiography, embolization procedures, and indwelling catheter placements. Radiation-induced skin injury occurs instantaneously following radiation exposure and is due to an impairment of functional stem cells, endothelial cell changes, inflammation, and epidermal cell apoptosis and necrosis.

Radiosensitizing agents act concomitantly to worsen skin damage. Pathophysiologic mechanisms leading to radiation-induced dermatitis can be classified as acute or chronic.

Acute Radiation Dermatitis

This occurs within 90 days of exposure. The patient may have changes ranging from faint erythema and dry desquamation to skin necrosis and ulceration, depending on the severity of the reaction. The National Cancer Institute has developed a four-stage criterion for the classification of acute radiation dermatitis:

- Grade 1—Faint erythema or dry desquamation.
- Grade 2—Moderate to brisk erythema or patchy, moist desquamation confined to skin folds and creases. Moderate edema.
- Grade 3—Confluent, moist desquamation greater than 1.5 cm diameter, which is not confined to the skin folds. Pitting edema.
- Grade 4—Skin necrosis or ulceration of full thickness dermis.

Chronic Radiation Dermatitis

This is an extension of the acute process and involves further inflammatory cytokines. Long-lasting impairment of the skin's ability to heal can be due to compromised cellular dysfunction. Fibroblasts may be permanently altered, leading to atrophy and fibrosis.

Onset may occur from 15 days to 10 years after the beginning of the procedure. There is no increased predilection for radiation injuries between men and women. The predominance in males of radiation dermatitis merely reflects the higher incidence of coronary artery disease and subsequent increased use of fluoroscopic procedures for therapeutic purposes.

Radiation Recall

This is a well-documented phenomenon that occurs at sites of previous radiation therapy, after an antineoplastic agent (e.g., methotrexate and etoposide) is given. The reaction may occur weeks to years after radiation. As in acute radiation dermatitis, it is graded according to the severity of the cutaneous reaction and ranges from erythema to necrosis, ulceration, and hemorrhage. It tends to occur when cytotoxic agents are used following the completion of radiotherapy. Radiation recall has also been seen after the use of drugs such as nonsteroidal antiestrogens, interferon alpha-2b, and antituberculosis drugs.

Risk factors for radiation dermatitis in the general population are as follows:

- Poor nutritional status
- Problems with skin integrity
- Overlapping skin folds
- Prolonged or multiple procedures requiring radiation exposure
- Increased exposure, especially in obese patients. (Larger patients require higher doses of radiation and are, therefore, more susceptible to developing skin changes.)
- Total radiation doses of greater than 55 Gy, or large individual doses per fraction (>3 to 4 Gy per dose)
- Concurrent cetuximab therapy in patients receiving radiation for head and neck malignancies

Certain diseases and syndromes increase the risk of radiation dermatitis:

- Connective tissue diseases (systemic lupus erythematosus, scleroderma, or mixed connective tissue diseases). Peripheral blood lymphocytes from patients with rheumatoid arthritis, systemic lupus erythematosus, and polymyositis are more radiosensitive and exhibit greater DNA damage after irradiation. Thus, the presence of connective tissue diseases is a contraindication to radiation therapy.
- Diseases with reduced cellular DNA capability, such as hereditary nevoid basal cell carcinoma.
- Diseases involving chromosomal breakage syndromes, like Fanconi anemia and Bloom syndrome.
- Homozygosity for the ataxia telangiectasia gene.
- Infectious diseases—Patients with HIV show a reduced tolerance of the skin and mucous membranes to treatment. Not only do they develop cutaneous changes at lower doses but they also cause more significant systemic problems.
- Diabetes mellitus
- Radiosensitizing drugs (e.g., paclitaxel or docetaxel) given before or up to 7 days after radiation therapy increase cellular damage.

Secondary cutaneous malignancy may also result from radiation therapy. The most common type occurring is basal cell carcinoma.

Immunocompromised Patient Considerations

An increased rate of cutaneous reactions, including bullous eruptions, has been reported in patients with HIV receiving radiotherapy.

Look For

Acute Radiation Dermatitis

The cutaneous changes seen here depend on the time that the symptoms appear. Signs will be localized to the site of radiation, but be sure to examine both sites of entry and exit portals.

Early changes (days to weeks)

- Erythema
- Dermal necrosis
- Edema and blister formation
- Desquamation
- Acute ulceration
- Epilation

Late changes (months to years)

- Hypopigmentation
- Hyperpigmentation
- Telangiectasia
- Skin induration
- Alopecia
- Epidermal atrophy, fragility
- Recurrent erosions
- Severe ulceration
- Scarring

Very late changes

- Necrosis
- Chronic ulceration
- Squamous cell carcinoma

Chronic Radiation Dermatitis

Symptoms may not appear for months to years after exposure. Some changes are temporary, such as the edematous peau d'orange appearance of breast skin following radiation. Other changes, such as postinflammatory hypopigmentation or hyperpigmentation, may persist or take longer to resolve (Figs. 4-493 and 4-494).

Signs of chronic radiation dermatitis

- Xerosis
- Hyperkeratosis
- Desquamation
- Telangiectasia

- Permanent loss of nail and skin appendages, including alopecia and/or decreased or absent sweating/loss of sweat glands
- Fibrosis leading to tissue retraction, limitation of movement, and pain

Diagnostic Pearls

- Radiation dermatitis typically shows a geometric pattern on the skin that follows the field of exposure. Circle and square shapes are common patterns.
- Changes may appear at both entry and exit portals.

Differential Diagnosis and Pitfalls

Acute

- Dermatitis
- Allergic contact dermatitis
- Cellulitis/erysipelas
- Carcinoma erysipeloids
- Primary/autoimmune blistering disease

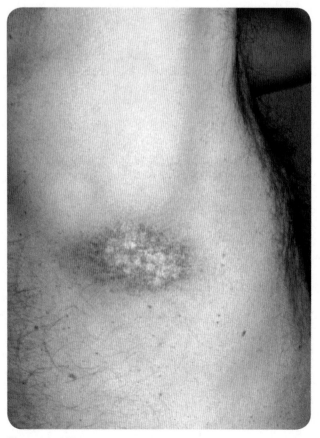

Figure 4-493 Atrophy and telangiectasias 10 years after radiation therapy for a skin lesion.

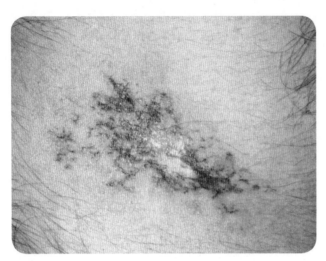

Figure 4-494 Poikiloderma with hypopigmentation and hyperpigmentation and telangiectasias 10 years after radiation therapy.

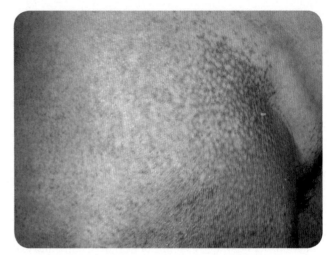

Figure 4-495 Poikiloderma vasculare atrophicans, often a precursor to mycosis fungoides, for comparison to radiodermatitis.

Chronic

- Poikilodermatous mycosis fungoides (Fig. 4-495)
- Morphea
- Lichen sclerosus et atrophicus
- Graft-versus-host disease (chronic and sclerodermatous)
- Carcinoma en cuirasse
- Scleredema
- Scleromyxedema
- Nephrogenic systemic fibrosis
- A prodromal nonspecific dermatitic eruption at the irradiation portal should not be interpreted as radiation dermatitis.

✓ Best Tests

- There are no specific tests for radiation dermatitis. Diagnosis is based on history, physical findings, and ruling out other conditions.
- Lab tests are generally done to rule out other diagnoses.
- Because connective tissue diseases are a predisposing factor, tests for antinuclear antibodies and rheumatoid factor should be obtained.

▲▲ Management Pearls

Radiation necrosis caused by high-dose radiotherapy is difficult to manage due to impaired healing and superinfection that occurs in these tissues.

Prevention

Skin damage may be prevented or minimized by the following actions:

- Continuous surveillance of X-ray dose
- Keeping irradiated areas as small as possible

Therapy

Treatment will vary according to the severity of skin injury and whether it is acute or chronic radiation dermatitis.

Acute Radiation Dermatitis

Early changes of erythema and dry desquamation should be treated symptomatically to prevent progression to moist desquamation. The site should be washed with either water alone or combined with a low-pH soap. Washing limits bacterial presence, thereby reducing chances of superantigen-induced inflammation. Petroleum-based emollients used to treat skin dryness are usually better tolerated than a cream form.

Later changes of erosions and ulcers involve the use of dressings, which serve the purpose of absorbing secretions, protecting against contamination, and pain control.

- Hydrocolloid dressing can be used for wounds that are minimally exudative.
- Alginate or foam dressings for wounds that are highly exudative.
- Radioemulsions (thought to be radioprotective), such as trolamine, act by being macrophage stimulators that remove necrotic tissue, promote fibroblast formation, and reduce vascular alteration and promote epithelial cell proliferation. Although controlled studies show no clinical radioprotective effect, patients express satisfaction with these ointments.
- Ionic silver pads or topical antibiotics may be used for infected wounds.

Avoid neomycin, a frequent cause of allergic contact dermatitis. Patients should limit the use of topical irritants such as perfumes and deodorants. They should wear clothes that fit well but do not stick to the skin.

Systemic treatment with pentoxyphylline 400 to 800 mg p.o. three times daily and/or pyridoxine 50 to 150 mg twice daily can be helpful.

Chronic Radiation Dermatitis

Debridement of the ulcer can be achieved in a number of ways:

- Mechanical debridement involves removing eschars with the patient under local anesthesia.
- Enzymatic debridement or autolytic dressings may also be used (DuoDERM or Tegasorb).
- Oral antibiotics may be necessary for infected wounds.
- Chronic fibrosis may be minimized by physical therapy and deep massage.
- Intramuscular injections of liposomal copper/zinc superoxide dismutase twice weekly for 2 weeks have shown some regression of fibrosis.
- Hyperbaric oxygen therapy leads to reepithelialization of small areas in addition to reducing pain, edema, erythema, and lymphedema.
- Pulsed-dye laser treatment may be used for radiation-induced telangiectasia.
- Deep ulceration may require surgical debridement with skin grafting.

Suggested Readings

Aistars J, Vehlow K. Radiation dermatitis. *Oncology* (*Williston Park*). 2007 Jul;21(8 Suppl.):41–43.

Frazier TH, Richardson JB, Fabré VC, et al. Fluoroscopy-induced chronic radiation skin injury: A disease perhaps often overlooked. *Arch Dermatol.* 2007 May;143(5):637–640.

Giro C, Berger B, Bölke E, et al. High rate of severe radiation dermatitis during radiation therapy with concurrent cetuximab in head and neck cancer: Results of a survey in EORTC institutes. *Radiother Oncol.* 2009 Feb;90(2):166–171.

Hivnor CM, Seykora JT, Junkins-Hopkins J, et al. Subacute radiation dermatitis. *Am J Dermatopathol.* 2004 Jun;26(3):210–212.

Jain S, Agarwal J, Laskar S, Gupta T, et al. Radiation recall dermatitis with gatifloxacin: a review of literature. *J Med Imaging Radiat Oncol.* 2008 Apr;52(2):191–193.

Smith ML. Environmental and sports-related skin diseases. In: Bolognia J, Jorizzo JL, Rapini RP, eds. *Dermatology.* 2nd Ed. St. Louis, MO: Mosby; 2008:1356–1357.

Smith KJ, Skelton HG, Tuur S, et al. Increased cutaneous toxicity to ionizing radiation in HIV-positive patients. Military Medical Consortium for the Advancement of Retroviral Research (MMCARR). *Int J Dermatol.* 1997 Oct;36(10):779–782.

Scleroderma

◼ Diagnosis Synopsis

Scleroderma, or systemic sclerosis, is an autoimmune connective tissue disease that involves sclerotic changes of the skin and internal organs. While the etiology remains unknown, the disease is characterized by autoantibody production, collagen deposition, and vascular dysfunction. The disease is observed in all ages and races but is slightly more common in blacks and three to four times more common in women. The age of onset is usually between 30 and 50 years.

Scleroderma can affect the connective tissue of any organ, including the skin, gastrointestinal tract, lungs, kidneys, joints, muscles, heart, and blood vessels. Pulmonary disease is the leading cause of mortality. Additional common clinical features include esophageal fibrosis and dysmotility, arthralgias, and Raynaud phenomenon. Less common manifestations include hypertensive renal crisis, pulmonary hypertension and interstitial lung disease, and cardiomyopathy.

The major diagnostic criterion for scleroderma is symmetric sclerosis of the skin proximal to the metacarpophalangeal or metatarsophalangeal joints. Minor criteria include bibasilar pulmonary fibrosis, sclerodactyly, substance loss of the finger pad, and digital pitting scars. Note that scleroderma is mainly a clinical diagnosis with one major criterion or two minor criteria satisfying the American College of Rheumatology classification scheme. Autoantibodies assist in the diagnosis. More than 90% of patients, limited or diffuse, will demonstrate elevated antinuclear antibodies (ANA) titers with a discrete speckled or nucleolar pattern. Additional autoantibodies include anti-Scl-70 antibody, which confers an increased risk for pulmonary involvement; anti-centromere antibodies, which are more often seen with limited disease; and anti-RNP antibodies, which are more often seen with diffuse disease.

There are two major subsets of scleroderma: limited scleroderma and diffuse scleroderma. Note that limited and diffuse refer to the degree of cutaneous involvement and that both subsets demonstrate internal organ involvement. Internal organ involvement occurs decades after initial diagnosis in the limited form and within 5 years in the diffuse form, carrying a worse prognosis.

Additional risk factors that confer a worse prognosis include internal organ involvement at presentation, male gender, sclerotic changes of the trunk, elevated ESR, black ethnicity, and older age at presentation.

Variants of limited scleroderma are the following:

- CREST syndrome (calcinosis, Raynaud phenomenon, esophageal dysmotility, syndactyly, and telangiectasias) refers to a subset of patients with limited scleroderma.
- Systemic sclerosis sine scleroderma refers to a subset of patients with limited scleroderma that demonstrate internal organ involvement and positive serologies but no cutaneous disease.

◉ Look For

Cutaneous changes include the following:

- Induration and taut, shiny skin.
- Pigmentary changes including diffuse hyperpigmentation as well as depigmentation with sparing of perifollicular skin, giving a salt-and-pepper appearance (Fig. 4-496). This is especially common on the back and legs.
- Telangiectasias that are most commonly seen on the lips, palms, and proximal nailfolds (Figs. 4-497 and 4-498). Of note, the telangiectasias are flat, in contrast to the raised telangiectasias observed in hereditary hemorrhagic telangiectasia.
- Calcinosis cutis of the fingers.
- Raynaud phenomenon resulting in cutaneous ulcers of the digits (Fig. 4-499). Acutely, this can appear as transient red, blue, or white changes in the skin of the fingers or toes (Fig. 4-500).
- The face may develop a characteristic "beak-like" appearance. There is a paucity of wrinkling.
- Sclerodactyly and joint contractures with the loss of skin creases.

Limited cutaneous scleroderma usually involves the distal extremities and may involve the face and neck. The diffuse form of scleroderma has additional sclerotic changes of the trunk and proximal extremities.

Diagnostic Pearls

Because many of the features of scleroderma are nonspecific, care must be taken to consider other clinical diseases that overlap with scleroderma. These include overlap

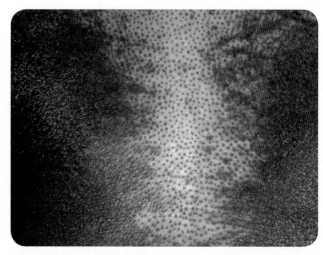

Figure 4-496 Scleroderma frequently has hypopigmented follicular areas surrounded by normal or hyperpigmented skin (salt and pepper pattern).

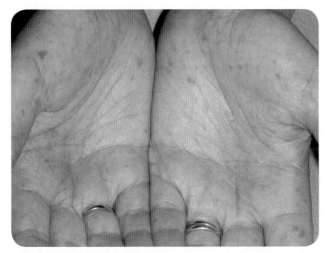

Figure 4-497 A form of scleroderma, CREST syndrome has prominent telangiectasias on the hands, face, and mucosal surfaces.

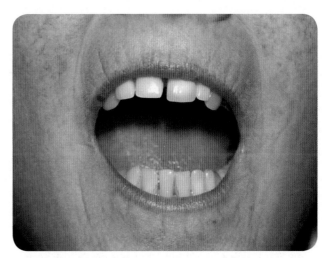

Figure 4-498 Linear furrows on the lips and decreased oral aperture are common in scleroderma.

with rheumatoid arthritis, systemic lupus erythematosus, polymyositis, and rarely vasculitis. Consideration of additional serologies is important if symptoms of these other conditions are present.

?? Differential Diagnosis and Pitfalls

- Generalized morphea—Asymmetric induration, no Raynaud phenomenon, no systemic involvement
- Scleredema—ANA negative, no Raynaud phenomenon, no systemic involvement
- Scleromyxedema—ANA and anticentromere negative, no Raynaud phenomenon, no sclerodactyly
- Generalized myxedema
- Graft-versus-host disease—ANA negative, vascular abnormalities such as Raynaud phenomenon absent

- Eosinophilic fasciitis—ANA negative, no Raynaud phenomenon, no facial involvement
- Nephrogenic fibrosing dermopathy—Look for the recent history of radiologic imaging with gadolinium-based intravenous contrast in patients with renal insufficiency or renal transplant patient; ANA negative, no sclerodactyly, no Raynaud phenomenon
- Stiff skin syndrome—Characteristic sparing of the hands and feet, develops during early childhood, systemic involvement rare
- Porphyria cutanea tarda
- Phenylketonuria
- Polyvinyl chloride exposure—ANA negative, cutaneous changes reverse with the cessation of exposure
- Carcinoid
- Cutaneous T-cell lymphoma
- Amyloidosis

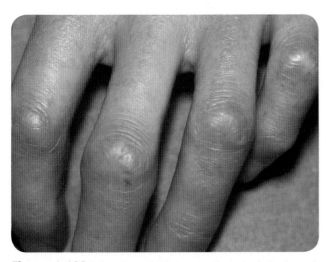

Figure 4-499 Sclerosis and tiny scars from healed ulcers in scleroderma.

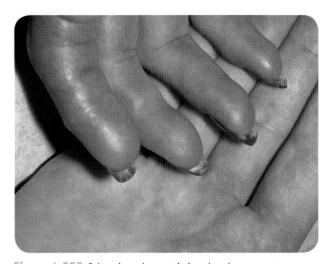

Figure 4-500 Sclerosis and cyanosis in scleroderma.

- Bleomycin toxicity
- Radiation effects
- Onchocerciasis can produce similar "salt-and-pepper" skin changes if a patient is from an endemic area.

✓ Best Tests

- A skin biopsy is not required for diagnosis but may help.
- ANAs are present in the majority of patients. Anti-centromere antibodies (more common in limited disease) and anti-Scl-70 antibodies (anti-topoisomerase I, only seen in diffuse disease) may be seen. Anti-Scl-70 is associated with pulmonary fibrosis but will be positive in only approximately 25% of patients. Other autoantibody tests may be useful, including anti-U3RNP, anti-fibrillin, and anti-PM-Scl. These antibodies are often associated with overlap syndromes.
- Additional screening to consider includes the following:
  - Urinalysis, BUN, creatinine clearance
  - Pulmonary function tests and high-resolution CT
  - Right heart catheterization
  - Echocardiogram
  - Esophagogastroduodenoscopy
  - Barium swallow

▲▲ Management Pearls

- The approach to the patient with scleroderma should be multidisciplinary. A rheumatologist should be involved. Depending on the manifestations and course of the disease, other specialties may need to be consulted (dermatology, nephrology, pulmonology, gastroenterology, or hand surgery).
- An experienced physician should be monitoring and treating internal organ involvement because effective therapies exist, particularly for early pulmonary and renal disease. Internal organ changes include the following:
  - Pulmonary hypertension and interstitial pulmonary fibrosis
  - Hypertensive renal crisis
  - Cardiomyopathy
  - Esophageal dysmotility
  - Sicca syndrome
  - Myositis
- Supportive measures are important. Patients should be kept warm to minimize Raynaud phenomenon. Any ulcers should be kept clean and dry. Encourage patients with dysphagia or reflux to eat smaller, more frequent meals. Advise smoking cessation, if applicable.
- Patients often require extensive occupational and physical therapy to maintain their range of motion and prevent contractures.
- Long-term follow-up is required to ensure a proper assessment of the extent of internal disease.

Therapy

Note that scleroderma is a challenging disease to treat, particularly the cutaneous manifestations. Therapies have demonstrated efficacy in treating the lungs and kidneys.

Corticosteroids:

- Prednisone 2.5 to 5 mg once daily; increase as needed

Immunomodulators:

- Azathioprine 50 to 150 mg p.o. daily

Immunosuppressants:

- Mycophenolate mofetil 1 to 1.5 mg p.o. twice daily
- Cyclophosphamide 50 to 150 mg p.o. daily

Antimetabolites:

- Methotrexate 7.5 to 25 mg weekly

Endothelin receptor antagonist:

- Bosentan 62.5 mg p.o. twice daily for 1 month, then increase to 125 mg p.o. twice daily
- Ambrisentan 5 mg p.o. daily; increase up to 10 mg p.o. daily, if tolerated

Statins:

- Atorvastatin 40 mg daily (helps prevent ulceration to the digits)

Phosphodiesterase type 5 inhibitor:

- Sildenafil 20 mg p.o. three times daily

Chelating agents:

- Penicillamine 750 mg p.o. daily

Cyclosporine (5 to 7 mg/kg daily) and etanercept (25 mg SQ twice weekly) have been used in a limited number of patients with success.

Extracorporeal photochemotherapy with psoralen and ultraviolet light A has helped some patients and is still under investigation.

Other treatments may be superior for managing internal organ involvement. For example, the best treatments for pulmonary disease are likely to be cyclophosphamide, endothelin receptor antagonists such as bosentan, and ambrisentan. Consult with a specialist experienced in treating the disease.

Important treatment adjuncts include the following:

- Nifedipine XL (30 mg p.o. daily) or a different calcium channel blocker, losartan (50 mg p.o. daily), oriloprost (IV) for Raynaud phenomenon

Emollients and antihistamines for pruritus include the following:

- Diphenhydramine (25 or 50 mg tablets or capsules) 25 to 50 mg nightly or every 6 h as needed
- Hydroxyzine (10 or 25 mg tablets) 12.5 to 25 mg every 6 h as needed
- Cetirizine (5 or 10 mg tablets) 5 to 10 mg per day
- Loratadine (10 mg tablets) once daily

Antacids (calcium carbonate), H2 blockers (ranitidine and famotidine), and proton-pump inhibitors (omeprazole and pantoprazole) can be used for gastroesophageal reflux symptoms.

Patients should be aggressively monitored for hypertension and placed on an ACE inhibitor as soon as it is detected to prevent a renal crisis.

Suggested Readings

Allanore Y, Avouac J, Wipff J, et al. New therapeutic strategies in the management of systemic sclerosis. *Expert Opin Pharmacother.* 2007 Apr;8(5):607–615.

Chung L, Lin J, Furst DE, Fiorentino D. Systemic and localized scleroderma. *Clin Dermatol.* 2006 Sep–Oct;24(5):374–392.

de Groote P, Gressin V, Hachulla E, et al. Evaluation of cardiac abnormalities by Doppler echocardiography in a large nationwide multicentric cohort of patients with systemic sclerosis. *Ann Rheum Dis.* 2008 Jan;67(1):31–36.

Denton CP, Black CM. Scleroderma (systemic sclerosis). In: Fitzpatrick TB, Wolff K, eds. *Fitzpatrick's Dermatology in General Medicine.* 7th Ed. New York, NY: McGraw-Hill; 2008:1553–1562.

Drake LA, Dinehart SM, Farmer ER, et al. Guidelines of care for scleroderma and sclerodermoid disorders. American Academy of Dermatology. *J Am Acad Dermatol.* 1996 Oct;35(4):609–614.

Gilliam AC. Scleroderma. *Curr Dir Autoimmun.* 2008;10:258–279.

Henness S, Wigley FM. Current drug therapy for scleroderma and secondary Raynaud's phenomenon: evidence-based review. *Curr Opin Rheumatol.* 2007 Nov;19(6):611–618.

Hoyles RK, Ellis RW, Wellsbury J, et al. A multicenter, prospective, randomized, double-blind, placebo-controlled trial of corticosteroids and intravenous cyclophosphamide followed by oral azathioprine for the treatment of pulmonary fibrosis in scleroderma. *Arthritis Rheum.* 2006 Dec;54(12):3962–3970.

Nihtyanova SI, Denton CP. Current approaches to the management of early active diffuse scleroderma skin disease. *Rheum Dis Clin North Am.* 2008 Feb;34(1):161–179; viii.

Sapadin AN, Fleischmajer R. Treatment of scleroderma. *Arch Dermatol.* 2002 Jan;138(1):99–105.

Steen VD. Treatment of systemic sclerosis. *Am J Clin Dermatol.* 2001;2(5):315–325.

Zandman-Goddard G, Tweezer-Zaks N, Shoenfeld Y. New therapeutic strategies for systemic sclerosis—a critical analysis of the literature. *Clin Dev Immunol.* 2005 Sep;12(3):165–173.

Steroid Atrophy

■■ Diagnosis Synopsis

Steroid atrophy presents as thinning of the skin and results from exposure to corticosteroids. Generalized thinning can occur as the result of long-term oral or inhaled steroid use. Localized thinning occurs following the direct application of topical agents to the skin. Steroid atrophy can be seen as early as 1 week after starting superpotent topical steroids under occlusion and as soon as 2 weeks with less potent agents. Atrophied skin may also be found over areas where intralesional steroids have been injected.

◉ Look For

Areas of thin, loose, fragile skin are localized to the area in which topical steroids were applied. Additionally, the skin appears shiny and transparent, with superficial blood vessels readily apparent (Figs. 4-501–4-504). Most common sites are the face, axilla, groin, medial thigh, and perirectal areas.

Diffuse thin, crepe paper-like, easily traumatized and bruised skin may be seen in those on systemic corticosteroids and is more marked in areas of chronic sun exposure (e.g., face, forearms, and legs).

Dark Skin Considerations

Striae may be prominent.

●● Diagnostic Pearls

Closely examine for marked erythema due to telangiectasia and even purpura. Striae may also be present.

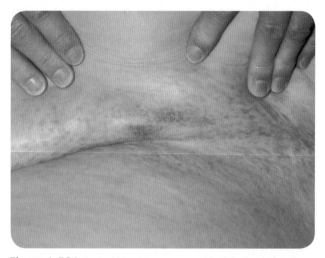

Figure 4-501 Topical steroids can cause skin thinning, dilated vessels, and hypopigmentation.

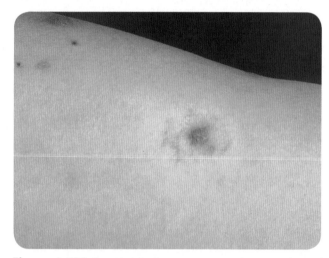

Figure 4-502 Steroid injections may cause deep atrophy and hypopigmentation.

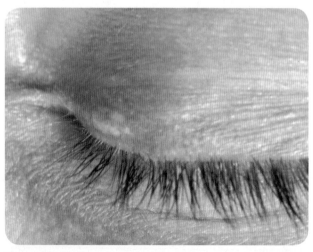

Figure 4-503 Redness and thinness of eyelid skin is common with prolonged steroid use in this location.

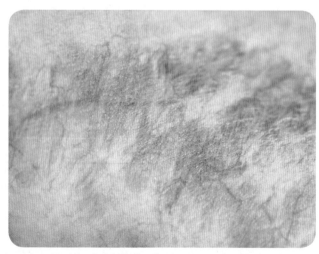

Figure 4-504 Steroid-induced atrophy with dilated small and large vessels.

?? Differential Diagnosis and Pitfalls

- Consider various possible causes (e.g., pregnancy, weight-lifting, rapid growth, topical or systemic steroids, and recent marked weight gain).
- Steroid atrophy has none of the epidermal scaling seen in inflammatory diseases.
- Radiation-induced changes
- Chronic sun damage
- Burn scar
- Lipoatrophy associated with insulin injections
- Morphea
- Lichen sclerosus et atrophicus

✓ Best Tests

This is a clinical diagnosis. Biopsy is rarely needed but can be used for confirmation if necessary.

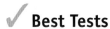 Management Pearls

- Discontinuation of the topical, systemic, or injected steroid is essential.
- Sun protection will reduce the added atrophy-inducing effects of ultraviolet light.

Therapy

Steroid atrophy is difficult to treat. Topical retinoids may be helpful in reversing some of the superficial changes (tretinoin 0.1% applied nightly).

Camouflage cosmetics may help improve appearance for some patients.

For deeper atrophic changes, fat transfer may be considered.

Suggested Readings

Cleary JD. Local atrophy following steroid injection. *Ann Pharmacother.* 2002 Apr;36(4):726.

Cossmann M, Welzel J. Evaluation of the atrophogenic potential of different glucocorticoids using optical coherence tomography, 20-MHz ultrasound and profilometry; a double-blind, placebo-controlled trial. *Br J Dermatol.* 2006 Oct;155(4):700–706.

Furue M, Terao H, Rikihisa W, et al. Clinical dose and adverse effects of topical steroids in daily management of atopic dermatitis. *Br J Dermatol.* 2003 Jan;148(1):128–133.

Striae

Diagnosis Synopsis

Striae (striae distensae), or stretch marks, are due to thinning or atrophic defects in the dermis, typically in areas of repeated or prolonged skin stretching. The etiology is probably multifactorial and may include mechanical stress, hormones, and genetics. They are commonly located on the abdomen, thighs, and buttocks and have been known to occur when the skin stretches excessively or when systemic or topical steroids have been used and have induced atrophy. Periods of rapid growth, such as puberty, pregnancy, and adolescent growth spurts, are common triggers. Striae occurring on the abdomen and breasts are most common in pregnancy. Other associated conditions include lactation, weight lifting, and rapid weight gain. Striae are slightly more common in whites and are twice as common in females than males. The skin findings themselves are only of cosmetic concern, but they may indicate an underlying disease state (such as Cushing syndrome). Striae tend to flatten and become less conspicuous over time.

Immunocompromised Patient Considerations

Patients treated with long-term systemic corticosteroids are at high risk of developing striae. Topical corticosteroid use, especially in flexural and intertriginous areas, is also a risk factor.

Protease inhibitor use in HIV patients is a well-recognized cause of lipoatrophy but has also been reported as a cause of striae.

Look For

Flat or depressed, wrinkle-like thinning of the skin in a longitudinal configuration, parallel to lines of skin relaxation (Figs. 4-505–4-508). Striae are often multiple and symmetric. The lesions are initially pink to violaceous and raised (striae rubra), then later become less colored and finally appear as a skin-colored, depressed scar (striae alba). When due to endogenous or exogenous corticosteroid excess, striae can be larger and widespread. In adolescent boys, they tend to occur on the thighs, shoulders, and lumbosacral region. In adolescent girls, they tend to occur on the proximal thighs, breasts, and buttocks.

Dark Skin Considerations

Striae can take on a deeply pigmented color in darker skin and a purplish hue in lighter skin.

Diagnostic Pearls

Striae due to Cushing syndrome are typically widespread, larger, and have a more violaceous color.

?? Differential Diagnosis and Pitfalls

- Anetoderma
- Lichen sclerosus et atrophicus
- Use of potent topical corticosteroids
- Linear focal elastosis

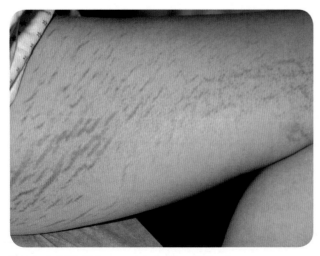

Figure 4-505 Striae associated with weight gain.

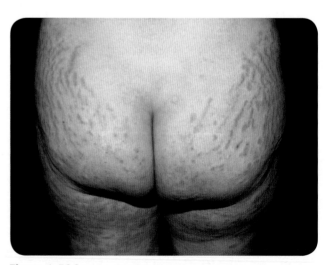

Figure 4-506 Striae associated with pregnancy.

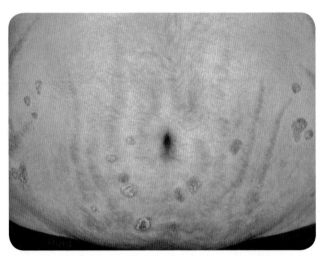

Figure 4-507 Striae associated with the use of high-potency corticosteroid to treat psoriasis.

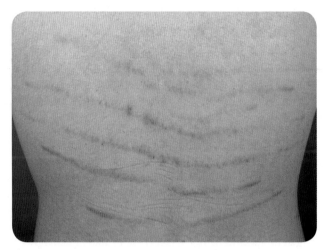

Figure 4-508 Parallel striae on the back are usually without a demonstrable cause.

Immunocompromised Patient Differential Diagnosis

- Systemic corticosteroid use
- Protease inhibitor use in HIV-infected patients

✓ Best Tests

- This is a clinical diagnosis based on history and physical exam.
- If there is concern for Cushing syndrome, consider obtaining a serum ACTH level, a 24-h urine-free cortisol level, and a plasma cortisol level.
- Skin biopsy is very rarely needed but will differentiate striae from linear focal elastosis.

▲▲Management Pearls

- Reassurance and observation are often all that are necessary in patients who are not overly concerned about the cosmetic appearance of their striae.
- In cases of steroid-induced striae, the offending medication should be decreased or withheld if it is safe to do so. Patients given high-potency topical corticosteroids should be warned of the risks of striae development at the outset of therapy.

Therapy

Striae are difficult to treat. Topical retinoids and laser treatments may improve the appearance.

Tretinoin cream has been shown to decrease the length and width of striae and improve their overall appearance. Apply a small quantity to affected skin once daily.

Pulsed dye laser therapy may decrease the erythema. Caution should be exercised in treating dark-skinned patients with laser therapy, given the risk of significant pigmentary alteration.

Alternative Treatments

- Excimer laser
- Intense pulsed light treatments
- Microdermabrasion
- Copper bromide laser
- Chemical peels containing glycolic acid

Suggested Readings

Darvay A, Acland K, Lynn W, et al. Striae formation in two HIV-positive persons receiving protease inhibitors. *J Am Acad Dermatol*. 1999 Sep;41 (3 Pt 1):467–469.

Harris D, Ridley CM. Striae from DEPO-PROVERA injections. *Clin Exp Dermatol*. 1996 Mar;21(2):172.

Maari C, Powell J. Atrophies of connective tissue. In: Bolognia J, Jorizzo JL, Rapini RP, eds. *Dermatology*. 2nd Ed. St. Louis, MO: Mosby; 2008: 1508–1509.

McDaniel DH. Laser therapy of stretch marks. *Dermatol Clin*. 2002 Jan;20(1):67–76, viii.

Spencer JM. Microdermabrasion. *Am J Clin Dermatol*. 2005;6(2):89–92.

Suh DH, Chang KY, Son HC, et al. Radiofrequency and 585-nm pulsed dye laser treatment of striae distensae: A report of 37 Asian patients. *Dermatol Surg*. 2007 Jan;33(1):29–34.

Yosipovitch G, DeVore A, Dawn A. Obesity and the skin: Skin physiology and skin manifestations of obesity. *J Am Acad Dermatol*. 2007 Jun;56(6): 901–916; quiz 917–920.

Diagnosis Synopsis

Factitial dermatitis (dermatitis artefacta) refers to a psychiatric condition in which patients self-induce skin lesions in order to satisfy an unconscious or conscious psychological need to assume the sick role. Patients will not admit to creating the lesions, which are usually more elaborate than simple excoriations. Factitial dermatitis should be differentiated from malingering, in which lesions are deliberately created for secondary gain, such as collecting disability or evading prosecution. Malingering is not a mental illness.

Dermatitis-like lesions, panniculitis, and vasculitis-like lesions may be seen. When an ulcer is present, the condition may more specifically be called a factitial ulcer. The diagnosis of self-abuse tends to occur more frequently in women and in those working in health care. The psychological profile of the patient with self-induced skin disease is the patient with a dependent and manipulative personality or borderline personality disorder.

The patient's typical lack of concern for how disfiguring the lesions appear is out of proportion to the reality of their presentation. The patient's history is inconsistent with the physical exam. This so-called hollow history is a characteristic of the disease. The lesions may be produced by scratching, picking, biting, cutting, burning (with heat or chemicals), injecting, and puncturing. More serious wounds can be complicated by gangrene, abscess formation, or other life-threatening infections. Treatment is often challenging and multidisciplinary.

Look For

A variety of unusual and bizarre lesions, often with geometric, linear, angular, or curving shapes (Figs. 4-509–4-512). Lesions are almost always in reach of the dominant

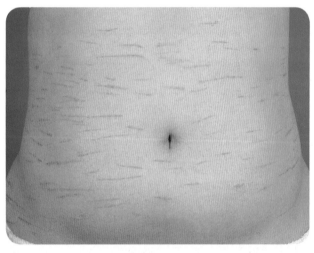

Figure 4-509 Multiple thin erosions in a uniform distribution consistent with self-induced disease.

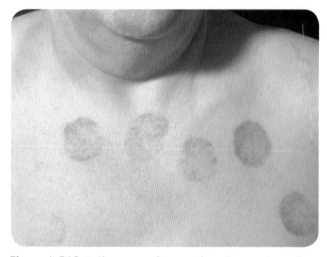

Figure 4-510 Uniform areas of purpura from therapeutic cupping.

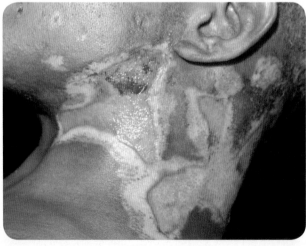

Figure 4-511 Sharply bordered geometric lesions strongly suggest self-induced disease.

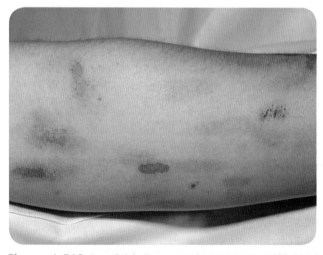

Figure 4-512 Superficial linear erosions suggest self-induced disease.

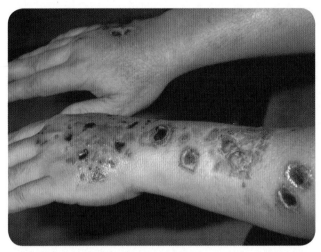

Figure 4-513 Self-induced ulcers may be more common on the left arm of a right-handed patient.

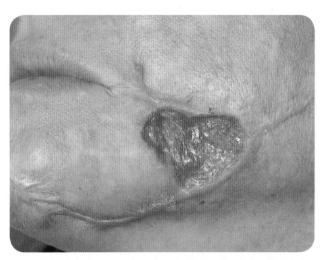

Figure 4-515 Ulcers with little inflammation are often suggestive of factitial lesions.

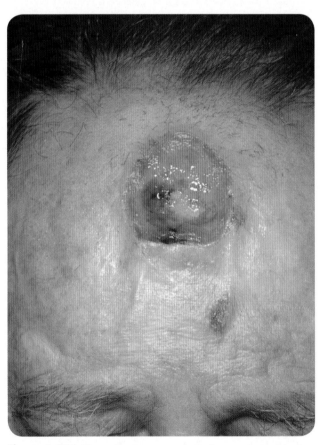

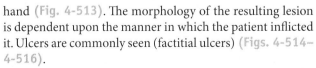

Figure 4-514 Ulceration in a scarred site in a patient with diagnosed psychosis.

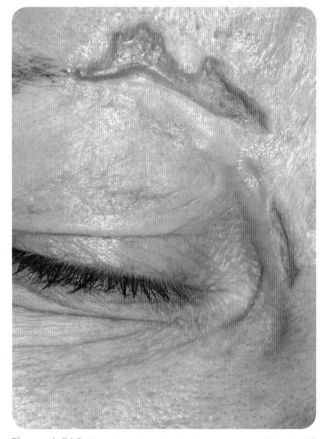

Figure 4-516 Arcuate and angular borders are suggestive of self-induced lesions.

hand (Fig. 4-513). The morphology of the resulting lesion is dependent upon the manner in which the patient inflicted it. Ulcers are commonly seen (factitial ulcers) (Figs. 4-514–4-516).

The patient will not tell you how he or she produces the lesions. The patient essentially creates the disease.

 ## Diagnostic Pearls

In factitial dermatitis, there is an absence of external incentives (e.g., financial gain, obtaining narcotics) for inducing the lesions.

?? Differential Diagnosis and Pitfalls

- Münchhausen syndrome by proxy is the intentional production or feigning of physical or psychological signs or symptoms by a patient's caregiver.
- Malingering
- Contact dermatitis—may also have a geometric arrangement but is not produced intentionally
- Acne excoriée
- Vasculitis
- Impetigo
- Arthropod reaction
- Delusions of parasitosis
- Lesch-Nyhan disease—self-mutilation by biting the lips, fingertips, and shoulders
- Burns
- Bullous diseases
- Abuse
- Neurotic excoriations
- Medical causes of pruritus
- Neuropathic ulcer—skin trauma in a patient with a neuropathy
- Pyoderma gangrenosum

✓ Best Tests

- If lesions heal when covered by an occlusive dressing and reappear when exposed, suspect the diagnosis.
- A skin biopsy will rule out organic dermatologic disease.
- Rule out malingering and identify any associated psychiatric disorders (e.g., depression).

▲▲ Management Pearls

- See these patients often for their skin disease. Do not confront them, as they will feel threatened and not follow up. Gradually gain their trust by treating their skin manifestations and by offering empathy and reassurance.
- Once a stable physician-patient relationship has been established, recommend consultation with a mental health professional.

- Carefully examine the patient for neuropathy. For example, in trigeminal neuralgia, where the ganglion has been destroyed by disease or therapy (such as injection with alcohol), the lack of sensation can predispose the tissue to destruction.

Therapy

Cover lesions with occlusive dressings (e.g., Unna boot).

Optimize the management of any secondary complications, such as infection.

Patients with factitial dermatitis benefit from psychiatric therapy and follow-up. However, most patients are resistant to being seen by a mental health professional. Broach the topic of psychiatric consultation once a trusting relationship has been established. Psychodynamic, behavioral, cognitive, or insight-oriented psychotherapies may be helpful.

Psychotropic medications, such as selective serotonin reuptake inhibitors (SSRIs) and pimozide or olanzapine (2.5 to 5 mg daily), may be useful in certain cases.

Suggested Readings

Antony SJ, Mannion SM. Dermatitis artefacta revisited. *Cutis*. 1995 Jun;55(6):362–364.

James WD, Berger TG, Elston DM. Pruritus and neurocutaneous dermatoses. In: James WD, Berger TG, Elston DM, Odom RB, eds. *Andrews' Diseases of the Skin: Clinical Dermatology*. 10th Ed. Philadelphia, PA: Saunders Elsevier; 2006:61–62.

Joe EK, Li VW, Magro CM, et al. Diagnostic clues to dermatitis artefacta. *Cutis*. 1999 Apr;63(4):209–214.

Koblenzer CS. Dermatitis artefacta. Clinical features and approaches to treatment. *Am J Clin Dermatol*. 2000 Jan–Feb;1(1):47–55.

Kwon EJ, Dans M, Koblenzer CS, et al. Dermatitis artefacta. *J Cutan Med Surg*. 2006 Mar–Apr;10(2):108–113.

Ugurlu S, Bartley GB, Otley CC, et al. Factitious disease of periocular and facial skin. *Am J Ophthalmol*. 1999 Feb;127(2):196–201.

Ecthyma

■■ Diagnosis Synopsis

Ecthyma is an ulcerative bacterial skin infection caused by group A beta-hemolytic streptococci and often secondarily associated with staphylococci. As ecthyma often begins superficially and extends into the dermis, it is often referred to as a deeper form of impetigo. Clinically, the lesions of ecthyma appear as vesicles or pustules that ulcerate and crust over. The lower extremities are sites of predilection. Immunosuppression, poor hygiene, overcrowding, malnutrition, humidity, and preexisting trauma to the tissues all predispose one to infection. It is more common in the extremes of age.

Immunocompromised Patient Considerations

In immunocompromised patients, ecthyma can be caused by pathogens other than group A beta-hemolytic streptococci. Pathogens reported to cause ecthyma-like lesions in immunocompromised hosts include *E. coli*, *Fusarium*, and *Mucor*.

◉ Look For

The lesions commonly begin as small, fluid-filled vesicles that are usually found on the shins, legs, or buttocks. As the vesicles enlarge, they rupture, and a thick gray-yellow crust covers the lesion (Figs. 4-517 and 4-518). If the crust is removed, a superficial ulcer is revealed that has a depressed, raw base and raised edge (Figs. 4-519 and 4-520).

The ulcers will heal within a few weeks but leave scarring. Variants include pustules and vesiculopustules evolving into superficial punched-out ulcers with overlying moist or greenish-yellow crust or eschars. There can be a violaceous border.

●● Diagnostic Pearls

- Lesions characteristically may persist for weeks to months with adherent crusts, especially on the lower legs. They may be few in number without other obvious signs of cellulitis.
- Regional lymphadenopathy is commonly present.

?? Differential Diagnosis and Pitfalls

- The disorder is similar to streptococcal impetigo but is differentiated by deeper components. Ecthyma should be differentiated from ecthyma gangrenosum, which is caused by *Pseudomonas* sepsis and is potentially life threatening and evolves over hours to days.
- Methicillin-resistant *Staphylococcus aureus* (MRSA) infections
- Pyoderma gangrenosum
- *Mycobacterium marinum* infection
- Leishmaniasis
- Insect bites/insect bite reactions
- Sporotrichosis
- Lymphomatoid papulosis
- Papulonecrotic tuberculids
- Tungiasis
- Venous or arterial ulcers

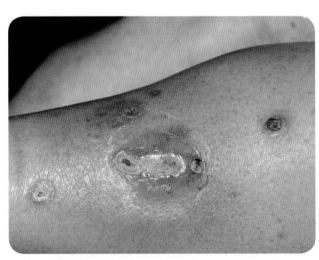

Figure 4-517 Lesion with very adherent crust and a band of peripheral erythema-ecthyma due to streptococcal infection.

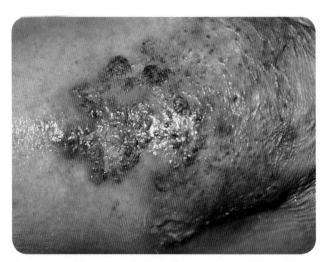

Figure 4-518 Ecthyma with eroded, red papules with accompanying erosions and crust.

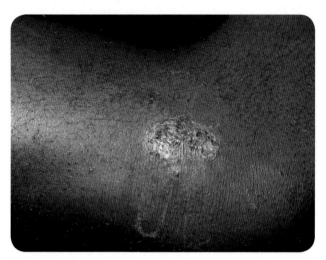

Figure 4-519 Superficial punched-out ulcers due to streptococcal infection.

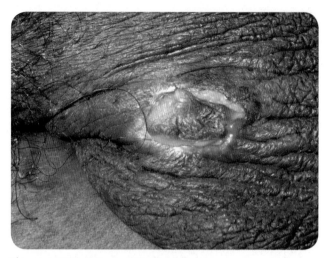

Figure 4-520 Ecthyma with scrotal ulcer.

Immunocompromised Patient Differential Diagnosis

Non-pseudomonal ecthyma gangrenosum caused by a variety of rare invasive pathogens including *Mucor, Candida, Fusarium, Metarrhizium anisopliae, Exserohilum,* and *Citrobacter freundii.*

✓ Best Tests

- Gram stain and culture of lesions will reveal Gram-positive cocci representing group A streptococci with or without *S. aureus.*
- Skin biopsy is rarely needed but, if performed, will show dermal necrosis and inflammation with a granulomatous perivascular infiltrate.

Immunocompromised Patient Considerations

A culture of skin biopsy is recommended in immunocompromised patients to rule out rare infectious pathogens that may mimic ecthyma.

▲▲ Management Pearls

- Manage with systemic antibiotics and aggressive saline soaks/wet compresses to remove crusts. Advise patient that lesions may leave atrophic scars.
- Proper hygiene is the most important measure in the prevention of ecthyma.

- Nonsuppurative complications of streptococcal skin infections include glomerulonephritis and scarlet fever.

Therapy

Treatment is similar to that for impetigo:

- Dicloxacillin—250 mg four times daily for 10 days
- ERYC—333 mg three times daily for 10 days
- Azithromycin—two tabs for 1 day then one tab per day for 4 days
- Cephalexin—250 mg four times daily for 10 days

Care for local wounds with gentle cleansing and the application of mupirocin ointment twice daily as adjunctive therapy.

Immunocompromised Patient Considerations

Consider empiric therapy with broad-spectrum antibacterials and antifungals in immunocompromised patients with ecthyma-like lesions. More directed antimicrobial therapy can be employed after obtaining culture results.

Suggested Readings

Dignani MC, Anaissie E. Human fusariosis. *Clin Microbiol Infect.* 2004 Mar;10(Suppl. 1):67–75.

Reich HL, Williams Fadeyi D, Naik NS, et al. Nonpseudomonal ecthyma gangrenosum. *J Am Acad Dermatol.* 2004 May;50(5 Suppl.):S114–S117.

Intertrigo

▪▪ Diagnosis Synopsis

Intertrigo is a chronic inflammatory condition of approximating or opposing skin surfaces (intertriginous skin) such as the axillae, groin, inframammary folds, abdominal folds, and/or labiocrural folds. Clinically, there is erythema and sometimes weeping, maceration, crusting, or erosions. The affected areas may itch or burn. Intertrigo is most frequently seen in obese and/or diabetic patients. It is induced or exacerbated by any conditions causing increased heat, wetness, and friction. It may be worse during hot and/or humid weather. Incontinence is a predisposing factor in intertrigo of the perineum and crural folds, and there is significant overlap with diaper dermatitis. Intertrigo may be initiated by superficial skin infection with yeast or bacteria. There is no ethnic or sex predilection. Intertrigo is seen more frequently at the extremes of age.

Immunocompromised Patient Considerations

An increased incidence of candidal intertrigo correlates with low CD4 counts and severe disease in HIV-infected patients.

◉ Look For

Erythema or erosions of opposing skin surfaces, such as the axillae, groin, perineum, inframammary creases, and abdominal folds (Figs. 4-521–4-524). There may be coexistent satellite pustular lesions in the case of intertrigo with candidal involvement. Linear fissuring and erosions may be present.

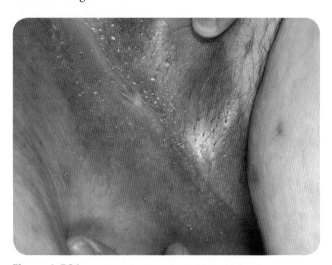

Figure 4-521 Lesions of intertrigo usually have color change but no papules, pustules, or plaques.

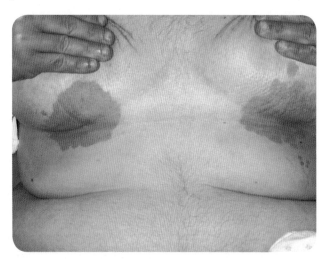

Figure 4-522 The perfect symmetry of lesions on both sides of the fold is an important clue to the diagnosis of intertrigo.

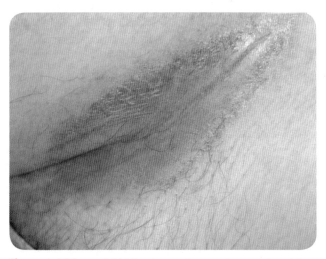

Figure 4-523 Crural fold showing erythema and maceration without papules or pustules, consistent with intertrigo.

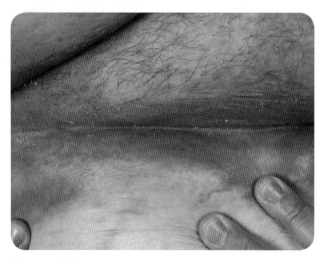

Figure 4-524 Inguinal fold is prone to intertrigo without papules or pustules.

Diagnostic Pearls

Look at other skin folds of the body for similar lesions.

?? Differential Diagnosis and Pitfalls

- Erythrasma
- Seborrheic dermatitis
- Allergic or irritant contact dermatitis (diaper dermatitis)
- Candidiasis
- Inverse psoriasis
- Lichen sclerosus et atrophicus
- Hailey-Hailey—rule out with biopsy
- Extramammary Paget disease—rule out with biopsy
- Group A β-hemolytic streptococci intertrigo
- Langerhans cell histiocytosis
- Inverse lichen planus

 ## Best Tests

- To rule out concomitant infection, perform a KOH preparation and bacterial culture.
- A Wood lamp examination may help rule out erythrasma.
- If the diagnosis is not straightforward, biopsy may be needed to rule out Paget disease, inverse psoriasis, etc.

▲▲▲ Management Pearls

- It is recommended to search for underling disease (e.g., diabetes) in cases of intertrigo that respond poorly to treatment.
- Conservative/preventative measures are aimed at eliminating friction, moisture, and heat. Patients should keep skin folds exposed to the air when feasible, or tuck cotton or linen towels or cloths between them. They should be instructed to avoid clothing that is too tight or chafes.
- Compresses with 1:40 Burow solution or dilute vinegar followed by fanning may help keep skin dry and soothe irritation. Castellani paint, another drying agent, may also be tried.
- Powders may increase skin irritation, and, therefore, should be used with caution.

Therapy

Conservative measures as above.

A low-potency corticosteroid (1% hydrocortisone, desonide) may be indicated to decrease inflammation; however, be careful with the use of topical steroids in occluded areas because this can lead to increased cutaneous side effects and increased systemic absorption. Lotrisone or other combination antifungal/topical steroid creams should be avoided for this reason.

Concomitant infection should be treated, if present. Topical antifungal agents (miconazole or clotrimazole cream) applied to the affected areas twice daily for several weeks may be helpful.

Several combination barrier creams are often used in the treatment of intertrigo, including the following:

- Desitin (zinc oxide, cod liver oil, and talc)
- Triple Paste (petrolatum, aluminum acetate, and zinc oxide)
- Vusion (miconazole, petrolatum, and zinc oxide)

A thick coat should be applied to the affected areas on an as-needed basis.

An adsorbent powder (Zeasorb) may be used to reduce moisture but should be rinsed off daily to avoid irritation.

Suggested Readings

Bernard P. Management of common bacterial infections of the skin. *Curr Opin Infect Dis*. 2008 Apr;21(2):122–128.

Farage MA, Miller KW, Berardesca E, et al. Incontinence in the aged: Contact dermatitis and other cutaneous consequences. *Contact Dermatitis*. 2007 Oct;57(4):211–217.

Hahler B. An overview of dermatological conditions commonly associated with the obese patient. *Ostomy Wound Manage*. 2006 Jun;52(6):34–36, 38, 40 passim.

Muñoz-Pérez MA, Rodriguez-Pichardo A, Camacho F, et al. Dermatological findings correlated with CD4 lymphocyte counts in a prospective 3 year study of 1161 patients with human immunodeficiency virus disease predominantly acquired through intravenous drug abuse. *Br J Dermatol*. 1998 Jul;139(1):33–39.

Yosipovitch G, DeVore A, Dawn A. Obesity and the skin: Skin physiology and skin manifestations of obesity. *J Am Acad Dermatol*. 2007 Jun;56(6): 901–916; quiz 917–920.

■■ Diagnosis Synopsis

Pitted keratolysis is a bacterial infection of the plantar stratum corneum caused by any of the following bacteria: *Micrococcus sedentarius* (*Kytococcus sedentarius*), *Dermatophilus congolensis*, or species of *Corynebacterium* or *Actinomyces*. The hands may rarely be affected. These lesions are generally asymptomatic but can emit a foul odor due to the production of isovaleric acid by the bacterial metabolism of the leucine in sweat. Rarely, pruritus, pain, or burning may be present. Predisposing factors are excessive sweating and prolonged occlusion in a warm, humid environment.

◉ Look For

Few to numerous shallow, rounded 1 to 3 mm pits present on the pressure-bearing areas of the soles with an occasional collarette of scale (Figs. 4-525–4-528). Lesions can coalesce to form furrows, and affected areas may become macerated.

●● Diagnostic Pearls

- Non-inflammatory, superficial, punched-out plantar pits are characteristic.
- May be more common in certain populations, such as male athletes and the homeless.

?? Differential Diagnosis and Pitfalls

- Tinea pedis is usually scaly and erythematous.
- Tinea nigra presents with a black pigmented patch.
- Dyshidrotic eczema presents with pruritus, scale, and pinpoint vesicles on the palms, soles, and lateral digits.
- Chronic hand and foot eczema tends to be more pruritic.
- Punctate keratoderma has firm keratotic papules.

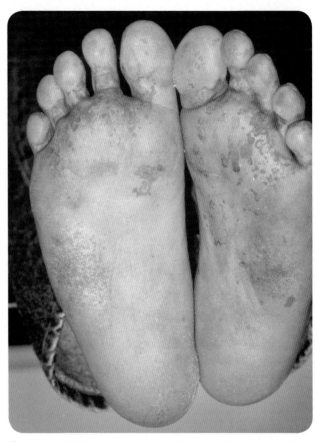

Figure 4-526 Pitted keratolysis with large erosions and hyperkeratosis accentuated in locations with pressure.

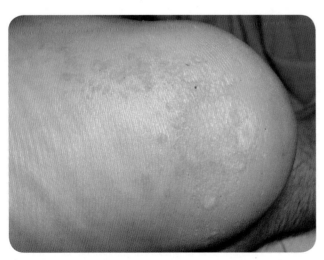

Figure 4-525 Pitted keratolysis. Discrete pitted erosions and hyperkeratotic plaque.

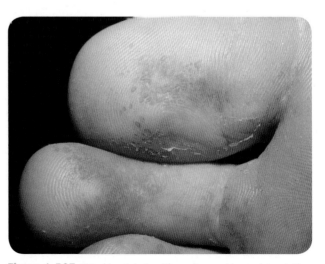

Figure 4-527 Pitted keratolysis with erosions and hyperpigmentation.

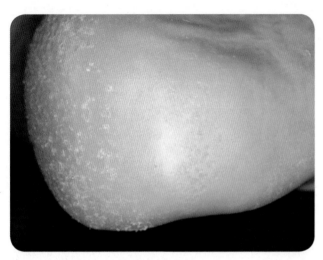

Figure 4-528 Pitted keratolysis with erosions and annular scale.

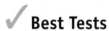 **Best Tests**

This is a clinical diagnosis, and skin biopsy is rarely necessary.

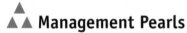 **Management Pearls**

Keep the feet dry with frequent sock changes, and, if needed, the addition of aluminum chloride 20% twice daily can reduce hyperhidrosis. For more severe cases of associated hyperhidrosis, botulinum toxin can be considered.

Therapy

Erythromycin 2% or clindamycin 1% topical solution applied twice daily for 2 to 4 weeks is the standard therapy. A combination of this with aluminum chloride 20% solution decreases the sweating.

Mupirocin ointment twice daily for 2 to 4 weeks will also eliminate the causative bacteria.

For severe cases, oral erythromycin 250 mg four times daily for 7 to 10 days.

Suggested Readings

Ara K, Hama M, Akiba S, et al. Foot odor due to microbial metabolism and its control. *Can J Microbiol.* 2006 Apr;52(4):357–364.

Halpern AV, Heymann WR. Bacterial diseases. In: Bolognia J, Jorizzo JL, Rapini RP, eds. *Dermatology.* 2nd Ed. St. Louis, MO: Mosby/Elsevier; 2008:1088–1089.

Omura EF, Rye B. Dermatologic disorders of the foot. *Clin Sports Med.* 1994 Oct;13(4):825–841.

Takama H, Tamada Y, Yano K, et al. Pitted keratolysis: Clinical manifestations in 53 cases. *Br J Dermatol.* 1997 Aug;137(2):282–285.

Vazquez-Lopez F, Perez-Oliva N. Mupirocine ointment for symptomatic pitted keratolysis. *Infection.* 1996 Jan–Feb;24(1):55.

Zaias N. Pitted and ringed keratolysis. A review and update. *J Am Acad Dermatol.* 1982 Dec;7(6):787–791.

Diagnosis Synopsis

Pyoderma gangrenosum (PG) is an inflammatory, noninfectious, ulcerative skin disease of uncertain etiology commonly misdiagnosed as an aggressive skin infection. Pustules form and give way to ulcers with a necrotic, undermined margin. PG can affect any age and take on a number of differing clinical presentations. The two primary variants are a classic ulcerative form, which often involves the lower extremities, and atypical PG, which is more superficial and tends to occur on the hands. Fever, toxicity, and pain can be associated with the onset of the skin lesions of PG. Extracutaneous manifestations may take the form of sterile neutrophilic abscesses, such as in the lungs, heart, GI tract, liver, eyes, CNS, and lymphatic tissue.

Though the exact cause is unknown, PG has associations with a number of systemic illnesses. In about 50% of cases, there is an association between PG and systemic diseases such as ulcerative colitis, Crohn disease, arthritis, myeloma, leukemia, monoclonal gammopathy, Wegener granulomatosis, collagen vascular disease, Behçet disease, and many other disorders. There is no racial or gender predilection. The disease occurs most often in middle-aged adults. PG tends to be self-limited, and although first-line therapies are widely accepted, alternative therapeutic recommendations are largely based on anecdotal evidence. Surgical intervention is a common exacerbating factor because skin trauma can lead to worsening disease. PG can have either an acute or chronic course and result in extensive scarring.

Look For

The skin lesions of PG typically begin as extremely painful, solitary nodules or deep-seated pustules that rupture and form a shaggy ulcer (Figs. 4-529–4-531). Often, there are pustules that do not progress to ulcerative lesions. The border of the ulcer has a deep violaceous or dusky color and is usually undermined. The ulcer extends peripherally with a bright erythematous or violaceous halo. Oral aphthae, ulcerative lesions of the oral mucosa, and ulcerative lesions of the vulva and eyes are possible. Necrosis is a common feature. As the ulcer progresses, a purulent coating commonly forms over the center of the ulcer. The ulcer may become secondarily infected and have a foul odor.

Variants of PG include pustular and bullous variants that can resemble Sweet syndrome. Vegetative forms have been described. Infrequently, PG can present in the form of suppurative panniculitis. With all variants, there may be eventual spontaneous healing with thin, atrophic scars.

The lesions of PG most commonly occur on the extremities.

Dark Skin Considerations

Black patients may heal with significant hypopigmentation or hyperpigmentation associated with the scarring.

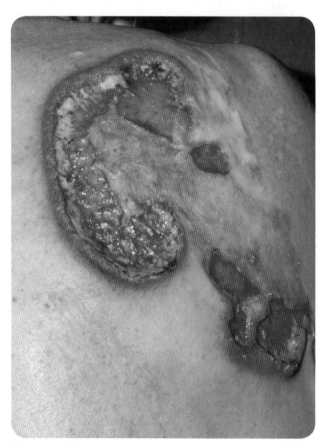

Figure 4-530 The border may not be a complete ring but is still usually undermined.

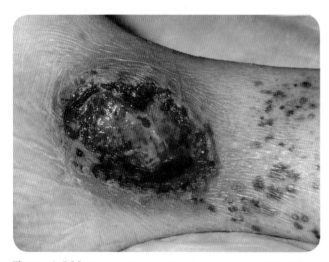

Figure 4-529 Ulcers with an undermined and purpuric border are characteristic of PG.

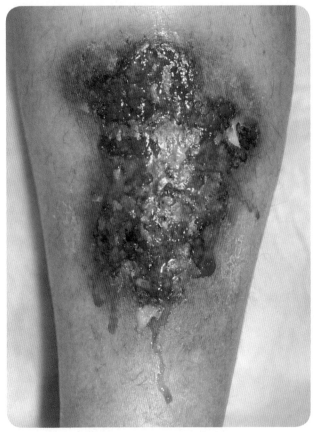

Figure 4-531 Combinations of deep and superficial ulcerations are often seen in PG.

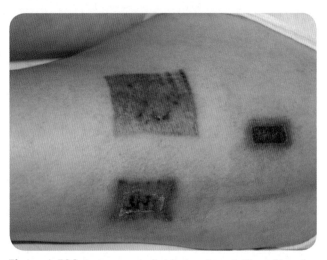

Figure 4-532 Lesions may be induced as sites of skin grafting done for therapy. This phenomenon of lesion induction by trauma or manipulation is called pathergy.

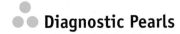

Diagnostic Pearls

The characteristic ulcer edge is undermined, and the base can be deep and is usually purulent. PG shares with Behçet disease and Sweet syndrome the occurrence of pathergy. Pathergy is the invocation of lesions by trauma to the skin such as a needle stick, biopsy procedure, or even insect bites (Fig. 4-532). Therefore, do *not* débride a PG ulcer because this will only result in increasing its size.

?? Differential Diagnosis and Pitfalls

Pustules/Nodules

- Cellulitis
- Folliculitis
- Furuncle
- Insect or spider bite
- Sporotrichosis
- *Mycobacterium marinum* infection
- Impetigo
- Panniculitis

- Sweet syndrome (acute febrile neutrophilic dermatosis)
- Bromoderma

Ulcers

Infectious causes of ulcers can mimic PG. PG is in the family of neutrophilic skin disorders, which includes Sweet syndrome, subcorneal pustular dermatosis, and Behçet disease. As many infectious processes can cause a similar picture (e.g., progressive bacterial synergistic gangrene, North American blastomycosis, other deep fungal infections, amebiasis, sporotrichosis, atypical mycobacteria, etc.), PG is a diagnosis of exclusion.

- Aphthous stomatitis
- Acute febrile neutrophilic dermatosis
- Calciphylaxis—rapidly progressive, can be associated with eschars
- Chancroid—usually present around genital skin
- Churg-Strauss syndrome
- Cutaneous anthrax—develops to an eschar and is a medical emergency
- Herpes simplex virus (HSV)—usually grouped, punched-out erosions
- Ecthyma
- Ecthyma gangrenosum
- Leukocytoclastic vasculitis
- Factitial ulcer—sharp geometric borders
- Factitial panniculitis
- Squamous cell carcinoma—associated with keratotic plaques
- Lymphoma
- Venous or arterial ulcerations
- Wegener granulomatosis

- Traumatic ulceration
- Necrobiosis lipoidica—usually associated with atrophic plaques
- Tertiary syphilis

If a patient has traveled to tropical countries within the last 6 months, diagnoses such as leishmaniasis, tropical ulcer, and Buruli ulcer must be considered.

Because PG may be a relapsing and remitting condition with treatment, atrophic, hyperpigmented, and hypopigmented scarring may occur. These scars may resemble scars from leukocytoclastic vasculitis or atrophie blanche.

Immunocompromised Patient Differential Diagnosis

- Chronic HSV
- Ulcerative Kaposi sarcoma

✓ Best Tests

PG is a diagnosis of exclusion; therefore, testing should be undertaken to rule out similar or associated disorders. Routine investigations to evaluate for systemic disease may include the following:

- CBC ± peripheral blood smear
- Serum electrolytes
- Liver function tests
- Urinalysis
- ANCA, ANA, antiphospholipid antibody and rheumatoid factor
- Serum and/or urine protein electrophoresis

Skin biopsy with culture for bacteria and fungi should be performed to rule out infectious etiologies. Cultures should be taken for analysis of viruses and atypical mycobacteria as well as bacteria and fungi. It is important to note that secondary infections in PG ulcers may lead to positive bacterial cultures, despite the fact that this infection is not the primary cause of the ulcers. Histopathology typically reveals a dense neutrophilic skin infiltrate, necrosis, and hemorrhage. Leukocytoclastic vasculitis may be observed in some biopsy specimens.

▲▲ Management Pearls

- Surgical therapy and elective surgeries should be avoided, if possible. Débridement should be avoided. If surgical therapy is required, it should be performed only in conjunction with immunosuppressive therapy. Autologous skin grafts should be avoided due to the risk of inducing PG at the donor sites.

- The inflammatory bowel disease that may be associated with PG can be subtle and requires a full evaluation, even in the absence of signs and symptoms. Referral to a gastroenterologist is indicated for possible endoscopy and management. The lesions of PG respond to the treatment of underlying rheumatoid arthritis or ulcerative colitis. An improvement of the underlying inflammatory disease may clear or make treatment of the PG easier.
- Other consultants may be needed: ophthalmologist, rheumatologist, oncologist, general, or plastic surgeon. Evaluate on a case-by-case basis.

Therapy

Effective treatment of any underlying medical condition will often ameliorate the lesions of PG. Referral to dermatology for management is often indicated for multiple lesions or widespread disease.

Systemic corticosteroids are the mainstay of therapy, as corticosteroids can arrest the rapid enlargement of the ulcers of PG.

First-line options include

- Prednisone 0.5 to 2 mg/kg p.o. divided two to four times daily; taper over weeks to months as symptoms resolve
- Methylprednisolone 0.5 to 1 mg/kg/day
- Methylprednisolone pulse dosing 1 g per day for 1 to 5 days (requires close inpatient monitoring)
- Cyclosporine-A (5 mg/kg/day divided twice daily)—often induces a rapid response and marked improvement in pain
- Combination of systemic steroids PLUS cyclosporine at the doses described above is also considered a good first-line therapy.

For mild disease, first-line agents include

- Intralesional corticosteroids (triamcinolone acetonide 10 mg/mL)
- High-potency topical corticosteroids (clobetasol propionate cream 0.05%)—not usually effective as standalone agents but can be used under occlusion to treat early lesions
- Topical tacrolimus (0.1% ointment) especially for peristomal PG

Alternate therapies include

- The tumor necrosis factor-alpha inhibitor infliximab may be used at 5 mg/kg and is infused at weeks 0, 2, 6, and every 8 weeks after that. Due to common

(Continued)

infusion reactions, systemic steroids (100 mg methyl-prednisolone IV) are recommended to be given concurrently. This therapy may be combined with oral steroids or other immunosuppressants such as methotrexate or azathioprine. Etanercept has been used as well at 50 mg given at home subcutaneously twice weekly, but there is far less supportive evidence for this medication than infliximab. Prior exposure to tuberculosis should be measured by a PPD before beginning these therapies.

- Dapsone 200 to 400 mg daily may be combined with systemic steroids in patients with normal glucose-6-phosphate dehydrogenase levels. CBC should be carefully monitored.
- Minocycline (100 mg twice daily)—usually as an adjunct to systemic steroids
- Sulfasalazine (0.5 to 2 g four times daily)
- Thalidomide (200 to 400 mg daily)—teratogenic, neuropathy side effects
- Clofazimine (300 to 400 mg daily)—side effects can include pigmentary changes
- Tacrolimus (FK506, 0.1 mg/kg/day)

As PG occasionally resolves sporadically, consideration should be given to local wound care in only those areas that are not cosmetically sensitive. In all cases, local wound care with saline-soaked dressings is recommended. Occlusive dressings are generally discouraged until the disease is controlled.

Suggested Readings

Brooklyn T, Dunnill G, Probert C. Diagnosis and treatment of pyoderma gangrenosum. *BMJ*. 2006 Jul;333(7560):181–184.

Brooklyn TN, Dunnill MG, Shetty A, et al. Infliximab for the treatment of pyoderma gangrenosum: A randomised, double blind, placebo controlled trial. *Gut*. 2006 Apr;55(4):505–509.

Gettler S, Rothe M, Grin C, et al. Optimal treatment of pyoderma gangrenosum. *Am J Clin Dermatol*. 2003;4(9):597–608.

Juillerat P, Christen-Zäch S, Troillet FX, et al. Infliximab for the treatment of disseminated pyoderma gangrenosum associated with ulcerative colitis. Case report and literature review. *Dermatology*. 2007;215(3):245–251.

Powell FC, Hackett BC. Pyoderma gangrenosum. In: Fitzpatrick TB, Wolff K, eds. *Fitzpatrick's Dermatology in General Medicine*. 7th Ed. New York, NY: McGraw-Hill; 2008:296–302.

Reichrath J, Bens G, Bonowitz A, et al. Treatment recommendations for pyoderma gangrenosum: An evidence-based review of the literature based on more than 350 patients. *J Am Acad Dermatol*. 2005 Aug;53(2):273–283.

Wollina U. Clinical management of pyoderma gangrenosum. *Am J Clin Dermatol*. 2002;3(3):149–158.

Wollina U. Pyoderma gangrenosum—a review. *Orphanet J Rare Dis*. 2007;2:19.

Ulcer, Pressure (Decubitus Ulcer)

◼◼ Diagnosis Synopsis

Pressure ulcers, previously termed decubitus ulcers, are also commonly referred to as pressure sores and bed sores. The ulcer is an area of ischemic ulceration or tissue necrosis that generally occurs over bony prominences in locations situated below the waist. Pressure ulcers affect from 1.5 to 3 million people in the United States at an annual cost of approximately 5 billion dollars.

They occur more commonly in certain subsets of patients such as the elderly (over the age of 70), patients who have had surgery for hip fracture, and patients with spinal cord injury.

Factors promoting pressure ulcer formation include the following:

- Pressure: This is the primary contributive factor leading to the formation of ulcers. The length of time over which high pressures are sustained is just as important as the degree of pressure. Thus, relieving pressure regularly prevents tissue damage or tissue death.
- Friction: This occurs when two surfaces resist movement at their interface, resulting in damage to superficial layers of skin. Intraepidermal blisters can result that then lead to superficial skin erosions. Friction can occur when a patient is dragged across a bed sheet or when a patient wears a badly fitting prosthetic device.
- Shearing forces: This is generated by the motion of bone and subcutaneous tissue relative to the skin, which is prevented from moving due to friction (as seen when the head of the bed is raised to more than 30 degrees or when a seated patient slides down a chair).
- Moisture: Moist surfaces predispose to ulcer formation in two ways. First, they increase the effects of pressure, friction, and shear. Second, they cause maceration of the skin, thereby increasing the incidence of ulcer formation fivefold. These conditions may arise due to perspiration, urinary or fecal incontinence, or leakage from a wound site.

Pressure ulcers are classified according to the extent of tissue damage:

- Stage I: Nonblanching erythema of intact skin.
- Stage II: Partial thickness skin loss, with loss of the epidermis and some of the dermis. No slough or necrotic tissue present.
- Stage III: Full thickness loss of skin, with the epidermis and dermis gone and damage to or necrosis of subcutaneous tissues. Damage extends down to but not through the underlying fascia.
- Stage IV: Full thickness loss of skin with extensive destruction, tissue necrosis, and damage to bone, muscle, or other supporting structures.

Recently, two more stages of pressure ulcer formation have been added (National Pressure Ulcer Advisory Panel; http://www.npuap.org/pr2.htm):

- Deep tissue injury: Localized area of discolored skin that is purple or maroon-red in color. It is nonblanching with an intact dermis, and skin has a boggy feel to it.
- Unstageable pressure ulcers: Full tissue thickness loss in which the base of the ulcer is covered by slough or an eschar, and therefore the true depth of the damage cannot be estimated until these are removed.

(**Note:** stable eschar—no erythema present, dry, and adherent—on the heels should not be removed, as it serves as a natural cover.)

Risk factors leading to pressure ulcer formation are as follows:

- Limited mobility
- Malnutrition
- Anemia
- Advanced age
- Fecal or urinary incontinence
- Smoking
- Dry skin
- Altered skin perfusion—decreased in cases of shock or increased if patient has fluid edema due to overhydration
- Acute illness leading to temporary immobility
- Chronic systemic illness
- Terminal illness
- Degenerative neurologic disease
- Increased weight
- Sudden decrease in weight
- Altered mental status
- Prolonged pressure

Simultaneous treatment with the following medications can also predispose to ulcer formation:

- Corticosteroids
- Sedatives
- Analgesics
- Antihypertensives

When a patient presents with a pressure ulcer, the following criteria should initially be followed:

1. Assess the stage of the ulcer and record it according to the ICD-9 codes.
2. Record the location according to the ICD-9 codes.
3. Carry out an assessment using the Braden or Norton scales. These are tools for predicting pressure ulcer risk; this should be done for patients who have not yet developed an ulcer but could be susceptible to one and those who have already developed one. This is an important assessment, as it determines the prevention measures taken and the type of pressure-reducing support surfaces consequently used.
4. Monitor the progress daily.

When assessing a pressure ulcer, take note of the following factors:

- Location of the ulcer.
- Size of the ulcer, including the length, width, and depth.
- Stage of the ulcer.
- Appearance of the ulcer bed, if visible. Observe the tissue color and whether it appears moist. The wound bed color for healthy granulating tissue is pink-red and cobblestone like. A red and smooth wound bed is indicative of clean but nongranulating tissue. Unhealthy granulation tissue is dark red and bleeds on contact.
- Wound edges—Look carefully at the edge of the ulcer for evidence of induration, maceration, rolling edges, and redness.
- Skin around the edges of the ulcer. The periwound skin should be assessed for color, texture, temperature, and integrity of the surrounding skin.
- Drainage—If exudate is present, note the color and amount.
- Presence of necrotic tissue or eschar.
- Presence of complicating features, such as undermining, tunneling, and tracts.
- Any odor emanating from the ulcer.
- Presence or absence of pain.

(●) Look For

Although the classic presentation of pressure ulcers is on the sacral areas and the heels of the patient, be sure to check for the presence of ulcers at other pressure points, such as the occiput, back of the ears, and elbows.

Clinical appearance will vary according to the stage of the ulcer:

- Stage I: Area of redness that does not resolve on removal of pressure. Epidermis appears normal. Site of the impending ulcer appears as an area of persistent redness in lighter-skinned people, whereas in darker-skinned individuals, the skin may appear as an area of persistent red-blue or purple tones (Fig. 4-533).
- Stage II: Epidermis is lost. Lesion appears as an abrasion, denuded blister, or superficial erosion.
- Stage III: Full thickness loss of skin extending into the subcutaneous tissue. May extend into the fascia but does not involve it. May be visible as a crater, and a little slough or necrotic tissue may be visible (Figs. 4-534 and 4-535).
- Stage IV: Full thickness loss of skin with extensive necrosis extending into muscle, bone, joint capsule, or tendon (Fig. 4-536).
- Deep tissue injury: Skin may appear as a localized area of purple or maroon discoloration or as a blood-filled blister due to damage of underlying soft tissue.
- Unstageable pressure ulcer: Full thickness tissue loss, but the base of the ulcer is covered by slough (yellow, green, and brown) or by eschar (black, brown, and tan).

Dark Skin Considerations

- Color variation may exist.
- Erythema may look grey on darker skin.
- Discoloration, warmth, induration, or hardness of skin may be the only signs of a stage I ulcer in people with darker skin.

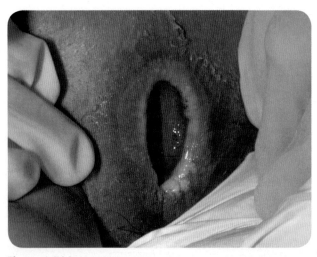

Figure 4-533 Most often, pressure ulcers have minimal inflammation.

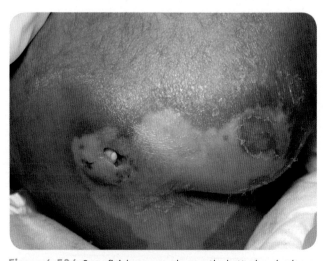

Figure 4-534 Superficial pressure ulcer on the buttock and a deeper ulcer over the coccyx.

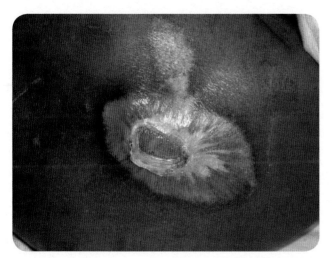

Figure 4-535 Recurrent pressure ulcers in a scarred location on the buttocks.

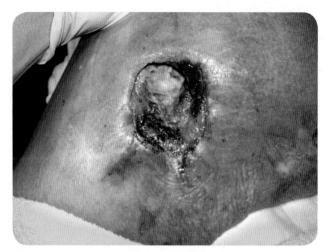

Figure 4-536 Stage IV pressure ulcer.

Diagnostic Pearls

Diagnosis of pressure ulcer is based on its location and the history of the patient. The presence of an ulcer at specific pressure points, such as the sacrum, heel, or occipital scalp, in conjunction with a history of hip fracture or being confined to bed either because of prolonged systemic illness or spinal cord injury should alert one to the diagnosis of pressure ulcer.

?? Differential Diagnosis and Pitfalls

- Pyoderma gangrenosum
- Squamous cell carcinoma
- Vasculitis
- Ecthyma gangrenosum
- Neurogenic (or diabetic) ulcer
- Stasis ulcer
- Ischemic ulcer
- Factitial ulcer
- Herpetic ulcer
- Basal cell carcinoma

Immunocompromised Patient Differential Diagnosis

Widespread ulcerative herpes simplex can commonly mimic pressure ulcers in immunocompromised patients.

✓ Best Tests

The diagnosis is based on a clinical assessment of the patient. However, the patient should undergo a full physical examination to identify any underlying factors that may be exacerbating wound development.

The following diagnostic studies should be carried out:

- CBC
- ESR
- HbA1c
- Nutritional assessment including
  - Albumin
  - Prealbumin
  - Transferrin levels
  - Serum protein
- Metabolic assessment including
  - Zinc levels
  - Copper levels
- Urinalysis

Wound cultures should be taken if there are signs of possible infection. The value of taking a wound culture, however, is debatable. If infection is suspected, treat with a broad-spectrum antibiotic.

Biopsy of the ulcer may be performed to rule out malignancy or an alternative diagnosis in the case of a long-standing ulcer.

Imaging studies may be employed to detect underlying complications such as osteomyelitis. This is particularly relevant in cases with deep pressure ulcer sores in which bone is exposed.

Viral culture for herpes simplex virus (HSV) or direct fluorescence antigen testing should be performed when erosive HSV infection is suspected.

▲▲ Management Pearls

Prevention is the best form of management:

- Turn patients at least every 2 h; rotate them to a 30-degree oblique position.

- Avoid elevation of the head of the bed to greater than 30 degrees.
- Patients who are chair bound should be properly positioned.
- Alleviate pressure over bony prominences, and protect skin from maceration secondary to incontinence or sweating.
- Patients at risk should be placed on a special pressure-reduction surface, not on an ordinary mattress.
- Maintain personal hygiene of patient.
- Ensure adequate nutrition and hydration of patient.
- Manage urinary and fecal incontinence by using a skin barrier cream to avoid the contamination of intact skin. Also, collecting pouches may be used or catheterization may be considered in incontinent patients.
- Avoid dragging the patient across the bed, and instead use lifting devices such as a bed linen or a trapeze.
- Massaging reddened areas over bony prominences should not be carried out, and this must be emphasized to the patient.

Continuous assessment of the pressure ulcer is imperative; assessment should be performed at least once a day. More frequent reassessment may be required if the patient does not show steady improvement.

The size of the ulcer may increase as it improves, especially if there was a lot of necrotic tissue at the base. This increase, however, should occur in the context of the ulcer looking healthier and cleaner.

If the ulcer worsens, multidisciplinary management is necessary, involving allied health professionals such as specialized wound care nurses, physical and occupational therapists, social workers, and dieticians. In addition, physicians in specialties such as geriatrics, general or plastic surgery, and rehabilitation may also be consulted.

Avoid the use of topical antibiotics that include neomycin. Allergic contact dermatitis is a frequent complication in the treatment of skin ulcers and erosions.

Therapy

Prevention Plan
Prevention is the single most important factor. Assess patients at risk for developing pressure ulcers using the Braden Scale (an assessment tool to identify hospitalized patients at risk for ulcer development). The protocols for management of the patient will vary according to their Braden Scale categorization.

The Braden Scale
Sensory perception: rated from 1 to 4, where 1 is completely limited perception and 4 is no impairment.

Moisture: rated from 1 to 4, where 1 is constantly moist and 4 is rarely moist.

Activity: rated from 1 to 4, where 1 is bedfast and 4 is walks frequently.

Mobility: rated from 1 to 4, where 1 is completely immobile and 4 is no limitation.

Nutrition: rated from 1 to 4, where 1 is very poor nutrition and 4 is excellent nutrition.

Friction and shear: rated from 1 to 3, where 1 is the presence of a problem and 3 is no apparent problem.

The scale determines the protocols for management. A score below 18 indicates a patient at risk.

Management protocols:
Not at risk (19 to 23)

At risk (score <15 to 18)

Frequent turning
Maximal remobilization
Protect heels
Manage moisture, nutrition, and friction and shear
Pressure-reduction support surfaces if bed or chair bound, and should include foam or gel mattress

Moderate risk (13 to 14)

Turning schedule
Use foam wedges for 30-degree lateral positioning
Pressure-reduction support surface can include either the foam or gel mattress or the alternating or low air loss system.
Maximal pressure reduction
Protect heels—elevate, use splint
Manage moisture, nutrition, friction, and shear

High risk (10 to 12)

Increase frequency of turning
Supplement with small shifts
Pressure-reduction support surface should include alternating or low air loss systems
Use foam wedges for 30-degree lateral positioning
Maximal remobilization
Protect heels—elevate, use splint
Manage moisture, nutrition, friction, and shear

Very high risk (9 or below)

All of the above plus the following: use pressure-relieving surface if patient has intractable pain or severe pain exacerbated by turning, or if there are additional risk factors.

The use of the air-fluidized bed, the Clinitron, is highly recommended.

General Management
Positioning
Patient should be positioned to avoid pressure over existing ulcers or over bony prominences. The pressure ulcer should be raised off the bed or chair using pillows or foam wedges. A pillow or foam should also be placed between the knees or ankles to prevent direct contact between these bony prominences. Optimal positioning for patients should be in a 30-degree oblique position to the left or the right, changing sides at least every 2 h. Maintain the head of the bed at the lowest elevation possible to minimize shearing forces.

Patients in a chair or wheelchair should use a pressure-relieving cushion to reduce pressure. They should be encouraged to shift position every 15 to 30 min to relieve pressure points and assisted hourly if unable to do so on their own.

Doughnut or ring cushions should be avoided, as they may precipitate ulcer formation.

Support Surfaces
Changing the support surface from that of a regular standard mattress may contribute to wound prevention and care. The following surfaces are used with the foam and fluid-filled products being used for low to moderate risk; the low air loss and alternating systems being used for moderate risk; and the air-fluidized bed, the Clinitron, being used for high-risk patients.

- Foam
- Fluid-filled products
- Low-air-loss systems (FlexiCair Eclipse)
- Alternating pressure systems
- Air fluidized beds (Clinitron)

Wound Management
1. Debridement—Necrotic tissue can be removed by sharp debridement or by mechanical, autolytic, or enzymatic means (papain/urea—Accuzyme, Panafil; collegenase—Santyl).
2. Cleansing—Keep the wound clean by gentle cleansing with saline. Avoid harsh cleaning agents such as povidone-iodine and hydrogen peroxide. If fecal or urinary contamination is a problem, consider catheterization or surgical diversion.
3. Infected wounds—Treat secondarily infected wounds with systemic antibiotics. A 2-week course of topical antibiotics may be used in cases where clean pressure ulcers have not healed or where purulent exudate is still present. The antibiotic should cover Gram-positive, Gram-negative, and anaerobic organisms. Topical agents such as Iodosorb, 1% silver sulfadiazine or silver impregnated dressings, gentamicin cream, or metronidazole gel may be considered for ulcers that appear to have a high bacterial burden.
4. Dressings—A moist (but not wet) environment will promote wound healing. Traditionally, wet-to-dry gauze dressings have been used, but occlusive dressings may be superior. Wet-to-dry dressings remain useful for mechanical debridement. The choice of wound dressing should be based on factors such as the amount of exudate, depth of ulceration, and presence of slough. Skin around the margin of the ulcer should be kept as dry as possible.

Examples of wound dressings that may be used:

- Semipermeable films (Tegaderm, OpSite Plus)—Best for flat, shallow wounds with a low to medium quantity of exudate.
- Hydrocolloids—Sheets such as DuoDERM and Tegasorb work best for cavities or flat, shallow wounds with a low to medium amount of exudate. Hydrofibers like Aquacel are highly absorbent and can be used in sinuses, flat wounds, cavities, and undermining wounds with a large amount of exudate.
- Hydrogels (Intrasite, Nu-Gel)—Suitable for flat wounds, cavities, and sinuses with slough or necrotic tissue and a low to medium quantity of exudate.
- Alginates (Tegagen, Sorbsan, AlgiSite)—Highly absorbent; for cavities, sinuses, and undermining wounds with a high amount of exudate.
- Foam (Allevyn brands)—Best for flat, shallow wounds. Several types of foam can be used based on the degree of exudate.
- Antimicrobial (Acticoat, AquacelAg, Arglaes, Iodosorb)—For locally infected wounds.

For deep ulcers, the dead space can first be filled in with alginate rope, hydrocolloid, or a hydrogel prior to covering with an occlusive dressing.

Nutritional Support
This is a very important aspect of management. A dietitian should be involved in ensuring that the patient is receiving adequate protein intake, with 1.25 to 1.5 g/kg of protein a day being the ideal level of intake. One study supports specific protein supplementation in long-term care residents.

(Continued)

Surgical Intervention

This may be necessary in the case of nonhealing ulcers and may take the form of muscular flaps to provide a skin covering.

In the case of a nonhealing ulcer, consider the possibility of osteomyelitis, and initiate treatment as appropriate.

Additional wound therapy such as hyperbaric oxygen, negative-pressure wound therapy, and electrical stimulation may be used if traditional methods fail.

Coexisting diseases or conditions should be managed simultaneously.

Ensure that the patient is receiving adequate pain management.

Suggested Readings

Armstrong DG, Ayello EA, Capitulo KL, et al. New opportunities to improve pressure ulcer prevention and treatment: Implications of the CMS inpatient hospital care present on admission indicators/hospital-acquired conditions policy: A consensus paper from the International Expert Wound Care Advisory Panel. *Adv Skin Wound Care*. 2008 Oct;21(10):469–478.

Enoch S, Grey JE, Harding KG. ABC of wound healing. Non-surgical and drug treatments. *BMJ*. 2006 Apr;332(7546):900–903.

Girouard K, Harrison MB, VanDenKerkof E. The symptom of pain with pressure ulcers: A review of the literature. *Ostomy Wound Manage*. 2008 May;54(5):30–40, 42.

Jones KR, Fennie K, Lenihan A. Evidence-based management of chronic wounds. *Adv Skin Wound Care*. 2007 Nov;20(11):591–600.

Kanj LF, Wilking SV, Phillips TJ. Pressure ulcers. *J Am Acad Dermatol*. 1998 Apr;38(4):517–536; quiz 537–538.

McInnes E, Bell-Syer SE, Dumville JC, et al. Support surfaces for pressure ulcer prevention. *Cochrane Database Syst Rev*. 2008 Oct;(4):CD001735.

Moore ZE, Cowman S. Risk assessment tools for the prevention of pressure ulcers. *Cochrane Database Syst Rev*. 2008 Jul;(3):CD006471.

Phillips TJ, Odo LM. Decubitus (pressure) ulcers. In: Fitzpatrick TB, Wolff K, eds. *Fitzpatrick's Dermatology in General Medicine*. 7th Ed. New York, NY: McGraw-Hill; 2008:878–886.

Pressure Ulcer Stages Revised by NPUAP. The National Pressure Ulcer Advisory Panel Web site. http://www.npuap.org/pr2.htm. Accessed 2008 Oct 29.

Reddy M, Gill SS, Kalkar SR, et al. Treatment of pressure ulcers: A systematic review. *JAMA*. 2008 Dec;300(22):2647–2662.

Stechmiller JK, Cowan L, Whitney JD, et al. Guidelines for the prevention of pressure ulcers. *Wound Repair Regen*. 2008 Mar–Apr;16(2):151–168.

Diagnosis Synopsis

Ischemic (or arterial) ulcers are a type of vascular ulcer caused by inadequate blood supply to the skin, usually the result of progressive atherosclerosis (peripheral vascular disease) or arterial embolization. They predominantly involve the feet but can occasionally be seen with upper extremity occlusive disease such as thoracic outlet syndrome or Raynaud disease.

Ischemic ulcers are often chronic in nature and are characteristically quite painful relative to other types of ulcers. Their occurrence may be precipitated by seemingly trivial trauma or localized pressure. The incidence of ischemic ulcers increases with advancing age; older individuals are also more likely to exhibit ulcers of mixed etiology. Patients with ischemic ulcers due to peripheral vascular disease will often give a history of claudication. Risk factors for the development of these ulcers include diabetes mellitus, smoking, hyperlipidemia, obesity, rheumatoid arthritis, coronary artery disease, hypertension, hyperhomocysteinemia, male gender, and sedentary lifestyle. The goals of therapy include pain relief, wound healing, avoidance of amputation via revascularization, and risk factor modification.

Critical limb ischemia is defined by the presence of greater than 2 weeks of limb pain at rest from ischemia, tissue loss due to ischemia, or ischemic ulceration. Clinicians of all types must be aware of the need for rapid revascularization, modifications in medical therapy, and wound care to minimize the loss of limbs and the loss of life in these patients.

Look For

An ulceration with a pale base and well-demarcated, "punched-out" appearing borders, most often involving the tips of the toes, the dorsal aspect of the foot, bony prominences, or the heel (Figs. 4-537–4-540). The ulcer bed may contain a small amount of grayish-white granulation tissue that bleeds only minimally upon manipulation. There may be dry eschar or gangrene. Exudate is not exuberant. Tendons and other deep structures may be exposed.

Associated skin findings may include persistent cyanosis or pallor, loss of hair, atrophy, or skin fissures. The extremities are often cool to the touch, distal pulses are diminished, and capillary refill is delayed (more than 3 to 4 s). Toenails may be thickened and dystrophic. Elevation pallor and dependency rubor are signs of limb ischemia.

Diagnostic Pearls

- The patient may report pain when supine, which is relieved by dependency of the extremity (e.g., dangling the affected limb off the edge of the bed).
- Elevation of the extremities (45 degrees for 1 min) will result in pallor, while lowering the limbs to a dependent position for 10 to 15 s leads to rubor.
- Ischemic ulcers tend to occur on the lateral malleoli, whereas venous ulcerations have a predilection for the medial malleoli.

?? Differential Diagnosis and Pitfalls

The differential diagnosis includes other disease processes in which ulceration is a prominent feature:

- Venous ulcers/venous insufficiency (approx. 70% to 80% of lower extremity ulcers)
- Neurogenic (diabetic) ulcers
- Pressure (decubitus) ulcers
- Infections (e.g., ecthyma, leishmaniasis, and cutaneous anthrax)
- Vasculitis (thromboangiitis obliterans, vasculitides associated with connective tissue diseases such as scleroderma or systemic lupus erythematosus, etc.)

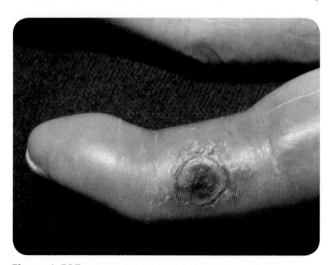

Figure 4-537 Arteriosclerotic ulcer in an elderly patient.

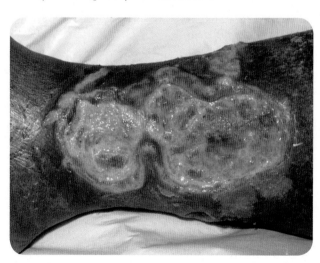

Figure 4-538 Diabetic patient with an arterial ulcer.

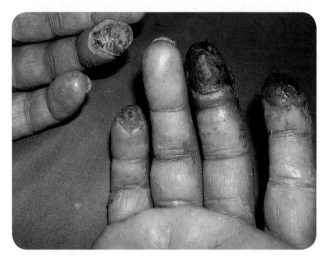

Figure 4-539 Ischemic ulcer due to Buerger disease in a 50-year-old smoker.

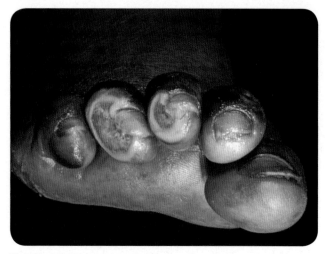

Figure 4-540 Toe ulcers in a man with Buerger disease.

- Hypercoagulable states and other hematologic diseases
- Panniculitis
- Necrobiosis lipoidica
- Frostbite
- Burn
- Trauma
- Pyoderma gangrenosum
- Neoplasms (basal cell carcinoma, squamous cell carcinoma, cutaneous T-cell lymphoma)
- Bites (e.g., brown recluse spider)
- Factitial ulcer
- Radiodermatitis

 Best Tests

Ankle-Brachial index (ABI): The ABI is a noninvasive tool used to diagnose peripheral arterial disease and will aid in differentiating arterial insufficiency from venous insufficiency. Specifically, the ABI measures the systolic blood pressures in the ankle and the arm using a Doppler probe and a blood pressure (BP) cuff.

How to Obtain the Brachial Systolic Blood Pressure

The patient should be at rest in the supine position for 5 min. Place the lower end of the BP cuff about 1 in. above the antecubital fossa. Locate the brachial artery and apply the probe gel over the artery. Place the tip of the probe into the gel until consistent and characteristic arterial sounds are heard. Inflate the BP cuff to 20 mm Hg above the blood pressure at which arterial sounds disappear. Slowly deflate the BP cuff until arterial sounds on Doppler are obtained. Repeat on the other arm. The higher of the two brachial systolic pressures will be used to calculate the ABI. In individuals with normal vascular anatomy, less than a 10 mm Hg difference between the two arms is observed.

How to Obtain the Ankle Systolic Blood Pressure

Place the lower end of the BP cuff about 2 in. above the medial malleolus. Locate the posterior tibial pulse and perform the same procedure as described above. Now identify the dorsalis pedis artery and perform the same procedure. Repeat on the other leg. The highest of the systolic pressures will be used to calculate the ABI.

ABI Calculation

There should now be three values for each side: a brachial, posterior tibialis, and dorsalis pedis artery systolic blood pressure for the right side and left side. Take the highest brachial artery value. This will be the denominator. For the lower extremity values, take the highest value, whether it is the posterior tibialis or the dorsalis pedis, of the right side, and divide it by the brachial value. Repeat for the left side.

Interpretation

- Normal ABI: 1.0 to as high as 1.3
- Noncompressible calcified vessel: values greater than 1.3
- Positive peripheral arterial disease: value less than 0.9

An ABI less than 0.9 has 100% specificity and 95% sensitivity for detecting angiogram-positive peripheral arterial disease. There is ≥50% stenosis in one or more major arteries.

An ABI of 0.40 to 0.90 indicates obstruction associated with claudication.

An ABI less than 0.4 represents severe ischemia.

Other Tests to Consider Include

- Duplex ultrasound
- Formal contrast angiography

- CT or MR angiography
- Consider obtaining a skin biopsy in particularly recalcitrant ulcers to rule out malignancy
- Glycosylated hemoglobin (HbA1c) determination (for occult diabetes)

▲▲ Management Pearls

- A biopsy of any leg ulcer should be undertaken with caution. Like the ulcer itself, the biopsy site will often experience difficulty with wound healing. Because carcinoma is in the differential, however, ulcers that do not heal after 4 to 6 months of optimal therapy should have a biopsy taken from the ulcer edge.
- Patients with ischemic ulcers typically require referral to a vascular surgeon and occasionally a plastic surgeon. Podiatry referrals are also indicated for foot ulcers.
- Patients may experience some relief of pain from raising the head of the bed 4 to 6 in. while resting.
- Avoid vasoconstrictive drugs such as nonselective beta-blockers.
- Compression should *not* be employed in the treatment of ischemic ulcers.

Therapy

General Principles

- Optimize the management or eliminate exacerbating factors (diabetes, smoking, hypertension, hyperlipidemia, etc.) and encourage exercise as tolerated
- Ensure measures to reduce risk of death from coronary artery disease and further morbidity from peripheral vascular disease:
  - Antiplatelet therapy with aspirin or clopidogrel
  - Selective beta-blockers
  - Lipid lowering therapy—goal LDL cholesterol <100 mg/dL and in very high risk patients <70 mg/dL
- Meticulous foot care
- Weight-offloading devices as directed by a podiatrist
- Antibiotics (topical or systemic) when clinically indicated for secondarily infected ulcers
- Any ulcer with extensive slough or necrotic tissue should be debrided, whether via surgical or enzymatic means:
  - Sharp surgical removal of nonviable tissues and surrounding callus
  - Remove thick eschar only when separating at wound edge
  - Topical collagenase preparations may be useful
- Pain control

Specific Treatments

- Wound dressings—As ischemic ulcers tend to have slough but low levels of exudate, hydrogel dressings that rehydrate wounds and promote autolytic debridement are most appropriate.
- Surgical revascularization, including endovascular procedures (angioplasty, stenting, and catheter-based plaque excision) or open lower extremity bypass, is the mainstay of therapy in patients who are acceptable surgical candidates. Nonhealing ulcerations and gangrene as well as rest pain and worsening claudication are indications for surgery.
- Skin graft and flap coverage of chronic ulcers often fail but are sometimes improved following surgical revascularization.
- Vacuum-assisted wound closure is useful for large wounds but is contraindicated in patients with friable, thin skin or neoplastic ulcers.
- Amputation is indicated in selected patients.
- The following modalities currently have limited evidence to support their use: oral zinc, hyperbaric oxygen, electrotherapy and electromagnetic therapy, biosurgery (myiasis) with sterile maggots, intermittent pneumatic compression in poor surgical candidates refusing amputation, and noncontact, low frequency ultrasound.

Note: Current data do not support the use of drugs such as pentoxifylline or iloprost.

Suggested Readings

Belch JJ, Topol EJ, Agnelli G, et al. Critical issues in peripheral arterial disease detection and management: A call to action. *Arch Intern Med.* 2003 Apr;163(8):884–892.

Hiatt WR. Medical treatment of peripheral arterial disease and claudication. *N Engl J Med.* 2001 May;344(21):1608–1621.

Holloway GA. Arterial ulcers: Assessment and diagnosis. *Ostomy Wound Manage.* 1996 Apr;42(3):46–48, 50–51.

Nelson EA, Bradley MD. Dressings and topical agents for arterial leg ulcers. *Cochrane Database Syst Rev.* 2007 Jan;(1):CD001836.

Phillips T. Ulcers. In: Bolognia J, Jorizzo JL, Rapini RP, eds. *Dermatology.* 2nd Ed. St. Louis, MO: Mosby/Elsevier; 2008:1597–1610.

Sambasivarao D, Sitaramam V. Characterization of mitochondrial membrane fragments resulting from spontaneous swelling: Novel stimulation of NADH-dependent respiration by carboxylic acids. *Indian J Biochem Biophys.* 1991 Aug;28(4):280–290.

Sieggreen MY, Kline RA. Arterial insufficiency and ulceration: Diagnosis and treatment options. *Adv Skin Wound Care.* 2004 Jun;17(5 Pt 1):242–251; quiz 252–253.

Slovut DP, Sullivan TM. Critical limb ischemia: Medical and surgical management. *Vasc Med.* 2008 Aug;13(3):281–291.

Takahashi PY, Kiemele LJ, Jones JP. Wound care for elderly patients: Advances and clinical applications for practicing physicians. *Mayo Clin Proc.* 2004 Feb;79(2):260–267.

Diagnosis Synopsis

Venous ulcers, or ulcers due to venous insufficiency/venous hypertension, are large, irregularly shaped, shallow ulcers that often demonstrate a yellow exudate covering the wound bed and are most commonly found in the medial malleolar region of the ankle. While the reported prevalence varies, it is estimated that approximately 0.05% to 1.52% of Americans suffer from venous ulcers. An increased prevalence is seen with age, and both sexes are affected equally. Additional risk factors include a history of thrombosis, phlebitis, leg injury such as fracture or trauma, and obesity.

The primary pathophysiology involves incompetent one-way venous valves or dysfunctional calf muscle pumping leading to insufficient venous blood return to the heart and chronic leg venous hypertension. This venous hypertension leads to aberrant tissue perfusion and subsequent decreased delivery of oxygen and nutrients, failure to remove metabolic byproducts, and tissue ischemia.

Additional commonly associated clinical features include leg and ankle edema, varicose veins, yellow-brown pigmentation secondary to hemosiderin deposition and extravasated red blood cells, eczematous changes with scaling and crusting (stasis dermatitis), and lymphedema. Lipodermatosclerosis is also seen and corresponds to fibrotic changes in subcutaneous tissue leading to a hard and indurated feel to the skin. An "inverted champagne bottle" leg indicates end stage lipodermatosclerosis and is caused by severe fibrotic changes in the distal leg and leg edema of the proximal leg. Atrophie blanche are smooth, ivory-colored atrophic plaques secondary to sclerosis seen in approximately 40% of patients with venous insufficiency.

Additional key points that the clinician should note are that stasis ulcers usually begin on the medial malleolus but may become circumferential over time. They may be painful, are difficult to treat, and frequently recur. They may become secondarily infected.

 Look For

Ulcers of varying depths occur on the medial ankles, depending upon the severity of the surrounding dermatitis and timeline of the process (Figs. 4-541–4-543). The ulcer bed usually contains a fibrinous base mixed with granulation tissue (Fig. 4-544). There is an irregular, sloping edge. Erythematous, scaly plaques involving the ankle and distal lower leg will typically surround the ulcer. Pitting edema of the lower extremities is often present. Nearby skin may be shiny (atrophic) and variably pigmented.

Diagnostic Pearls

- Venous insufficiency is the most common cause of lower leg ulcers. Pulses are usually normal, and the ulcers tend to be minimally painful.
- Look for other signs of chronic venous insufficiency, such as stasis dermatitis, lipodermatosclerosis, atrophie blanche, varicose veins, lymphedema, decreased hair growth on the legs, and ankle edema.
- Ankle-Brachial index (ABI): The ABI is a noninvasive tool used to diagnose peripheral arterial disease and will aid in differentiating arterial insufficiency from venous insufficiency. Specifically, the ABI measures the systolic blood pressures in the ankle and the arm using a Doppler probe and a blood pressure (BP) cuff.

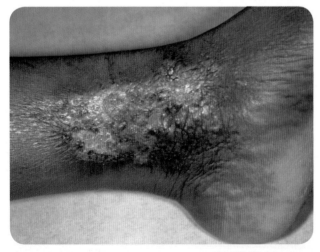

Figure 4-541 Edema and erythema around the medial malleolus are typical for a stasis ulcer.

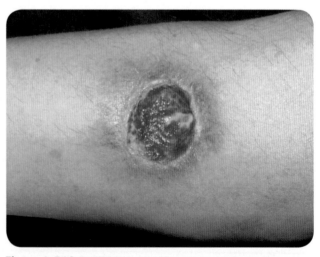

Figure 4-542 Stasis ulcers may have minimal inflammation.

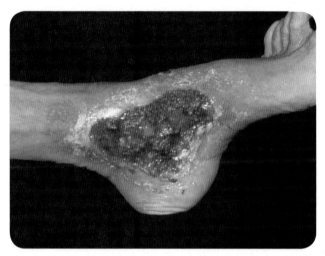

Figure 4-543 Minimal inflammation around a large stasis ulcer.

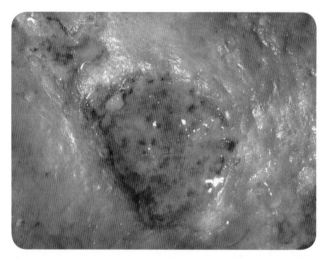

Figure 4-544 Fibrosis is common around a stasis ulcer and may slow healing.

How to Obtain the Brachial Systolic Blood Pressure

The patient should be at rest in the supine position for 5 min. Place the lower end of the BP cuff about 1 in. above the antecubital fossa. Locate the brachial artery and apply the probe gel over the artery. Place the tip of the probe into the gel until consistent and characteristic arterial sounds are heard. Inflate the BP cuff to 20 mm Hg above the blood pressure at which arterial sounds disappear. Slowly deflate the BP cuff until arterial sounds on Doppler are obtained. Repeat on the other arm. The higher of the two brachial systolic pressures will be used to calculate the ABI. In individuals with normal vascular anatomy, less than a 10 mm Hg difference between the two arms is observed.

How to Obtain the Ankle Systolic Blood Pressure

Place the lower end of the BP cuff about 2 in. above the medial malleolus. Locate the posterior tibial pulse and perform the same procedure as described above. Now identify the dorsalis pedis artery and perform the same procedure. Repeat on the other leg. The highest of the systolic pressures will be used to calculate the ABI.

ABI Calculation

There should now be three values for each side: a brachial, posterior tibialis, and dorsalis pedis artery systolic blood pressure for the right side and left side. Take the highest brachial artery value. This will be the denominator. For the lower extremity values, take the highest value, whether it is the posterior tibialis or the dorsalis pedis, of the right side, and divide it by the brachial value. Repeat for the left side.

Interpretation

- Normal ABI: 1.0 to as high as 1.3
- Noncompressible calcified vessel: values greater than 1.3
- Positive peripheral arterial disease: value less than 0.9

An ABI less than 0.9 has 100% specificity and 95% sensitivity for detecting angiogram positive peripheral arterial disease. There is ≥50% stenosis in one or more major arteries.

An ABI of 0.40 to 0.90 indicates obstruction associated with claudication.

?? Differential Diagnosis and Pitfalls

- Arterial ulcers—Weak or absent distal pulses, do not have surrounding areas of dermatitis, have a punched-out appearance; located anteriorly or laterally on the lower extremity consistent with pressure sites.
- Neurogenic (diabetic) ulcer—Almost invariably has peripheral neuropathy with decreased sensation and HgbA1C that is elevated; look for punched-out ulcers that are in pressure sites.
- Pyoderma gangrenosum—Look for very painful ulcers that have an irregular necrotic, undermined, overhanging border; these can occur anywhere.
- Thromboangiitis obliterans—Weak or absent distal pulses. Patients almost invariably have a history of smoking. Upper limb involvement is also seen.
- Cryofibrinogenemia—Look for associated livedo reticularis and purpura.
- Acroangiodermatitis—Although they do not often ulcerate, they are commonly seen in conjunction with venous hypertension and manifest as violaceous patches and plaques that appear on the extensor surfaces of the distal lower extremities.

- Trauma
- Bullous impetigo
- Squamous cell carcinoma
- Deep fungal infection
- Atypical mycobacterium infection
- Panniculitis with ulceration

✓ Best Tests

- This diagnosis is made clinically, but imaging and laboratory investigations are often ordered to evaluate the severity of venous disease. Skin biopsy can also be done if the diagnosis is in doubt.
- ABIs should be performed to determine if there is mixed arterial and venous disease. This is significant because compression stockings are a treatment option for venous disease but will worsen arterial disease. A vascular surgeon should subsequently evaluate any patient with a decrease in ABI.
- Duplex ultrasound is the test of choice for the evaluation of venous insufficiency.
- Magnetic resonance venography and direct contrast venography can be employed in challenging cases.

▲▲ Management Pearls

- Compressive leg stockings are a necessary long-term measure. Patients should be warned to remove the garments if they notice any side effects of numbness, pain, tingling, or dusky toes.
- Consultations with vascular or plastic surgeons may be indicated. Such surgeons may be able to ameliorate venous hypertension or address wound debridement and coverage.

Therapy

The main goal of treatment is to restore venous blood pressure and reverse the effects of venous hypertension.

Leg elevation and compression stockings (e.g., Jobst) are mainstays of treatment and should be tailored to fit the patient and the degree of venous insufficiency. Recommended pressure gradients are as follows:

- 15 to 20 mm Hg—indicated for mild varicose veins and minor leg swelling
- 20 to 30 mm Hg—indicated for moderate edema and moderate to severe varicosities

- 30 to 40 mm Hg—indicated for chronic venous insufficiency, severe edema, DVT and post-thrombotic syndrome, venous ulceration, lymphedema, and orthostatic hypotension

Optimize the patient's nutritional status. Supplementation may be indicated. Some clinicians advocate supplementation with ascorbic acid and/or zinc, although this remains to be proven in clinical trials.

Correct or maximize the treatment of other underlying factors, such as diabetes mellitus, peripheral vascular disease, anemia, obesity, or tobacco abuse. Exercise as safely tolerated should be encouraged. Minimize trauma to the area. Patients should be instructed to keep their legs elevated when at rest.

Keep the wound clean by gentle cleansing with saline. Treat secondarily infected wounds with systemic antibiotics. A bacterial culture of any frank purulent exudate may be helpful, but cultures of ulcers may be of limited utility due to colonization with skin commensals. Additional signs of infection include pain; foul odor; fever; tissue breakdown; and local erythema, warmth, and swelling. Empiric therapy should cover common skin pathogens (e.g., *Staphylococcus aureus*, streptococci) and may be changed based on the clinical scenario, response, and available culture data.

A moist (but not wet) environment will promote wound healing. Traditionally, wet-to-dry gauze dressings have been used, but occlusive dressings may be superior. Wet-to-dry dressings remain useful for mechanical debridement. The choice of wound dressing should be based on factors such as the amount of exudate, the depth of the ulceration, and the presence of slough, etc. Periulcer skin should be kept dry as much as possible. Examples of types of wound dressings are

- Semipermeable films (Tegaderm and OpSite Plus)—Best for flat, shallow wounds with a low to medium quantity of exudate.
- Hydrocolloids—Sheets such as DuoDERM and Tegasorb work best for cavities or flat, shallow wounds with a low to medium amount of exudate. Hydrofibers like Aquacel are highly absorbent and can be used in sinuses, flat wounds, cavities, and undermining wounds with a large amount of exudate.
- Hydrogels (IntraSite and Nu-Gel)—Suitable for flat wounds, cavities, and sinuses with slough or necrotic tissue and a low to medium quantity of exudate.

- Alginates (Tegagen, Sorbsan, and AlgiSite)—Highly absorbent; for cavities, sinuses, and undermining wounds with a high amount of exudate.
- Foam (Allevyn brands)—Best for flat, shallow wounds. Several different types of foam can be chosen based on the degree of exudate.
- Antimicrobial (Acticoat, Aquacel Ag, Arglaes, and Iodosorb)—For locally infected wounds.

Ulcers (except heel ulcers) with extensive slough or necrotic tissue should be debrided, whether via mechanical, surgical, or enzymatic (papain/urea—Accuzyme, Panafil; collagenase—Santyl, for noninfected wounds only) means.

Acute cases of associated stasis dermatitis require mid- to high-potency topical corticosteroids applied twice daily. Fill the ulcer with petroleum jelly to prevent exposure of the ulcer to the corticosteroid.

High-potency topical corticosteroids (class 2)

- Fluocinonide cream, ointment—apply twice daily (15, 30, 60, 120 g)
- Desoximetasone cream, ointment—apply twice daily (15, 60, 120 g)
- Halcinonide cream, ointment—apply twice daily (15, 60, 240 g)
- Amcinonide ointment—apply twice daily (15, 30, 60 g)

Mid-potency topical corticosteroids (classes 3 and 4)

- Triamcinolone cream, ointment—apply twice daily (15, 30, 60, 120, 240 g)
- Mometasone cream, ointment—apply twice daily (15, 45 g)
- Fluocinolone cream, ointment—apply twice daily (15, 30, 60 g)

Use steroid ointments that have fewer preservatives if an allergic contact dermatitis develops with multiple topical medications.

Surgical therapy is considered after medical treatment options have been exhausted. Surgical options include punch grafts, split-thickness grafts, epidermal or dermal engineered grafts, and saphenous vein surgery.

Suggested Readings

Al-Kurdi D, Bell-Syer SE, Flemming K. Therapeutic ultrasound for venous leg ulcers. *Cochrane Database Syst Rev.* 2008 Jan;(1):CD001180.

Carr SC. Diagnosis and management of venous ulcers. *Perspect Vasc Surg Endovasc Ther.* 2008 Mar;20(1):82–85.

Etufugh CN, Phillips TJ. Venous ulcers. *Clin Dermatol.* 2007 Jan–Feb; 25(1):121–130.

Heit JA, Rooke TW, Silverstein MD, et al. Trends in the incidence of venous stasis syndrome and venous ulcer: A 25-year population-based study. *J Vasc Surg.* 2001 May;33(5):1022–1027.

Hiatt WR. Medical treatment of peripheral arterial disease and claudication. *N Engl J Med.* 2001 May;344(21):1608–1621.

Jones KR, Fennie K, Lenihan A. Evidence-based management of chronic wounds. Adv *Skin Wound Care.* 2007 Nov;20(11):591–600.

Jones JE, Nelson EA. Skin grafting for venous leg ulcers. *Cochrane Database Syst Rev.* 2007 Apr;(2):CD001737.

O'Meara S, Al-Kurdi D, Ovington LG. Antibiotics and antiseptics for venous leg ulcers. *Cochrane Database Syst Rev.* 2008 Jan;(1):CD003557.

Robson MC, Cooper DM, Aslam R, et al. Guidelines for the prevention of venous ulcers. *Wound Repair Regen.* 2008 Mar–Apr;16(2):147–150.

Sieggreen MY, Kline RA. Recognizing and managing venous leg ulcers. *Adv Skin Wound Care.* 2004 Jul–Aug;17(6):302–311; quiz 312–313.

Takahashi PY, Kiemele LJ, Jones JP. Wound care for elderly patients: Advances and clinical applications for practicing physicians. *Mayo Clin Proc.* 2004 Feb;79(2):260–267.

Yosipovitch G, DeVore A, Dawn A. Obesity and the skin: Skin physiology and skin manifestations of obesity. *J Am Acad Dermatol.* 2007 Jun;56(6): 901–916; quiz 917–920.

Cellulitis

▪▪ Diagnosis Synopsis

Cellulitis is a common bacterial infection of the dermis and subcutaneous tissue characterized by erythema, pain, warmth, and swelling. Cellulitis occurs at any age, in both sexes, and in any ethnicity, but it is most commonly found in males aged 45 to 65. Causes of cellulitis are strongly correlated with age and immune status and include the following:

- Immunocompetent adults: *Staphylococcus aureus* (methicillin sensitive or methicillin resistant) and *Streptococcus pyogenes*
- Immunocompromised individuals, including those with diabetes, venous insufficiency, or decubitus ulcers: mixture of Gram-positive cocci and Gram-negative aerobes.

The most common routes of bacterial seeding in immunocompetent and immunocompromised individuals are direct bacterial inoculation and hematogenous seeding, respectively. Risk factors include minor skin trauma, body piercing, tinea pedis infection, injection drug use, animal bites, peripheral vascular disease, chronic systemic steroid use, neutropenia, intravenous drug use, lymph node dissection, radiation therapy, and vein harvest for coronary artery bypass surgery.

Fevers, chills, and malaise often precede the onset of cellulitis. Poorly defined borders, erythema, swelling, tenderness, and warmth characterize typical cellulitis lesions. In adults, the extremities are the most common sites affected. In more severe cases, additional clinical features may include vesicle and bulla formation, pustules, and necrosis. Complications are not common but can include glomerulonephritis, lymphadenitis, and subacute bacterial endocarditis.

Of note, a rising prevalence of methicillin-resistant *S. aureus* (MRSA) has been identified as a pathogen of skin and soft tissue infections in otherwise healthy individuals lacking the aforementioned risk factors for cellulitis. In a recent study of emergency room visits for purulent skin and soft tissue infections, MRSA was identified as the etiologic agent in 59% of cases in multiple locations nationwide. It is not currently known if nonpurulent skin infections like cellulitis are more frequently caused by MRSA today.

Immunocompromised Patient Considerations

In immunosuppressed individuals, cellulitis can progress rapidly, leading to large abscesses, necrosis, myositis, hematogenous dissemination, and sepsis. Additional causes of cellulitis in immunosuppressed individuals include *Streptococcus pneumoniae, Campylobacter jejuni, Bacteroides fragilis, Yersinia enterocolitica, Citrobacter, Escherichia coli, Bacillus cereus, Helicobacter cinaedi*, and the fungi *Paecilomyces* and *Cryptococcus*.

In HIV-infected individuals, *S. aureus* was the most common pathogen, followed by *Pseudomonas* spp., *E. coli*, and *S. pyogenes*. Polymicrobial infection was present in approximately 38% of cases. In addition, sepsis occurred in 25% of cellulitis episodes.

◉ Look For

- Unilateral erythematous, warm to hot, tender patches (Figs. 4-545–4-547)
- Unilateral extremity edema
- Lymphangitis and inflammation of regional lymph nodes
- Vesicles, bullae, ecchymoses, and petechiae in severe cases (Fig. 4-548)

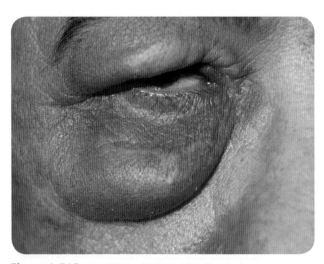

Figure 4-545 Periorbital cellulitis with edema and redness.

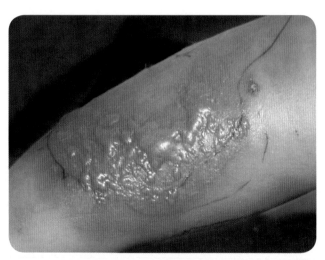

Figure 4-546 Streptococcal cellulitis can have edema and even purpura.

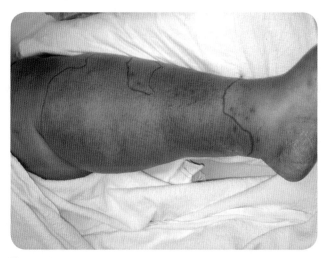

Figure 4-547 Unilateral erythematous, indurated, tender plaque on the leg with somewhat poorly defined borders.

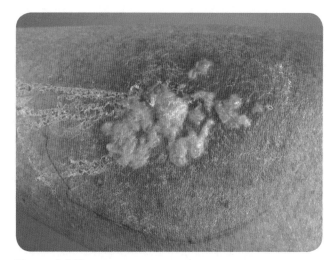

Figure 4-548 Cellulitis with erythema and opaque vesicles.

Diagnostic Pearls

Distinguishing cellulitis from necrotizing fasciitis is critical but clinically challenging. In contrast to cellulitis, which most commonly requires only antibiotics, necrotizing fasciitis requires immediate surgical intervention. The following clinical features suggest a deep necrotizing infection:

- Constant pain that is quite severe, and pain is out of proportion to physical exam
- Presence of bullae
- Skin necrosis or ecchymosis that precedes necrosis
- Gas (crepitus or crackling sounds) in the soft tissues
- Edema extending beyond areas of erythema
- Signs of systemic toxicity including fever, delirium, renal failure, hypotension, and tachycardia
- Cutaneous anesthesia
- Rapid progression despite antibiotic therapy

Crepitant and gangrenous cellulitis may be seen when *Clostridia* and other anaerobes are involved.

A tender and edematous extremity with minimal overlying erythema strongly suggests a process affecting deeper tissues. Rule out necrotizing infection if there is significant pain and rule out deep venous thrombosis (DVT).

?? Differential Diagnosis and Pitfalls

- Cellulitis can be caused by many different bacterial pathogens, but the diagnosis of typical cellulitis is usually made clinically.
- Necrotizing fasciitis—Look for a violaceous hue, bullae or necrosis, and severe localized pain. Pain is out of proportion to physical exam and extends beyond the area of erythema. Anesthesia and malodorous fluid are associated features. Does not respond to antibiotics alone, and requires surgical debridement. Rapidly progressive. Consider an MRI to delineate soft tissue involvement.
- Erysipelas—Well-defined erythematous plaque, associated with fever, chills, and malaise.
- Deep vein thrombosis—Rule out with ultrasound, decreased unilateral distal pulses, pain with ambulation, and less erythema.
- Stasis dermatitis—No systemic signs; commonly bilateral with pigmentary changes and chronic course.
- Panniculitis—Tender, indurated, less superficial, and epidermal changes.
- Lipodermatosclerosis—Look for signs of chronic venous hypertension. Biopsy, lack of response to antibiotics, and studies demonstrating venous dysfunction support this diagnosis.
- Thrombophlebitis—No fever, tenderness and erythema overlying a palpable cord.
- Impetigo—Honey-colored serous crusting.
- Atopic dermatitis—Chronic course; pruritic and scaly.
- Contact dermatitis—Look for well-demarcated, weeping erythematous and pruritic plaques. Vesicles and bullae can be present. Usually no associated systemic signs.
- Myonecrosis (gas gangrene)—Rapidly progressive; commonly occurs post surgical intervention; *C. perfringens* isolated in over 80% of cases.
- Toxic shock syndrome—High grade fevers (>38.9°C [102°F]), severe systemic symptoms including vomiting and diarrhea. Hypotension quickly ensues. Diffuse scarlatiniform exanthem that starts on the trunk.
- Herpes zoster—Painful and burning. Unilateral and usually dermatomal. Grouped vesicles on an erythematous base.
- Erythema migrans—Non-tender, slow spreading.

409

✓ Best Tests

- Diagnosis is most often made clinically
- Gram stain and tissue culture
- White blood cell count is normal or elevated
- Blood cultures are usually negative in immunocompetent patients
- Biopsy can be performed on atypical presentations
- An MRI can be performed to evaluate deeper tissue involvement

▲▲ Management Pearls

Mark the leading edge of erythema with pen or marker, and check every 4 to 6 h. If progressive after 24 h of therapy, consider more aggressive therapy or other etiologies. Surgical consultation is recommended if necrotizing fasciitis is a possibility.

Precautions: Standard and Contact. (Isolate patient, wear gloves and a gown, limit patient transport, and avoid sharing patient-care equipment.)

Therapy

In the majority of cases, antibiotics should include *S. aureus* and *S. pyogenes* coverage. The majority of patients develop mild cellulitis, and oral antibiotics can be administered. Antibiotics with MRSA coverage should be administered in patients with recurrent infections, a history of MRSA, and in immunocompromised individuals. Note that patients should be evaluated frequently to determine appropriate response to therapy.

- Dicloxacillin
  - Adults: 500 mg p.o. every 6 h
  - Children: 50 mg/kg/day p.o. divided every 6 h
- Cephalexin
  - Adults: 500 mg p.o. every 6 h
  - Children: 50 mg/kg/day p.o. divided every 6 h
- Ceftriaxone
  - Adults: 1 to 2 g IV/IM daily or divided twice daily
  - Children: 50 to 75 mg/kg/day IV/IM divided twice daily
- Nafcillin
  - Adults: 2 g IV/IM every 4 h
  - Children: 150 mg/kg/day IV/IM divided every 6 h
- Vancomycin: 30 mg/kg/day IV divided twice daily

- Cefazolin
  - Adults: 1 g IV/IM every 8 h
  - Children: 20 mg/kg IV/IM every 8 h
- Imipenem and cilastatin: 500 mg IV every 6 h, 50 mg/kg/day IV divided every 6 h
- Linezolid: 400 to 600 mg p.o./IV every 12 h for 10 to 14 days

Suggested Readings

Abrahamian FM, Moran GJ. Methicillin-resistant *Staphylococcus aureus* infections. *N Engl J Med*. 2007 Nov;357(20):2090; author reply 2090.

Bernard P. Management of common bacterial infections of the skin. *Curr Opin Infect Dis*. 2008 Apr;21(2):122–128.

Björnsdóttir S, Gottfredsson M, Thórisdóttir AS, et al. Risk factors for acute cellulitis of the lower limb: A prospective case-control study. *Clin Infect Dis*. 2005 Nov;41(10):1416–1422.

Chambers HF, Moellering RC Jr, Kamitsuka P. Clinical decisions. Management of skin and soft-tissue infection. *N Engl J Med*. 2008 Sep; 359(10):1063–1067.

Cohen PR. The skin in the gym: A comprehensive review of the cutaneous manifestations of community-acquired methicillin-resistant *Staphylococcus aureus* infection in athletes. *Clin Dermatol*. 2008 Jan–Feb;26(1):16–26.

Halpern J, Holder R, Langford NJ. Ethnicity and other risk factors for acute lower limb cellulitis: A U.K.-based prospective case-control study. *Br J Dermatol*. 2008 Jun;158(6):1288–1292.

Kroshinsky D, Grossman ME, Fox LP. Approach to the patient with presumed cellulitis. *Semin Cutan Med Surg*. 2007 Sep;26(3):168–178.

Madaras-Kelly KJ, Remington RE, Oliphant CM, et al. Efficacy of oral beta-lactam versus non-beta-lactam treatment of uncomplicated cellulitis. *Am J Med*. 2008 May;121(5):419–425.

Moran GJ, Krishnadasan A, Gorwitz RJ, et al.; EMERGEncy ID Net Study Group. Methicillin-resistant *S. aureus* infections among patients in the emergency department. *N Engl J Med*. 2006 Aug;355(7):666–674.

Rogers RL, Perkins J. Skin and soft tissue infections. *Prim Care*. 2006 Sep;33(3):697–710.

Ruhe JJ, Menon A. Tetracyclines as an oral treatment option for patients with community onset skin and soft tissue infections caused by methicillin-resistant *Staphylococcus aureus*. *Antimicrob Agents Chemother*. 2007 Sep;51(9):3298–3303.

Ruhe JJ, Smith N, Bradsher RW, et al. Community-onset methicillin-resistant *Staphylococcus aureus* skin and soft-tissue infections: Impact of antimicrobial therapy on outcome. *Clin Infect Dis*. 2007 Mar;44(6):777–784.

Stevens DL, Bisno AL, Chambers HF, et al.; Infectious Diseases Society of America. Practice guidelines for the diagnosis and management of skin and soft-tissue infections. *Clin Infect Dis*. 2005 Nov;41(10):1373–1406.

Swartz MN. Clinical practice. Cellulitis. *N Engl J Med*. 2004 Feb;350(9): 904–912.

Dermatomyositis

◼◼ Diagnosis Synopsis

Dermatomyositis is a multisystem autoimmune connective tissue disease that is most often characterized by a symmetric proximal extensor inflammatory myopathy, a characteristic violaceous cutaneous eruption, and pathogenic circulating autoantibodies. Dermatomyositis demonstrates a bimodal incidence, with the adult form most commonly seen in individuals aged 45 to 60, and the juvenile form found in children aged 10 to 15 years. A 2:1 female-to-male incidence ratio exists in adults.

While the etiology remains unclear, some evidence suggests that genetically susceptible individuals with certain HLA types mount aberrant cellular and humoral responses after exposure to malignancy, infection, or drug ingestion.

Clinical features of dermatomyositis can be categorized into cutaneous and systemic manifestations. Cutaneous features are quite characteristic and include a violaceous poikilodermic eruption seen around the eyes (heliotrope rash) and the extensor surfaces, including the knuckles (Gottron sign), elbows, and knees. Periorbital edema is often seen with violaceous plaques. Poikilodermic features include hypopigmentation and hyperpigmentation, telangiectasias, and epidermal atrophy. Nailfold changes are commonly observed and include chronically inflamed cuticles with ragged edges, nailfold telangiectasias, and occasionally calcinosis cutis. Pruritus is also a common associated feature.

Systemic manifestations of dermatomyositis include fatigue, malaise, myalgias, and the following:

- Musculoskeletal—Proximal extensor muscle group inflammation (triceps and quadriceps) that leads to muscle pain and weakness. Patients may have difficulty getting up from a sitting position without assistance.
- Gastrointestinal—Dysphagia can be seen in patients with scleroderma overlap.
- Pulmonary—Some level of pulmonary involvement will be present in 15% to 30% of patients. Diffuse interstitial fibrosis and acute respiratory distress syndrome are manifestations of pulmonary involvement. Antisynthetase syndrome includes pulmonary involvement and autoantibodies to aminoacyl-tRNA synthetase (anti-Jo-1, anti-PL-7, anti-PL-12, anti-OJ, and anti-EJ).
- Cardiac—Although usually asymptomatic, arrhythmias can be seen.

In addition, the clinician should be aware of several key points in patients with dermatomyositis:

- Malignancy—Up to 40% of patients with the adult form may have an occult malignancy. Initial cancer screening and vigilant serial monitoring for 2 to 3 years after diagnosis is strongly recommended. Chest, abdomen, and pelvis CT scanning—even in the absence of symptoms—should be considered. Commonly found malignancies include colon, ovarian, breast, pancreatic, lung, and gastric cancers and lymphoma. The juvenile form does not share this risk.
- Autoimmune disease overlap—Dermatomyositis can occur in conjunction with SLE, mixed-connective tissue disease, Sjögren syndrome, scleroderma, and rheumatoid arthritis.
- CREST syndrome—The most common overlap syndrome seen with dermatomyositis. Scleroderma, Raynaud phenomenon, esophageal dysmotility, sclerodactyly, and telangiectasias.
- Antisynthetase syndrome—Fever, Raynaud phenomenon, "mechanic's hands," interstitial pulmonary fibrosis, a polyarthritis, and autoantibodies to aminoacyl-tRNA synthetase.
- Variants—Dermatomyositis sine myositis is the amyopathic form where dermatomyositis is limited to cutaneous involvement.

With proper therapy, 75% of patients can be disease free within 3 years.

◉ Look For

- A heliotrope rash, a violaceous edematous periorbital erythema that may be slightly scaly, is considered pathognomonic for dermatomyositis (Figs. 4-549–4-551).
- Gottron papules appear as red to purple, scaly, flat-topped papules on the dorsal knuckles. They may be telangiectatic and may eventually atrophy (Fig. 4-552).
- Muscle strength should be serially graded. In addition, MRI of the proximal muscle groups can demonstrate an increased T2-weighted signal density and correlates with inflammation.
- Erythema and telangiectasias at the base of the nails are seen with some capillary loops exaggerated. Thickening,

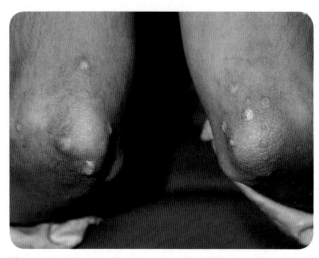

Figure 4-549 Calcinosis cutis is seen in both juvenile and adult dermatomyositis.

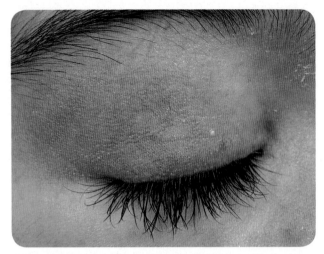

Figure 4-550 Dermatomyositis with heliotrope eruption on eyelids.

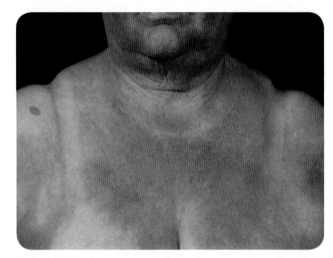

Figure 4-551 Dermatomyositis may have profound photosensitivity with sparing under heavily clothed locations.

Evaluation for myositis should be sought and includes the following:

- Electromyogram (EMG)
- MRI or ultrasound
- Serum levels of creatine kinase (CK) and aldolase
- Triceps muscle biopsy (gold standard)

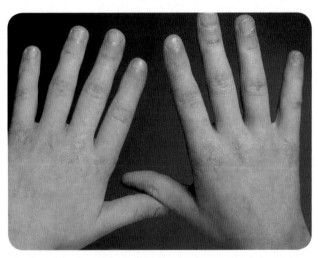

Figure 4-552 Atrophic plaques (Grotton papules) over hand joints are characteristic of dermatomyositis.

roughness, hyperkeratosis, and irregularity of the cuticle with little or no redness are frequent.
- "Mechanic's hands" refers to the hyperkeratosis, scaling, fissuring, and hyperpigmentation on the ulnar aspect of the thumb and radial side of the fingers.
- Other cutaneous manifestations include vesicles, bullae, lichenoid papules, and calcinosis cutis.
- Scalp involvement may be present in the majority of patients but is frequently misdiagnosed as psoriasis or seborrheic dermatitis. Scalp lesions generally appear as diffuse, atrophic, erythematous, scaly plaques, often with some degree of alopecia.

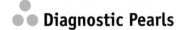 Diagnostic Pearls

A skin biopsy should be performed in a patient with cutaneous features consistent with dermatomyositis.

?? Differential Diagnosis and Pitfalls

- Lupus erythematosus—Violaceous color and extensor-limited skin disease not seen in lupus erythematosus. Check anti-ds DNA, anti-Sm if considering lupus erythematosus.
- CREST syndrome—Can have overlap with dermatomyositis. Refers to a subset of patients with limited scleroderma.
- Polymorphous light eruption—Most lesions resolve within several days' time. Skin lesions are located on all sun-exposed areas, not just extensors. Violaceous color not characteristic.
- Seborrheic dermatitis—No systemic findings. Erythema and scale in sebaceous distribution.
- Scleroderma—Check for anticentromere antibodies and anti-Scl-70 antibodies. Typified by sclerotic changes in skin not seen in dermatomyositis.
- Graft-versus-host disease—Occurs after allogeneic stem-cell transplantation.
- Mixed connective tissue disease—Check for anti-U1RNP antibody. Most patients are positive for this in mixed connective tissue disease.
- Generalized morphea—Asymmetric induration, no Raynaud phenomenon, no systemic involvement.
- Polymyositis—Without cutaneous findings.
- Acute lesions of erythropoietic protoporphyria may have similar locations, especially on the dorsum of the hands, but usually there is no weakness.

- For patients with myositis, one must rule out scleroderma, polymyositis, mixed connective tissue disease, and lupus erythematosus.

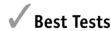 **Best Tests**

Muscle

- EMG —Look for altered electrical conduction.
- MRI (has been replacing triceps muscle biopsy)—Look for increased T2-weighted signal density of triceps of quadriceps.
- Serum levels of CK and aldolase—Look for elevated levels during exacerbations.
- Triceps muscle biopsy (gold standard)—Look for type II muscle fiber atrophy, lymphocytes in perifascicular and perivascular distribution, necrosis, sarcolemmal nuclei that are centrally placed.

Skin

- Skin biopsy—Mucin deposition in the dermis, lymphocytic infiltrate, epidermal atrophy, vacuolar changes of the basal keratinocytes.

Pulmonary

- High-resolution CT—Look for interstitial pulmonary fibrosis.
- Pulmonary function tests
- Check anti-Jo-1 antibody—Can identify those at risk of pulmonary involvement and the antisynthetase syndrome.

Cardiac

- ECG for conduction and rhythm aberrancies
Additional studies should be performed based on symptoms. For example, dysphagia and a barium swallow.

Once a diagnosis of dermatomyositis is confirmed, all adults should be screened for underlying malignancy. In two large studies, 30% to 40% of patients with dermatomyositis had an occult malignancy that was detected with CT scanning or other screening methods. Cancer screening studies can include CT scan of the chest, abdomen, and pelvis as well as colonoscopy, mammography, stool occult blood test, and CBC.

▲▲▲ Management Pearls

- In the adult form, serial cancer screening is of paramount importance. This includes serial history and physical examinations, laboratory evaluations, and chest, abdomen, and pelvic CT scans.

- Patients can contact the Myositis Support Group. The care of patients with dermatomyositis is multidisciplinary, including a rheumatologist and/or a neurologist. Patients may benefit from the expertise of a physical or occupational therapist.

Therapy

Treatment strategy should be primarily dictated by the degree of muscle disease and additional internal organ involvement.

Treatment of Skin Disease
Note that cutaneous disease in dermatomyositis is notoriously difficult to treat. Sun avoidance and appropriate protection remain key interventions. Sunscreens that contain both UVB and UVA blockers (Parsol 1789 or titanium dioxide) should be used.

Hydroxychloroquine: 200 to 400 mg p.o. daily
Chloroquine: 250 to 500 mg p.o. daily for adults

High-potency topical corticosteroids (class 2)

- Fluocinonide cream, ointment—apply twice daily (15, 30, 60, 120 g)
- Desoximetasone cream, ointment—apply twice daily (15, 60, 120 g)
- Halcinonide cream, ointment—apply twice daily (15, 60, 240 g)
- Amcinonide ointment—apply twice daily (15, 30, 60 g)

Mid-potency topical corticosteroids (classes 3 and 4)

- Triamcinolone cream, ointment—apply twice daily (15, 30, 60, 120, 240 m)
- Mometasone cream, ointment—apply twice daily (15, 45 m)
- Fluocinolone ointment, cream—apply twice daily (15, 30, 60 m)

Treatment of Muscle Disease
- Prednisone: 1 to 2 mg/kg p.o. daily with very slow taper
- Methotrexate: 10 to 30 mg p.o. or SC weekly
- Azathioprine: 2 to 3 mg/kg p.o. daily
- Mycophenolate: 1 to 1.5 g p.o. daily
- Rituximab: 375 mg/m2 IV weekly for four doses
- Intravenous Immunoglobulin (IVIg): 1 g/kg/daily IV for 2 days, then 400 mg/kg IV every month for 6 months

Suggested Readings

András C, Ponyi A, Constantin T, et al. Dermatomyositis and polymyositis associated with malignancy: A 21-year retrospective study. *J Rheumatol.* 2008 Mar;35(3):438–444. Epub 2008 Jan 15.

Callen JP. Dermatomyositis. *Lancet*. 2000 Jan;355(9197):53–57.

Callen JP. When and how should the patient with dermatomyositis or amyopathic dermatomyositis be assessed for possible cancer? *Arch Dermatol*. 2002 Jul;138(7):969–971.

Callen JP. Immunomodulatory treatment for dermatomyositis. *Curr Allergy Asthma Rep*. 2008 Jul;8(4):348–353.

Callen JP, Wortmann RL. Dermatomyositis. *Clin Dermatol*. 2006 Sep–Oct; 24(5):363–373.

Dourmishev AL, Dourmishev LA. Dermatomyositis and drugs. *Adv Exp Med Biol*. 1999;455:187–191.

Drake LA, Dinehart SM, Farmer ER, et al. Guidelines of care for dermatomyositis. American Academy of Dermatology. *J Am Acad Dermatol*. 1996 May;34(5 Pt 1):824–829.

Hayashi S, Tanaka M, Kobayashi H, et al. High-resolution computed tomography characterization of interstitial lung diseases in polymyositis/dermatomyositis. *J Rheumatol*. 2008 Feb;35(2):260–269.

Hirakata M, Suwa A, Takada T, et al. Clinical and immunogenetic features of patients with autoantibodies to asparaginyl-transfer RNA synthetase. *Arthritis Rheum*. 2007 Apr;56(4):1295–1303.

Iorizzo LJ III, Jorizzo JL. The treatment and prognosis of dermatomyositis: An updated review. *J Am Acad Dermatol*. 2008 Jul;59(1):99–112.

Klein RQ, Teal V, Taylor L, et al. Number, characteristics, and classification of patients with dermatomyositis seen by dermatology and rheumatology departments at a large tertiary medical center. *J Am Acad Dermatol*. 2007 Dec;57(6):937–943. Epub 2007 Oct 17.

Krathen MS, Fiorentino D, Werth VP. Dermatomyositis. *Curr Dir Autoimmun*. 2008;10:313–332.

Manlhiot C, Liang L, Tran D, et al. Assessment of an infectious disease history preceding juvenile dermatomyositis symptom onset. *Rheumatology (Oxford)*. 2008 Apr;47(4):526–529.

Sontheimer RD. The management of dermatomyositis: Current treatment options. *Expert Opin Pharmacother*. 2004 May;5(5):1083–1099.

Sparsa A, Liozon E, Herrmann F, et al. Routine vs. extensive malignancy search for adult dermatomyositis and polymyositis: A study of 40 patients. *Arch Dermatol*. 2002 Jul;138(7):885–890.

Diagnosis Synopsis

There are more than 80 specific cutaneous drug reaction patterns in the skin. Adverse cutaneous drug reactions are seen in 2% to 3% of inpatients. This synopsis summarizes simple drug eruptions with minimal systemic involvement. Complex drug eruptions with systemic manifestations such as drug hypersensitivity syndrome, Stevens-Johnson syndrome, toxic epidermal necrolysis, and serum sickness-like reaction are discussed in greater detail elsewhere. Drug-induced eruptions should always be considered in the differential diagnosis of any patient on medication presenting with a sudden "rash," particularly in individuals who are on multiple medications or have recently started a new drug or drug preparation.

Drug eruptions are often of unknown etiology and mechanism but always constitute an adverse effect. They may be immunologic or nonimmunologic; not all drug eruptions imply allergy. Possible other causes include metabolic reaction, drug accumulation or overdosage, combined manifestation with a coexistent disease, or interactions with other medications. The most common morphologies seen are morbilliform (95%) and urticarial (5%). Pustular, bullous, and papulosquamous morphologies also occur but are less common. Drug reactions may cause pruritus without an obvious cutaneous manifestation. They occur more commonly in inpatients, the elderly, females, and the immunocompromised.

Drugs and classes of medications frequently reported to cause a simple exanthem include antibiotics (penicillins, cephalosporins, trimethoprim-sulfamethoxazole, quinolones, gentamicin), nonsteroidal anti-inflammatory drugs (NSAIDs), ACE inhibitors, sulfonamides, anticonvulsants, allopurinol, thiazides, isoniazid, thalidomide, and nelfinavir.

Immunocompromised Patient Considerations

In the immunocompromised patient, drug eruptions are more common and often more severe. The incidence of drug eruptions increases as the patient becomes more immunocompromised; however, the mechanism is unknown. In the patient with HIV, sulfonamides frequently cause a minor or a severe reaction such as Stevens-Johnson syndrome or toxic epidermal necrolysis. Patients with HIV on multidrug therapy present with a spectrum of drug-induced dermatoses such as bullous, lichenoid, fixed drug, and exanthematous reactions.

Transplant patients receiving chemotherapy and antibiotics frequently develop cutaneous and oral mucosal lesions. These presentations can be difficult to distinguish between graft-versus-host disease, viral exanthem, and a drug eruption. A dermatology consult should be requested in this setting.

Drug eruptions should always be on the differential diagnosis list of any immunocompromised patient presenting with a rash.

Look For

Red macules or papules, erythema, urticaria, vesicles, pustules, or bullae occur a few days to weeks after the use of a new medication (Figs. 4-553–4-556). In the classic morbilliform exanthem, lesions often begin in intertriginous areas (such as the skin folds of the axillae or groin) or the trunk and spread centrifugally to involve the extremities. Involvement of the face (especially with edema of the central face) is worrisome for a more systemic, complicated adverse drug reaction.

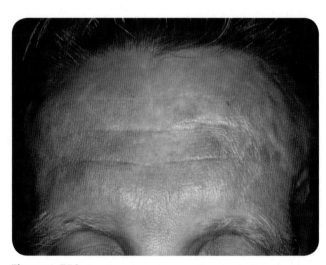

Figure 4-553 Exanthematous drug eruption due to itraconazole.

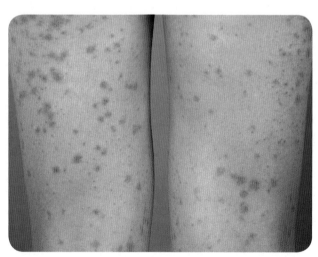

Figure 4-554 Exanthematous drug eruption due to amoxicillin.

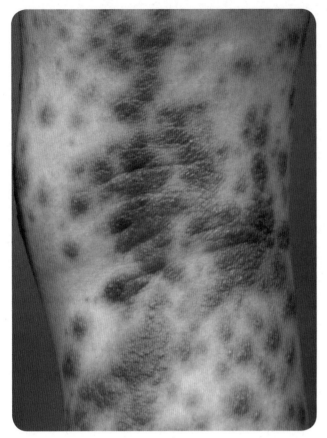

Figure 4-555 Vesiculobullous eruption associated with cephalexin.

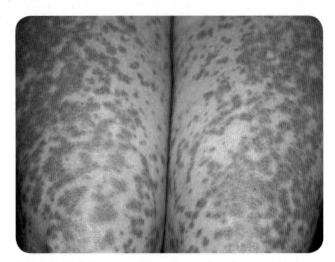

Figure 4-556 Papular eruption due to rofecoxib.

Recurring solitary plaques or patches are seen in fixed drug eruptions, discussed in more detail in this chapter.

Dark Skin Considerations

Lesions may have more of a hyperpigmented component, and erythema may be less obvious.

Diagnostic Pearls

- Patients with a simple drug eruption complain of itching.
- Warning signs of a potential serious drug reaction include systemic signs and symptoms (e.g., fever), blisters and erosions, angioedema, palpable purpura, skin necrosis, and a positive Nikolsky sign. Elevated eosinophils, BUN/creatinine, and liver function tests are worrisome for systemic involvement.

?? Differential Diagnosis and Pitfalls

- If lesions are painful and the patient appears ill or toxic, consider impending erythema multiforme, Stevens-Johnson syndrome, or toxic epidermal necrolysis.

Immunocompromised Patient Considerations

Blacks with AIDS have an increased incidence of drug eruptions with sulfa derivatives.

If there is fever, the degree of erythema is associated with a higher relative risk. Itching is common for many drug eruptions. If lesions are painful or tender, this may be worrisome for impending erythema multiforme, Stevens-Johnson syndrome, or toxic epidermal necrolysis.

- Viral exanthems (coxsackievirus, CMV, enteroviruses, adenoviruses, EBV, measles, HHV-6, parvovirus and B-19, and HIV)
- Graft-versus-host disease
- Eruption of lymphocyte recovery
- Bacterial infection (streptococcal, meningococcal, and rickettsial)
- Kawasaki disease
- Porphyria cutanea tarda
- Other causes of urticaria (e.g., physical stimuli)
- Acne
- Pityriasis rosea
- Lichen planus
- Contact dermatitis
- Sweet syndrome
- Scarlet fever
- Syphilis
- Leukocytoclastic vasculitis

Immunocompromised Patient Differential Diagnosis

Graft-versus-host disease should always be in the differential diagnosis for any transplant recipient.

✓ Best Tests

- Complete history and physical exam is often sufficient to make the diagnosis. A high index of clinical suspicion is needed.
- A skin biopsy is often used for additional information. However, it does not reliably distinguish between drug eruptions, viral exanthems, and graft-versus-host disease. The skin biopsy also does not help identify the culprit drug. Traditionally, it was believed that the presence of eosinophils suggested a diagnosis of a drug eruption; however, this is now controversial.
- If the patient has a severe eruption or systemic signs and/or symptoms, further testing may be needed. A CBC may show leukopenia, thrombocytopenia, or eosinophilia in a drug reaction. Serum chemistry studies, including tests of renal and liver function, should be ordered. Serologic tests are used infrequently (anti-histone antibodies in cases of drug-induced systemic lupus erythematosus [SLE]). Drug-induced SLE rarely presents with skin involvement.
- Cultures may be needed to rule out a primary or secondary infection.
- Patients with suspected vasculitis should additionally have a chest X-ray, a urinalysis, and fecal occult blood testing.

▲▲▲ Management Pearls

- Identify and eliminate the culprit medication, and clearly label the patient's medical record. If multiple medications are suspected, then stopping all agents (if possible) is best.
- A drug chart is often a valuable tool in identifying the culprit medication. A spreadsheet may be used with a vertical column for all medications used in the 2 to 3 weeks preceding the onset of the eruption, a horizontal row labeling the specific dates. An "X" may be marked for each day that the patient received every drug. This format is often helpful for inpatients and other patients on multiple agents.
- If the eruption is mild and the medication is essential with no suitable alternatives, the drug may be continued with careful monitoring.
- It often takes between days to weeks after discontinuing a drug to see a response in the skin.
- Skin tests, patch tests, and oral rechallenges are of limited diagnostic value and may be hazardous.

Therapy

Identify and eliminate the responsible drug(s), as outlined above. Counsel the patient regarding avoiding this medication and its related compounds.

Most simple drug eruptions are self-limited once the causative agent is withdrawn. Therefore, treatment is largely symptomatic. Antihistamines and topical corticosteroids are used to ameliorate pruritus and skin inflammation.

Antihistamines

- Diphenhydramine hydrochloride (25, 50 mg tablets or capsules): 25 to 50 mg nightly or every 6 h, as needed
- Hydroxyzine (10, 25 mg tablets): 12.5 to 25 mg, every 6 h, as needed
- Cetirizine hydrochloride (5, 10 mg tablets): 5 to 10 mg/day
- Loratadine (10 mg tablets): 10 mg tablet once daily

Topical corticosteroids may help with erythema and pruritus. Choice of potency should be body-site specific. Use lowest potency preparation needed to achieve the desired effect. High-potency topical corticosteroids should be reserved for truncal and extremity skin.

High-potency topical corticosteroids (class 2)

- Fluocinonide cream, ointment—apply twice daily (15, 30, 60, 120 g)
- Desoximetasone cream, ointment—apply twice daily (15, 60, 120 g)
- Halcinonide cream, ointment—apply twice daily (15, 60, 240 g)
- Amcinonide ointment—apply twice daily (15, 30, 60 g)

Mid-potency topical corticosteroids (classes 3 and 4)

- Triamcinolone cream, ointment—apply twice daily (15, 30, 60, 120, 240 g)
- Mometasone cream, ointment—apply twice daily (15, 45 g)
- Fluocinolone ointment, cream—apply twice daily (15, 30, 60 g)

Use mild-potency topical steroids on thinner skin and class 6 and 7 steroids on the face and intertriginous areas (desonide cream, lotion, or ointment twice daily).

If bullous lesions arise, use topical antibiotics occluded with Telfa or Vigilon to eroded sites. Change daily. Extensive blistering often requires hospitalization, aggressive wound care, and monitoring for infection, dehydration, electrolyte disturbances, and end-organ compromise. Extensive blistering would likely indicate a more systemic reaction, for which the treatment is discussed in toxic epidermal necrolysis, discussed in more detail in this chapter.

Oral corticosteroids are not indicated in simple drug eruptions with no systemic involvement.

Suggested Readings

Babu KS, Belgi G. Management of cutaneous drug reactions. *Curr Allergy Asthma Rep*. 2002 Jan;2(1):26–33.

Coopman SA, Johnson RA, Platt R, et al. Cutaneous disease and drug reactions in HIV infection. *N Engl J Med*. 1993 Jun;328(23):1670–1674.

Drake LA, Dinehart SM, Farmer ER, et al. Guidelines of care for cutaneous adverse drug reactions. American Academy of Dermatology. *J Am Acad Dermatol*. 1996 Sep;35(3 Pt 1):458–461.

Knowles SR, Shear NH. Recognition and management of severe cutaneous drug reactions. *Dermatol Clin*. 2007 Apr;25(2):245–253, viii.

Marra DE, McKee PH, Nghiem P. Tissue eosinophils and the perils of using skin biopsy specimens to distinguish between drug hypersensitivity and cutaneous graft-versus-host disease. *J Am Acad Dermatol*. 2004 Oct;51(4):543–546.

Nellen RG, van Marion AM, Frank J, et al. Eruption of lymphocyte recovery or autologous graft-versus-host disease? *Int J Dermatol*. 2008 Nov;47(Suppl. 1):32–34.

Roujeau JC, Stern RS. Severe adverse cutaneous reactions to drugs *N Engl J Med*. 1994 Nov;331(19):1272–1285.

Shear NH, Knowles SR, Shapiro L. Cutaneous reactions to drugs. In: Fitzpatrick TB, Wolff K, eds. *Fitzpatrick's Dermatology in General Medicine*. 7th Ed. New York, NY: McGraw-Hill; 2008:355–362.

Sullivan JR, Shear NH. Drug eruptions and other adverse drug effects in aged skin. *Clin Geriatr Med*. 2002 Feb;18(1):21–42.

Wintroub BU, Stern R. Cutaneous drug reactions: Pathogenesis and clinical classification. *J Am Acad Dermatol*. 1985 Aug;13(2 Pt 1):167–179.

Wyatt AJ, Leonard GD, Sachs DL. Cutaneous reactions to chemotherapy and their management. *Am J Clin Dermatol*. 2006;7(1):45–63.

■ Diagnosis Synopsis

Drug hypersensitivity syndrome (DHS), or drug reaction with eosinophilia and systemic symptoms (DRESS), is a serious multisystem drug reaction. It is an idiosyncratic reaction consisting of fever, rash, eosinophilia, and internal organ involvement, usually hepatitis. It tends to occur between 1 and 3 weeks after starting a new medication but may develop months later. A rash is present in over 80% of cases. Additional findings include pharyngitis, lymphadenopathy, facial edema, and nephritis.

The most commonly implicated drug groups causing DHS include anticonvulsants, sulfonamides, and nonsteroidal anti-inflammatory drugs (NSAIDs). Anticonvulsants include phenytoin, carbamazepine, phenobarbital, and lamotrigine. Sulfonamide-induced DHS is typically related to sulfonamide antibiotics and has an earlier onset than hypersensitivity syndromes caused by other classes, appearing as early as 7 to 14 days after the initiation of therapy. Minocycline, allopurinol, metronidazole, dapsone, antiretroviral agents (e.g., nevirapine), clopidogrel, and ticlopidine are other known causes of DHS.

It is imperative to withdraw the suspect medication(s) as soon as possible as there is a 10% mortality associated with this syndrome.

◉ Look For

There is a rash in over 80% of cases. A morbilliform or measles-like eruption is common, with macules and papules ranging in color from faint pink to dark red distributed symmetrically and spreading from the face downward (Figs. 4-557–4-559) Pustules may also be seen. Lymphadenopathy is another common finding and can be striking, leading to a misdiagnosis of lymphoma or mononucleosis. Facial edema is common.

Some patients will have urticarial plaques that may resemble erythema multiforme. Others will have manifestations of Stevens-Johnson syndrome, with atypical targetoid lesions, vesicles, and mucosal involvement, which progress to toxic epidermal necrolysis (TEN). Erythroderma is an additional serious manifestation of this syndrome.

Dark Skin Considerations

In dark-skinned individuals, the rash may present with deep red to brown macules and papules that are also distributed in a symmetrical fashion starting at the face and spreading downward.

●● Diagnostic Pearls

The liver, kidneys, and the hematologic system are the most commonly involved internal organ systems, but, rarely, pneumonitis, pericarditis, or myocarditis may be seen.

Immunocompromised Patient Considerations

Cases with nevirapine during anti-HIV therapy are commonly reported.

?? Differential Diagnosis and Pitfalls

- Infectious mononucleosis
- Cytomegalovirus infection
- Roseola
- Measles

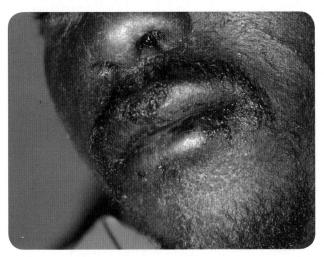

Figure 4-557 DRESS due to phenytoin.

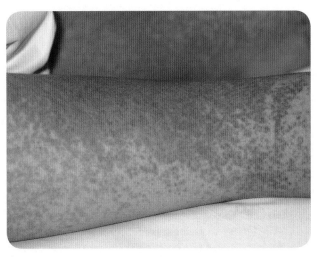

Figure 4-558 DRESS with multiple papules due to phenytoin.

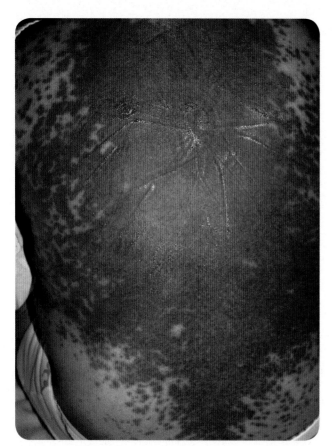

Figure 4-559 DRESS with linear vesiculations in a child due to phenytoin.

- Other viral exanthems
- Leukemia or lymphoma
- Drug eruption NOS
- Erythema multiforme
- Rocky Mountain spotted fever
- Rickettsialpox
- Secondary syphilis
- Meningococcemia

✓ Best Tests

It is important to identify any internal organ involvement.

Laboratory Studies

- Liver function tests
- CBC with differential—Look for the presence of leukocytosis with eosinophilia and atypical lymphocytes.
- Urinalysis and renal function tests

Chest X-ray and/or EKG can be ordered if symptoms of cough or chest discomfort are present.

A skin biopsy may show evidence of a common drug eruption but may include keratinocyte necrosis indicative of erythema multiforme, Stevens-Johnson syndrome, or TEN.

▲▲ Management Pearls

- The inciting drug must be identified and immediately stopped. Counsel the patient regarding avoidance of the drug and related compounds in the future, and clearly mark the patient's medical record. Conduct a thorough search for signs of systemic involvement.
- Patients with DHS warrant hospitalization and may require treatment in an intensive care setting, with meticulous attention paid to wound care, temperature regulation, nutrition, and fluid and electrolyte balance.
- Aromatic anticonvulsants (phenobarbital, carbamazepine, phenytoin) cross-react; therefore, all related compounds should be strictly avoided as well. Valproic acid and levetircetam are safe alternative options.
- Oral rechallenge tests and skin testing may be harmful and are, therefore, not recommended.
- Patients who have had DHS are at an increased risk for becoming hypothyroid. This usually occurs 4 to 12 weeks after the reaction.
- Consultations may be needed with dermatology, critical care, gastroenterology, ophthalmology (for patients with TEN), or nephrology.

Therapy

Many patients will recover spontaneously, although slowly. Optimize supportive care for any specific organ dysfunction.

The use of systemic corticosteroids has been advocated in patients with signs and symptoms of internal organ involvement. The dose of steroids depends on the severity of the reaction, but a dose of 1 to 2 mg/kg of prednisone daily is a good starting point. Tapering of the steroids should be done slowly (over 4 to 6 weeks)

In cases with a TEN-type picture, aggressive supportive care and the addition of intravenous immune globulin may be helpful (1 g/kg daily for 3 to 4 days). Patients with an extensive skin sloughing or erythroderma often need intravenous fluids, warming blankets, ophthalmic care, and topical antiseptics, emollients, and/or corticosteroids. Burn unit protocols are often used.

Monitor for and promptly treat any complicating infections.

Suggested Readings

Bachot N, Roujeau JC. Differential diagnosis of severe cutaneous drug eruptions. *Am J Clin Dermatol*. 2003;4(8):561–572.

Seth D, Kamat D, Montejo J. DRESS syndrome: A practical approach for primary care practitioners. *Clin Pediatr (Phila)*. 2008 Nov;47(9):947–952.

Shalom R, Rimbroth S, Rozenman D, et al. Allopurinol-induced recurrent DRESS syndrome: Pathophysiology and treatment. *Ren Fail*. 2008;30(3):327–329.

Tas S, Simonart T. Management of drug rash with eosinophilia and systemic symptoms (DRESS syndrome): An update. *Dermatology*. 2003;206(4):353–356.

Ecthyma Gangrenosum

Diagnosis Synopsis

Ecthyma gangrenosum (EG) is a cutaneous manifestation of *Pseudomonas aeruginosa* bacteremia. EG typically develops in immunocompromised patients (see below). Though most commonly caused by *P. aeruginosa*, it can less frequently be caused by other organisms. In the context of bacteremia, purpuric or black, painful eschars develop on the skin.

Severe complications such as nephritis and osteomyelitis may occur. The course depends on the underlying disease, but once manifestations of shock appear, the patient may quickly and irreversibly decline. Disseminated intravascular coagulation (DIC) may appear with Gram-negative sepsis. Most patients are systemically ill and have associated fever, chills, and hypotension. Diabetic patients, however, may have few symptoms early on in the disease. EG is seen in approximately 25% of patients with *P. aeruginosa* sepsis. The mortality rate ranges from 18% to 96%.

Immunocompromised Patient Considerations

EG typically develops in immunocompromised patients, including those with hematologic malignancies, immunodeficiency syndromes, neutropenia, pancytopenia, severe burns, malnutrition, recent chemotherapy, immunosuppressive therapy, and diabetes mellitus.

Look For

Initially, the lesions present as painless erythematous or purpuric macules. Within 12 to 24 h, the lesions become painful and develop into hemorrhagic vesicles or bullae. The lesions rupture, leaving a gangrenous ulcer with a central black necrotic eschar (Figs. 4-560–4-563). There may be one or multiple lesions. Within a 24-h period, the lesions can rapidly increase in size from 1 cm to greater than 10 cm. EG most commonly presents on the buttock or extremities but can also be noted in the axilla or on the trunk.

Immunocompromised Patient Considerations

In immunocompromised patients, the lesions of EG are similar to those in immunocompetent adults. However, they may be more rapidly progressive or more widespread depending on the level of immunosuppression.

Diagnostic Pearls

Pseudomonal sepsis occurs frequently after surgical procedures, especially urologic procedures. Chronic indwelling urinary catheters and long-term intravenous catheters have also been associated with EG. Prolonged use of antibiotic therapy targeting non-pseudomonal organisms may promote overgrowth of *P. aeruginosa*.

?? Differential Diagnosis and Pitfalls

- Pyoderma gangrenosum
- Necrotizing vasculitis
- Cryoglobulinemia
- Disseminated meningococcemia
- Polyarteritis nodosa

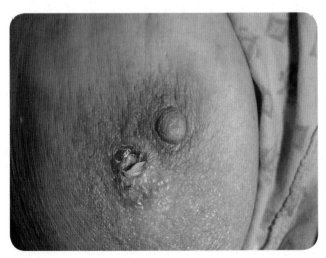

Figure 4-560 Early lesion of EG with ruptured vesicle and erythema.

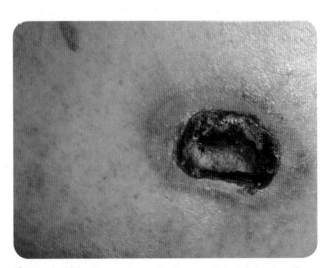

Figure 4-561 Adherent hemorrhagic crust with peripheral erythema in EG.

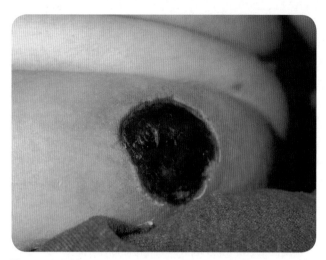

Figure 4-562 Hemorrhagic crusts with a wide peripheral band of erythema in EG.

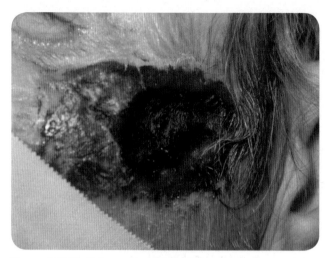

Figure 4-563 EG in a patient with AIDS.

Clinically indistinguishable lesions can occur with disseminated infections caused by other *Pseudomonas* species, *Aeromonas* species, *Citrobacter freundii*, *Serratia* species, *Staphylococcus aureus*, *Stenotrophomonas maltophilia*, *Candida* species, and fungi, including *Aspergillus, Mucor,* and *Fusarium* species.

✓ Best Tests

- Gram stain, blood and tissue cultures, and skin biopsy should be performed. Gram stain of vesicle fluid or skin biopsy will show numerous Gram-negative rods (GNRs), and on skin biopsy numerous GNR will be present around necrotic vessels with the extravasation of erythrocytes and edema.
- Despite the fact that EG commonly occurs in the setting of bacteremia or sepsis, in HIV patients, EG may be detected early at the port of entry by culture of the lesion and before dissemination occurs.

▲▲ Management Pearls

Therapy must be initiated immediately based on a high clinical index of suspicion for EG, as patients can rapidly decline.

Therapy

Therapy should be initiated empirically based on clinical suspicion with antipseudomonal intravenous antibiotics.

Initial treatment should be with an aminoglycoside (tobramycin, gentamicin, or amikacin) combined with an antipseudomonal penicillin (carbenicillin, piperacillin, or ticarcillin), a cephalosporin (ceftazidime or cefepime), or carbapenem (meropenem).

Granulocyte-macrophage colony-stimulating factor (GMCSF) may adjunctively be used in neutropenic patients and those with myeloid dysplasia.

- Ceftazidime—2 g IV every 8 h
- Cefepime—2 g IV every 12 h
- Ticarcillin—3 g IV every 4 h
- Piperacillin—4 g IV every 4 h
- Gentamicin and tobramycin—3 to 5 mg/kg in two to three divided doses daily
- Amikacin—7.5 mg/kg IV every 12 h
- Meropenem—0.5 g every 8 h or imipenem 0.5 g every 6 h

For patients with beta-lactam allergies

- Aztreonam—1.5 g every 6 h
- Piperacillin-tazobactam—3.375 g every 4 h

Suggested Readings

Downey DM, O'Bryan MC, Burdette SD, et al. Ecthyma gangrenosum in a patient with toxic epidermal necrolysis. *J Burn Care Res.* 2007 Jan–Feb;28(1):198–202.

James WD, Berger TG, Elston DM. Bacterial infections. In: James WD, Berger TG, Elston DM, Odom RB, eds. *Andrews' Diseases of the Skin: Clinical Dermatology.* 10th Ed. Philadelphia, PA: Saunders Elsevier; 2006:271–272.

Reich HL, Williams Fadeyi D, Naik NS, et al. Nonpseudomonal ecthyma gangrenosum. *J Am Acad Dermatol.* 2004 May;50(5 Suppl.):S114–S117.

Solowski NL, Yao FB, Agarwal A, et al. Ecthyma gangrenosum: A rare cutaneous manifestation of a potentially fatal disease. *Ann Otol Rhinol Laryngol.* 2004 Jun;113(6):462–464.

Erysipelas

■■ Diagnosis Synopsis

Erysipelas is a superficial bacterial infection of the skin most often caused by beta-hemolytic group A streptococci (*Streptococcus pyogenes*). It involves the lymphatics of the superficial dermis. Erysipelas usually occurs in isolation and has a predilection for the extremes of age, debilitated patients, and patients with poor lymphatic drainage. Historically, erysipelas occurred on the face, but, at the present time, this infection is more commonly seen on the lower extremities of patients with venous insufficiency and stasis dermatitis. There are some who view erysipelas as an extreme form of cellulitis.

Clinically, it presents as strikingly red, well-demarcated plaques that are very tender. Burning paresthesias may be present. Commonly involved areas are the face, extremities, and penis. Cutaneous findings are usually preceded by abrupt onset of fever, chills, nausea, and malaise. Lymphadenopathy is almost always present. Trauma to the skin is thought to be an important factor in the development of erysipelas; therefore, a concomitant dermatophyte infection, surgical incision, ulceration, insect bite, or inflammatory skin condition may provide a portal of entry for bacteria. The nasopharynx is often the reservoir in cases of facial erysipelas. Additional predisposing factors for erysipelas include alcoholism, diabetes, an immunocompromised state, and nephrotic syndrome.

Penile erysipelas responds to treatment with antibiotics but tends to recur, causing a progressive, chronic lymphedema with permanent swelling of the penis (elephantiasis). Elephantiasis may also develop in the lower extremities from recurring bouts of erysipelas.

Immunocompromised Patient Considerations

An immunocompromised state predisposes for the development of erysipelas. In addition, immunocompromised patients can develop erysipelas-like eruptions from organisms that seldom cause erysipelas in immunocompetent hosts.

◉ Look For

Sharply demarcated, fiery red plaques with warmth and tenderness (Fig. 4-564). The plaques will continue to progress if untreated. Overlying bullae and vesicles and purpura (bleeding into the skin) within the lesions can occur (Fig. 4-565). Lymphangitic streaking and regional lymphadenopathy are usually seen. The infection is generally preceded by trauma to the skin that may or may not be apparent on examination, but searching for a portal of entry is important to both diagnosis and management. Lesions heal with dry desquamation and occasionally postinflammatory dyspigmentation.

Penile erysipelas starts with erythema, itching, and tingling, which are followed by swelling and pain. Black, necrotic areas may appear within the lesion (Fig. 4-566). The lesion may spread to the pubic area. Erysipelas may involve the scrotum and be limited to it.

●● Diagnostic Pearls

- Erysipelas is differentiated from angioedema or contact dermatitis of the face by the presence of pain, fever, and an elevated leukocyte count (with left shift). ASO titers are often positive.
- If infection appears to involve the eyelids and there are signs of proptosis and/or ophthalmoplegia, consider orbital cellulitis rather than erysipelas. Conduct a prompt ophthalmologic exam; orbital cellulitis can lead to vision loss, cavernous sinus thrombosis, abscess formation, and meningitis.

?? Differential Diagnosis and Pitfalls

- Unilateral facial erysipelas can be confused with zoster.
- Acute contact dermatitis is usually pruritic.
- Orbital cellulitis
- Burn
- Cellulitis
- Deep venous thrombosis
- Polyarteritis nodosa
- Inflammatory carcinoma of the breast
- Eosinophilic cellulitis (Well syndrome)
- Necrotizing fasciitis

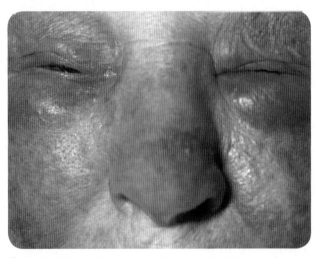

Figure 4-564 Facial erysipelas with edema involving the soft tissue around the eye.

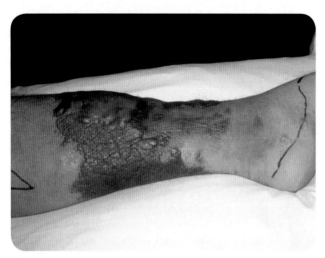

Figure 4-565 Erysipelas with vesicles and purpura. Note the raised edge of the plaque.

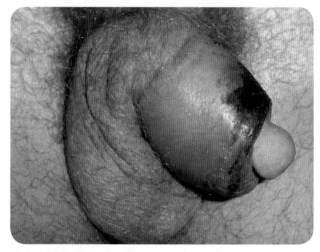

Figure 4-566 Erysipelas of the penis with edema and necrosis.

- Angioedema
- Urticaria
- Erysipeloid
- Sweet syndrome
- Familial Mediterranean fever
- Vasculitis
- Stasis dermatitis

 Best Tests

This is a clinical diagnosis.

Immunocompromised Patient Considerations

In the immunocompetent patient, routine blood and tissue cultures are not recommended because they have a low yield, and the results ultimately have minimal impact on management. However, in immunosuppressed patients, culture will help identify a nonbacterial or unusual bacterial etiologic agent.

Management Pearls

- Hospitalization for intravenous antibiotics is recommended in severe cases, in the immunocompromised, and in patients at the extremes of age (infants and the elderly).
- Consider using a penicillinase-resistant antibiotic to cover for *Staphylococcus aureus* in cases of erysipelas not responding appropriately to penicillin.
- In the United States, infections due to invasive group A streptococcus are reportable in many states.

Therapy

Penicillin is first-line therapy:

- Penicillin V 250 to 500 mg p.o. four times daily for 10 to 14 days; penicillin G procaine 0.6 to 1.2 MU IM twice daily for 10 days

Dicloxacillin:

- 250 to 500 mg p.o. four times daily for 10 days

Erythromycin (for penicillin-allergic patients):

- 250 to 500 mg p.o. four times daily for 10 days
- Cold sterile saline dressings may relieve pain, especially with bullous disease.

Penile erysipelas also requires treatment with steroids (prednisone) to prevent chronic lymphedema and subsequent elephantiasis.

Consider daily prophylaxis with penicillin in patients with multiple recurrent bouts of erysipelas who have poor lymphatic drainage.

Suggested Readings

Bisno AL, Stevens DL. Streptococcal infections of skin and soft tissues. *N Engl J Med.* 1996 Jan;334(4):240–245.

Cox NH. Oedema as a risk factor for multiple episodes of cellulitis/erysipelas of the lower leg: A series with community follow-up. *Br J Dermatol.* 2006 Nov;155(5):947–950.

Dompmartin A, Troussard X, Lorier E, et al. Sweet syndrome associated with acute myelogenous leukemia. Atypical form simulating facial erysipelas. *Int J Dermatol.* 1991 Sep;30(9):644–647.

Edwards J, Green P, Haase D. A blistering disease: Bullous erysipelas. *CMAJ.* 2006 Aug;175(3):244.

Guberman D, Gilead LT, Zlotogorski A, et al. Bullous erysipelas: A retrospective study of 26 patients. *J Am Acad Dermatol.* 1999 Nov;41(5 Pt 1):733–737.

Horrevorts AM, Huysmans FT, Koopman RJ, et al. Cellulitis as first clinical presentation of disseminated cryptococcosis in renal transplant recipients. *Scand J Infect Dis.* 1994;26(5):623–626.

Koster JB, Kullberg BJ, van der Meer JW. Recurrent erysipelas despite antibiotic prophylaxis: An analysis from case studies. *Neth J Med.* 2007 Mar;65(3):89–94.

Krasagakis K, Samonis G, Maniatakis P, et al. Bullous erysipelas: Clinical presentation, staphylococcal involvement and methicillin resistance. *Dermatology.* 2006;212(1):31–35.

Leclerc S, Teixeira A, Mahé E, et al. Recurrent erysipelas: 47 cases. *Dermatology.* 2007;214(1):52–57.

Mokni M, Dupuy A, Denguezli M, et al. Risk factors for erysipelas of the leg in Tunisia: A multicenter case-control study. *Dermatology.* 2006;212(2):108–112.

Petit A, Callot C, Dellion S, et al. Leg cellulitis caused by Aeromonas hydrophila. Medical treatment. *Ann Dermatol Venereol.* 1992;119(10): 749–752.

Török L. Uncommon manifestations of erysipelas. *Clin Dermatol.* 2005 Sep–Oct;23(5):515–518.

Zeglaoui F, Dziri C, Mokhtar I, et al. Intramuscular bipenicillin vs. intravenous penicillin in the treatment of erysipelas in adults: Randomized controlled study. *J Eur Acad Dermatol Venereol.* 2004 Jul;18(4):426–428.

Hand-Foot-and-Mouth Disease

■■ Diagnosis Synopsis

Hand-foot-and-mouth disease (HFMD) is an acute, self-limited viral illness caused most commonly by Coxsackie virus A16, though it can be caused by other coxsackie viruses and enteroviruses. It predominantly affects children, but adults can also develop the disease. The incubation period is short, ranging from 3 to 6 days. The illness begins with a mild fever, sore throat and mouth, cough, headache, malaise, diarrhea, and occasionally arthralgias. One or two days after the onset of fever, small oral vesicles develop. Later, vesicles appear on the hands, feet, and, occasionally, the buttocks.

The disease is highly contagious and often spreads via aerosolized droplets, nasal or oral secretions, or fecal material. Epidemic outbreaks usually occur from June to October. Though HFMD is typically self-limited, it can be complicated by encephalitis and other life-threatening complications. These include interstitial pneumonia, myocarditis, meningoencephalitis, and spontaneous abortion. Complications more commonly arise when the infectious agent is an enterovirus.

◉ Look For

Small erythematous macules appear on the oropharynx, later developing into 1 to 3 mm vesicles, which ulcerate easily (Figs. 4-567 and 4-568). Shallow ulcerations may involve the palate, tongue, gingiva, or buccal mucosa, and they are often painful. On average, approximately five to ten ulcers may be present.

Lesions on the extremities begin as erythematous macules and then develop a central, yellow-gray, oval or football-shaped vesicle on an erythematous base (Figs. 4-569 and 4-570).

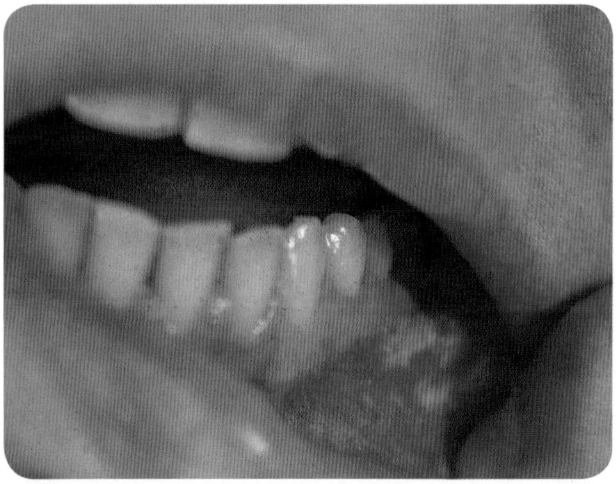

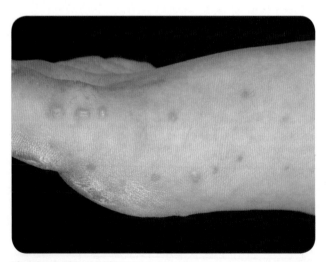

Figure 4-567 One or more painful aphthous ulcers are characteristic of HFMD.

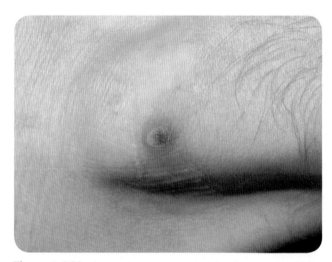

Figure 4-568 The lesion in HFMD may briefly be a papule, but then it forms a vesicle, which in this case raised the differential diagnosis of erythema multiforme minor.

Figure 4-569 A few to many clear vesicles with minimal inflammation on the hands and feet are characteristic of HFMD.

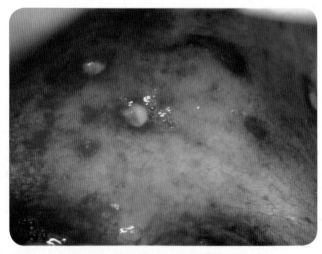

Figure 4-570 Intact vesicles and red macules on the palate in HFMD.

Lesions are most prevalent on the palms and soles, but they can also be seen on the lateral and dorsal surfaces of fingers and toes as well as on the buttocks. Another helpful finding is that lesions tend to be oriented parallel to skin lines.

 ## Diagnostic Pearls

Patients may have cervical or submandibular lymphadenopathy.

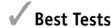 ## Differential Diagnosis and Pitfalls

- Varicella
- Erythema multiforme minor

For oral lesions, consider

- Herpes stomatitis
- Aphthous ulcers
- Streptococcal infection
- Candidal infection
- Herpangina

For lesions on the hands, consider

- Disseminated herpes simplex virus (HSV)/zoster
- Papular acrodermatitis of childhood
- Meningococcemia—purpura and pustules
- Rocky Mountain spotted fever—purpura, not vesicular or eroded
- Subacute bacterial endocarditis—purpura
- Gonococcemia—pustular and purpuric

✓ ## Best Tests

- HFMD disease is usually a clinical diagnosis, and, generally, no tests are required.

- If a CBC with differential is performed, white blood cell counts may be slightly elevated, and atypical lymphocytes may be present.
- The virus can be cultured from swabs of vesicles or mucosal surfaces and from stool specimens.
- Neutralizing antibodies may be detected during the acute phase of the illness, and complement-fixing antibodies can be isolated from convalescent sera.

 ## Management Pearls

This is a self-limited viral infection that needs to be treated only symptomatically.

Therapy

Supportive therapy and reassurance are generally all that is required. Oral pain may interfere with alimentation, and topical oral anesthetics (combination mouth rinses with diphenhydramine elixir, viscous lidocaine, and over-the-counter liquid antacids [all mixed 1:1:1]) are often needed. Encourage adequate hydration.

Suggested Readings

Kushner D, Caldwell BD. Hand-foot-and-mouth disease. *J Am Podiatr Med Assoc.* 1996 Jun;86(6):257–259.

Ooi MH, Solomon T, Podin Y, et al. Evaluation of different clinical sample types in diagnosis of human enterovirus 71-associated hand-foot-and-mouth disease. *J Clin Microbiol.* 2007 Jun;45(6):1858–1866.

Stalkup JR, Chilukuri S. Enterovirus infections: A review of clinical presentation, diagnosis, and treatment. *Dermatol Clin.* 2002 Apr;20(2):217–223.

Thomas I, Janniger CK. Hand, foot, and mouth disease. *Cutis.* 1993 Nov;52(5):265–266.

Henoch-Schönlein Purpura (HSP)

■■ Diagnosis Synopsis

Henoch-Schönlein purpura (HSP) is a small vessel vasculitis of uncertain etiology characterized by IgA-immune complex and C3 deposition in venules, capillaries, and arterioles. Approximately half of patients report a preceding upper respiratory tract infection 1 to 2 weeks prior to presentation. The classic tetrad of clinical manifestations includes hematuria, colicky abdominal pain, arthritis, and palpable purpura. HSP occurs predominantly in children, but it may be seen in adults and is more common in males. HSP is also seasonal, with most cases occurring during winter.

Additional symptoms include fever, malaise, headache, vomiting, hematemesis, diarrhea, hematochezia, melena, and scrotal pain. An individual episode may persist for 3 to 6 weeks, and recurrences are frequent. Occasionally, inflammation of the bowel may lead to appendicitis, ileus, and intussusception. Arthritic complaints most commonly involve the ankles and knees.

Renal involvement is common but is usually self-limited, with only a small fraction of patients progressing to chronic renal failure. The risk of renal failure is higher in adult patients and in those presenting with nephrotic or nephritic syndrome.

◉ Look For

Palpable purpura (violaceous erythematous nonblanchable papules) most commonly distributed on the legs and buttocks but occasionally involving the upper extremities, face, and trunk (Figs. 4-571–4-573). Urticarial wheals may occur early in the course. Lesions may develop necrotic centers (Fig. 4-574). Localized soft tissue edema of the hands, feet, scalp, ears, or scrotum may also be present.

●● Diagnostic Pearls

Palpable purpura over dependent areas such as the buttocks and legs and over pressure points, in the setting of a recent upper respiratory tract infection.

?? Differential Diagnosis and Pitfalls

- Other small vessel vasculitides (urticarial vasculitis, erythema elevatum diutinum, and acute hemorrhagic edema of infancy).

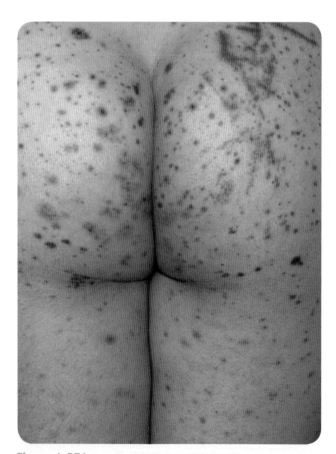

Figure 4-571 Symmetrical areas of papules. Some linear areas of purpura suggestive of the cutaneous vasculitis of HSP.

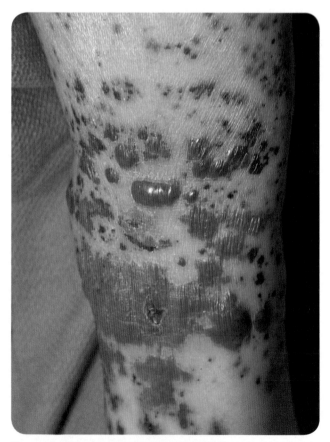

Figure 4-572 HSP with some purpuric vesicles.

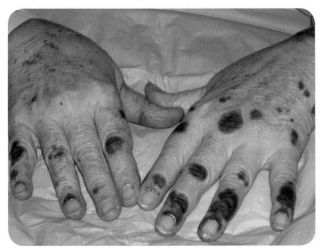

Figure 4-573 HSP with hemorrhagic lesions occurring bilaterally on the hands.

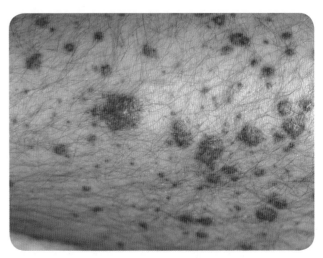

Figure 4-574 Raised purpuric lesions with some necrosis in HSP.

- Urticarial vasculitis is characterized by painful urticarial lesions.
- Erythema elevatum diutinum initially presents with palpable purpura over extensor surfaces that later become fibrotic.
- Pigmented purpura consists of nonblanchable macules with no associated vessel inflammation.
- Erythema multiforme has erythematous, targetoid plaques most commonly acrally distributed. Systemic lupus erythematosus has associated photosensitivity.
- Meningococcemia may result in purpura fulminans characterized by necrotic, nonblanchable palpable purpura on predominantly acral areas.
- In disseminated intravascular coagulation (DIC), patients are more systemically ill and present with petechiae (nonblanchable, nonpalpable macules).
- Endocarditis can present with characteristic Osler nodes and Janeway lesions (palpable purpura) over acral areas.
- Thrombocytopenic purpura presents like DIC with petechiae.
- Cryoglobulinemia has palpable purpura commonly in the setting of hepatitis C.
- Rickettsial infections have characteristic purpura on the hands and feet, and patients are systemically ill.

✓ Best Tests

- This is largely a clinical diagnosis. However, several tests may help aid in the diagnosis.
- Commonly ordered laboratory tests include a urinalysis, CBC with differential, ESR, BUN, creatinine, coagulation studies, antistreptolysin-O (ASO) titers, and fecal occult blood testing.
- Leukocytosis, an elevated ESR, hematuria, proteinuria, and a positive stool Hemoccult test are often seen. BUN

and creatinine may also be elevated. An elevated serum IgA is suggestive.
- Skin biopsy and direct immunofluorescence studies are diagnostic.
- Abdominal and/or testicular ultrasounds may be conducted to rule out intussusception or testicular torsion.

▲▲▲ Management Pearls

- Second episodes may be common despite adequate therapy.
- Close follow-up with repeat urinalyses is necessary to exclude associated renal nephritis and renal failure.

Therapy

HSP is usually benign and self-limited, and treatment is often supportive, including rest and adequate hydration. Nonsteroidal anti-inflammatory drugs (NSAIDs)—ibuprofen 600 mg p.o. every 6 h, naproxen 250 to 500 mg p.o. twice daily—may be used for joint pain when renal disease has been excluded.

Systemic corticosteroids (approx. 1 mg/kg p.o. daily) have been used to treat the associated vasculitis, nephritis, abdominal pain, and subcutaneous edema. However, steroids do not prevent the recurrence of skin lesions.

Systemic corticosteroids have also been combined with cyclophosphamide (2 mg/kg/day), and azathioprine in cases of severe renal disease. Cyclosporine, dipyridamole, high-dose IV IgG, fish oil, and plasmapheresis have also been used.

Suggested Readings

Chung L, Kea B, Fiorentino DF. Cutaneous vasculitis. In: Bolognia JL, Jorizzo JL, Rapini RP, eds. *Dermatology*. 2nd Ed. St. Louis, MO: Mosby; 2008:351–353.

Diehl MP, Harrington T, Olenginski T. Elderly-onset Henoch-Schonlein purpura: A case series and review of the literature. *J Am Geriatr Soc.* 2008 Nov;56(11):2157–2159.

Rashtak S, Pittelkow MR. Skin involvement in systemic autoimmune diseases. *Curr Dir Autoimmun.* 2008;10:344–358.

Diagnosis Synopsis

Systemic lupus erythematosus (SLE) is a multisystem autoimmune disease that affects the skin and internal organs and is characterized by pathogenic circulating autoantibodies. Sex and ethnicity are the strongest risk factors for developing SLE, with a 6:1 female-to-male ratio, and black women demonstrating a fourfold higher incidence when compared to whites. Women of child-bearing potential are most commonly affected.

The etiology of SLE is poorly understood, but there is a strong association with autoantibodies and SLE. For example, even though the autoantibodies are not organ specific, only certain organs in a given patient demonstrate end-organ damage. It is hypothesized that a complex interplay between genetic proclivity and environmental influences leads to a perpetuated autoimmune response. Autoantibodies play significant roles in the diagnosis, management, and prognosis of SLE. They are as follows:

- Anti-dsDNA—Highly specific for SLE. Rising levels correlate with an increased SLE activity and an increased risk for SLE nephritis. Seen in approximately 55% to 65% of SLE patients.
- Anti-Sm—Highly specific for SLE. Seen in approximately 25% to 30% of SLE patients. Considerable diagnostic value, but levels do not correlate with disease activity.
- Anti-RNP—Highly specific for SLE. Seen in approximately 5% of SLE patients.
- ANA—Highly sensitive for SLE. Seen in approximately 99% of SLE patients. In other words, it is very rare for an SLE individual to have a negative ANA. Considerable screening value, but levels do not correlate with disease activity.
- Anti-histones—Highly specific for drug-induced SLE.

The organ systems most commonly affected in SLE are the skin, renal, pulmonary, CNS, hematologic, and joints. Fever, myalgias, weight loss, and lymphadenopathy are very common nonspecific constitutional findings. Of note, SLE patients often require a multidisciplinary team and, hence, efforts should be made to clarify the level and location of involvement to assist the various disciplines.

In regard to classifying cutaneous lesions, specific and nonspecific types exist. Within the group of specific lesions, there are three main subtypes based on chronicity, association with SLE, and location/depth of inflammatory infiltrate. They are as follows:

- Acute cutaneous lupus erythematosus (ACLE)
  - Transient cutaneous findings typified by malar erythema without scarring
  - Strongly associated with systemic findings
  - Inflammatory infiltrate seen in the superficial dermis on biopsy

- Subacute cutaneous lupus erythematosus
  - Photosensitive cutaneous eruption lasting longer than ACLE but without scarring
  - 10% to 15% of patients go on to have systemic findings
  - Inflammatory infiltrate seen in the upper dermis on biopsy
- Chronic cutaneous lupus erythematosus
  - Also known as discoid lupus erythematosus (DLE)
  - Chronic discoid lesions with permanent disfiguring scars
  - 5% to 10% of patients go on to develop systemic findings
  - Significant inflammatory infiltrate seen in superficial and deep dermis as well as prominent involvement of the adnexal structures on biopsy

While investigatory efforts have led to promising novel drug targets for SLE, antimalarial therapy remains the gold standard. Hydroxychloroquine is the most commonly used antimalarial.

Dark Skin Considerations

Pneumonitis, nephritis, hypocomplementemia, and discoid lesions are more common in blacks. Black women have an earlier onset of SLE and nephritis.

Look For

The classic cutaneous finding in SLE is the malar or "butterfly" blush (Fig. 4-575). Erythema covering the nose and medial cheeks can occur after sun exposure and precede the systemic symptoms by weeks. The erythema often develops into fine, scaling, coalesced papules (Fig. 4-576).

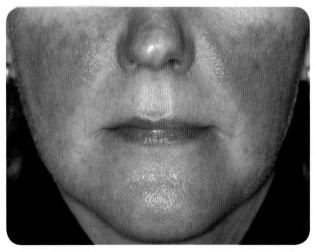

Figure 4-575 The malar butterfly rash of lupus usually spares the nasolabial folds.

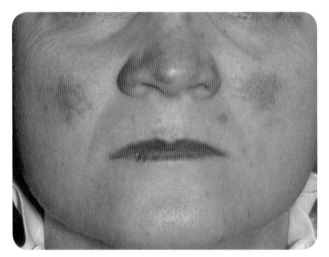

Figure 4-576 SLE with red plaques on the cheeks, nose, and upper lips.

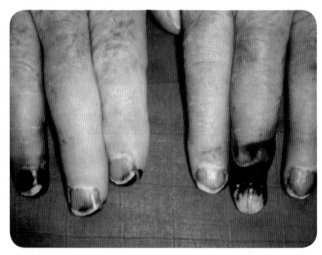

Figure 4-577 SLE with vasculitis causing digital necrosis.

The erythema can become intense, and small infarcts and necrosis can develop in fulminant cases.

A photodistributed cutaneous eruption can develop with prominence on the dorsa of the hands, arms, and trunk. Nail fold erythema and even necrosis can occur (Fig. 4-577). Small mucous membrane ulcers, especially on the palate, can develop (Fig. 4-578). Livedo reticularis is common.

DLE lesions can also be seen in conjunction with other cutaneous findings or alone. If SLE does not start within the first few (often 2) years of the disease, there is a low probability of SLE. Variants also include bullous lupus erythematosus. Purpura can occur secondary to vasculitis and is usually found on the extremities. Lupus profundus is a panniculitis rarely seen in patients with SLE. Some patients with SLE will have psoriasiform or annular lesions in a photodistribution (subacute cutaneous lupus).

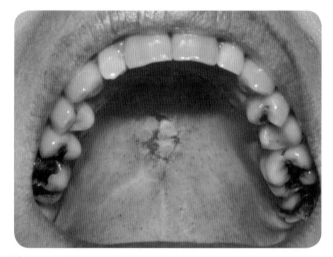

Figure 4-578 Oral hard palate ulceration in SLE.

Dark Skin Considerations

The malar or "butterfly" blush is not as prevalent in blacks. Photosensitivity is also less common.

Diagnostic Pearls

The American College of Rheumatology 1982 Revised Criteria for Classification of Systemic Lupus Erythematosus. Any 4 or more of the 11 criteria are present, simultaneously or serially, during any given interval of clinical observation.

The criteria for SLE include four of the following at any time during a patient's history:

- Malar rash
- Discoid rash
- Photosensitivity
- Oral ulcers
- Arthritis
- Serositis
- Renal disorder
- Neurologic disorder
- Hematologic disorder
- Immune disorder
- Presence of anti-nuclear antibodies

Dark Skin Considerations

Alopecia is 1.5 times more common in blacks when compared to whites.

?? Differential Diagnosis and Pitfalls

- Dermatomyositis—Characteristic heliotrope rash (violaceous plaques surrounding eyes), photodistributed cutaneous eruption, and nailfold changes. Look for elevated serum creatine kinase (CK) levels and proximal symmetric extremity weakness.
- Erythema multiforme major—Characteristic target lesions, prominent systemic symptoms, but ANA and direct immunofluorescene (DIF) negative.
- Antiphospholipid antibody/lupus anticoagulant—Can overlap with SLE; associated with recurrent thromboses and spontaneous abortions, elevated PT time.
- Polymorphous light eruption (PMLE)—Most lesions resolve within several days; skin lesions are located primarily on sun-exposed areas (SLE can occur on sun-exposed and sun-protected areas). Note that previous studies have shown that up to 19% of patients with PMLE can be ANA positive. Hence, an ANA alone may not be sufficient in differentiating PMLE from SLE.
- Drug-related photosensitivity—Look for drug history; will be ANA negative.
- Granuloma faciale—Histology is different than seen in SLE.
- Rosacea—ANA negative.
- Seborrheic dermatitis—Sebaceous distribution affecting the nasolabial folds where SLE usually spares this area. Will also be ANA negative.
- Tinea faciale—Check KOH; will also be ANA negative.

✓ Best Tests

- Diagnosis is made on clinical and serologic grounds, using the American Rheumatologic Association (ARA) criteria for diagnosis.
- ARA criteria meet at least 4 of the following: malar rash, discoid rash, photosensitivity, oral ulcers, arthritis, serositis, renal disorder, neurologic disorder, hematologic disorder, immunologic disorder, and presence of antinuclear antibody.
- ANA and anti-DNA antibodies are found in a majority of patients.
- Skin biopsy can be diagnostic for lupus, as well as biopsy of uninvolved skin for direct immunofluorescence (DIF—lupus band test). DIF can be very useful when conventional histopathology is not discerning and will demonstrate granular deposition of IgG, IgA, or IgM at the dermal–epidermal junction.
- Check BUN/Cr, liver urinalysis, function tests, and serum complement (CH50). Slight elevations in PTT and PT might suggest the presence of the lupus anticoagulant. Patients with the lupus anticoagulant are at higher risk for stroke and thrombosis.

▲▲ Management Pearls

Consultation with multiple specialists is mandatory for patients with SLE.

Therapy

Antimalarials
- Hydroxychloroquine: 200 to 400 mg p.o. daily
- Chloroquine: 125 to 250 mg p.o. daily

Glucocorticoids
- Prednisone: 5 to 60 mg p.o. daily or divided two to four times daily; taper over 2 weeks

Immunosuppressives
- Cyclophosphamide: 10 to 20 mg/kg IV every 3 to 4 weeks or 1.5 to 2.5 mg/kg p.o. daily
- Azathioprine: 1.5 to 3 mg/kg p.o. daily, maintenance dose of 1 to 2 mg/kg/day
- Mycophenolate mofetil: 500 mg p.o. twice daily, increase over several weeks to 1,500 mg p.o. twice daily
- Arthritis, arthralgias, and myalgias can be managed with nonacetylated salicylates (choline magnesium trisalicylate 500 mg to 1.5 g p.o. two to three times daily) and nonsteroidal anti-inflammatory drugs (NSAIDs)—ibuprofen 400 to 600 mg p.o. every 4 to 6 h, as needed.

Suggested Readings

Bertsias G, Gordon C, Boumpas DT. Clinical trials in systemic lupus erythematosus (SLE): Lessons from the past as we proceed to the future–the EULAR recommendations for the management of SLE and the use of end-points in clinical trials. *Lupus.* 2008;17(5):437–442.

Bertsias G, Ioannidis JP, Boletis J, et al.; Task Force of the EULAR Standing Committee for International Clinical Studies Including Therapeutics. EULAR recommendations for the management of systemic lupus erythematosus Report of a Task Force of the EULAR Standing Committee for International Clinical Studies Including Therapeutics. *Ann Rheum Dis.* 2008 Feb;67(2):195–205.

Costner ML, Sontheimer RD. Lupus erythematosus. In: Fitzpatrick TB, Wolff K, eds. *Fitzpatrick's Dermatology in General Medicine.* 7th Ed. New York, NY: McGraw-Hill; 2008:1515–1535.

Guidelines for referral and management of systemic lupus erythematosus in adults. American College of Rheumatology Ad Hoc Committee on Systemic Lupus Erythematosus Guidelines. *Arthritis Rheum.* 1999 Sep;42(9):1785–1796.

Majeski C, Ritchie B, Giuffre M, et al. Pincer nail deformity associated with systemic lupus erythematosus. *J Cutan Med Surg.* 2005 Jan;9(1):2–5.

Munoz LE, van Bavel C, Franz S, et al. Apoptosis in the pathogenesis of systemic lupus erythematosus. *Lupus.* 2008;17(5):371–375.

Petri M. Review of classification criteria for systemic lupus erythematosus. *Rheum Dis Clin North Am.* 2005 May;31(2):245–254, vi.

Rahman A, Isenberg DA. Systemic lupus erythematosus. *N Engl J Med.* 2008 Feb;358(9):929–939.

Rhodes B, Vyse TJ. The genetics of SLE: An update in the light of genome-wide association studies. *Rheumatology (Oxford).* 2008 Nov;47(11):1603–1611.

Diagnosis Synopsis

Infection with the Gram-negative bacterium *Neisseria meningitidis* is responsible for acute meningococcemia, a severe illness that typically occurs in small epidemics. It is transmitted from person to person by respiratory droplets; the human nasopharynx is the only known reservoir. Between 5% and 10% of people in the United States are carriers at any given time.

The distribution is worldwide; infections are commonly caused by serogroups A, B, C, Y, and W-135 and are more common in crowded areas (such as army barracks and college dormitories) and within contacts of infected family members. Increased risk is linked to deficiencies of complement, immunoglobulins and properdin, asplenia, liver disease, systemic lupus erythematosus, enteropathies, and the nephrotic syndrome. Acute meningococcemia has been reported in patients coinfected with HIV and hepatitis C. In the immunocompetent, acute meningococcemia is seen in children aged younger than 4 years and also in teenagers (and, rarely, in persons of all ages, especially during epidemics).

The clinical picture consists of headache, nausea, vomiting, and myalgias quickly leading to obtundation and a septic-appearing patient. Patients may report a preceding upper respiratory tract infection. Petechiae are the most common cutaneous sign, seen in one-third to one-half of affected patients. Altered mental status, nuchal rigidity, seizures, and gait disturbance can also occur. In asplenic patients, fulminant meningococcemia can lead to sepsis, hypotension, shock, and death in a matter of hours. Complications of acute meningococcemia include pericarditis/myocarditis, disseminated intravascular coagulation (DIC), meningitis and permanent neurologic sequelae, septic arthritis, osteomyelitis,

adrenal hemorrhage (Waterhouse-Friderichsen syndrome), gangrene, and death. The overall mortality rate is between 5% and 10%; however, meningococcemia associated with DIC has a mortality rate exceeding 90%.

Chronic meningococcemia is characterized by a persistent low fever, rash, and arthralgias, and it is commonly mistaken for gonococcemia.

Immunocompromised Patient Considerations

The risk of meningococcemia is increased in patients with asplenia and deficiencies of complement, immunoglobulins, or properdin. Hepatic dysfunction leading to low complement synthesis may be a predisposing factor to invasive infection.

Look For

The very early rash is reported to resemble a viral exanthem with erythematous macules and papules; this morbilliform eruption is not seen in the majority of patients. Thirty to fifty percent of patients present with a petechial eruption on the trunk and the distal extremities. Pustules, vesicles, and bullae, which may have central infarcts, quickly follow (Fig. 4-579). Stellate purpura with a central gray or dusky hue is characteristic of meningococcemia (Fig. 4-580). This central discoloration is sometimes referred to as "gun-metal gray."

In severe cases, gangrenous purpura develops (purpura fulminans), which is indicative of concurrent DIC (Figs. 4-581 and 4-582). Mucosal surfaces, such as the oral cavity and the conjunctiva, may also be affected.

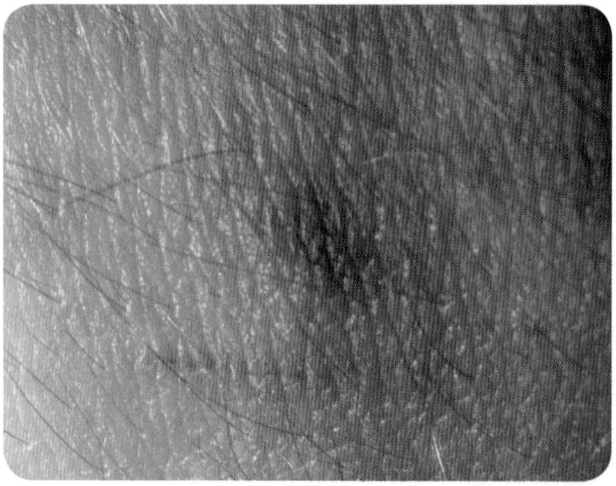

Figure 4-579 Early lesion of acute meningococcemia with a deep red plaque with central purpura.

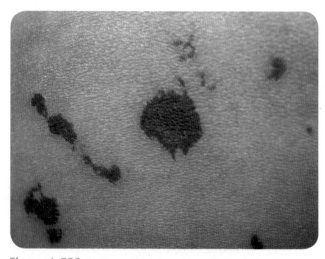

Figure 4-580 Acute meningococcemia with necrotic annular and linear purpura.

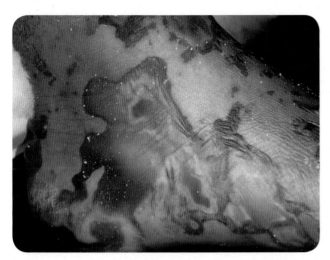

Figure 4-581 Hemorrhagic and necrotic lesions of meningococcemia with DIC.

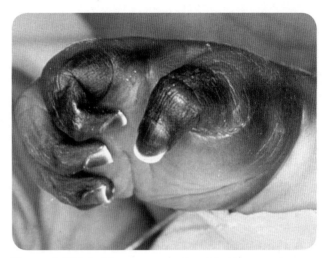

Figure 4-582 Peripheral gangrene from DIC due to meningococcemia.

Dark Skin Considerations

The petechiae of meningococcemia typically have gray or dusky centers and are slightly vesicular in appearance. Chronic cases can be associated with terminal complement deficiencies.

Diagnostic Pearls

Larger lesions will have complex arcuate and geographic or maple leaf–like borders.

?? Differential Diagnosis and Pitfalls

- Subacute bacterial endocarditis usually does not have as many skin lesions.
- Rocky Mountain spotted fever (RMSF) lesions appear first distally on the extremities, including the wrists, ankles, palms, and soles; exposure to RMSF usually occurs in an endemic region.
- Other rickettsial infection
- Hypersensitivity vasculitis
- Septic vasculitis
- Thrombotic thrombocytopenic purpura
- Disseminated intravascular coagulation
- Enteroviral infections (echo and adenovirus)
- Leptospirosis
- Erythema multiforme
- Toxic shock syndrome

- Disseminated gonococcal infection
- Other causes of bacterial sepsis
- Meningitis, other
- Typhoid fever
- Q fever
- Typhus
- Fulminant hepatitis, other
- Hantavirus hemorrhagic fever with renal syndrome
- Shigellosis
- Hemolytic-uremic syndrome
- In patients traveling abroad or recent immigrants to the United States:
  - Marburg virus
  - Ebola
  - Dengue hemorrhagic fever
  - Malaria
  - Kyasanur forest disease
  - Yellow fever
  - Viral hemorrhagic fever, other
  - Crimean-Congo hemorrhagic fever

✓ Best Tests

- On CBC, leukocytosis or thrombocytopenia may be seen.
- Meningococci may be seen in skin specimens (scrapings, lesional aspirates, or punch biopsies) using a Brown-Hopp–modified Gram stain.
- Blood cultures should be performed, although results will not be available for 12 to 24 h.
- Lumbar puncture for latex agglutination of soluble antigens in cerebrospinal fluid (CSF); CSF Gram stain and

culture. Look for increased CSF protein and polymorpho-nuclear leukocytes and decreased CSF glucose.

- Throat culture should be obtained, bearing in mind that only asymptomatic colonization may be detected.
- Sensitivities should be obtained for all meningococcal isolates.
- An MRI can be used to detect muscle or bone involvement.
- Chest X-ray can evaluate for the adult respiratory distress syndrome or pneumonia.
- Echocardiography is indicated when pericarditis or other cardiac sequelae are suspected.
- Evaluate for end-organ damage with the appropriate laboratory investigations (e.g., liver and renal function tests).

▲▲ Management Pearls

- If you are thinking of this diagnosis, do not wait for the results of confirmatory tests to initiate therapy, as this can be a life-threatening illness.
- In addition to antibiotics, many patients will require intensive supportive care, including aggressive IV fluid resuscitation, close monitoring of vital signs, electrolytes and end organ function, and ventilatory and/or inotropic support. An involvement of intensivists and infectious disease physicians is often indicated. General or plastic surgical consultation may be needed for amputation, the debridement of necrotic tissue, and possible flaps or grafts. A complication of acute meningococcemia is DIC, requiring multispecialty management in the intensive care unit.
- Close contacts of all patients with invasive disease should receive chemoprophylaxis with rifampin (600 mg p.o. twice daily for 2 days), ciprofloxacin (500 mg p.o. single dose), or ceftriaxone (250 mg IM single dose) within 24 hours of diagnosis of the primary case. A quadrivalent vaccine (Menomune A/C/Y/W-135, 0.5 mL SC single dose) is available that protects against certain serogroups of *N. meningitidis*. It is recommended for military recruits and patients with terminal complements deficiencies or asplenia. Affected patients treated with IV antibiotics may subsequently receive a single dose of ciprofloxacin 500 mg p.o. to eradicate nasal carriage.

Precautions: Standard, Droplet. (Isolate patient, wear a mask, and limit patient transport.)

Therapy

Intravenous penicillin G is the drug of choice for susceptible isolates:

- 300,000 U/kg IV daily divided every 4 h. Many adult patients are begun at a dose of 4 MU IV every 4 h. Continue administration for 5 to 7 additional days after the patient's temperature has returned to normal.

Intravenous chloramphenicol should be used in patients highly allergic to penicillin:

- 1 g IV every 6 h. Administer for 5 to 7 additional days after the patient's temperature has returned to normal.

Third generation cephalosporins (cefotaxime and ceftriaxone) may be used as a third alternative and may be considered for initial therapy in areas of the world with penicillin-resistant strains (e.g., the United Kingdom and Spain) or in septic patients while the diagnosis is being confirmed.

- Cefotaxime 2 g IV every 4 h
- Ceftriaxone 2 g IV/IM every 12 h
- Administer for 5 to 7 additional days after the patient's temperature has returned to normal.

Prevention: There are vaccines available.

Suggested Readings

Bilukha OO, Rosenstein N; National Center for Infectious Diseases, Centers for Disease Control and Prevention (CDC). Prevention and control of meningococcal disease. Recommendations of the Advisory Committee on Immunization Practices (ACIP). *MMWR Recomm Rep.* 2005 May;54(RR-7):1–21.

Cartwright KA, Jones DM. ACP Broadsheet 121: June 1989. Investigation of meningococcal disease. *J Clin Pathol.* 1989 Jun;42(6):634–639.

de Filippis I, do Nascimento CR, Clementino MB, et al. Rapid detection of *Neisseria meningitidis* in cerebrospinal fluid by one-step polymerase chain reaction of the nspA gene. *Diagn Microbiol Infect Dis.* 2005 Feb;51(2):85–90.

James WD, Berger TG, Elston DM. Bacterial infections. In: James WD, Berger TG, Elston DM, Odom RB, eds. *Andrews' Diseases of the Skin: Clinical Dermatology.* 10th Ed. Philadelphia, PA: Saunders Elsevier; 2006:278–279.

Nelson CG, Iler MA, Woods CW, et al. Meningococcemia in a patient coinfected with hepatitis C virus and HIV. *Emerg Infect Dis.* 2000 Nov-Dec;6(6):646–648.

Ramesh V, Mukherjee A, Chandra M, et al. Clinical, histopathologic & immunologic features of cutaneous lesions in acute meningococcaemia. *Indian J Med Res.* 1990 Jan;91:27–32.

Razminia M, Salem Y, Elbzour M, et al. Importance of early diagnosis and therapy of acute meningococcal myocarditis: A case report with review of literature. *Am J Ther.* 2005 May–Jun;12(3):269–271.

Rompalo AM, Hook EW, Roberts PL, et al. The acute arthritis-dermatitis syndrome. The changing importance of *Neisseria gonorrhoeae* and *Neisseria meningitidis. Arch Intern Med.* 1987 Feb;147(2):281–283.

Sapadin A, Gordon M, Bottone EJ. Acute meningococcemia. *Mt Sinai J Med.* 1997 Sep–Oct;64(4–5):353.

Tappero JW, Reporter R, Wenger JD, et al. Meningococcal disease in Los Angeles County, California, and among men in the county jails. *N Engl J Med.* 1996 Sep;335(12):833–840.

van Deuren M, van Dijke BJ, Koopman RJ, et al. Rapid diagnosis of acute meningococcal infections by needle aspiration or biopsy of skin lesions. *BMJ.* 1993 May;306(6887):1229–1232.

Vincent Halpern A, Heymann WR. Bacterial diseases. In: Bolognia J, Jorizzo JL, Rapini RP, eds. *Dermatology.* 2nd Ed. St. Louis, MO: Mosby; 2008: 1091–1092.

von Gottberg A, du Plessis M, Cohen C, et al. Emergence of endemic serogroup W135 meningococcal disease associated with a high mortality rate in South Africa. *Clin Infect Dis.* 2008 Feb;46(3):377–386.

▦ Diagnosis Synopsis

Necrotizing fasciitis is a deep and often devastating bacterial infection that tracks along fascial planes and expands well beyond any outward cutaneous signs of infection (i.e., erythema). It occurs from the extension of infection at the site of a skin lesion such as an abrasion, furuncle, or insect bite in 80% of cases. Classically, group A β-hemolytic streptococci is associated with necrotizing fasciitis, but many other organisms including *Staphylococcus aureus*, *Vibrio vulnificus*, Enterobacteriaceae, and *Bacteroides* spp. have been reported. Polymicrobial infection is frequent. Group A *Streptococcus* and *S. aureus*, in particular, should be considered in necrotizing fasciitis resulting after a varicella infection.

Patients with necrotizing fasciitis are acutely ill. They are often thought to have cellulitis that is not responding to standard antibiotic therapy. Pain is out of proportion to physical findings. There is often associated skin necrosis and bullae formation. Signs of systemic illness such as fever, lethargy, hypotension, and tachycardia are present; these may progress to multi-organ failure. Predisposing factors for necrotizing fasciitis include recent surgery, diabetes mellitus, malignancy, and alcoholism.

The mortality of necrotizing fasciitis is high. Treatment includes broad-spectrum intravenous antibiotics and immediate surgical debridement of infected and devitalized tissue. Therefore, if you are considering this diagnosis, stop reading this and contact a surgeon now.

When necrotizing fasciitis is localized to the lower abdominal wall, perineum, or genitals, it is known as Fournier gangrene. Diabetic patients are particularly susceptible to Fournier gangrene, which is often polymicrobial with mixed anaerobic organisms.

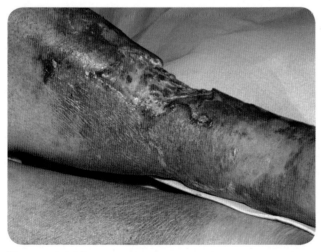

Figure 4-583 Necrotizing fasciitis with full-thickness skin ulceration.

Immunocompromised Patient Considerations

Patients who are immunocompromised from an underlying disease state (e.g., HIV and malignancy) as well as patients undergoing iatrogenic immunosuppression (prevention of transplant rejection or for treatment of an autoimmune/inflammatory condition) are at a significantly higher risk for developing necrotizing fasciitis. These patients also have a higher likelihood of developing necrotizing fasciitis from uncommon infectious agents, making cultures of debrided tissue valuable in directing adjuvant antimicrobial therapy. Rare infectious causes of necrotizing fasciitis in immunocompromised hosts include *Cryptococcus*, *V. vulnificus*, *Mucor*, *Mycobacterium tuberculosis*, *Serratia marcescens*, *Histoplasma capsulatum*, and multiple *Salmonella* species.

Although necrotizing fasciitis caused by methicillin-resistant *S. aureus* (MRSA) is rare, it has been observed in patients with HIV/AIDS and may be on the rise in this patient population.

◉ Look For

Early on, there is erythema and edema typical of cellulitis in the setting of a patient who appears severely ill. Despite standard antibiotic therapy, the edema progresses and can become associated with bullae, cyanosis, and eventual gangrene (Figs. 4-583–4-587). Crepitus may be present. The subcutaneous tissues will often have a hard, wooden feel.

Diagnostic Pearls

Distinguishing necrotizing fasciitis from a cellulitis that does not require surgical intervention may be challenging. The following clinical features suggest a deep necrotizing infection:

- Constant pain that is often quite severe and is out of proportion with visible skin changes
- Presence of bullae
- Skin necrosis or ecchymosis that precedes necrosis
- Gas in the soft tissues
- Edema extending beyond areas of erythema
- Systemic toxicity (fever, delirium, renal failure, hypotension, and tachycardia)
- Cutaneous anesthesia
- Rapid spread despite antibiotic therapy

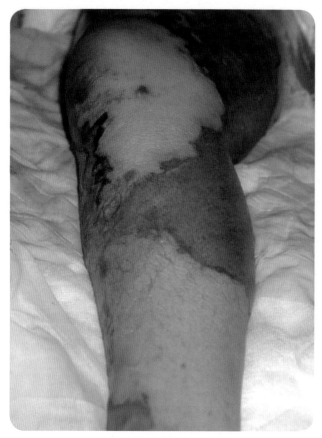

Figure 4-584 Necrotizing fasciitis with full-thickness skin necrosis before ulceration.

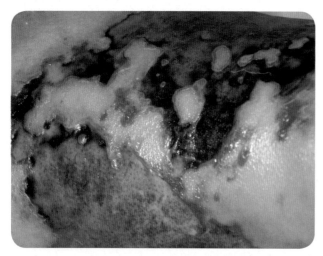

Figure 4-585 Extension of the necrosis in Figure 4-584.

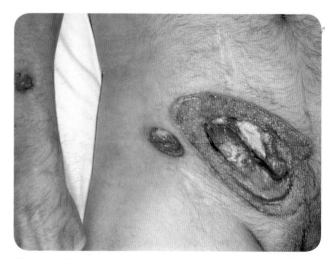

Figure 4-586 Deep skin ulceration after necrotizing fasciitis.

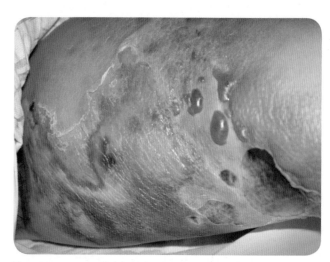

Figure 4-587 Bullae, necrosis, and surrounding erythema in necrotizing fasciitis. A clinical clue to the diagnosis may be anesthesia in of the affected area.

?? Differential Diagnosis and Pitfalls

- Cellulitis
- Erysipelas
- Purpura fulminans compliciating varicella

- Vasculitis
- Calciphylaxis
- Ecthyma gangrenosum
- Disseminated intravascular coagulation
- Staphylococcal scalded skin syndrome
- Insect bite (e.g., brown recluse spider)
- Toxic shock syndrome
- Gas gangrene (clostridial myonecrosis)
- Sweet syndrome
- Pyoderma gangrenosum (PG)

It can sometimes be difficult to differentiate necrotizing fasciitis from PG. This is especially true in the pustular variant of PG that may not develop into frank ulceration. Relatively rapidly progressing soft tissue inflammation not responding to broad-spectrum antibiotics and surgical debridement should be promptly evaluated by a dermatologist to rule out PG.

✓ Best Tests

- This diagnosis is made on clinical grounds. Immediate surgical intervention is required. Therefore, if you are considering this diagnosis, **contact a surgeon now**. To confirm suspected necrotizing fasciitis, a small, exploratory incision can be made at the site of maximum suspicion. In cases of necrotizing fasciitis, there will often be a thin, brownish exudate with extensive undermining of the surrounding tissues, which dissect easily with a blunt instrument or gloved finger. The fascia will be swollen and gray, with areas of necrosis.
- CT scan or MRI may demonstrate edema extending along fascial planes, and plain films may demonstrate gas in the tissues. However, definitive treatment of this disease should not be delayed in order to obtain radiologic studies.
- Obtain blood cultures, tissue, and exudate specimens for Gram stain and culture (aerobic and anaerobic) from the deep tissues at the time of surgery.

▲▲ Management Pearls

- Necrotizing fasciitis is a medical and surgical emergency, which often requires a tertiary medical center and supportive treatment in an ICU setting. In addition to debridement and intravenous antibiotics, patients will require wound care and careful attention to fluid and electrolyte balance, nutrition, and temperature regulation. Patients may need ventilatory and/or hemodynamic support.
- Commonly needed consultations (in addition to general surgery) include infectious disease, critical care, and plastic surgery.
- There is an association between the nonsteroidal anti-inflammatory drug (NSAID) use and the development of necrotizing fasciitis. Although no studies have been able to show a causative role, it is generally accepted that NSAIDs mask the symptoms and potentially delay diagnosis. Thus, NSAIDs should be avoided in patients suspicious of having necrotizing fasciitis.

Therapy

Therapy requires immediate surgical intervention in addition to antibiotics. Antibiotics alone are of little benefit because of the ischemia found in these infections. All infected and devitalized tissue must be removed. Often, patients will need multiple (if not daily) trips to the operating room to accomplish this.

Initial choice of antibiotic therapy can be directed by Gram stain(s) taken at the time of the initial operation. Antibiotics will need to be continued until such time as operative procedures are no longer needed and the patient has been afebrile for 2 to 3 days.

Polymicrobial Infection

- Ampicillin-sulbactam 1.5 to 3.0 g IV every 6 to 8 h
- Piperacillin-tazobactam 3.375 g IV every 6 to 8 h plus clindamycin 600 to 900 mg IV every 8 h plus ciprofloxacin 400 mg IV every 12 h
- Imipenem/cilastatin 1 g IV every 6 to 8 h
- Meropenem 1 g IV every 8 h
- Ertapenem 1 g IV every 24 h

Streptococcal Infection

- Clindamycin is recommended as additional therapy in cases of group A streptococcal disease to block toxin production
- Penicillin 2 to 4 MU IV every 4 to 6 h plus clindamycin 600 to 900 mg IV every 8 h

S. aureus Infection

- Nafcillin or oxacillin 1 to 2 g IV every 4 h
- Cefazolin 1 g IV every 8 h
- Vancomycin (for MRSA) 30 mg/kg/day IV divided in two doses

Clostridial Infection

- Penicillin 2 to 4 MU IV every 4 to 6 h
- Clindamycin 600 to 900 mg IV every 8 h

Patients will require aggressive fluid resuscitation.

Suggested Readings

Anaya DA, Dellinger EP. Necrotizing soft-tissue infection: Diagnosis and management. *Clin Infect Dis*. 2007 Mar;44(5):705–710.

Andriessen MJ, Kotsopoulos AM, Bloemers FW, et al. Necrotizing fasciitis caused by Salmonella enteritidis. *Scand J Infect Dis*. 2006;38(11–12): 1106–1107.

Harada AS, Lau W. Successful treatment and limb salvage of mucor necrotizing fasciitis after kidney transplantation with posaconazole. *Hawaii Med J*. 2007 Mar;66(3):68–71.

Kaul R, McGeer A, Low DE, et al. Population-based surveillance for group A streptococcal necrotizing fasciitis: Clinical features, prognostic indicators, and microbiologic analysis of seventy-seven cases. Ontario Group A Streptococcal Study. *Am J Med*. 1997 Jul;103(1):18–24.

Miller LG, Perdreau-Remington F, Rieg G, et al. Necrotizing fasciitis caused by community-associated methicillin-resistant *Staphylococcus aureus* in Los Angeles. *N Engl J Med*. 2005 Apr;352(14):1445–1453

Olsen RJ, Burns KM, Chen L, et al. Severe necrotizing fasciitis in a human immunodeficiency virus-positive patient caused by methicillin-resistant *Staphylococcus aureus*. *J Clin Microbiol*. 2008 Mar;46(3):1144–1147. Epub 2008 Jan 16.

Salcido RS. Necrotizing fasciitis: Reviewing the causes and treatment strategies. *Adv Skin Wound Care.* 2007 May;20(5):288–293; quiz 294–295.

Souyri C, Olivier P, Grolleau S, et al; French Network of Pharmacovigilance Centres. Severe necrotizing soft-tissue infections and nonsteroidal anti-inflammatory drugs. *Clin Exp Dermatol.* 2008 May;33(3):249–255. Epub 2008 Feb 2.

Stebbings AE, Ti TY, Tan WC. Necrotizing fasciitis—an unusual presentation of miliary mycobacterium tuberculosis. *Singapore Med J.* 1997 Sep;38(9):384–385.

Young MH, Engleberg NC, Mulla ZD, et al. Therapies for necrotising fasciitis. *Expert Opin Biol Ther.* 2006 Feb;6(2):155–165.

Diagnosis Synopsis

Rocky Mountain spotted fever (RMSF) is caused by the Gram-negative bacterium *Rickettsia rickettsii*. It is the most severe rickettsial illness of humans; without treatment, the case fatality rate is 20% to 30%.

The disease is transmitted most commonly via the tick bite of the *Dermacentor*, *Rhipicephalus*, or *Amblyomma* ticks. Mucosal transmission can occur when contaminated by a crushed tick or by tick fecal matter. RMSF occurs over a wide distribution in the United States: the eastern two-thirds of United States, Pacific Coast, Rocky Mountain states, and southwestern United States. RMSF can also be seen in northern Mexico and Central and South America. Over 90% of cases occur during April through September. The disease is more frequent in males and children. The incidence of RMSF has been steadily increasing to an estimated 2,000 cases per year.

Early clinical manifestations of RMSF include high fever, severe headache, myalgias, nausea, and vomiting. Later manifestations include rash, photophobia, confusion, ataxia, seizures, cough, dyspnea, arrhythmias, jaundice, and severe abdominal pain. Thrombocytopenia and hyponatremia may also be seen. Long-term sequelae include CNS deficits and amputations.

RMSF can be prevented by the use of protective clothing and repellants, avoidance of tick-infested areas, and thorough tick inspections after periods of outdoor activity.

Look For

Signs and symptoms of RMSF begin 2 to 14 days after infection. Fever, myalgias, and headache are almost always present. The rash of RMSF (seen in about 90% of patients) may not be apparent until 2 to 5 days after onset of fever. It begins as 1 to 5 mm macules, typically on the ankles, wrists, and forearms, spreading centripetally to the trunk. The face is usually spared. The palms and soles are commonly affected. Lesions progress from papules to petechiae (Figs. 4-588–4-591), which may eventually coalesce into ecchymoses. The rash may be asymmetric or localized.

In severe cases, necrotic ulcerations and distal gangrene can be seen, resulting in amputations.

Dark Skin Considerations

In dark-skinned patients, the rash can be subtle, resulting in delayed diagnosis.

Diagnostic Pearls

- A palm and sole petechial eruption in the setting of high fever, myalgias, and headache is characteristic of RMSF.
- Involvement of the scrotum or vulva is a clue for RMSF.
- In areas with high concentrations of disease, consider RMSF as a cause of unexplained fever in spring or summer.
- Travel to endemic areas should be considered.

?? Differential Diagnosis and Pitfalls

- Meningococcemia typically occurs in the late winter to early spring with fever and rash appearing within 24 h of infection. There is also marked lymphadenopathy.
- Measles typically occurs in the winter to spring and has associated symptoms of cough, coryza, conjunctivitis, and Koplik spots.
- Enteroviral infections typically occur in the summer to fall. The fever and rash often appear together. Sick contacts are common.

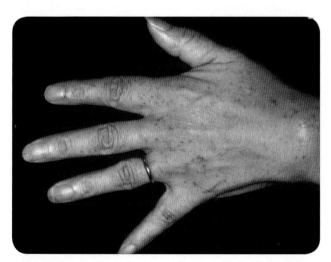

Figure 4-588 Lesions of purpura on the dorsum of the hand consistent with RMSF.

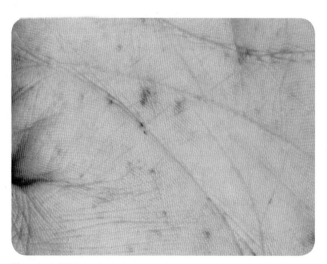

Figure 4-589 Typical palmar petechiae of RMSF.

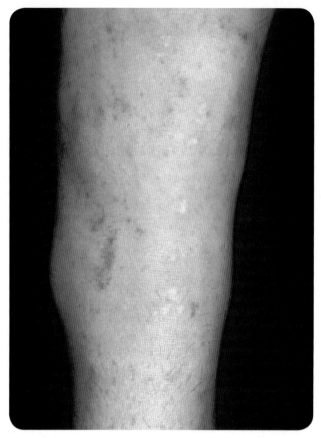

Figure 4-590 Scattered petechiae of larger areas of purpura in RMSF.

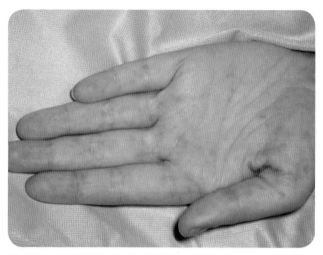

Figure 4-591 Palmar petechiae in RMSF.

- Dengue fever, also known as "breakbone fever," has severe arthralgias.
- Vasculitis is marked by palpable purpura rather than petechiae.
- Drug eruptions will have a history of exposure.
- Secondary syphilis can also present with a palm and sole rash; occasionally, the rash imparts a rust-colored hue.
- Gonococcemia may present with asymmetric monoarticular arthritis and a pustular or petechial rash.
- Viral or bacterial enterocolitis presents with nausea and vomiting.
- Acute surgical abdomen has severe abdominal pain.
- Hepatitis presents with jaundice.
- Meningitis has prominent neurological signs.
- Immune thrombocytopenic purpura presents with a petechial rash.
- Thrombotic thrombocytopenic purpura is characterized by fever, anemia, thrombocytopenia, renal impairment, and neurological deficits.

✓ Best Tests

Serology

- Indirect immunofluorescence assay (IFA)
- ELISA

Treatment should be initiated immediately with high clinical suspicion. Early in infection, serologic assays may be unreliable, but any delays in diagnosis may result in death. In the first week of illness, 85% of patients lack diagnostic titers, and up to 50% may lack diagnostic titers 7 to 9 days after onset of illness. It is important to test acute and convalescent samples 2 to 4 weeks apart in order to confirm infection. A fourfold rise in IFA titers is confirmatory. ELISA is not quantitative.

Skin biopsy with direct immunofluorescence may help confirm diagnosis in the acute setting with a sensitivity of 70%.

Immunohistochemical staining, polymerase chain reaction (PCR), and electron microscopy may aid in diagnosis.

▲▲ Management Pearls

- Rapid diagnosis and treatment prevent deaths.
- Removal of the tick within 6 h of bite may prevent transmission. However, exposure to a crushed tick or to tick fecal matter may result in immediate transmission. Antimicrobial prophylaxis following a tick bite is not recommended and may, in fact, delay the onset of disease.

Therapy

Doxycycline is the drug of choice for treatment of all tick-borne rickettsial disease in children and adults. The risks of significant morbidity from RMSF outweigh the low risk of dental staining in children from doxycycline. Therefore, doxycycline is recommended in children of all ages if RMSF is suspected. Clinical response time is typically within 24 to 72 h. Other broad-spectrum antimicrobials are usually ineffective.

Adults or children greater than 45 kg: Doxycycline 100 mg twice daily p.o. or IV

Pregnant adult or tetracycline allergic: Chloramphenicol 500 mg four times per day IV. Complicated cases in pregnant women should be treated with doxycycline 100 mg daily p.o. or IV.

IV therapy is frequently indicated for hospitalized patients. Oral therapy is acceptable for patients considered to be in early stages of the disease and for those who can be managed as outpatients.

The optimal duration of therapy has not been established, but current recommendations are to treat for at least 3 days after the fever subsides and when evidence of clinical improvement is noted. Severe or complicated disease might require longer treatment courses.

Suggested Readings

Centers for Disease Control and Prevention (CDC). Fatal cases of Rocky Mountain spotted fever in family clusters—three states, 2003. *MMWR Morb Mortal Wkly Rep.* 2004 May;53(19):407–410.

Chapman AS, Bakken JS, Folk SM, et al.; Tickborne Rickettsial Diseases Working Group, CDC. Diagnosis and management of tickborne rickettsial diseases: Rocky Mountain spotted fever, ehrlichioses, and anaplasmosis—United States: A practical guide for physicians and other health-care and public health professionals. *MMWR Recomm Rep.* 2006 Mar;55(RR-4):1–27.

Donovan BJ, Weber DJ, Rublein JC, et al. Treatment of tick-borne diseases. *Ann Pharmacother.* 2002 Oct;36(10):1590–1597.

Holman RC, Paddock CD, Curns AT, et al. Analysis of risk factors for fatal Rocky Mountain spotted fever: Evidence for superiority of tetracyclines for therapy. *J Infect Dis.* 2001 Dec;184(11):1437–1444.

Masters EJ, Olson GS, Weiner SJ, et al. Rocky Mountain spotted fever: A clinician's dilemma. *Arch Intern Med.* 2003 Apr;163(7):769–774.

Sexton DJ, Kaye KS. Rocky Mountain spotted fever. *Med Clin North Am.* 2002 Mar;86(2):351–360, vii–viii.

■■ Diagnosis Synopsis

Scarlet fever is an acute erythrogenic toxin-mediated disease caused by infection with Group A beta-hemolytic strepto-cocci (*Streptococcus pyogenes*). Most cases follow a strep-tococcal pharyngitis or tonsillitis. However, streptococcal sepsis, cellulitis, puerperal infection, or surgical infection can initiate scarlet fever. Scarlet fever is most common in children aged younger than 10, but it can affect adults as well. A 2 to 5 day incubation period precedes the onset of rash. Associated prodromal symptoms include fever, nausea, vomiting, myalgias, headache, and malaise. The characteris-tic rash begins within 12 to 48 h of fever onset. Generalized lymphadenopathy is common.

Once a fatal disease in the preantibiotic era, associated complications are now fortunately rare with the existence of effective antibiotic therapy. However, meningitis, otitis, sinusitis, pneumonia, arthritis, rheumatic fever, and glom-erulonephritis can still rarely occur.

◉ Look For

Scarlet fever is characterized by a "sandpaper-like" exanthem with minute (1 to 2 mm), blanchable papules on an ery-thematous base resembling "a sunburn with goose bumps" (Figs. 4-592–4-594). The lesions begin on the neck and then spread inferiorly to the trunk and extremities. The rash is accentuated in skin folds and flexural areas.

When streptococcal pharyngitis or tonsillitis is the evok-ing infection, the tonsils are beefy red and enlarged with a purulent exudate with associated tender submandibular ade-nopathy. Initially, the tongue is white with red papilla, giving it a characteristic "white strawberry" appearance. Eventually the tongue becomes bright red ("red strawberry tongue") (Fig. 4-595).

Flushed cheeks with circumoral pallor is characteristic as well as palatal petechiae.

The rash typically lasts for 4 to 5 days. During resolution, desquamation begins on the head and neck and progresses to the acral regions over 2 to 6 weeks.

●● Diagnostic Pearls

- Classic sandpaper rash following acute pharyngitis or tonsillitis.
- White strawberry or red strawberry tongue.
- Pastia lines (linear petechiae in the antecubital, axillary, and inguinal areas) are classic findings in more severe cases.

?? Differential Diagnosis and Pitfalls

- Toxic shock syndrome originates from *Staphylococcus aureus* infections arising in the setting of super absorbent tampons, nasal packing, or surgical site infections. Patients are systemically ill and eventually desquamate.
- Staphylococcal scalded skin syndrome usually occurs in young children following an *S. aureus* infection—Affected skin is notably tender.

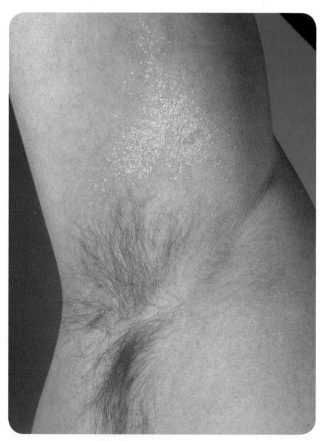

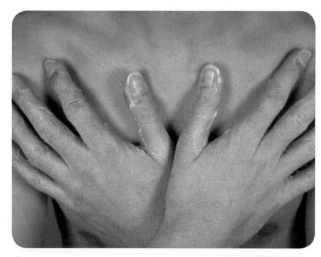

Figure 4-592 Acral erythema and scaling of scarlet fever.

Figure 4-593 Redness and fine desquamation of scarlet fever.

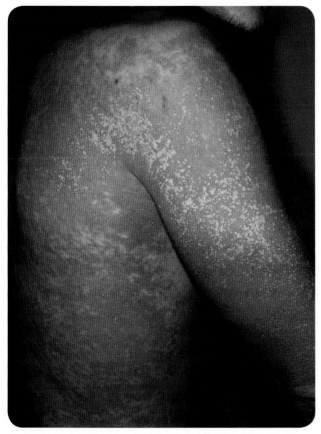

Figure 4-594 Erythema and scaling along with some islands of normal skin in scarlet fever.

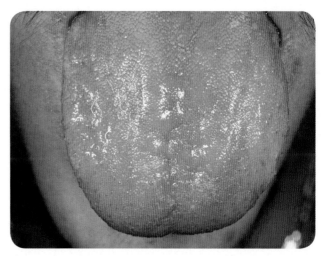

Figure 4-595 Red depapillated tongue in a patient with scarlet fever. Same patient as in Figure 4-593.

- Kawasaki disease is characterized by "strawberry tongue," conjunctival injection, cervical lymphadenopathy, and rash—This is also more common in children.
- Drug eruptions will have a history of exposure.
- Sunburns occur after sun exposure and are photodistributed.
- Photodrug eruptions are photodistributed.
- Photocontact dermatitis is photodistributed.
- Rubeola has associated cough, coryza, conjunctivitis, and Koplik spots.
- Rubella has occipital and post-auricular lymphadenopathy.
- Rat-bite fever
- Infectious mononucleosis has associated lymphadenopathy.
- Primary HIV infection is characterized by lymphadenopathy and rash.
- Lupus erythematosus has associated photosensitivity.

✓ Best Tests

The diagnosis is usually made on clinical grounds and supported by a rising antistreptolysin-O (ASO) titer and positive throat or wound cultures for *Streptococcus*.

▲▲ Management Pearls

- Because of the potential for complications, do not delay the treatment of suspected scarlet fever while waiting for laboratory confirmation.
- Should patients develop complications or if they are found to have a serious source of infection (i.e., osteomyelitis), further workup and treatment is warranted.

Therapy

Group A beta-hemolytic streptococci remains sensitive to penicillin, making it the drug of choice:

- Penicillin G benzathine—1.2 MU IM single dose or Penicillin VK 250 mg p.o. three to four times daily for 10 days

Alternatives include the following:

- Erythromycin 333 mg p.o. every 8 h for 10 days for penicillin-allergic patients
- Amoxicillin 250 to 500 mg p.o. three times daily for 10 days
- Cephalexin 250 to 500 mg p.o. three times daily for 10 days

Suggested Readings

Bialecki C, Feder HM, Grant-Kels JM. The six classic childhood exanthems: a review and update. *J Am Acad Dermatol.* 1989 Nov;21(5 Pt 1):891–903.

Davies RJ, de Bono JP. A young rash on old shoulders—scarlet fever in an adult male. *Lancet Infect Dis.* 2002 Dec;2(12):750.

Serum Sickness and Serum Sickness–Like Reaction

Diagnosis Synopsis

Serum Sickness

Serum sickness is a type III immune-complex disease resulting from exposure to therapeutic heterologous (classically nonhuman) serum or certain medications. The reaction is also rarely observed after blood transfusions. Serum sickness typically occurs 7 to 21 days after exposure to exogenous proteins or chemicals. Antigens induce antibody production resulting in circulating antigen-antibody complexes, complement activation, and then initiation of symptoms that include urticaria (often first noticed at the site of injection), fever, myalgia, arthralgia, arthritis, and lymphadenopathy. The disease is usually self-limited and lasts less than a week. Renal and neurologic sequelae occur rarely. Previously sensitized hosts can see an accelerated onset of symptoms occurring 1 to 3 days after exposure to the antigen.

Serum Sickness–Like Reaction

Serum sickness–like reaction (SSLR) is a drug reaction that manifests several of the clinical findings of serum sickness disease but lacks the immune complex formation, complement activation, and vasculitic changes characteristic of the latter. Most reactions occur between 5 and 30 days after drug initiation and present with urticarial or exanthematous rash, arthralgia, fever, and sometimes with lymphadenopathy. Most reactions are mild and self-limited and resolve after drug withdrawal within several days to weeks. Upper airway edema may lead to life-threatening respiratory compromise.

Beta-lactam antibiotics, cephalosporins (particularly cefaclor), penicillin, minocycline, and sulfa antibiotics are among the most frequent offenders. Bupropion and propranolol are also recognized causes. Newer biologic therapies, especially chimeric antibodies such as rituximab and infliximab, are emerging causes recently described in the literature.

Immunocompromised Patient Considerations

Up to 30% of organ transplant recipients may receive polyclonal antibodies as part of induction therapy or treatment of acute graft rejection. Often these heterologous antibodies may precipitate serum sickness, usually 1 to 3 weeks after administration.

Look For

Serum Sickness

Urticarial plaques and papules (especially on the sides of the hands and feet) or a morbilliform-like rash (Figs. 4-596 and 4-597). Urticaria may be both pruritic and painful. Large urticarial plaques often appear centrally dusky. Purpura may be present, often predominant on the lower extremities.

Serum Sickness–Like Reaction

Rash, usually urticarial, but may be exanthematous with associated fever and arthralgias 1 to 2 weeks after the initiation of the causative drug.

Diagnostic Pearls

Serum Sickness

This is a clinical diagnosis based on an examination, prior exposure to a serum or drug (with between 8 and 12 days between the exposure and the onset of the rash), and the constellation of symptoms and rash.

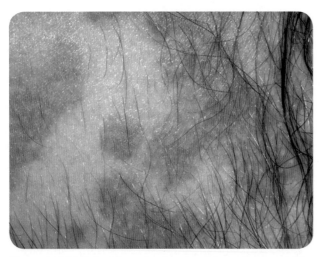

Figure 4-596 Urticarial eruption in serum sickness due to penicillin.

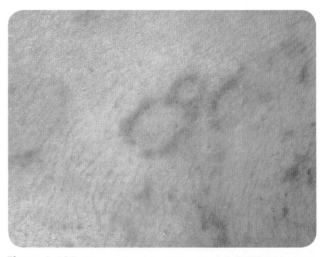

Figure 4-597 Polyarcuate urticarial eruption in serum sickness.

446

Serum Sickness–Like Reaction

This is a clinical diagnosis based on examination and the constellation of symptoms and rash. Causative agents are typically nonprotein drugs, opposed to true serum-sickness reaction.

?? Differential Diagnosis and Pitfalls

Serum Sickness

- Systemic lupus erythematosus
- SSLR (incited by nonprotein drugs)
- Rocky Mountain spotted fever
- Leukocytoclastic vasculitis
- Morbilliform drug eruption
- Drug rash with eosinophilia and systemic symptoms (DRESS)
- Erythema multiforme
- Urticaria multiforme
- Infective endocarditis
- Cryoglobulinemia
- Mononucleosis
- Urticarial vasculitis
- Henoch-Schönlein purpura

Serum Sickness–Like Reaction

- Urticaria
- Cellulitis
- Morbilliform drug eruption
- Systemic lupus erythematosus
- Hereditary angioedema
- Still disease
- Parvovirus B19 infection
- Rheumatic fever
- Acute hepatitis B infection

✓ Best Tests

Serum Sickness

- Serum complement levels. Look for low C3 and C4 levels, and nadir at 7 to 10 days.
- WBC may be either elevated or decreased. Peripheral eosinophilia may be present.
- Erythrocyte sedimentation rate (ESR) is usually elevated.
- Cryoglobulins may be present.
- Urinalysis may reveal mild proteinuria or hematuria; serum creatinine may be transiently elevated.
- Skin biopsy for H&E and direct immunofluorescence.

Serum Sickness–Like Reaction

- This is a clinical diagnosis.

▲▲ Management Pearls

Serum Sickness

- Make sure there is no compromising of respiration in the larynx or at the bronchial level.
- Patients should be warned that re-exposure to the offending agent may provoke a more serious response.

Serum Sickness–Like Reaction

Make sure that there is no compromising of respiration in the larynx or at the bronchial level. If oral steroids are required, a taper over 2 weeks may prevent the relapse of symptoms. Re-exposure to the offending agent should be avoided.

Therapy

Serum Sickness
Serum sickness is self-limited. Avoidance and/or withdrawal of the inciting agent is indicated. Symptomatic therapy consists of antihistamines and nonsteroidal anti-inflammatory agents. Systemic corticosteroids (1 mg/kg/day) for 10 to 14 days may be needed for severe reactions.

Antihistamines
- Diphenhydramine hydrochloride—25 to 50 mg every 6 to 8 h as needed
- Hydroxyzine—25 mg every 6 h as needed
- Cetirizine hydrochloride—5 to 10 mg daily
- Loratadine—one 10 mg tablet daily

Non-Steroidal Anti-Inflammatory Agents
- Ibuprofen—200 to 800 mg p.o. four times daily, not to exceed 3,200 mg per day
- Naproxen sodium—550 mg p.o. twice daily

Serum Sickness–Like Reaction
Self-limited. Symptomatic therapy with antihistamines and antipruritics. For severe reactions, systemic corticosteroids (prednisone 40 to 60 mg per day) for short courses (1 to 2 weeks).

Immunocompromised Patient Considerations

Plasma exchange therapy has been used successfully in organ transplant patients with serum sickness poorly responsive to systemic corticosteroids.

Suggested Readings

Bielory L, Gascon P, Lawley TJ, et al. Human serum sickness: A prospective analysis of 35 patients treated with equine anti-thymocyte globulin for bone marrow failure. *Medicine (Baltimore)*. 1988 Jan;67(1):40–57.

Jackson R. Serum sickness. *J Cutan Med Surg*. 2000 Oct;4(4):223–225.

Katta R, Anusuri V. Serum sickness-like reaction to cefuroxime: A case report and review of the literature. *J Drugs Dermatol*. 2007 Jul;6(7):747–748.

Lawley TJ, Bielory L, Gascon P, et al. A prospective clinical and immunologic analysis of patients with serum sickness. *N Engl J Med*. 1984 Nov;311(22):1407–1413.

Lazoglu AH, Boglioli LR, Taff ML, et al. Serum sickness reaction following multiple insect stings. *Ann Allergy Asthma Immunol*. 1995 Dec;75(6 Pt 1):522–524.

Mehsen N, Yvon CM, Richez C, et al. Serum sickness following a first rituximab infusion with no recurrence after the second one. *Clin Exp Rheumatol*. 2008 Sep–Oct;26(5):967.

Peloso PM, Baillie C. Serum sickness-like reaction with bupropion. *JAMA*. 1999 Nov;282(19):1817.

Revuz J, Valeyrie-Allanore L. Drug reactions. In: Bolognia J, Jorizzo JL, Rapini RP, eds. *Dermatology*. 2nd Ed. St. Louis, MO: Mosby; 2008:314.

Todd DJ, Helfgott SM. Serum sickness following treatment with rituximab. *J Rheumatol*. 2007 Feb;34(2):430–433.

Yerushalmi J, Zvulunov A, Halevy S. Serum sickness-like reactions. *Cutis*. 2002 May;69(5):395–397.

Staphylococcal Scalded Skin Syndrome

■ Diagnosis Synopsis

Staphylococcal scalded skin syndrome (SSSS), or Ritter disease, is a toxin-mediated infection that is characterized by skin tenderness, flaccid bullae, and skin detachment. A prodrome of fever, sore throat, malaise, and irritability accompanied by purulent rhinorrhea and/or conjunctivitis often occurs prior to the onset of bullae and desquamation. SSSS is mainly a disease of infants and in children younger than 6 years, with a higher incidence seen in males. Among adults, risk factors for SSSS include immunosuppression and chronic renal insufficiency.

In the United States, phage group II staphylococci are the most common toxin-producing strains. These phage group II strains can be methicillin sensitive and resistant and produce exotoxins (epidermolytic toxins A and B, ETA and ETB) that cause cleavage within the epidermis with subsequent superficial epidermal sloughing. Specifically, ETA and ETB are serine proteases that cleave the extracellular domain of desmoglein 1, an adhesion molecule that holds keratinocytes together. Note that bullous impetigo and toxic shock syndrome are also toxin-mediated diseases that are considered within the same spectrum of SSSS.

The natural history of SSSS is characterized by the following:

- Prodromal symptoms and/or purulent rhinorrhea and/or conjunctivitis
- Facial erythema that generalizes to the body in less than 48 h
- Bullae development, positive Nikolsky sign, very tender skin
- Skin wrinkling and epidermal sloughing within 48 h after bullae develop

- Desquamation continues for up to 5 days
- Reepithelialization, without scarring, completed over following 2 weeks

With appropriate antibiotics, SSSS can resolve over 1 to 2 weeks. However, many adults who suffer from SSSS have underlying medical problems like renal insufficiency, and mortality rates are estimated at 60% or even higher in immunocompromised patients.

Immunocompromised Patient Considerations

When SSSS does occur in adults, it is most frequently associated with the immunocompromised or a patient with renal insufficiency. In these patients, there is significant morbidity and mortality.

◉ Look For

The skin findings begin as a scarlatiniform eruption. Flaccid blisters may develop within 24 to 48 h (Figs. 4-598–4-600). Nikolsky sign (disrupting the epidermal barrier with firm rubbing) is positive, and large sheets of epidermis are shed (Fig. 4-601). Circumoral erythema becomes crusted after a few days. Mild facial edema, lip fissuring, and purulent conjunctivitis can occur. The erythema is accentuated in periorificial and flexural areas.

Involvement is generally widespread.

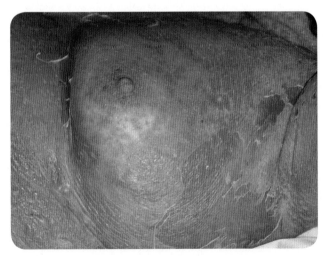
Figure 4-598 Multiple large erosions in an adult with SSSS.

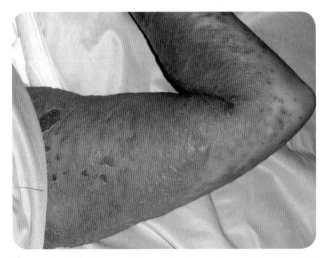
Figure 4-599 Intact vesicles and erythema in an adult with SSSS. Same patient as in Figure 4-598.

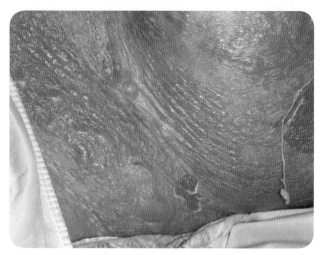

Figure 4-600 Intact vesicles may be more common in adults with SSSS because of the thicker epidermis in adults than in children.

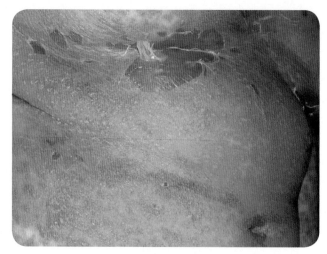

Figure 4-601 Extensive peeling of the skin in SSSS in an adult.

Diagnostic Pearls

- SSSS is mainly a clinical diagnosis.
- Fluid from bullae is normally sterile.
- *Staphylococcus aureus* can be isolated from the nasopharynx, conjunctiva, blood, or any pyogenic focus on the skin.
- White blood cell count can be elevated or normal.
- Diagnosis can be confirmed with ELISA test for the toxin or frozen section biopsy.

?? Differential Diagnosis and Pitfalls

- Bullous impetigo—localized with honey-colored crusted plaques, bacteria present in bullae
- Toxic shock syndrome—high fevers and severe systemic symptoms including vomiting and diarrhea; hypotension quickly ensues; diffuse scarlatiniform exanthem that starts on the trunk (in contrast to face in SSSS)
- Kawasaki disease—Fever lasting more than 5 days with oral mucosal changes, conjunctival injection, and cervical lymphadenopathy
- Sunburn
- Drug eruption
- Cellulitis
- Toxic epidermal necrolysis (TEN)—drug induced, high fevers, skin tenderness, mucosal erosions, and skin detachment about 1 to 3 weeks after the inciting medication is started
- Stevens-Johnson syndrome—drug induced, high fevers, skin tenderness, mucosal erosions, and skin detachment about 1 to 3 weeks after the inciting medication is started
- Scarlet fever—1 mm erythematous papules, always elevated WBC with left shift, eosinophilia in up to 20% of patients

- Physical abuse
- Erysipelas
- Necrotizing fasciitis—rapidly progressing necrosis of fascia and subcutaneous fat

✓ Best Tests

- The erythrocyte sedimentation rate (ESR) is elevated; WBC may be normal or elevated.
- Clumps of Gram-positive cocci by Gram stain, culture of presumed sites of infection; consider nasal and throat swabs (plus any other suspicious areas) to determine the source of the infection.
- The skin biopsy or histologic examination of the roof of a blister provides a rapid diagnosis; epidermal cleavage is superficial in SSSS and deeper in TEN.
- The toxins responsible for SSSS can be identified by ELISA, latex agglutination assays, or PCR.

▲▲ Management Pearls

- Use parenteral penicillinase-resistant antistaphylococcal antibiotics, supportive skin care, IV fluids, and admission to the ICU or burn unit depending on severity.
- Approximately 20% to 40% of the population is an asymptomatic carrier of *S. aureus* (nares, axillae, and perineum). These individuals may be responsible for outbreaks (e.g., in the neonatal intensive care unit), and, in such cases, efforts should be made to identify and treat carriers.

Precautions: Standard and Contact. (Isolate patient, wear gloves and a gown, limit patient transport, and avoid sharing patient-care equipment.)

Therapy

Use only nonadherent dressings, such as petroleum-impregnated gauze, on areas of denuded epidermis.

Identify susceptibility of organism when possible. If susceptibility is unknown, use a penicillinase-resistant penicillin such as nafcillin or methicillin. Use penicillin G if the organism is susceptible. Use macrolides or aminoglycosides in patients with penicillin allergy. Mode of administration (oral versus parenteral) is dictated by degree of severity.

- Nafcillin or oxacillin (150 mg/kg/day IV in four divided doses) for 5 to 7 days
- A macrolide such as azithromycin (500 mg IV daily for 2 days, then 250 to 500 mg p.o. daily to complete a course of 7 to 10 days) is an alternative
- Vancomycin IV: 2 to 3 g per day (20 to 45 mg/kg/day) in divided doses every 6 to 12 h; maximum 3 g per day; **Note:** dose requires adjustment in renal impairment

Change to oral penicillins after 1 to 2 days to avoid possible phlebitis: amoxicillin or dicloxacillin 500 mg p.o. four times daily

Suggested Readings

Amagai M, Matsuyoshi N, Wang ZH, et al. Toxin in bullous impetigo and staphylococcal scalded-skin syndrome targets desmoglein 1. *Nat Med.* 2000 Nov;6(11):1275–1277.

Amagai M, Yamaguchi T, Hanakawa Y, et al. Staphylococcal exfoliative toxin B specifically cleaves desmoglein 1. *J Invest Dermatol.* 2002 May;118(5):845–850.

Farrell AM. Staphylococcal scalded-skin syndrome. *Lancet.* 1999 Sep;354(9182):880–881.

Ladhani S. Recent developments in staphylococcal scalded skin syndrome. *Clin Microbiol Infect.* 2001 Jun;7(6):301–307.

Murray RJ. Recognition and management of *Staphylococcus aureus* toxin-mediated disease. *Intern Med J.* 2005 Dec;35(Suppl. 2):S106–S1019.

Patel GK. Treatment of staphylococcal scalded skin syndrome. *Expert Rev Anti Infect Ther.* 2004 Aug;2(4):575–587.

Patel GK, Finlay AY. Staphylococcal scalded skin syndrome: Diagnosis and management. *Am J Clin Dermatol.* 2003;4(3):165–175.

Stanley JR, Amagai M. Pemphigus, bullous impetigo, and the staphylococcal scalded-skin syndrome. *N Engl J Med.* 2006 Oct;355(17):1800–1810.

Travers JB, Mousdicas N. Gram-positive infections associated with toxin production. In: Fitzpatrick TB, Wolff K, eds. *Fitzpatrick's Dermatology in General Medicine.* 7th Ed. New York, NY: McGraw-Hill; 2008: 1710–1714.

Stevens-Johnson Syndrome

■■ Diagnosis Synopsis

Stevens-Johnson syndrome (SJS) and toxic epidermal necrolysis (TEN) are two rare severe drug reactions that are characterized by high fevers, skin tenderness, mucosal erosions, and skin detachment about 1 to 3 weeks after the inciting medication is started. SJS and TEN should be considered the same disease on opposite ends of the spectrum, with the level of skin detachment differentiating these two entities. SJS is characterized by less than 10% of body surface area (BSA), while TEN involves greater than 30% BSA. SJS–TEN overlap occurs when 10% to 30% BSA is involved. Note that SJS can rapidly evolve into TEN, and both can have an unpredictable clinical course. Even expert groups may identify patients in the overlap area, and this can complicate decision making for therapy.

While the molecular events and etiology of SJS and TEN are not well defined, a medication history is strongly associated with their development in greater than 80% of cases. The three main classes that have most frequently been implicated include nonsteroidal anti-inflammatory drugs (NSAIDs), antibiotics, and anticonvulsants. Investigations over the past decade have provided strong evidence that SJS and TEN are secondary to the host's inability to detoxify drug metabolites. This results in a cell-mediated immune response that activates cytotoxic T-cells and subsequent induction of keratinocyte apoptosis via cell surface death receptor signaling (membrane-bound or soluble CD95–CD95 ligand interaction). Additional causes, albeit rare, include immunizations and infections.

SJS/TEN can affect all ages and races, with a slight preponderance seen in women (1.5:1) and an increasing incidence with age. Risk factors that confer a worse prognosis include extent of BSA involved at the time of diagnosis, older age, cancer or hematological malignancy, AIDS, number of medications, and elevated serum urea, glucose, and creatinine levels.

SJS and TEN run an unpredictable clinical course. The primary lesions include dusky red macules of irregular size and shape that start on the trunk and spread to the proximal extremities, neck, and face. The onset of disease occurs 1 to 3 weeks after the ingestion of an antibiotic or within the first 2 months of anticonvulsant treatment. Within hours to days, the epidermis can detach from the dermis, with serosanguineous fluid filling the space and subsequent flaccid blister formation. Ocular, oral, and genital mucosa will be affected in more than 90% of cases. Mucosal symptoms that should be screened for include painful eyes, painful swallowing, dysuria, and diarrhea.

SJS carries a 1% to 5% mortality risk, may or may not have systemic symptoms, and involves the trunk and face with many isolated lesions. TEN involves greater than 30% of BSA, carries a 25% to 35% mortality risk, invariably has systemic symptoms, and the lesions on the trunk and face are largely coalesced.

Rapid identification and withdrawal of the offending drug and transfer to a burn unit with aggressive supportive care are the most critical steps in the management.

◉ Look For

Specifically for SJS:

- Less than 10% BSA.
- Isolated, irregularly shaped, dusky red macules on the trunk, face, and palms/soles.
- Atypical target lesions may also be seen; they are atypical in the sense that they do not have the characteristic three concentric rings seen in erythema multiforme (EM).
- Erosions and ulcerations with underlying bleeding dermis exposed (Fig. 4-602).
- Flaccid bullae due to epidermal-dermal detachment (Fig. 4-603).

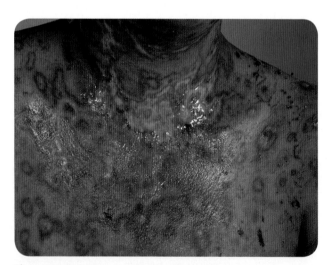

Figure 4-602 Plaques with ulceration in SJS.

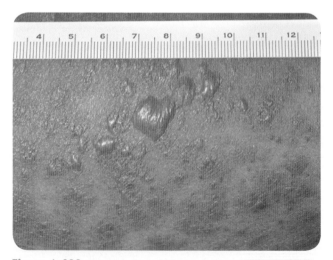

Figure 4-603 Flaccid bullae within a red plaque with a suggestion of a target lesion in SJS.

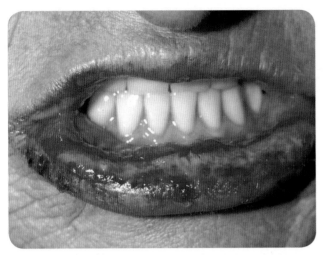

Figure 4-604 Ulcerations on the mucosal surface of the lower lip in SJS.

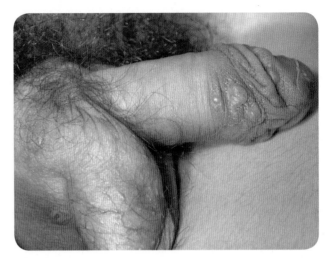

Figure 4-605 Penile vesicles and crusts are common in SJS.

- Nikolsky sign—Tangential mechanical pressure of an erythematous macule leads to epidermal-dermal detachment.
- Mucosal involvement including the eyes, lips (Fig. 4-604), mouth, and genitalia (Fig. 4-605).
- Look for hemorrhagic crust, bullae, and denudation in these areas.
- Systemic symptoms are commonly present but not invariably (as seen with TEN).

Diagnostic Pearls

The clinician should be aware of nonvisual signs of mucosal involvement including painful swallowing, painful micturition, and diarrhea. In addition, there are characteristic features of SJS/TEN blisters. The blisters are flaccid, break easily, and can be extended laterally by slight tangential pressure (Asboe-Hansen sign).

?? Differential Diagnosis and Pitfalls

- EM—Histologic features may not differentiate EM from SJS/TEN. Clinically, however, EM has characteristic target lesions (three concentric colors that are round and well demarcated) that occur on the extremities more often than the trunk. Precipitating factors are usually infectious (HSV, mycoplasma, etc.) and not medications. Lesions may be papular. Note that EM is not considered within the same disease spectrum as SJS/TEN and confers no risk in progressing to TEN. Nikolsky sign negative.
- Staphylococcal scalded skin syndrome—Usually occurs in newborns, infants, and young children; mucous

membranes and palms/soles are spared. The exfoliated skin is significantly more superficial (subcorneal versus epidermal-dermal). Also look for purulent discharge from the nose, and histologically very different from SJS/TEN. Nikolsky sign can be positive.
- Acute generalized exanthematic pustulosis (AGEP)—Look for neutrophilia, eosinophilia, almost confluent erythema with overlying non-follicular pustules. Nikolsky sign can be positive. Histology will clearly differentiate AGEP from SJS/TEN.
- Generalized fixed drug eruption—Look for erythematous plaques that develop on the lips, face, distal extremities, and genitalia 1 to 2 weeks after drug ingestions. Oral mucosa can be involved. Histology will differentiate fixed drug from SJS/TEN.
- Linear IgA disease—Look for tense blisters; histology will help differentiate Linear IgA from SJS/TEN. Direct immunofluorescence will demonstrate linear IgA deposition. DIF is negative in SJS/TEN.
- Toxic shock and toxic-shock–like syndrome—Look for the sudden onset of exanthematous eruption. Histology will help differentiate TSS and SJS/TEN.
- Drug reaction with eosinophilia and systemic symptoms (DRESS)—Look for facial edema (hallmark of DRESS), eosinophilia, hepatitis, and other viscera.
- Bullous pemphigoid—Widespread bullae, usually in older patients
- Pemphigus vulgaris
- Paraneoplastic pemphigus—Significant involvement of the vermillion border
- Dermatitis herpetiformis—Extremely pruritic
- Sweet syndrome
- Acute graft-versus-host disease—Look for history of bone marrow transplant

✓ Best Tests

- A skin biopsy will largely aid in confirming the diagnosis. Early stage biopsy demonstrates apoptotic keratinocytes throughout the epidermis. Late stage biopsy demonstrates subepidermal blisters and full thickness epidermal necrosis.
- Patients with SJS/TEN require ongoing biochemical and microbiological monitoring for infection, end-organ damage, and electrolyte disturbances. This level of vigilance requires frequent determinations of serum labs such as CBC, comprehensive serum electrolytes, BUN and creatinine, transaminases, and urine output. Swabs from potentially infected areas, blood and urine cultures, and information from blood gases are also needed. Baseline chest films and GI studies are needed to follow possible respiratory and GI tract involvement.

▲▲ Management Pearls

Patients with SJS/TEN require intensive care level or a burn unit level care. The primary goals are to provide fluid/nutritional support, pain control, and monitoring for infection. The use of systemic corticosteroids is controversial. Many authorities believe that they offer no clinical benefit and may increase the rate of complications. Consultations are needed and include a dietician, dermatologist, ophthalmologist, and/or a burn or wound care specialist. There is no role for prophylactic antibiotics, but monitor for and promptly treat any identified infections.

A severity-of-illness score that estimates mortality in TEN has been developed (SCORTEN) with the following factors:

- Age > 40
- HR > 120 bpm
- Malignancy
- Involved BSA > 10%
- BUN > 10 mEq/L
- Serum bicarbonate < 20 mEq/L
- Blood glucose > 252 mg/dL

Mortality estimates are based on the number of above criteria met:

- 0 to 1 factor ≥ 3.2%
- 2 factors ≥ 12.1%
- 3 factors ≥ 35.3%
- 4 factors ≥ 58.3%
- 5 or more factors ≥ 90%

Therapy

Early diagnosis of SJS/TEN and rapid identification and discontinuation of the inciting drug is of paramount importance. The faster the inciting drug is discontinued, the more favorable the prognosis. Supportive therapy in a burn unit is the mainstay of treatment. No universally accepted specific therapies exist. Consultation with a dermatologist or other experienced specialist is recommended.

Supportive Care

- Wound care—Consider nanocrystalline gauze materials containing silver ions (non-adherent) or petrolatum-based gauze pads.
- Fluid and electrolyte management—Correct for transepidermal water loss.
- Nutritional supplementation—Consider nutritional support via nasogastric tube. Request nutrition consult.
- Temperature management—Heat loss via epidermal loss can be significant, and the patient should be treated like a burn victim. Consider increasing the room temperature to 30°C to 32°C (86°F to 89.6°F).
- Superinfections—Patients with SJS/TEN are at high risk for sepsis and infection. Patient should be pancultured (skin, blood, urine, and any arterial lines and catheters) routinely throughout hospital stay. Note that systemic antibiotics are not used prophylactically.
- Ocular care—Vigorous lubrication and lysis of any adhesions that develop. Immediately request an ophthalmologic consult to decrease risk of irreversible ocular damage.

Specific Therapies

- Corticosteroids—Data regarding the use of steroids are mixed, and their use remains controversial.
- Intravenous immunoglobulin (IVIg)—Data regarding the use of IVIg are also mixed, but this therapy is still considered effective. Strongly consider with a specialist or physician experienced with SJS/TEN. Dosing is usually 0.8 g/kg/day for 3 to 4 days. Coagulopathies, acute renal failure, anaphylaxis, and aseptic meningitis can be rare, severe side effects of therapy. If timing permits, check IgA levels because anaphylaxis can ensue in patients with IgA deficiency.
- Plasmapheresis—Mixed findings; consider adjunct with IVIg.

Most patients have considerable pain. The use of opioid analgesics is often required. There may be considerable pruritus as the skin reepithelializes. This can be controlled with antihistamines:

- Diphenhydramine hydrochloride (25, 50 mg tablets or capsules): 25 to 50 mg nightly or every 6 h as needed.
- Hydroxyzine (10, 25 mg tablets): 12.5 to 25 mg every 6 h as needed.
- Cetirizine (5, 10 mg tablets): 5 to 10 mg per day.
- Loratadine (10 mg tablets): 10 mg tablet once daily.

Suggested Readings

Bachot N, Roujeau JC. Differential diagnosis of severe cutaneous drug eruptions. *Am J Clin Dermatol.* 2003;4(8):561–572.

Coursin DB. Stevens-Johnson syndrome: Nonspecific parasensitivity reaction?. *JAMA.* 1966 Oct;198(2):113–116.

Fromowitz JS, Ramos-Caro FA, Flowers FP, University of Florida. Practical guidelines for the management of toxic epidermal necrolysis and Stevens-Johnson syndrome. *Int J Dermatol.* 2007 Oct;46(10):1092–1094.

Hazin R, Ibrahimi OA, Hazin MI, et al. Stevens-Johnson syndrome: Pathogenesis, diagnosis, and management. *Ann Med.* 2008;40(2):129–138.

Khalili B, Bahna SL. Pathogenesis and recent therapeutic trends in Stevens-Johnson syndrome and toxic epidermal necrolysis. *Ann Allergy Asthma Immunol.* 2006 Sep;97(3):272–280; quiz 281–283, 320.

Lee HY, Pang SM, Thamotharampillai T. Allopurinol-induced Stevens-Johnson syndrome and toxic epidermal necrolysis. *J Am Acad Dermatol.* 2008 Aug;59(2):352–353.

Mockenhaupt M, Viboud C, Dunant A, et al. Stevens-Johnson syndrome and toxic epidermal necrolysis: Assessment of medication risks with emphasis on recently marketed drugs. The EuroSCAR-study. *J Invest Dermatol.* 2008 Jan;128(1):35–44.

Palmieri TL, Greenhalgh DG, Saffle JR, et al. A multicenter review of toxic epidermal necrolysis treated in U.S. burn centers at the end of the twentieth century. *J Burn Care Rehabil.* 2002 Mar–Apr;23(2):87–96.

Pereira FA, Mudgil AV, Rosmarin DM. Toxic epidermal necrolysis. *J Am Acad Dermatol.* 2007 Feb;56(2):181–200.

Rzany B, Correia O, Kelly JP, et al. Risk of Stevens-Johnson syndrome and toxic epidermal necrolysis during first weeks of antiepileptic therapy: A case-control study. Study Group of the International Case Control Study on Severe Cutaneous Adverse Reactions. *Lancet.* 1999 Jun;353(9171):2190–2194.

Valeyrie-Allanore L, Roujeau JC. Epidermal necrolysis (Stevens-Johnson syndrome and toxic epidermal necrolysis). In: Fitzpatrick TB, Wolff K, eds. *Fitzpatrick's Dermatology in General Medicine.* 7th Ed. New York, NY: McGraw-Hill; 2008:349–355.

Subacute Bacterial Endocarditis

Diagnosis Synopsis

Bacterial endocarditis can be divided into either acute or subacute disease. Acute bacterial endocarditis (ABE) refers to the abrupt onset of symptoms occurring for less than 2 weeks, whereas subacute bacterial endocarditis (SBE) evolves over several weeks or months. Overall, streptococci cause the majority of valvular endocarditis. Staphylococci cause the majority of disease in IV drug abusers, and a combination of staphylococci and streptococci causes a significant number of late prosthetic valve endocarditis.

Clinically, the patient may appear acutely ill or chronically ill and wasted. There are two major cutaneous findings: Osler nodes and Janeway lesions. Osler nodes are painful erythematous nodules located on the fingertips. Janeway lesions are nontender hemorrhagic macules and papules on the palms. Both findings are thought to result from septic embolization from a source of infective endocarditis. Other cutaneous findings include palpable purpura (cutaneous small vessel vasculitis) and splinter hemorrhages. Most patients will have a cardiac murmur at some stage, although in early stages, and especially with right-sided ABE, up to 15% of patients will have no murmur. Splenomegaly is seen in about 30% to 50% of patients.

The number of patients with prior cardiac surgery, immunosuppression, and drug abuse has increased. Mitral valve prolapse is a risk factor for endocarditis only when associated with a precordial systolic murmur. In recent years, an increase in endocarditis in males and elderly patients, acute endocarditis, and endocarditis caused by Gram-negative bacteria, fungi, and miscellaneous microbes has occurred. Endocarditis may be "culture-negative" when caused by *Candida* or *Aspergillus*. Tricuspid valvular disease is associated with IV drug abuse. Veterinarians in California have been shown to be at risk for Q fever endocarditis.

Immunocompromised Patient Considerations

HIV-infected patients with advanced immunosuppression are more likely to develop infective endocarditis and have higher morbidity and mortality.

Look For

Petechiae or palpable purpura on the palms (Fig. 4-606), soles, distal extremities, fingers (Fig. 4-607), and toes (Fig. 4-608). Splinter hemorrhages will be 1 to 3 mm purpuric macules in the nail bed. These are best seen by transilluminating the distal volar finger with a flashlight. Janeway lesions are erythematous, nontender macules on the palms and soles of a few patients with SBE. Osler nodes occur in 10% to 20% of patients and are tender, erythematous nodules often located on the fingertips (Fig. 4-609). Retinal hemorrhages are found in 10% to 25% of patients with SBE and ABE. Roth spots have an ivory or white center surrounded by a red halo.

Diagnostic Pearls

Petechiae are often discrete. 2–5 mm "splinter petechiae" on distal extremities.

Differential Diagnosis and Pitfalls

- Other causes of endocarditis include *Coxiella burnetii* (the cause of Q fever), mycobacteria, and chlamydia.

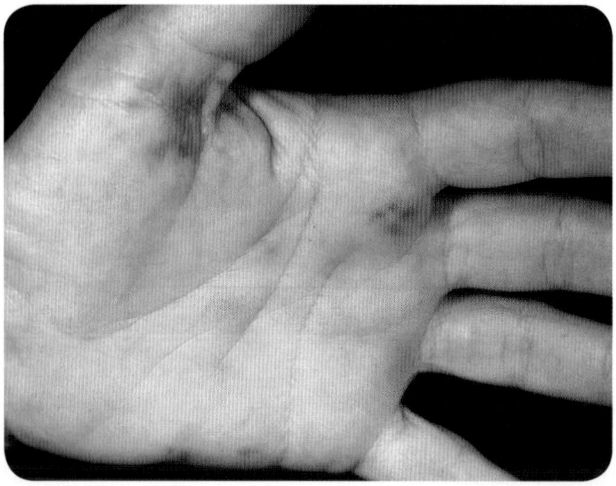

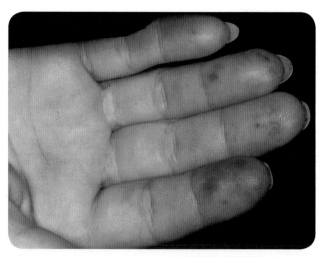

Figure 4-606 Palmar petechiae and purpura in ABE.

Figure 4-607 Petechiae and purpura in ABE.

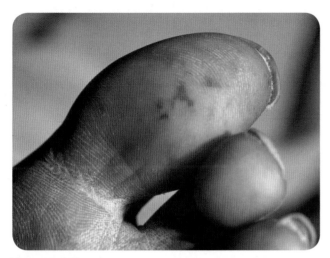

Figure 4-608 Distal purpuric papules in SBE.

- Bacterial sepsis
- Candidemia
- Ecthyma gangrenosum
- Leukocytoclastic vasculitis from another cause
- Rocky Mountain spotted fever

Immunocompromised Patient Considerations

Disseminated fungal infection

✓ Best Tests

- Blood cultures, obtained as recommended in three venous cultures on the first hospital day, and two more venous cultures on the second day if clinically indicated. On the third day, if indicated, draw two more venous cultures and one arterial culture. Blood cultures are positive in the majority of patients, with multiple blood cultures sometimes needed before the organism is grown.
- Transesophageal echocardiography is useful in detecting perivalvular abscesses and vegetations.
- Positive tourniquet test may be present.
- Anemia, mild leukocytosis, elevated erythrocyte sedimentation rate (ESR)—almost always, hematuria, RBC casts in urine, biological false-positive syphilis tests, and elevated gamma globulins may occur.

▲▲ Management Pearls

Patients may have their course complicated by arrhythmias and myocarditis. Close monitoring is advised. Obtain blood cultures early in therapy to insure the efficacy of therapy. Monitor blood levels of drug.

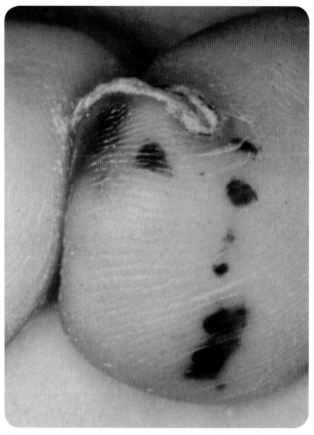

Figure 4-609 Vasculitis lesions on the volar surface (Osler nodes) in SBE.

Therapy

Prolonged administration of relatively high intravenous doses of bactericidal antibiotics based on culture results and sensitivities.

Suggested Readings

Bauer A, Jabs WJ, Süfke S, et al. Vasculitic purpura with antineutrophil cytoplasmic antibody-positive acute renal failure in a patient with Streptococcus bovis case and Neisseria subflava bacteremia and subacute endocarditis. *Clin Nephrol.* 2004 Aug;62(2):144–148.

Eisert J. Skin manifestations of subacute bacterial endocarditis. Case report of subacute bacterial endocarditis mimicking Tappeiner's angioendotheliomatosis. *Cutis.* 1980 Apr;25(4):394–395, 400.

Falcone PM, Larrison WI. Roth spots seen on ophthalmoscopy: Diseases with which they may be associated. *Conn Med.* 1995 May;59(5):271–273.

Gebo KA, Burkey MD, Lucas GM, et al. Incidence of, risk factors for, clinical presentation, and 1-year outcomes of infective endocarditis in an urban HIV cohort. *J Acquir Immune Defic Syndr.* 2006 Dec;43(4):426–432.

Suhge d'Aubermont PC, Honig PJ, Wood MG. Subacute bacterial endocarditis presenting with necrotic skin lesions. *Int J Dermatol.* 1983 Jun;22(5):295–299.

Verhagen DW, Vedder AC, Speelman P, et al. Antimicrobial treatment of infective endocarditis caused by viridans streptococci highly susceptible to penicillin: Historic overview and future considerations. *J Antimicrob Chemother.* 2006 May;57(5):819–824.

Sweet Syndrome (Acute Febrile Neutrophilic Dermatosis)

■■ Diagnosis Synopsis

Sweet syndrome, or acute febrile neutrophilic dermatosis, is an inflammatory disorder manifesting as multiple painful erythematous plaques that are usually associated with fever. The plaques are usually located on the extremities but can also occur on the head, neck, or trunk. The disease may be seen in patients of all ages, but it is more common in women aged between 20 and 60. Although the exact etiology is still unclear, Sweet syndrome has been considered a reactive process and has been associated with a number of inflammatory, infectious, and malignant diseases. These include inflammatory bowel disease, streptococcal pneumonia, and hematologic malignancies (especially myeloid leukemias). It can also occur during pregnancy and with the use of certain drugs (sulfamethoxazole-trimethoprim, minocycline, and G-CSF). Most cases are idiopathic or associated with benign conditions; about 15% to 20% are associated with malignancy.

While many of the features of the disease are quite distinct, Sweet syndrome is one subtype of the larger category of sterile neutrophilic diseases that includes pyoderma gangrenosum, subcorneal pustular dermatosis, erythema elevatum diutinum, neutrophilic eccrine hidradenitis, leukocytoclastic vasculitis, and others. These conditions share significant features including overlap presentations, sterile collections of normal neutrophils on histologic examination, extracutaneous manifestations, association with systemic illnesses, and responsiveness to a similar set of therapeutic agents.

Sweet syndrome itself frequently includes extracutaneous manifestations. Symptoms such as fever, headaches, myalgias, malaise, and arthralgias are frequently present. Fever often precedes the appearance of lesions. The respiratory system is the most common organ system involved, with cough and infiltrates on chest X-ray. Other sites that may be affected include the gastrointestinal tract, the musculoskeletal system, the kidneys, the heart, and the central nervous system. Conjunctivitis, episcleritis, and oral mucosal lesions have been reported. Sweet syndrome often responds quite well to systemic corticosteroids, but recurrences are common.

◉ Look For

Deep red, thick, sharply demarcated plaques or nodules that appear vesiculated but have no expressible fluid (Figs. 4-610 and 4-611). The lesions may have pustules within them. The plaques are nonscarring. Ulcers and bullae may occur; however, these lesions are associated more often with underlying malignancy (Fig. 4-612). Subcutaneous forms may mimic erythema nodosum.

The plaques are typically distributed asymmetrically on the extremities, face, neck, and upper trunk. On occasion, lesions may be predominantly distributed over the dorsum of the hands and fingers; some experts consider this to be an anatomically limited subset of Sweet syndrome (neutrophilic dermatosis of the dorsal hands).

Mucosal lesions are infrequent. When present, they usually consist of ulcerations.

Formal diagnosis of Sweet syndrome proceeds from identifying two major and two of four minor diagnostic criteria:

Major Criteria

1. Typical skin lesions—abrupt onset of painful erythematous plaques and nodules
2. Typical histopathology—sterile, dense collections of neutrophils without leukocytoclastic vasculitis

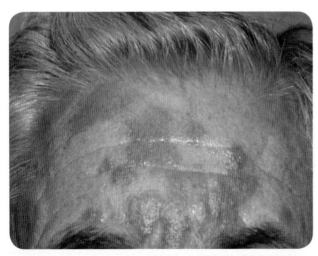

Figure 4-610 Thick, red plaques characteristic of Sweet syndrome.

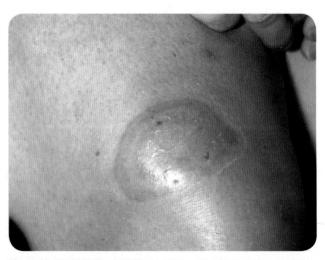

Figure 4-611 Sweet syndrome with deep purpuric center and annular rings of erythema.

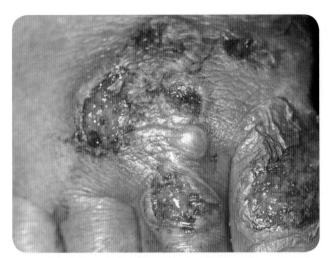

Figure 4-612 Sweet syndrome with vesicles and an erosion and a border, with some undermining suggestive of pyoderma gangrenosum.

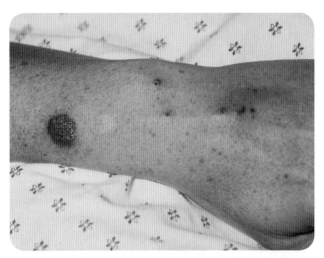

Figure 4-613 Sweet syndrome with lesion induction at a venipuncture site: the pathergy phenomenon.

Minor Criteria

1. Pyrexia more than 38°C (100.4°F) with constitutional symptoms
2. Excellent response to corticosteroids or potassium iodide
3. Association with an underlying hematologic or visceral malignancy, inflammatory disease, or pregnancy, OR preceded by an upper respiratory or gastrointestinal infection or vaccination
4. Abnormal laboratory values at presentation (3 of 4): erythrocyte sedimentation rate > 20 mm/h; positive C-reactive protein; >8,000 leukocytes; >70% neutrophils

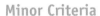

Diagnostic Pearls

Fever often precedes skin lesions.

Lesions may occur in areas of skin trauma (pathergy) (Fig. 4-613). Lesions may form at sites of IV insertion in patients on chemotherapy for hematologic malignancies.

Oral lesions may occur as well as conjunctivitis and episcleritis.

Drug-induced Sweet syndrome is defined by lesions with characteristic clinical and histologic morphology, temperature greater than 38°C (100.4°F), and temporal relationship to treatment with a specific drug and resolution subsequent to the discontinuation of a suspected drug.

Neutrophilic eccrine hidradenitis is sometimes seen with chemotherapy and has a neutrophilic infiltrate; it should not be confused with Sweet syndrome.

?? Differential Diagnosis and Pitfalls

- Sweet-like lesions have been seen at sites of erythropoietin injections. Lesions are sometimes mistaken for the infiltration of the underlying hematologic malignancy.

- Pyoderma gangrenosum—rolled border around purulent ulcers
- Neutrophilic eccrine hidradenitis
- Bowel-associated dermatosis—arthritis syndrome
- Well syndrome
- Erythema multiforme—targetoid lesions
- Drug eruption
- Urticarial vasculitis
- Erythema elevatum diutinum—primarily over extensor surfaces
- Cutaneous small vessel vasculitis—palpable purpura
- Behçet disease—associated with oral or genital ulcers
- Bromoderma or iododerma
- Bacterial infections (furunculosis and cellulitis)
- Deep fungal infection
- Erythema nodosum—primarily over the shins
- Atypical mycobacterial infection
- Leishmaniasis—recent travel to endemic areas
- Lymphoma/leukemia cutis
- Metastatic carcinoma

✓ Best Tests

Skin biopsy is used to confirm the diagnosis and will show a dense neutrophilic infiltrate in the lower dermis.

Consider a medical workup to narrow the differential or elucidate the underlying cause of the condition, such as an infection or hematologic malignancy. Such investigations may include

- CBC with differential
- Erythrocyte sedimentation rate and/or C-reactive protein level
- Pregnancy test
- Cultures of lesions
- Comprehensive age and gender appropriate screening for malignancy

- Chest X-ray
- PET scan, ultrasound, CT, or MRI for malignancy
- Bone marrow biopsy

▲▲ Management Pearls

- Consultations with the following specialties may be indicated: dermatology, hematology/oncology.
- If possible, withdraw any suspected triggering medication.

Therapy

Maximize the treatment of any identified underlying condition.

Corticosteroids, either systemically (prednisone 0.5 to 1.0 mg/kg p.o. daily and tapered over 4 to 6 weeks) or locally (clobetasol propionate 0.05% twice daily or intralesional injections of triamcinolone 3 to 10 mg/mL) are first-line treatment. In patients receiving oral prednisone, an additional 2 to 3 months of low-dose therapy may be useful to suppress recurrences. Pulsed dosing of intravenous methylprednisolone (up to 1 g daily for 3 to 5 days) is an alternative.

Topical calcineurin inhibitors (tacrolimus or pimecrolimus) are alternatives to topical steroids in localized disease.

Oral saturated solution of potassium iodide (SSKI or Lugol solution) is another commonly used agent. Begin SSKI at 5 drops in orange juice three times daily and advance daily 1 drop, as tolerated, to 15 drops three times daily. An alternative is potassium-iodide enteric-coated tablets 900 mg daily. In long-term use, monitor thyroid function.

Colchicine (0.5 to 0.6 mg p.o. two to three times daily).

Dapsone (100 to 200 mg p.o. daily), indomethacin (100 to 150 mg p.o. daily), and clofazimine (100 to 200 mg p.o. daily) have also been tried with some success. Doxycycline, cyclosporine, chlorambucil, metronidazole, etretinate, cyclophosphamide, etanercept, and interferon alpha have been used as well. Combination therapy may be useful.

Suggested Readings

Cohen PR. Sweet's syndrome—a comprehensive review of an acute febrile neutrophilic dermatosis. *Orphanet J Rare Dis.* 2007;2:34.

Cohen PR, Kurzrock R. Sweet's syndrome: A review of current treatment options. *Am J Clin Dermatol.* 2002;3(2):117–131.

Fukae J, Noda K, Fujishima K, et al. Successful treatment of relapsing neuro-Sweet's disease with corticosteroid and dapsone combination therapy. *Clin Neurol Neurosurg.* 2007 Dec;109(10):910–913.

Moschella SL, Davis MD. Neutrophilic dermatoses. In: Bolognia J, Jorizzo JL, Rapini RP, eds. *Dermatology.* 2nd Ed. St. Louis, MO: Mosby; 2008: 380–383.

Neoh CY, Tan AW, Ng SK. Sweet's syndrome: A spectrum of unusual clinical presentations and associations. *Br J Dermatol.* 2007 Mar;156(3):480–485.

Ratzinger G, Burgdorf W, Zelger BG, Zelger B. Acute febrile neutrophilic dermatosis: A histopathologic study of 31 cases with review of literature. *Am J Dermatopathol.* 2007 Apr;29(2):125–133.

Ritter S, George R, Serwatka LM, et al. Long-term suppression of chronic Sweet's syndrome with colchicine. *J Am Acad Dermatol.* 2002 Aug;47(2):323–324.

Thompson DF, Montarella KE. Drug-induced Sweet's syndrome. *Ann Pharmacother.* 2007 May;41(5):802–811.

von den Driesch P. Sweet's syndrome (acute febrile neutrophilic dermatosis). *J Am Acad Dermatol.* 1994 Oct;31(4):535–556; quiz 557–560.

Wallach D, Vignon-Pennamen MD. From acute febrile neutrophilic dermatosis to neutrophilic disease: Forty years of clinical research. *J Am Acad Dermatol.* 2006 Dec;55(6):1066–1071.

Toxic Epidermal Necrolysis (Lyell Disease)

■■ Diagnosis Synopsis

Toxic epidermal necrolysis (TEN) and Stevens-Johnson syndrome (SJS) are two rare severe drug reactions that are characterized by high fevers, skin tenderness, mucosal erosions, and skin detachment about 1 to 3 weeks after the inciting medication is started. SJS and TEN should be considered the same disease on opposite ends of the spectrum, with the level of skin detachment differentiating these two entities. SJS is characterized by less than 10% of body surface area (BSA), while TEN involves greater than 30% BSA. SJS–TEN overlap occurs when 10% to 30% BSA is involved. Note that SJS can rapidly evolve into TEN, and both may follow an unpredictable clinical course. Even expert groups may identify patients in the overlap area, and this can complicate decision making for therapy.

While the molecular events and etiology of SJS and TEN are not entirely defined, a drug history is strongly associated with their development in greater than 80% of cases. The three main classes that have been most frequently implicated include nonsteroidal anti-inflammatory drugs (NSAIDs), antibiotics, and anticonvulsants. There is some evidence that SJS and TEN are due to the host's inability to detoxify drug metabolites, resulting in a cell-mediated immune response that activates cytotoxic T-cells and subsequent induction of keratinocyte apoptosis via cell surface death receptor signaling (membrane-bound or soluble CD95-CD95 ligand interaction). Additional rare causes include immunizations and infections.

SJS/TEN can affect all ages and races, with a slight preponderance seen in women (1.5:1) and an increasing incidence with age. Risk factors that confer a worse prognosis include extent of BSA involved at the time of diagnosis, older age, cancer or hematological malignancy, AIDS, number of medications, and elevated serum urea, glucose, and creatinine levels.

Primary lesions include dusky red macules of irregular size and shape that start on the trunk and spread to the proximal extremities, neck, and face. The onset of disease occurs 1 to 3 weeks after the ingestion of an antibiotic or within the first 2 months of anticonvulsant treatment. Within hours to days, the epidermis can detach from the dermis, with serosanguineous fluid filling the space and subsequent flaccid blister formation. Ocular, oral, and genital mucosa will be affected in more than 90% of cases. Mucosal symptoms that should be screened for include painful eyes, painful swallowing, dysuria, and diarrhea.

SJS carries a 1% to 5% mortality risk, may or may not have systemic symptoms, and involves the trunk and face with many isolated lesions. TEN involves greater than 30% BSA, carries a 25% to 35% mortality risk, invariably has systemic symptoms, and the lesions on the trunk and face are largely coalesced.

Rapid identification and withdrawal of the offending drug and transfer to a burn unit with aggressive supportive care are the most critical steps in the management. The fatality rate of TEN approaches 35%. Death is usually due to sepsis, adult respiratory distress syndrome, gastrointestinal bleeding, or pulmonary embolism. A few days after the epidermis is sloughed, reepithelialization begins. Most of the epidermis is reepithelialized after 2 to 3 weeks with no scarring over most areas. Mucous membrane erosions may persist for months, however.

◉ Look For

Specifically for TEN:

- Greater than 30% BSA.
- Irregularly shaped, dusky red macules on the trunk and face and palms/soles largely coalescing.
- Atypical target lesions may also be seen (i.e., atypical in the sense that they do not have the characteristic three concentric rings seen in erythema multiforme [EM]).
- "Scalded"-appearing skin—epidermal detachment with underlying dermis exposed (Figs. 4-614–4-617).
- Flaccid bullae due to epidermal–dermal detachment.
- Nikolsky sign—tangential mechanical pressure of an erythematous macule leads to epidermal–dermal detachment.
- Mucosal involvement including the eyes, lips, mouth, and genitalia—Look for hemorrhagic crust, bullae, and denudation. Mucous membrane changes occur at these sites in descending order of frequency: the oropharynx, eyes, genitalia, and anus. Greater than 90% of patients experience mucous membrane involvement with painful erosions. In one-third of cases, mucous membrane changes precede cutaneous changes by 1 to 3 days. Pseudomembranous conjunctival erosions (Fig. 4-618) and hemorrhagic crusting of the lips are common findings.
- Systemic symptoms are invariably present.

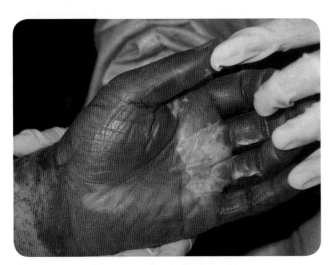

Figure 4-614 TEN with separation of palmar skin.

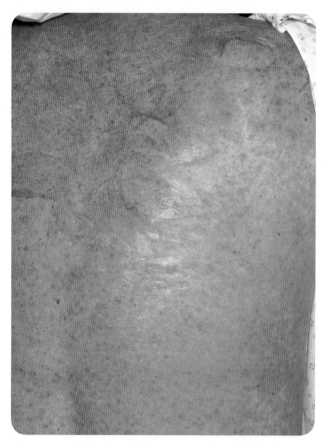

Figure 4-615 Sheet-like separation of portions of the upper back without discreet inflammatory lesions.

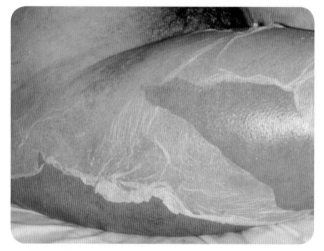

Figure 4-617 Sheet-like skin separation in TEN secondary to carbamazepine.

 Diagnostic Pearls

In evaluating the patient, the clinician should be aware of nonvisual signs of mucosal involvement including painful swallowing, painful micturition, and diarrhea. In addition,

462

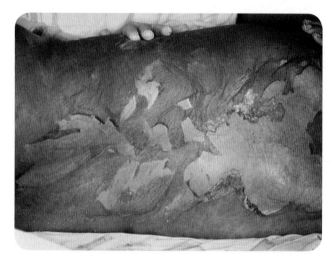

Figure 4-616 Large sites of epidermal separation on the back in TEN.

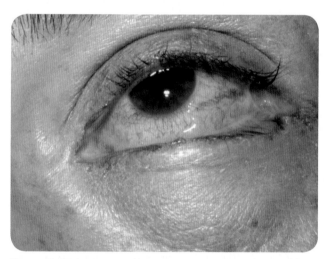

Figure 4-618 Conjunctival involvement from TEN in a patient with AIDS.

there are characteristic features of SJS/TEN blisters. The blisters are flaccid, break easily, and can be extended laterally by slight tangential pressure (Asboe-Hansen sign).

?? **Differential Diagnosis and Pitfalls**

- EM—Histologic features may not differentiate EM from SJS/TEN. Clinically, however, EM has characteristic target lesions (three concentric colors that are round and well demarcated) and occurs on the extremities more often than the trunk. Precipitating factors are usually infectious (HSV, mycoplasma, etc.) and not medications. Lesions may be papular. Note that EM is not considered within the same disease spectrum as SJS/TEN and confers no risk in progressing to TEN. Nikolsky sign negative.

- Staphylococcal scalded skin syndrome—Usually occurs in newborns, infants, and young children; mucous membranes and palms/soles are spared. The exfoliated skin is significantly more superficial (subcorneal versus epidermal–dermal). Also look for purulent discharge from nose, and histologically very different from SJS/TEN. Nikolsky sign can be positive.
- Acute generalized exanthematic pustulosis (AGEP)—Look for neutrophilia, eosinophilia, almost confluent erythema with overlying nonfollicular pustules. Nikolsky sign can be positive. Histology will clearly differentiate AGEP versus SJS/TEN.
- Generalized fixed drug eruption—Look for erythematous plaques that develop on the lips, face, distal extremities, and genitalia 1 to 2 weeks after drug ingestions. Oral mucosa can be involved. Histology will differentiate fixed drug versus SJS/TEN.
- Linear IgA disease—Look for tense blisters; histology will help differentiate linear IgA versus SJS/TEN; direct immunofluorescence will demonstrate linear IgA deposition. Immunofluorescence is negative in SJS/TEN.
- Toxic shock and toxic shock-like syndrome—Look for sudden onset of exanthematous eruption. Histology will help differentiate TSS and SJS/TEN.
- Drug reaction with eosinophilia and systemic symptoms (DRESS)—Look for facial edema (hallmark of DRESS), eosinophilia, hepatitis, and other visceral involvement.
- Bullous pemphigoid—widespread bullae, usually in older patients.
- Pemphigus vulgaris
- Paraneoplastic pemphigus—significant involvement of the vermillion border
- Dermatitis herpetiformis—extremely pruritic
- Sweet syndrome
- Acute graft-versus-host disease—Look for history of bone marrow transplant

✓ Best Tests

- A skin biopsy will largely aid in confirming the diagnosis. Early stage biopsy demonstrates apoptotic keratinocytes throughout the epidermis. Late stage biopsy demonstrates subepidermal blisters and full-thickness epidermal necrosis.
- Patients with SJS/TEN require ongoing biochemical and microbiological monitoring for infection, end-organ damage, and electrolyte disturbances. This level of vigilance requires frequent determinations of serum labs such as CBC, comprehensive serum electrolytes, BUN and creatinine, transaminases, and urine output. Swabs from potentially infected areas, blood and urine cultures, and information from blood gases are also needed.
- Baseline chest films and GI studies are needed to follow possible respiratory and GI tract involvement.

▲▲▲ Management Pearls

Patients with SJS/TEN require intensive care level or a burn unit level care. The primary goals are to provide fluid/nutritional support, pain control, and monitoring for infection. The use of systemic corticosteroids is controversial. Many authorities believe that they offer no clinical benefit and may increase the rate of complications. Consultations are needed and include a dietician, dermatologist, ophthalmologist, and/or a burn or wound care specialist. There is no role for prophylactic antibiotics, but monitor for and promptly treat any identified infections.

A severity-of-illness score that estimates mortality in TEN has been developed (SCORTEN) with the following factors:

- Age > 40
- HR > 120 bpm
- Malignancy
- Involved BSA > 10%
- BUN > 10 mEq/L
- Serum bicarbonate < 20 mEq/L
- Blood glucose > 252 mg/dL

Mortality estimates are based on the number of above criteria met:

- 0 to 1 factor ≥ 3.2%
- 2 factors ≥ 12.1%
- 3 factors ≥ 35.3%
- 4 factors ≥ 58.3%
- 5 or more factors ≥ 90%

Therapy

Early diagnosis of SJS/TEN and rapid identification and discontinuation of the inciting drug is of paramount importance. The faster the inciting drug is discontinued, the more favorable the prognosis. Supportive therapy in a burn unit is the mainstay of treatment. No universally accepted specific therapies exist. Consultation with a dermatologist or other experienced specialist is recommended.

Supportive Care
- Wound care—Consider nanocrystalline gauze materials containing silver ions (nonadherent) or petrolatum-based gauze pads.
- Fluid and electrolyte management—Correct for transepidermal water loss.
- Nutritional supplementation—Consider nutritional support via nasogastric tube. Request nutrition consult.
- Temperature management—Heat loss via epidermal loss can be significant, and the patient should be

(Continued)

treated like a burn victim. Consider increasing the room temperature to 30°C to 32°C (86°F to 89.6°F).

- Superinfections—Patients with SJS/TEN are at high risk for sepsis and infection. Patient should be routinely pan-cultured (skin, blood, urine, and any arterial lines and catheters) throughout hospital stay. Note that systemic antibiotics are not used prophylactically.
- Ocular care—Vigorous lubrication and lysis of any adhesions that develop. Request an ophthalmologic consult immediately to decrease risk of irreversible ocular damage.

Specific Therapies

- Corticosteroids—Data regarding the use of steroids is mixed, and their use remains controversial.
- Intravenous immunoglobulin (IVIg)—Data regarding the use of IVIg are also mixed but is still considered effective. Strongly consider with a specialist or physician experienced with SJS/TEN. Dosing is usually 0.8 g/kg/day for 3 to 4 days. Coagulopathies, acute renal failure, anaphylaxis, and aseptic meningitis can be rare, severe side effects of therapy. If timing permits, check IgA levels, as anaphylaxis can ensue in patients with IgA deficiency.
- Plasmapheresis—Mixed findings; consider adjunct with IVIg.
- Most patients have considerable pain. The use of opioid analgesics is often required. There may be considerable pruritus as the skin reepithelializes. This can be controlled with antihistamines:
- Diphenhydramine hydrochloride (25, 50 mg tablets or capsules)—25 to 50 mg nightly or every 6 h as needed
- Hydroxyzine (10, 25 mg tablets)—12.5 to 25 mg every 6 h as needed
- Cetirizine (5,10 mg tablets)—5 to 10 mg per day
- Loratadine (10 mg tablets)—10 mg tablet once daily

Suggested Readings

Atiyeh BS, Dham R, Yassin MF, et al. Treatment of toxic epidermal necrolysis with moisture-retentive ointment: A case report and review of the literature. *Dermatol Surg*. 2003 Feb;29(2):185–188.

Bachot N, Roujeau JC. Differential diagnosis of severe cutaneous drug eruptions. *Am J Clin Dermatol*. 2003;4(8):561–572.

Borchers AT, Lee JL, Naguwa SM, et al. Stevens-Johnson syndrome and toxic epidermal necrolysis. *Autoimmun Rev*. 2008 Sep;7(8):598–605.

Chave TA, Mortimer NJ, Sladden MJ, et al. Toxic epidermal necrolysis: Current evidence, practical management and future directions. *Br J Dermatol*. 2005 Aug;153(2):241–253.

Fromowitz JS, Ramos-Caro FA, Flowers FP, University of Florida. Practical guidelines for the management of toxic epidermal necrolysis and Stevens-Johnson syndrome. *Int J Dermatol*. 2007 Oct;46(10):1092–1094.

Guégan S, Bastuji-Garin S, Poszepczynska-Guigné E, et al. Performance of the SCORTEN during the first five days of hospitalization to predict the prognosis of epidermal necrolysis. *J Invest Dermatol*. 2006 Feb;126(2):272–276.

Hazin R, Ibrahimi OA, Hazin MI, et al. Stevens-Johnson syndrome: Pathogenesis, diagnosis, and management. *Ann Med*. 2008;40(2):129–138.

Palmieri TL, Greenhalgh DG, Saffle JR, et al. A multicenter review of toxic epidermal necrolysis treated in U.S. burn centers at the end of the twentieth century. *J Burn Care Rehabil*. 2002 Mar–Apr;23(2):87–96.

Pereira FA, Mudgil AV, Rosmarin DM. Toxic epidermal necrolysis. *J Am Acad Dermatol*. 2007 Feb;56(2):181–200.

Roujeau JC, Kelly JP, Naldi L, et al. Medication use and the risk of Stevens-Johnson syndrome or toxic epidermal necrolysis. *N Engl J Med*. 1995 Dec;333(24):1600–1607.

Rzany B, Correia O, Kelly JP, et al. Risk of Stevens-Johnson syndrome and toxic epidermal necrolysis during first weeks of antiepileptic therapy: A case-control study. Study Group of the International Case Control Study on Severe Cutaneous Adverse Reactions. *Lancet*. 1999 Jun;353(9171):2190–2194

Saiag P, Caumes E, Chosidow O, et al. Drug-induced toxic epidermal necrolysis (Lyell syndrome) in patients infected with the human immunodeficiency virus. *J Am Acad Dermatol*. 1992 Apr;26(4):567–574.

Schneck J, Fagot JP, Sekula P, et al. Effects of treatments on the mortality of Stevens-Johnson syndrome and toxic epidermal necrolysis: A retrospective study on patients included in the prospective EuroSCAR Study. *J Am Acad Dermatol*. 2008 Jan;58(1):33–40.

Valeyrie-Allanore L, Roujeau JC. Epidermal necrolysis (Stevens-Johnson syndrome and toxic epidermal necrolysis). In: Fitzpatrick TB, Wolff K, eds. *Fitzpatrick's Dermatology in General Medicine*. 7th Ed. New York, NY: McGraw-Hill; 2008:349–355.

■■ Diagnosis Synopsis

Toxic shock syndrome (TSS) is a severe exotoxin-mediated bacterial infection that is characterized by high fevers, headache, pharyngitis, vomiting, diarrhea, and hypotension. Two subtypes of TSS exist, based on the bacterial etiology: *Staphylococcus aureus* and group A streptococci. Significantly, the severity of TSS can range from mild disease to rapid progression to shock and end-organ failure. The dermatologic manifestations of TSS include the following:

- Erythema of the palms and soles that desquamates 1 to 3 weeks after the initial onset (Figs. 4-619 and 4-620)
- Diffuse scarlatiniform exanthem that begins on the trunk and spreads toward the extremities (Fig. 4-621)
- Erythema of the mucous membranes (strawberry tongue and conjunctival hyperemia)

TSS was identified in and most commonly affected menstruating young white females using tampons in the 1980s. Current TSS cases are seen in post-surgical interventions. Staphylococcal TSS is caused by *S. aureus* strains that can produce the toxic shock syndrome toxin-1 (TSST-1). TSST-1 is believed to cause disease via direct noxious effects on end organs, impairing clearance of gut flora derived endotoxins, and TSST-1 acting as a superantigen leading to massive non-specific activation of T-cells and subsequent inflammation and vascular leakage. In this form of TSS, risk factors include lacking an antibody to TSST-1, surgical packing, abscesses, surgical mesh, and tampon use.

Streptococcal TSS is also caused by exotoxins that cause massive stimulation of T-cells via a superantigen mechanism. Clinically, the most common presenting symptom is severe pain in an extremity with or without underlying soft tissue infection. A prodrome of fever, diarrhea, and myalgias is often seen. The macular exanthem seen in staphylococcal TSS is much less commonly found in streptococcal TSS. Approximately 48 to 72 h after the initial onset, shock and multiorgan failure follow. In this form of TSS, risk factors include varicella infection, bites, and lacerations.

Both forms of TSS can result in confusion and coma, renal impairment, liver impairment, adult respiratory distress syndrome, and disseminated intravascular coagulation (Fig. 4-622). Supportive measures (intravenous fluids, vasopressors, etc.) and appropriate antibiotics are the mainstays of treatment.

◉ Look For

Staphylococcal TSS

- Diffuse macular erythroderma
- Desquamation of palms/soles 1 to 3 weeks after onset of symptoms

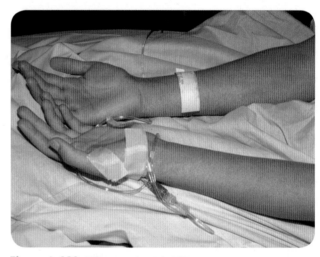

Figure 4-620 Diffuse erythema in TSS.

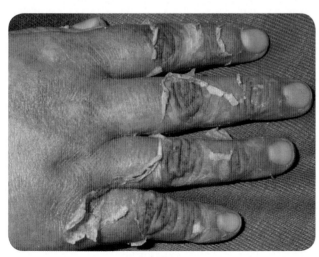

Figure 4-619 Desquamation phase of TSS.

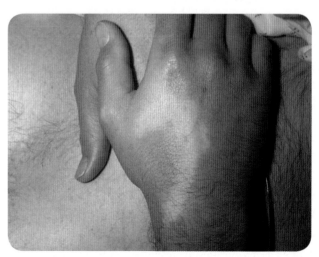

Figure 4-621 Early phase of TSS with edema and erythema.

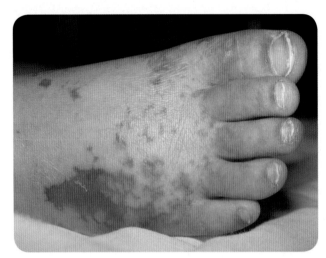

Figure 4-622 Purpura from disseminated intravascular coagulation with TSS.

- High grade fever
- Hypotension
- Multiorgan involvement

Streptococcal TSS

- Severe localized pain in an extremity
- Prodromal symptoms
- Desquamation of palms/soles 1 to 3 weeks after onset of symptoms
- Hypotension within 48 to 72 h of initial onset of symptoms
- Multiorgan involvement

Note that there are significant differences between staphylococcal and streptococcal TSS. They are as follows:

- Diffuse macular erythroderma is commonly seen in staphylococcal TSS but not in streptococcal TSS.
- Soft tissue infections are rare in staphylococcal TSS but common in streptococcal TSS.
- Positive blood cultures are seen in less than 15% of staphylococcal TSS cases but in over 50% of streptococcal TSS.
- Mortality rates are approximately 3% in staphylococcal TSS and 30% to 60% in streptococcal TSS.

Group A streptococci can be isolated from blood, CSF, tissue biopsy, surgical wound, sputum, throat, vagina, and superficial skin lesion.

 Diagnostic Pearls

The CDC diagnostic criteria for TSS are as follows:

- Fever, hypotension, and characteristic rash
- Involvement of three or more organ systems

No serologic evidence of the following: Rocky Mountain spotted fever, measles, leptospirosis, syphilis, Epstein-Barr virus, hepatitis B, or antinuclear antibodies (ANA).

?? Differential Diagnosis and Pitfalls

- Staphylococcal scalded skin syndrome (SSSS)
- Scarlet fever—1 mm erythematous papules, always elevated WBC with left shift, eosinophilia in up to 20% of patients
- Necrotizing fasciitis—violaceous hue, bullae or necrosis, and severe localized pain
- Drug eruption
- Stevens-Johnson syndrome—drug induced, high fevers, skin tenderness, mucosal erosions, and skin detachment about 1 to 3 weeks after the inciting medication is started
- Toxic epidermal necrolysis—drug induced, high fevers, skin tenderness, mucosal erosions, and skin detachment about 1 to 3 weeks after the inciting medication is started
- Kawasaki disease—fever lasting for more than 5 days with oral mucosal changes, conjunctival injection, and cervical lymphadenopathy
- Meningococcemia—rapid decompensation, characteristic petechial eruption caused by *N. meningitidis*
- Rocky Mountain spotted fever—characteristic retiform purpura; check for serologies

Best Tests

The clinical picture and examination are more important than any test and should prompt the initiation of therapy as soon as possible. The following tests and findings support the diagnosis:

- Blood cultures
- Culture of any potentially infected site (e.g., skin lesions, throat)
- CBC—leukocytosis, occasionally thrombocytopenia and/or anemia
- Electrolyte abnormalities, including azotemia
- Liver function tests—often bilirubin and/or transaminases will be elevated
- Coagulation studies—PTT and fibrin split products may be elevated
- Arterial blood gas—metabolic acidosis
- Creatine kinase may be increased
- Urinalysis may be abnormal, with myoglobulin or casts
- Serologic testing as mentioned in Diagnostic Pearls may be performed to rule out other causes of the clinical findings.

Depending on the clinical scenario, further testing will be needed to investigate or monitor possible complications and may include

- ECG/continuous cardiac monitoring
- Invasive hemodynamic monitoring
- Chest radiographs

466

- Echocardiogram
- Plain films, CT, or MRI of any suspected site of infection
- Lumbar puncture

 ## Management Pearls

Supportive care in a tertiary medical center (if possible) is necessary for a successful outcome.

Therapy

Immediate intervention for shock and systemic antistaphylococcal/streptococcal antibiotics is essential. Aggressive fluid support will be needed. Cardiovascular, pulmonary, and metabolic intervention/support may be necessary.

Nafcillin or oxacillin 2 g IV every 4 h OR:

- Cefazolin 1 g IV every 8 h
- Clindamycin 600 to 900 mg IV every 8 h (covers streptococci and some methicillin-resistant *S. aureus* [MRSA])

Also for MRSA or penicillin-allergic patients:

- Vancomycin 30 mg/kg/day IV divided twice daily
- Linezolid 600 mg IV every 12 h

Continue antibiotics for a total of 10 to 14 days.

Immune globulin (400 mg/kg over 2 to 3 h) contains antibody to TSS and may be used for patients with refractory foci of infection.

Suggested Readings

Annane D, Clair B, Salomon J. Managing toxic shock syndrome with antibiotics. *Expert Opin Pharmacother.* 2004 Aug;5(8):1701–1710.

Bach MC. Dermatologic signs in toxic shock syndrome—clues to diagnosis. *J Am Acad Dermatol.* 1983 Mar;8(3):343–347.

Parsonnet J, Hansmann MA, Delaney ML, et al. Prevalence of toxic shock syndrome toxin 1-producing *Staphylococcus aureus* and the presence of antibodies to this superantigen in menstruating women. *J Clin Microbiol.* 2005 Sep;43(9):4628–4634.

Proft T, Fraser JD. Streptococcal superantigens. *Chem Immunol Allergy.* 2007;93:1–23.

Soper DE. Abortion and clostridial toxic shock syndrome. *Obstet Gynecol.* 2007 Nov;110(5):970–971.

Varicella (Chickenpox)

Diagnosis Synopsis

Varicella, also known as chickenpox, is a self-limited viral infection caused by varicella zoster virus (VZV), a member of the *Herpesviridae* family. Prior to the clinical implementation of the varicella vaccine, more than 99% of adults aged 40 and older had evidence of previous infection. Transmission occurs via airborne respiratory droplets or direct contact with vesicular fluid. The incubation period ranges from 10 to 20 days.

Varicella is characterized by a prodrome of malaise, myalgias, and mild fever that is followed by an acute eruption of pruritic, erythematous macules and papules that start on the face, oral mucosa, and scalp, and spread to the trunk and extremities. The lesions rapidly evolve into 1 to 3 mm vesicles with clear serous fluid on an erythematous background. The hallmark of chickenpox is the presence of lesions in various stages of development. Older lesions will evolve to form pustules and serous crusts that heal within 10 days of time.

In healthy individuals, the clinical course is most commonly benign and self-limited. From a clinical standpoint, it is important to note that varicella is highly contagious, and the infected individual has the potential to infect others until all cutaneous lesions have completely crusted over. The most common complication in otherwise healthy individuals is secondary bacterial infection with subsequent scarring. In immunocompromised individuals, varicella can cause significant morbidity and mortality, and patients often present with more hemorrhagic and purpuric lesions. Complications in immunocompetent and immunocompromised individuals include the following:

- Central nervous system: encephalitis, Reye syndrome, acute cerebellar ataxia
- Pulmonary: varicella pneumonia and acute respiratory distress syndrome
- Hepatic: viral hepatitis
- Cutaneous: herpes zoster and postherpetic neuralgia
- Additional rare complications include myocarditis, pancreatitis, glomerulonephritis, uveitis, optic neuritis, and vasculitis.

Congenital varicella infection can cause a wide range of fetal abnormalities, with the highest risk of abnormalities seen in the first trimester. Congenital abnormalities include the following: ocular abnormalities, cortical atrophy, low birth weight, cicatricial skin lesions, hypoplastic limbs, and psychomotor retardation.

Since widespread use of the varicella vaccine in 1995 for children, incidence of varicella infection has decreased in the United States, and cases that do occur tend to be milder than in those who have not been vaccinated.

Immunocompromised Patient Considerations

Varicella may be severe in HIV-infected and immunocompromised individuals (particularly those with lymphoma and those receiving immunosuppressive therapy, including systemic steroid therapy), with a 7% to 10% mortality rate. These patients often have a more extensive and atypical eruption (often with purpura and hemorrhagic vesicles) as well as visceral involvement (CNS, lung, liver). HIV-infected patients have a 7 to 15 times greater risk of developing herpes zoster.

Maternal varicella in the first 20 weeks of pregnancy is associated with a 2% risk of fetal damage. If maternal varicella occurs near the time of delivery, the neonate is at risk for severe varicella.

Look For

- Erythematous macular eruption that evolves to papules and then vesicles with a surrounding halo of erythema, known as "dewdrops on a rose petal." Tens to hundreds of lesions can be present on one individual (Fig. 4-623).
- Mucous membranes, palms, and soles can be involved, but the disease burden is greater on the face, scalp, and trunk.
- Vesicles are usually discrete (Fig. 4-624), unlike the clustered vesicles seen in herpes simplex or in herpes zoster.
- Simultaneous appearance of lesions in different stages of evolution is the hallmark of varicella infection (Fig. 4-625).
- Vesicles become cloudy appearing (pustular) and then crust over, with healing completed within 1 to 3 weeks (Fig. 4-626).

Diagnostic Pearls

The vesicle is classically described as "a dewdrop on a rose petal." The vesicle is thin walled and easily broken.

Differential Diagnosis and Pitfalls

- Herpes simplex virus (HSV)—Grouped vesicles on an erythematous base. Request direct fluorescence antigen (DFA) testing—DFA HSV, in contrast to DFA VZV—and viral culture. Look for more localized lesions in HSV at the site of primary infection.
- Hand-foot-and-mouth disease (Coxsackie virus)—Look for vesicular eruption of palms and soles.
- ECHO virus

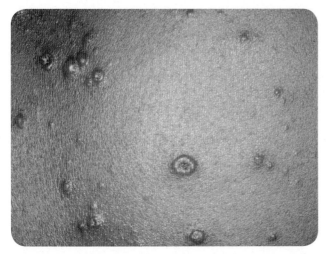

Figure 4-623 Varicella with umbilicated vesicles with hemorrhagic centers.

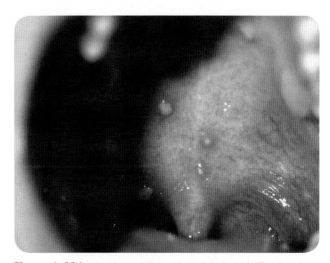

Figure 4-624 Discrete vesicle on the palate in varicella.

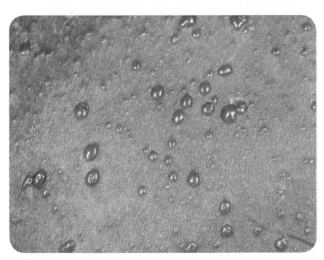

Figure 4-625 Varicella with multiple umbilicated and early non-umbilicated vesicles.

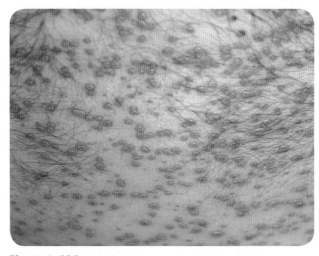

Figure 4-626 Varicella with numerous crusted vesicles.

- Impetigo—Honey-colored crusts with larger plaques and erosions.
- Rickettsialpox—Check serologies, transmitted by the house mite.
- Pityriasis lichenoides et varioliformis acuta (PLEVA)—Asymptomatic crops of erythematous papules that spontaneously resolve within weeks and recur at a later time.
- Drug eruption—Often present with urticarial, exanthematous, or vesicular/bullous lesions. Eosinophilia on CBC and histology are often seen (but not an invariable finding). Look for nonsteroidal anti-inflammatory drugs (NSAIDs), sulfonamides, and penicillin medication history.
- Gianotti-Crosti syndrome (in children)—Lesions are monomorphic edematous papules (in contrast to various stages of lesions seen with PLEVA).
- Contact dermatitis—Does not have prodromal symptoms and will be localized to site of contact (in contrast to disseminated distribution seen in VZV).

- Vasculitis—Check for RF, ANA, anti-ds DNA, ANCA, cryoglobulins. C3, C4 levels, and clinical course that does not resolve over several weeks.
- Eczema herpeticum—Hemorrhagic crusted papules and vesicles overlying eczematous skin, usually on the face.

✔ Best Tests

- This diagnosis can often be made clinically, but a number of investigations are available to confirm the clinical impression.
- DFA testing of skin lesion scrapings is more sensitive and specific than a Tzanck preparation, although the Tzanck will give more immediate results. Tzanck smears may be positive in 100% of cases, but false positives can be a problem. DFA is a rapid (<24 h) and sensitive test for HSV-1, HSV-2, and VZV. This test is performed by vigorously scraping the

469

base of a vesicle with a sterile cotton-tipped swab or no. 15 blade and smearing the cells onto a glass slide from a DFA kit. The slide is then fixed (usually contained in a kit) and sent for immunofluorescence analysis. Individual slides must be sent for each virus suspected. Slides can be stored at room temperature for 24 h after fixation if needed.

- Viral culture of vesicular fluid.
- Serologic studies are often used to confirm past infection and to assess current susceptibility. Among these are a latex agglutination assay, an enzyme-linked immunosorbent assay (ELISA), an indirect fluorescent antibody test, a radioimmunoassay, a neutralization test, and a fluorescent antibody to membrane antigen test.
- Consider obtaining a chest X-ray with respiratory signs and symptoms and, likewise, perform a lumbar puncture on patients with neurologic signs and/or symptoms.
- PCR can be used to detect viral DNA in the cerebrospinal fluid.

▲▲ Management Pearls

The pruritus can lead to atrophic scars if excoriated. If pruritus is intense, systemic antihistamines (e.g., hydroxyzine or diphenhydramine) are more effective than the traditional calamine lotion.

Note: The CDC Advisory Committee on Immunization Practices recommends that all health care workers must ensure that they are immune to varicella as nosocomial transmission of varicella is a well-recognized problem. If susceptible persons must enter the room of a patient known or suspected to have varicella, they should wear respiratory protection (N95 respirator). Persons immune to varicella need not wear respiratory protection.

Nonimmune pregnant women who have had contact with a person with varicella should receive varicella zoster immune globulin (VZIG) for post-exposure prophylaxis.

Consult with an infectious disease specialist in complicated cases. Certain patients may require hospitalization.

Precautions: Standard and Airborne. (Isolate patient in a negative pressure room, wear respiratory protection [N95 mask], and limit patient transport.)

Therapy

Symptomatic treatment consists of antipyretics (acetaminophen), cool compresses and baths, calamine lotion, and systemic antihistamines:

- Diphenhydramine hydrochloride (25, 50 mg tablets or capsules): 25 to 50 mg nightly or every 6 h as needed
- Hydroxyzine (10, 25 mg tablets): 12.5 to 25 mg every 6 h as needed

- Cetirizine (5, 10 mg tablets): 5 to 10 mg per day
- Loratadine (10 mg tablets): 10 mg once daily

Acyclovir and related compounds can lessen the severity of acute infection and decrease the incidence of complications. Consideration should be given to the administration of these agents in adults and especially those with risk factors such as chronic lung disease or immunosuppression.

- Acyclovir 800 mg p.o. five times daily for 7 days
- Famciclovir 500 mg p.o. three times daily for 7 days
- Valacyclovir 1,000 mg p.o. three times daily for 7 days
- Foscarnet 40 mg/kg IV every 8 h for 10 days given as an infusion over 1 h for patients who have developed resistance to acyclovir

A live, attenuated varicella vaccine imparts protective antibody formation in 96% of patients immunized (0.5 mL SC twice in adults; second dose is given 4 to 8 weeks after the first).

Treat any secondarily infected lesions with the appropriate topical or systemic antibiotics.

Immunocompromised Patient Considerations

Prevention: Varicella vaccine is a live vaccine and is contraindicated in immunocompromised patients. It can, however, be used in patients with HIV if the CD4+ T-cell count is greater than 200.

Suggested Readings

Gardella C, Brown ZA. Managing varicella zoster infection in pregnancy. *Cleve Clin J Med*. 2007 Apr;74(4):290–296.

Heininger U, Seward JF. Varicella. *Lancet*. 2006 Oct;368(9544):1365–1376.

Kaneko T, Ishigatsubo Y. Varicella pneumonia in adults. *Intern Med*. 2004 Dec;43(12):1105–1106.

Kimberlin DW, Whitley RJ. Varicella-zoster vaccine for the prevention of herpes zoster. *N Engl J Med*. 2007 Mar;356(13):1338–1343.

Marin M, G. Prevention of varicella: Recommendations of the Advisory Committee on Immunization Practices (ACIP). *MMWR Recomm Rep*. 2007 Jun;56(RR-4):1–40.

Snoeck R, Andrei G, De Clercq E. Current pharmacological approaches to the therapy of varicella zoster virus infections: A guide to treatment. *Drugs*. 1999 Feb;57(2):187–206.

Straus SE, Oxman ME, Schmader KE. Varicella and herpes zoster. In: Fitzpatrick TB, Wolff K, eds. *Fitzpatrick's Dermatology in General Medicine*. 7th Ed. New York, NY: McGraw-Hill; 2008:1885–1898.

Tunbridge AJ, Breuer J, Jeffery KJ, British Infection Society. Chickenpox in adults—clinical management. *J Infect*. 2008 Aug;57(2):95–102.

Wallace MR, Bowler WA, Murray NB, Brodine SK, Oldfield EC. Treatment of adult varicella with oral acyclovir. A randomized, placebo-controlled trial. *Ann Intern Med*. 1992 Sep;117(5):358–363.

Diagnosis Synopsis

A number of viruses can cause a viral exanthem. Viral exanthems have a variety of presentations and distributions. They can be widespread, localized, dermatomal, morbilliform, scarlatiniform, urticarial, petechial, purpuric, macular, macular and papular, or vesicular. Rubeola, rubella, echovirus, Epstein-Barr virus, cytomegalovirus (CMV), HIV, togavirus, parvovirus, and herpes viruses are most commonly responsible for viral exanthems. Common associated clinical findings include fever, myalgias, gastrointestinal symptoms, and malaise.

It is important to rule out rubella, CMV, herpes, and parvovirus in the gravid female due to secondary complications that may affect the developing fetus or viability of pregnancy.

Immunocompromised Patient Considerations

Viral exanthems are extremely common and should be considered within the differential diagnosis of the immunocompromised patient presenting with a widespread erythematous eruption.

Human herpes viruses 6 and 7 (HHV-6 and HHV-7) are particularly associated with HIV and immunosuppressed patients after organ transplant.

HIV acute retroviral syndrome presents with lymphadenopathy and a cutaneous eruption resembling acute mononucleosis.

CMV infection may lead to complications including hemolytic anemia, meningoencephalitis, pneumonia, and thrombocytopenia.

 Look For

Nonspecific widespread, erythematous eruptions can be seen in a variety of viral exanthems (Figs. 4-627–4-631).

Rubeola (measles) presents with a macular exanthem that spreads from the head downward. On the oral mucosa, some patients have Koplik spots, which are 1 to 3 mm red macules with a central white or blue spot. Patients may also have cough, coryza, and conjunctivitis.

Rubella (German measles) presents with occipital and postauricular lymphadenopathy and a macular exanthem that spreads from the head downward.

Mononucleosis presents with a nonspecific macular exanthem and associated pharyngitis and adenopathy. If given ampicillin or amoxicillin, almost all patients develop a diffuse macular or papular skin eruption.

Parvovirus presents in adults with a lacy, reticulated macular exanthem on the trunk and extremities and associated arthralgias. Papular-purpuric gloves and socks syndrome may also be present.

Targetoid macules are observed in herpes-associated erythema multiforme eruptions.

A vesicular eruption may indicate herpes zoster (shingles) when in a dermatomal distribution or varicella (chickenpox) when diffusely distributed with lesions in various stages of evolution (erythematous papules, vesicles, and crusted papules).

Pityriasis rosea (suspected HHV-7 infection) has finely scaled patches in a "Christmas tree" pattern on the trunk, preceded by a herald patch.

Diagnostic Pearls

The patient does not appear toxic, and the rash is often the most significant finding. Viral exanthems are rarely pruritic, compared with drug exanthems that are commonly pruritic.

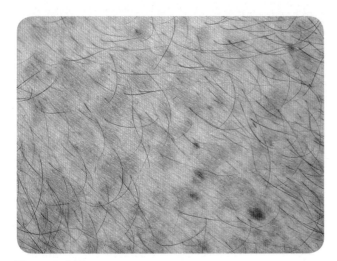

Figure 4-627 Pink papules in a viral exanthem.

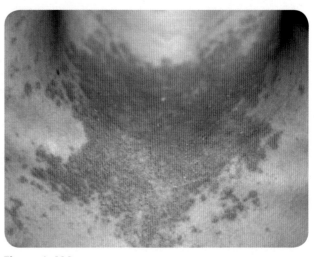

Figure 4-628 Viral exanthem with discrete and confluent papules.

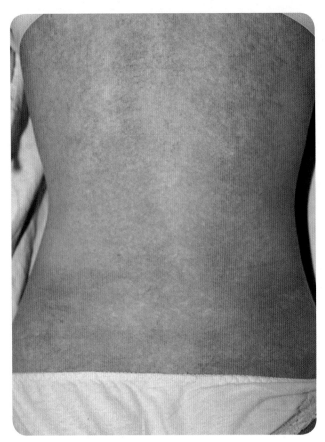

Figure 4-629 Macules and papules in infectious mononucleosis.

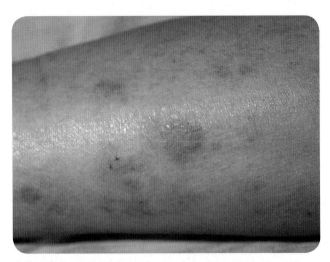

Figure 4-630 Urticarial plaque in cytomegalic infection.

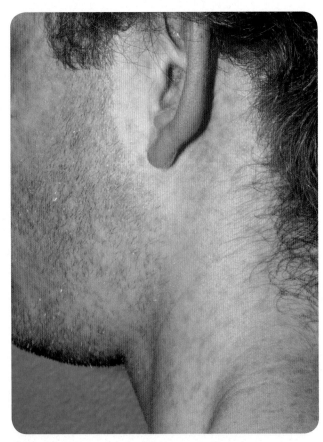

Figure 4-631 Macules and papules around the ears in rubella.

?? Differential Diagnosis and Pitfalls

Medication-associated exanthems have a history of exposure to medication with associated pruritus.

Immunocompromised Patient Considerations

Acute seroconversion with HIV can present with mononucleosis-like symptoms and an exanthematous rash. Consider this diagnosis in those at risk.

Graft-versus-host disease can also present with a variety of cutaneous eruptions resembling viral exanthems.

✓ Best Tests

- History is important to help distinguish between viral exanthems, drug eruptions, and immunocompromised-associated conditions.
- A biopsy is helpful and often necessary when the clinical diagnosis is in doubt.
- Most laboratory tests are nonspecific. Eosinophilia is typically absent in viral exanthems, but it may be present in drug exanthems and may help to distinguish between these clinical entities.
- Chest X-ray may be obtained when suspecting pulmonary involvement.

▲▲ Management Pearls

- Symptomatic relief.
- Parvovirus may be associated with a hemolytic anemia in some patients.
- Nearly all patients with infectious mononucleosis who receive a β-lactam antibiotic (e.g., ampicillin or amoxicillin) will develop a macular or papular skin eruption.

Immunocompromised Patient Considerations

HIV test if suspecting acute retroviral syndrome.

Therapy

Many of the nonspecific viral exanthems are self-limited. Treatment is mainly for the symptomatic relief of associated fevers and arthralgias.

Treatment of varicella-zoster- or herpes-associated erythema multiforme includes antivirals (acyclovir, valacyclovir, etc.).

Suggested Readings

Belazarian L, Lorenzo ME, Pace NC, et al. Exanthematous viral diseases. In: Fitzpatrick TB, Wolff K, eds. *Fitzpatrick's Dermatology in General Medicine.* 7th Ed. New York, NY: McGraw-Hill; 2008:1851–1872.

Drago F, Rampini E, Rebora A. Atypical exanthems: Morphology and laboratory investigations may lead to an aetiological diagnosis in about 70% of cases. *Br J Dermatol.* 2002 Aug;147(2):255–260.

Scott LA, Stone MS. Viral exanthems. *Dermatol Online J.* 2003 Aug;9(3):4.

Yamanishi K, Okuno T, Shiraki K, et al. Identification of human herpesvirus-6 as a causal agent for exanthem subitum. *Lancet.* 1988 May;1(8594):1065–1067.

Abscess

▪▪ Diagnosis Synopsis

An abscess is a localized inflammatory process in which the white blood cells accumulate at the site of infection in the dermis and/or subcutaneous tissue, creating a collection of pus. Commonly associated pathogens are *Staphylococcus aureus,* streptococci, and normal skin flora. Trauma or any break in the skin barrier predisposes to abscess formation. Lesions evolve over days to 1 or 2 weeks. They are usually painful/tender, erythematous, warm, and fluctuant masses that are sometimes associated with fever. A tender subcutaneous nodule with overlying erythema but minimal fluctuance may be an early presentation. Incision and drainage is the mainstay of therapy. In an otherwise healthy, ambulatory patient, the addition of antibiotics is not indicated. Indications for further antibiotics may include patients who are systemically ill, have a high burden of disease (indicated by concomitant widespread folliculitis or associated cellulitis), or have failed incision and drainage.

Methicillin resistant *S. aureus* (MRSA) first emerged as an important nosocomial pathogen in the 1960s. In more recent years, community-acquired outbreaks of MRSA (CA-MRSA) have increasingly been described among healthy individuals lacking the traditional risk factors for such infections (IV drug use, incarceration, participation in contact sports, etc.). These strains have a propensity for causing abscesses, furunculosis, and folliculitis and have a unique antibiotic susceptibility profile from health care–associated strains of MRSA (HA-MRSA).

In a recent study of emergency room visits for purulent skin and soft tissue infections, MRSA was identified as the etiologic agent in the majority (59%) of cases in multiple locations nationwide. Furthermore, this study determined that 57% of patients with MRSA did not receive the appropriate initial antibiotic therapy.

Immunocompromised Patient Considerations

Abscesses can be caused by a number of bacterial or fungal organisms in the immunocompromised patient. HIV-infected individuals who are intravenous drug users are at particular risk for skin abscesses. Perirectal abscesses are more common in the immunocompromised patient and are likely due to the blockage of anal mucous glands and infection with aerobic and anaerobic bacteria. Bacteremia, sepsis, and fistula formation are common complications of perirectal abscesses. Lesions evolve over days to 1 or 2 weeks. They are usually painful and are sometimes associated with fever. In the immunocompromised patient, such as the intravenous drug abuser with HIV/AIDS, skin abscesses are associated with a risk of bacterial endocarditis.

◉ Look For

A tender, erythematous, warm, fluctuant mass (Figs. 4-632–4-635). The pus is not generally seen at the skin level but sometimes appears as a multi-headed pustule. The abscess may have multiple loculated or interconnected areas, especially in the back of the neck.

Dark Skin Considerations

The associated erythema may be less pronounced in darker skin types.

Immunocompromised Patient Considerations

In the intravenous drug abuser, abscesses tend to occur on the extremities at sites of "skin popping."

◉◉ Diagnostic Pearls

Gentle pressure often reveals an opaque white core. If the lesion is on the scalp, look for signs of scalp dermatophyte infection such as broken hairs (black dot fungus) or fine scales to suggest dermatophyte infection rather than an abscess.

Immunocompromised Patient Considerations

In the immunosuppressed patient, inflammation may be decreased or absent.

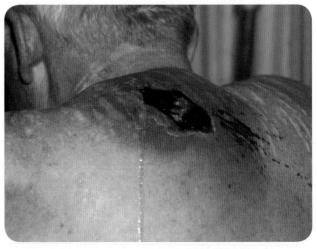

Figure 4-632 Draining abscess with overlying skin necrosis.

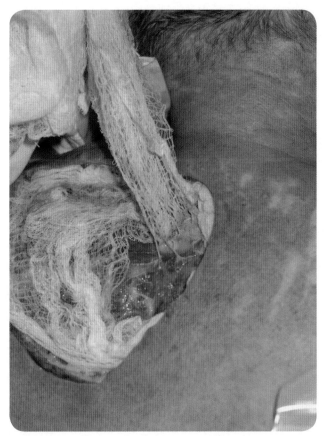

Figure 4-633 Abscess after debriding and packing; follow-up of Figure 4-632.

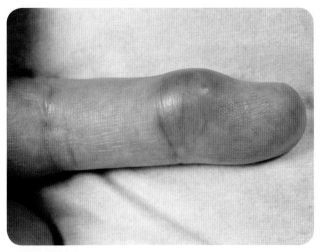

Figure 4-635 Abscess on the finger. It does not have the multiple grouped vesicles of herpetic whitlow.

?? Differential Diagnosis and Pitfalls

- Kerions on the scalp are fungal-induced hypersensitivity reactions, commonly associated with adenopathy, and difficult to differentiate from bacterial-induced abscesses.

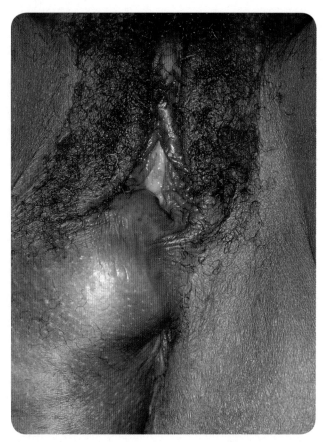

Figure 4-634 Vulval abscess.

- Mycobacterial infections present as a "cold abscess" (little to no erythema or warmth) in a normal host
- Ruptured epidermoid cysts
- Foreign body reactions or foreign body granulomas
- Hidradenitis suppurativa
- Necrotizing fasciitis—if considered, this is a medical emergency
- Pyomyositis
- Panniculitis—infectious or noninfectious causes of panniculitis
- Pseudolymphoma

Immunocompromised Patient Differential Diagnosis

The differential diagnosis of a tender, erythematous dermal or subcutaneous nodule in the immunosuppressed host must include both bacterial, fungal, and mycobacterial organisms. These cannot be differentiated clinically and must be cultured to determine the causative organism.

✓ Best Tests

- In the otherwise healthy patient, an abscess can usually be diagnosed clinically. If in doubt, needle aspiration or a small nick can be made in the overlying skin in an attempt to express purulent material. Rarely, ultrasound or other imaging modalities, such as CT scan, may be needed to determine the extent of soft tissue involvement or precise location of deeper abscesses.

- Gram, fungal, and acid-fast stains of the exudate or aspirate may yield an immediate microbiologic diagnosis. Cultures will take a few days (bacterial) or weeks (fungal, mycobacterial).
- Sensitivities should be performed on all infectious isolates to determine the appropriate antimicrobial.

▲▲▲ Management Pearls
. . . .

- In cases where antibiotics are indicated, given the prevalence of MRSA, maintain a high index of suspicion for this diagnosis and make the initial choice of empiric antibiotic therapy accordingly. It is helpful to be aware of patterns of antimicrobial resistance within your community.
- The eradication of MRSA nasal carriage may be accomplished with application of 2% mupirocin cream to the nares. The combination of rifampin plus trimethoprim-sulfamethoxazole (TMP–SMX) has also been shown to eradicate MRSA colonization.

Precautions: Standard and Contact (Isolate patient, wear gloves and a gown, limit patient transport, and avoid sharing patient-care equipment.)

Immunocompromised Patient Considerations

Systemic antibiotics for sufficient time are necessary for the resolution of a lesion. Perirectal and other deep abscesses may require treatment within the operating suite with the patient adequately anesthetized.

Sensitivities should be performed on all infectious isolates to determine the appropriate antimicrobial.

Therapy

Incision and drainage is the mainstay of therapy. Locally anesthetize with 1% lidocaine, and use a no. 11 blade to incise the fluctuant mass. Probing may be necessary if there is a suggestion of a foreign body or to break up any loculations. Consider using a ribbon of iodoform gauze to pack the cavity if it is large. Adequately drained simple abscesses do not require further antibiotics in an otherwise well patient. If there are systemic symptoms, evidence of concomitant cellulitis, multiple lesions, gangrene, or if the patient is immunosuppressed in any way, antimicrobial therapy is indicated.

Mild infections in otherwise healthy patients can initially be managed on an outpatient basis with incision and drainage and close follow-up. Home nursing care may be needed for dressing/packing changes.

Antibiotic Regimens
For patients with high burden of disease such as concomitant folliculitis, suggested initial outpatient antibiotic regimens include

- Dicloxacillin or cephalexin 500 mg p.o. four times daily for 10 to 14 days
- Patients should frequently be assessed (every 24 to 72 h) to determine appropriate response to therapy

Patients exhibiting signs or symptoms of systemic involvement or with rapidly progressing infections or significant comorbidities (i.e., immunosuppressed) should be hospitalized for observation and parenteral antibiotic administration. Suggested regimens include nafcillin or oxacillin 1 to 2 g IV every 4 h or cefazolin 1 g IV every 8 h.

Standard cephalosporins and penicillins are of no benefit in treating MRSA. In recent studies, CA-MRSA has demonstrated a high degree of susceptibility to TMP-SMX and rifampin (100%), clindamycin (95%), and tetracycline (92%). Inducible resistance to clindamycin should be excluded by performing a D-zone disk-diffusion test on any isolates.

Possible antibiotic regimens for MRSA include

- Clindamycin 600 mg IV every 8 h or 300 to 450 mg p.o. three times daily, TMP-SMX 1 to 2 double strength tabs p.o. twice daily.

Critically ill patients with MRSA or suspected MRSA should receive vancomycin or linezolid:

- Vancomycin 30 mg/kg/day IV divided twice daily or linezolid 600 mg IV or p.o. every 12 h

Immunocompromised Patient Considerations

Customize therapy to the immune status of the patient and organism sensitivities.

Based on recent clinical trials, daptomycin and tigecycline are likely reasonable alternatives to these drugs. A long-acting glycopeptide, dalbavancin, may also be considered.

Suggested Readings

Cohen PR. Community-acquired methicillin-resistant Staphylococcus aureus skin infections: Implications for patients and practitioners. *Am J Clin Dermatol.* 2007;8(5):259–270.

Elston DM. Community-acquired methicillin-resistant Staphylococcus aureus. *J Am Acad Dermatol.* 2007 Jan;56(1):1–16; quiz 17–20.

Fowler VG Jr, Boucher HW, Corey GR, et al. Daptomycin versus standard therapy for bacteremia and endocarditis caused by Staphylococcus aureus. *N Engl J Med.* 2006 Aug;355(7):653–665.

Frazee BW, Lynn J, Charlebois ED, et al. High prevalence of methicillin-resistant Staphylococcus aureus in emergency department skin and soft tissue infections. *Ann Emerg Med.* 2005 Mar;45(3):311–320.

Mody L, Kauffman CA, McNeil SA, et al. Mupirocin-based decolonization of Staphylococcus aureus carriers in residents of 2 long-term care facilities: A randomized, double-blind, placebo-controlled trial. *Clin Infect Dis.* 2003 Dec;37(11):1467–1474.

Moran GJ, Krishnadasan A, Gorwitz RJ, et al.; EMERGEncy ID Net Study Group. Methicillin-resistant S. aureus infections among patients in the emergency department. *N Engl J Med.* 2006 Aug;355(7):666–674.

Rajendran PM, Young D, Maurer T, et al. Randomized, double-blind, placebo-controlled trial of cephalexin for treatment of uncomplicated skin abscesses in a population at risk for community-acquired methicillin-resistant Staphylococcus aureus infection. *Antimicrob Agents Chemother.* 2007 Nov;51(11):4044–4048. Epub 2007 Sep 10.

Weigelt J, Itani K, Stevens D, et al.; CSSTI Study Group. Linezolid versus vancomycin in treatment of complicated skin and soft tissue infections. *Antimicrob Agents Chemother.* 2005 Jun;49(6):2260–2266.

Ziglam H. Daptomycin and tigecycline: A review of clinical efficacy in the antimicrobial era. *Expert Opin Pharmacother.* 2007 Oct;8(14):2279–2292.

Acrochordon (Skin Tag)

▪▪ Diagnosis Synopsis

Acrochordons, also known as skin tags, are common benign cutaneous growths. They present as small flesh-colored, pedunculated, fleshy papules, most commonly found on the eyelids, neck, axillary, and inguinal areas. They are usually asymptomatic but can become irritated by clothing or jewelry. They may spontaneously fall off if their blood supply becomes strangulated. Acrochordons are associated with increasing age, diabetes, and obesity. Men and women are affected equally.

Acrochordons can also be a feature of the autosomal dominantly inherited Birt-Hogg-Dube syndrome. They are increased in number in acromegaly and are sometimes associated with acanthosis nigricans.

◉ Look For

Soft, pedunculated (having a stalk) papules, commonly found on the eyelids, neck, groin, and axillae (Figs. 4-636–4-638). They are often flesh colored or slightly hyperpigmented. They range in size from 1 to 6 mm.

Acrochordons may also occur on the oral, anal, or vulvovaginal mucosa.

●● Diagnostic Pearls

Fleshy pedunculated growths in the flexural areas. If strangulated, they will occasionally become tender and erythematous, eventually necrosing and falling off spontaneously (Fig. 4-639).

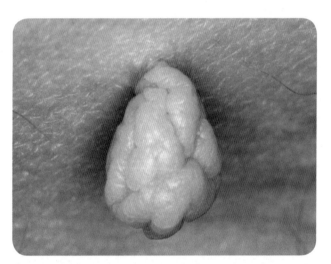

Figure 4-636 Large acrochordon with a broad base.

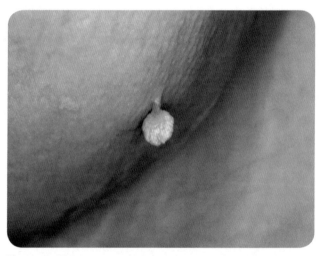

Figure 4-637 Acrochordon with a narrow pedunculated stalk.

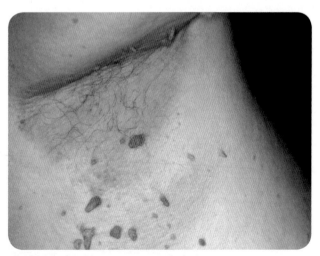

Figure 4-638 Multiple acrochordons are common in the axilla.

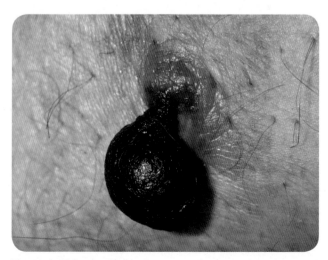

Figure 4-639 Pedunculated acrochordons may spontaneously infarct and become hemorrhagic.

?? Differential Diagnosis and Pitfalls

- Seborrheic keratoses have a "stuck-on" appearance and are usually hyperpigmented.
- Verruca vulgaris tends to have a more verrucous or roughened surface.
- Pedunculated neurofibromas usually have a firmer texture.
- In basal cell nevus syndrome, the basal cell carcinomas can be tan to brown and pedunculated, greatly resembling skin tags.
- Intradermal melanocytic nevus

✓ Best Tests

This is a clinical diagnosis. If there is doubt or concern for malignancy, a skin biopsy is diagnostic.

▲▲ Management Pearls

- Observation is acceptable if the lesion is not irritated or cosmetically concerning for the patient.
- When removing lesions with scissors, take care to use sharp surgical scissors and rapid cutting to avoid extensive pain.

Therapy

If lesions become symptomatic, they can be removed by mechanical snipping (fine iris or gradle scissors), shave excision, cryotherapy, or electrodesiccation. Smaller lesions can easily be "snipped" without anesthesia, and aluminum chloride or simple pressure will provide hemostasis. Larger lesions may require cauterization.

Suggested Readings

Levine N. Brown patches, skin tags on axilla. Are this patient's velvety plaques related to his obesity and diabetes? *Geriatrics*. 1996 Oct;51(10):27.

Monfrecola G, Riccio G, Viola L, et al. A simple cryo-technique for the treatment of cutaneous soft fibromas. *J Dermatol Surg Oncol*. 1994 Feb;20(2):151–152.

Schaffer JV, Gohara MA, McNiff JM, et al. Multiple facial angiofibromas: A cutaneous manifestation of Birt-Hogg-Dubé syndrome. *J Am Acad Dermatol*. 2005 Aug;53(2 Suppl. 1):S108–S111.

Welsch MJ, Krunic A, Medenica MM. Birt-Hogg-Dubé Syndrome. *Int J Dermatol*. 2005 Aug;44(8):668–673.

Yosipovitch G, DeVore A, Dawn A. Obesity and the skin: skin physiology and skin manifestations of obesity. *J Am Acad Dermatol*. 2007 Jun;56(6):901–916; quiz 917–920.

◼◼◼ Diagnosis Synopsis

Spiders are members of the Arachnida class, which also includes ticks, mites, and scorpions. The jaws of spiders have fangs that deliver venom via a small hole at the tips. Composition, potency, and clinical effects of venom vary among the different spider species.

Almost all species of spiders are venomous, but only a few dozen can harm humans. Of the few spiders that are of medical importance, envenomation can cause a range of clinical manifestations from skin lesions to systemic illness and in rare cases, even death. Though tarantulas have venom, they usually cause illness from their urticating hairs.

The severity of a spider bite depends on the type of spider, the amount of venom injected, the site of the bite, and the health and age of the patient.

Spiders of medical importance include the following:

Widow Spiders*

Spiders of the *Latrodectus* genus are found worldwide and have neurotoxic venoms, with α-latrotoxin as the major component. The black widow spider, *L. mactans,* is the most common widow spider in the United States and is found in woodpiles. Neurotoxic venoms cause systemic symptoms relating to cholinergic and catecholamine excesses. The bite is often very painful, and systemic symptoms develop, which include hypertension, tachycardia, palpitations, diaphoresis, anxiety, shortness of breath, hyperthermia or hypothermia, excessive salivation, nausea, vomiting, and severe abdominal pain. The abdominal pain may be misdiagnosed as appendicitis or acute abdomen. The bite may have noticeable fang marks with the development of a halo-like lesion around the bite. Female black widow spiders can easily be identified by the characteristic red hour-glass figure present on their ventral abdomen.

Recluse Spiders*

Spiders of the *Loxosceles* genus are found worldwide in temperate and tropical regions. Envenomation can cause local necrosis and, rarely, severe systemic symptoms due to a cytotoxic venom composed of the phospholipase enzyme, sphingomyelinase D. Cytotoxic venoms cause local tissue injury and necrosis. The bite is often initially painless. Pain, swelling, bullae, and ischemia develop minutes to hours later. Lesions may eventually ulcerate and become necrotic and gangrenous. Though systemic toxicity is rare, disseminated intravascular coagulation (DIC) may occur. The brown recluse spider, *L. recluse,* is regularly and erroneously blamed as the cause of necrotic lesions throughout the United States, although this spider is most commonly found in the Midwest and Southern states. It can be identified by the characteristic violin-shaped figure spanning its dorsal head and thorax.

Funnel-Web Spiders*

In the Pacific Northwest, the **hobo spider** (*Tegenaria agrestis*), commonly known as the aggressive house spider, is often blamed as the cause of necrotic skin lesions. However, there is only one documented case of hobo spider envenomation causing tissue necrosis. *Atrax/Hadronyche* species in Australia include the most dangerous spider, the **Sydney funnel-web spider** (*Atrax robustus*). The venom of this spider is neurotoxic, capable of producing severe pain at the bite site and systemic symptoms that can rarely be fatal within minutes.

Tarantulas*

Tarantulas, of the family Theraphosidae, have relatively harmless bites. However, they can disperse urticating hairs from their abdomens, resulting in local skin reactions, ocular problems, and allergic rhinitis.

Other spiders that less commonly cause significant skin irritation or dermal necrosis are as follows:

Yellow sac spiders of the *Cheiracanthium* genus are found in North America, Europe, Africa, Asia, Australia, and the Pacific Islands.

Wolf spiders of the *Lycosa* genus are common spiders found worldwide. **Banana spiders** of the *Phoneutria* genus, of Central and South America, have extremely potent venom that is neurotoxic and can be lethal.

Six-eyed crab spiders of the *Sicarius* genus are found in Africa and South America and are considered to be extremely venomous but, fortunately, live in remote areas. Their venom is proteolytic.

*For More Information, See the Following Diagnoses in VisualDx

- Hobo Spider Envenoming
- Latrodectism (Widow Spider Envenoming)
- Loxoscelism (Recluse Spider Envenoming)
- Tarantula Envenoming
- Wolf Spider Envenoming

⊙ Look For

Common spider bites usually present with erythema and edema. A necrotic or dusky center within a red, inflammatory plaque is characteristic (Fig. 4-640).

In brown recluse spider bites, vesicles and bullae can present early (Fig. 4-641). Between 12 and 24 h after envenomation, a large plaque consisting of erythema, ischemia, and necrosis ("red, white, and blue" sign) develops (Fig. 4-642).

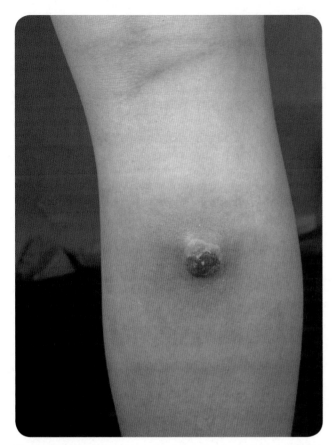

Figure 4-640 Spider bite with hemorrhagic eroded papule with peripheral erythema.

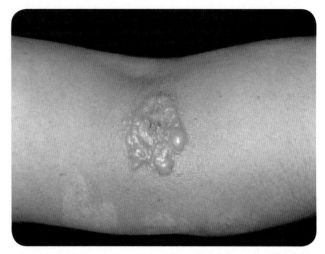

Figure 4-641 Central necrosis and peripheral vesicles in a brown recluse spider bite.

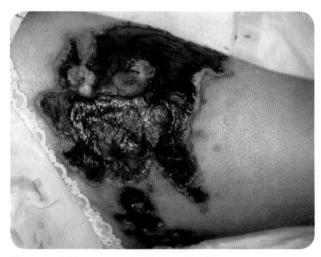

Figure 4-643 Necrosis 20 days after a brown recluse spider bite.

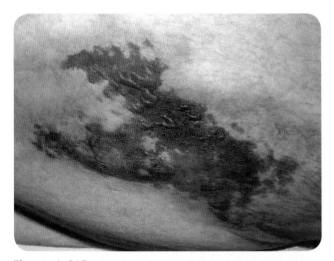

Figure 4-642 Brown recluse spider bite with thrombosis and necrosis.

Later, these lesions can progress into painful, full-thickness necrotic plaques (Fig. 4-643).

Patients with black widow bites have local sweating, piloerection, redness, and mild edema. The systemic symptoms of muscle pain, cramps, abdominal pain, salivation, lacrimation, sweating, and tremors are more prominent than the skin findings.

If the victim brings in the spider, seek out a trained arachnologist or entomologist for accurate identification.

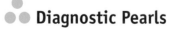 **Diagnostic Pearls**

- Look closely for two small puncta, the fang marks of the spider.
- Most suspected spider bites seen in the United States turn out to be the result of other causes, most commonly cellulitis or furunculosis. Unless the spider has specifically been identified as the etiology of the symptoms, be cautious about narrowing your differential diagnosis.

?? Differential Diagnosis and Pitfalls

- Acute coronary syndrome
- Acute abdomen:
  - Abdominal aneurysm
  - Acute appendicitis
  - Mesenteric ischemia
  - Ectopic pregnancy
  - Pancreatitis
- Allergic reaction
- Anaphylaxis
- Anxiety
- Caterpillar envenomation
- Cellulitis
- Centipede envenomation
- Contact dermatitis
- Ecthyma
- Ecthyma gangrenosum
- Diabetic ulcer
- Factitial ulcer
- Furuncle (consider MRSA)
- Hymenoptera stings
- Insect bites
- Iritis
- Lyme disease
- Medication-induced drug reactions:
  - Stevens-Johnson syndrome
  - Toxic epidermal necrolysis
- MRSA skin infection
- Muscle spasms
- Necrotizing fasciitis
- Priapism
- Pyoderma gangrenosum
- Skin cancer
- Skin infections caused by:
  - *Bacillus anthracis* (anthrax)
  - *Staphylococcus* (particularly CA-MRSA)
  - *Streptococcus*
  - Sporotrichosis
  - Herpes zoster (shingles)
  - Herpes simplex virus
- Tetanus
- Tularemia
- Uveitis
- Vasculitis such as emboli, ergotism, and cryoglobulins

✓ Best Tests

- The diagnosis of a spider bite is primarily made on history. There are no tests in widespread clinical use to diagnose spider envenomation.
- If systemic involvement due to a brown recluse spider bite is suspected, check for evidence of hemolysis. If systemic involvement is present, serial hemoglobin and plasma-free haptoglobin levels should be followed. Monitor for rhabdomyolysis, renal failure, and DIC.

▲▲ Management Pearls

- Given the difficulty in confirming spider envenomation, always consider other causes of bite wounds, necrotic lesions, and systemic symptoms, and manage them accordingly. Any serous or purulent drainage should be cultured to rule out an MRSA infection.
- Most brown spider bites heal in 2 to 3 months without medical treatment.

Therapy

Treatment includes:

- Collection and identification of spider, if possible.
- Wound irrigation.
- Rest, cold compresses, elevation of the affected extremity.
- Symptomatic treatment as indicated.
- Tetanus prophylaxis as indicated.
- Conservative local debridement of clearly necrotic tissue.
- Antivenom as indicated.
- Symptomatic treatment as indicated.
- For necrotic lesions, treatment with dapsone within the first 36 h has been advocated by some. However, this remains controversial due to the serious rare side effects of dapsone administration and lack of clear evidence of significant improvement with this therapy.

Suggested Readings

Carbonaro PA, Janniger CK, Schwartz RA. Spider bite reactions. *Cutis.* 1995 Nov;56(5):256–259.

Isbister GK, Gray MR. A prospective study of 750 definite spider bites, with expert spider identification. *QJM.* 2002 Nov;95(11):723–731.

James WD, Berger TG, Elston DM. Parasitic infestations, stings, and bites. In: James WD, Berger TG, Elston DM, Odom RB, eds. *Andrews' Diseases of the Skin: Clinical Dermatology.* 10th Ed. Philadelphia, PA: Saunders Elsevier; 2006:455–456.

Steen CJ, Carbonaro PA, Schwartz RA. Arthropods in dermatology. *J Am Acad Dermatol.* 2004 Jun;50(6):819–842, quiz 842–844.

Steen CJ, Schwartz CA. Arthropod bites and stings. In: Fitzpatrick TB, Wolff K, eds. *Fitzpatrick's Dermatology in General Medicine.* 7th Ed. New York, NY: McGraw-Hill; 2008:2054–2063.

Wilson JR, Hagood CO, Prather ID. Brown recluse spider bites: A complex problem wound. A brief review and case study. *Ostomy Wound Manage.* 2005 Mar;51(3):59–66.

Wilson DC, King LE. Spiders and spider bites. *Dermatol Clin.* 1990 Apr;8(2):277–286.

Bowen Disease (SCC In Situ)

▪▪ Diagnosis Synopsis

Bowen disease is squamous cell carcinoma (SCC) in situ (i.e., malignant keratinocytes are limited to the epidermis). This epidermal malignancy is primarily seen in older adults and frequently occurs on sun-exposed skin. The development of Bowen disease has also been associated with radiation exposure, arsenic ingestion, and human papillomavirus. There is no gender predilection. If left untreated, lesions can progress to invasive SCC.

Erythroplasia of Queyrat refers specifically to Bowen disease of the glans penis and prepuce, most commonly seen in uncircumcised individuals. It is typically a red, moist, velvety, or smooth plaque.

Immunocompromised Patient Considerations

Multiple SCC in situ lesions are more likely to occur in immunocompromised patients and are more likely to transform into invasive SCC.

◉ Look For

A red, scaly, well-demarcated superficial plaque or plaques. Plaques slowly expand, have a slightly scaly appearance with a red base, and can have a round or annular shape (Figs. 4-644–4-647).

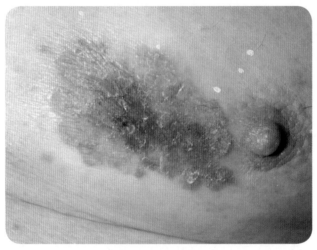

Figure 4-644 Plaque-like lesion with satellites of SCC in situ. Paget disease would be in the differential diagnosis.

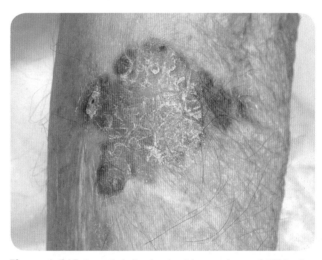

Figure 4-645 Irregularly bordered red-brown plaque of SCC in situ.

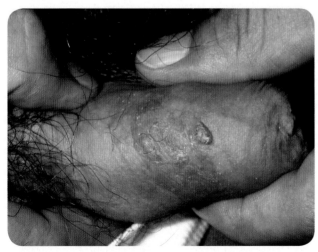

Figure 4-646 Plaque of SCC in situ on the penis with small nodules.

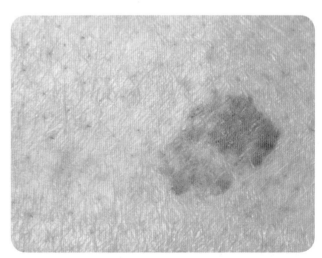

Figure 4-647 Red atrophic plaque of SCC in situ. Superficial basal cell carcinoma is within the differential diagnosis.

Bowen disease may occur anywhere on the body, but it is slightly more common in sun-exposed areas.

Dark Skin Considerations

The pigmented variant of SCC in situ is more commonly present in dark-skinned patients.

Diagnostic Pearls

Bowen disease usually presents with red plaques. The presence of any pigment suggests pigmented SCC in situ, melanoma, or basal cell carcinoma.

Differential Diagnosis and Pitfalls

- Superficial basal cell carcinoma
- SCC
- Psoriasis
- Actinic keratosis
- Seborrheic keratosis
- Paget disease
- Tinea
- Nummular dermatitis
- Melanoma
- Lichen planus
- Verruca vulgaris
- Bowenoid papulosis
- Lichen simplex
- Discoid lupus erythematosus
- Subacute cutaneous lupus erythematosus

Best Tests

Diagnosis is made by skin biopsy.

Management Pearls

- If untreated, Bowen disease can evolve into invasive SCC. Treatment is often a superficial process. Frequently, the removal or destruction can be performed easily and without referral to a surgeon. Dermatologists often remove these tumors by three cycles of electrodesiccation and curettage or by cryotherapy (destruction with liquid nitrogen). Patients will require routine follow-up to assess for recurrence.

- With the exception of anogenital Bowen disease associated with a genitourinary carcinoma, there is little evidence that Bowen disease in other locations is associated with internal malignancy. Therefore, only a routine medical workup should be performed, not an extensive search for occult malignancy.

Immunocompromised Patient Considerations

Immunocompromised patients may have more aggressive SCC in situ tumors and also have increased rates of recurrence.

Therapy

Treatment is usually via surgical excision, aggressive cryosurgery, or electrodesiccation and curettage. Mohs micrographic surgery achieves a lower rate of recurrence than simple excision.

Small plaques may be treated with topical 5-fluorouracil alone (5FU, 5% cream applied twice daily) or in combination with tretinoin cream 0.05% added prior to the twice daily application of 5% 5FU. Other treatment modalities that have been used successfully include photodynamic therapy, 5% imiquimod cream, and laser ablation (CO_2, 810-nm diode lasers).

Suggested Readings

Braathen LR, Szeimies RM, Basset-Seguin N, et al.; International Society for Photodynamic Therapy in Dermatology. Guidelines on the use of photodynamic therapy for nonmelanoma skin cancer: an international consensus. International Society for Photodynamic Therapy in Dermatology, 2005. *J Am Acad Dermatol.* 2007 Jan;56(1):125–143.

Cox NH, Eedy DJ, Morton CA; Therapy Guidelines and Audit Subcommittee, British Association of Dermatologists. Guidelines for management of Bowen's disease: 2006 update. *Br J Dermatol.* 2007 Jan;156(1):11–21.

Duncan KO, Geisse JK, Leffell DJ. Epithelial precancerous lesions. In: Fitzpatrick TB, Wolff K, eds. *Fitzpatrick's Dermatology in General Medicine.* 7th Ed. New York, NY: McGraw-Hill; 2008:1007–1027.

Kossard S, Rosen R. Cutaneous Bowen's disease. An analysis of 1001 cases according to age, sex, and site. *J Am Acad Dermatol.* 1992 Sep;27(3):406–410.

Patel GK, Goodwin R, Chawla M, et al. Imiquimod 5% cream monotherapy for cutaneous squamous cell carcinoma in situ (Bowen's disease): A randomized, double-blind, placebo-controlled trial. *J Am Acad Dermatol.* 2006 Jun;54(6):1025–1032.

Pontén F, Lundeberg J, Asplund A. Principles of tumor biology and pathogenesis of BCCs and SCCs. In: Bolognia JL, Jorizzo JL, Rapini RP, eds. *Dermatology.* 2nd Ed. St. Louis, MO: Mosby; 2008:1646–1647.

Calcinosis Cutis

Diagnosis Synopsis

Calcinosis cutis, or cutaneous calcification, is the deposition of insoluble calcium salts in the skin due to the local dysregulation of calcium metabolism. Disorders of calcium metabolism can be broadly categorized into 4 main groups: dystrophic, metastatic, idiopathic, and iatrogenic. Calcinosis cutis can be viewed as a type of dystrophic calcification, where serum calcium and phosphorus levels are normal, but previously damaged skin leads to altered calcium metabolism and subsequent calcium salt deposition.

It is most commonly seen in autoimmune connective tissue diseases, especially in the CREST form of scleroderma and juvenile dermatomyositis. Approximately 50% to 60% of juvenile dermatomyositis children will develop calcinosis cutis or some form of cutaneous calcification; about 20% of patients with adult dermatomyositis experience this condition. In addition, affected sites in dermatomyositis and CREST scleroderma differ: knees, elbows, fingers in the former, and hands, upper arms, and bony prominences in the latter. Note, however, that calcinosis cutis can occur anywhere on the body and that local trauma, infections (particularly parasitic), pancreatic disease, lupus profundus, and lymphoma have been associated with calcinosis cutis.

The most common clinical presentations include painful irregularly surfaced nodules. In addition, patients can experience the extrusion of chalk-like substance from their calcified nodules and secondary infection.

Look For

Small, firm, white-to-yellow papules, plaques, or nodules that may ulcerate and extrude a white chalk-like substance. Lesions typically occur at the tips of fingers and over bony prominences (Figs. 4-648–4-650). Calcinosis universalis

is the most severe variant where deposition of calcium salts occurs diffusely along fascial planes (Fig. 4-651).

Common locations:

- Dermatomyositis—knees, elbows, fingers
- CREST or scleroderma—hands, upper arms, bony prominences, and tendons

Diagnostic Pearls

Palpation will demonstrate firm lesions. X-ray will demonstrate characteristic densities.

Differential Diagnosis and Pitfalls

- Gout
- Calcified epidermoid cysts
- Milia
- Xanthomas
- Molluscum contagiosum
- Warts
- Osteoma cutis
- Subepidermal calcified nodule (usually solitary—head in children; extremities in adults)
- Scrotal calcinosis (often multiple)
- Pseudoxanthoma elasticum

Best Tests

Histopathologic examination of skin biopsy specimens will be diagnostic, but an underlying cause of the disorder should be sought:

- Calcium, phosphate, parathyroid hormone, vitamin D3 serum levels
- BUN, creatinine, AST, ALT, alkaline phosphatase, lipase, amylase serum levels

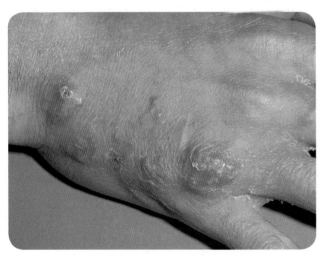

Figure 4-648 Calcinosis cutis secondary to an IV line.

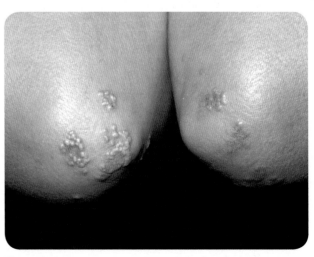

Figure 4-649 Calcinosis cutis in pseudopseudohypoparathyroidism.

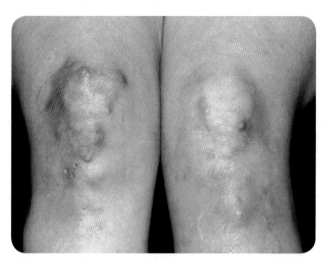

Figure 4-650 Calcinosis cutis in a patient with evidence of scleroderma in other skin locations.

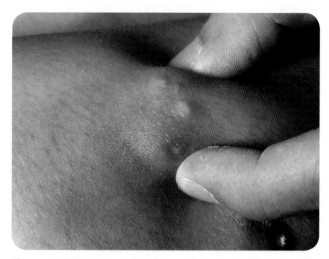

Figure 4-651 Calcinosis cutis in a patient with calcinosis universalis.

- CBC with differential
- Autoantibodies (ANA, anti-SCL-70, anti-dsDNA, anti-Jo-1) if suspecting autoimmune connective tissue disease
- Serum levels of muscle enzymes including aldolase, CK, lactate dehydrogenase if suspecting dermatomyositis
- Aldolase and amylase
- Soft tissue radiograph may assist in delineating the extent of tissue involvement

▲▲ Management Pearls

- Consultations are sought on the basis of the underlying disease and may include a nephrologist, hematologist/ oncologist, or rheumatologist.
- Consider dietary modifications such as a low phosphate or calcium diet, when appropriate.
- Small lesions can be excised if symptomatic or interfering with patient function. There is a risk that calcification will recur in the surgical scar.

Therapy

Treatment of the underlying disorder is the first line of therapy. Limited cases with a benign etiology can be observed and may heal spontaneously.

The vast majority of therapies for calcinosis cutis have only been described in case reports. The following treatments have been tried with varied success:

- Diltiazem (60 mg p.o. daily initially, slowly increased to 360 mg p.o. daily)
- Surgical excision
- Colchicine (1 mg p.o. daily)
- Probenecid (250 mg p.o. daily)
- Aluminum hydroxide (320 to 1,800 mg p.o. before every meal)
- Intralesional corticosteroids (triamcinolone acetonide 25 mg/mL) monthly
- Bisphosphonates (etidronate 10 mg/kg p.o. daily)

Suggested Readings

Cousins MA, Jones DB, Whyte MP, et al. Surgical management of calcinosis cutis universalis in systemic lupus erythematosus. *Arthritis Rheum.* 1997 Mar;40(3):570–572.

Federico A, Weinel S, Fabre V, et al. Dystrophic calcinosis cutis in pseudoxanthoma elasticum. *J Am Acad Dermatol.* 2008 Apr;58(4):707–710.

Vinen CS, Patel S, Bruckner FE. Regression of calcinosis associated with adult dermatomyositis following diltiazem therapy. *Rheumatology (Oxford).* 2000 Mar;39(3):333–334.

Walsh JS, Fairley JA. Cutaneous mineralization and ossification. In: Fitzpatrick TB, Wolff K, eds. *Fitzpatrick's Dermatology in General Medicine.* 7th Ed. New York, NY: McGraw-Hill; 2008:1293–1297.

Calciphylaxis

■■ Diagnosis Synopsis

Calciphylaxis is the diffuse deposition of insoluble calcium salts in the skin due to the systemic dysregulation of calcium metabolism. Disorders of calcium metabolism can be broadly categorized into four main groups: dystrophic, metastatic, idiopathic, and iatrogenic. Calciphylaxis is the most severe form of metastatic calcification and is most commonly associated with chronic renal failure, patients on hemodialysis, and secondary hyperparathyroidism.

While the exact pathogenesis is unclear, characteristic pathologic findings include progressive medial calcification of cutaneous blood vessels and subsequent ischemic necrosis of the skin. In addition, the process is believed to be triggered by chronic hypocalcemia from a decreased intestinal absorption of calcium; this leads to increased levels of parathyroid hormone (PTH) and subsequent recruitment of calcium and phosphate from bone.

Painful, violaceous patches are initially seen clinically, followed by necrosis, ulcers, and/or gangrene. Mortality from calciphylaxis is high (60% to 87%) and is secondary to sepsis from large, nonhealing ulcers.

Risks for developing calciphylaxis include female gender, diabetes, obesity, and calcium-based phosphate binders. The condition has also been observed in patients with breast cancer treated with chemotherapy, systemic lupus erythematosus, end-stage liver disease, and Crohn disease.

◉ Look For

Initially, look for livedo reticularis (net-like erythema or violaceous patches) and deep, painful, red or purple nodules or plaques. Tissue necrosis, ulcers, and thrombosis occur secondary to arterial vessel occlusion (Figs. 4-652–4-655).

Most common body locations include the thighs, buttocks, trunk, and upper extremities.

Dark Skin Considerations

In darker-skinned individuals, livedo reticularis may appear as dark brown or violaceous reticular patches or net-like erythema, and deep, painful, red or purple, indurated plaques may be present.

●● Diagnostic Pearls

Scrotal or penile involvement is common.

?? Differential Diagnosis and Pitfalls

- Cholesterol emboli
- Cryoglobulinemia
- Cellulitis
- Antiphospholipid syndrome
- Coumadin necrosis—indurated, necrotic areas on the breasts, thighs, and buttocks
- Vasculitis
- Disseminated intravascular coagulation
- Nephrogenic systemic fibrosis
- Lupus profundus lesions may have calcification on X-ray.
- Dermatomyositis and CREST syndrome may have associated calcification.
- Myxoma emboli
- Pancreatic panniculitis
- Peripheral atherosclerotic vascular disease
- Pyoderma gangrenosum
- Wegener granulomatosis

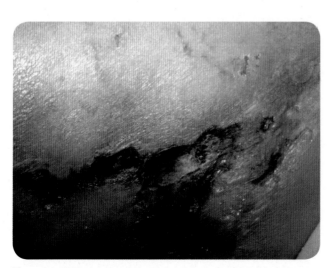

Figure 4-652 Necrosis 2 days after a blister began in a patient on hemodialysis.

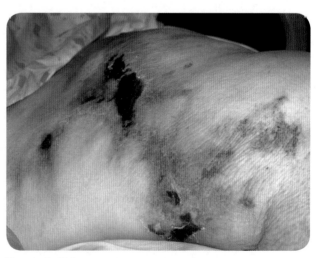

Figure 4-653 Petechiae, purpura, and frank necrosis in a patient with calciphylaxis.

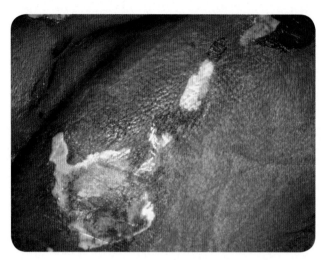

Figure 4-654 After 7 years of dialysis, there were subcutaneous nodules, blisters, and then necrosis with calciphylaxis.

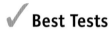 Best Tests

Note that there are no laboratory findings that are specific for calciphylaxis. Some but not all patients demonstrate elevated calcium–phosphate product and/or elevated parathyroid hormone.

Labs

- Calcium, phosphate, parathyroid hormone, and vitamin D3 serum levels
- Coagulation factors (PT, PTT, protein C and S levels, anti-cardiolipin antibody, lupus anticoagulant, and factor V Leiden)
- Cryoglobulin, cryofibrinogen, and hepatitis C antibody
- CBC with differential

Radiologic

- Plain radiographs
- High-resolution CT
- Three-phase technetium 99m methylene diphosphate bone scintigraphy

▲▲▲ Management Pearls

- Aggressive wound care
- Pain management
- Surgical consultation is often necessary for wound debridement and/or parathyroidectomy
- Nutritional consult
- Patients often require a multidisciplinary team of specialists including a nephrologist, an internist/critical care expert, a surgeon, a dermatologist, and a pain specialist.

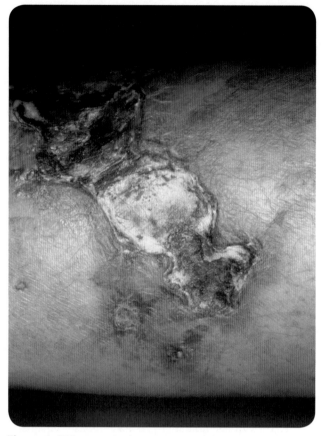

Figure 4-655 Hemorrhagic necrosis with calciphylaxis.

Therapy

Treatment is largely supportive, with aggressive wound care and management of the underlying disease.

First-Line Treatments

- Aggressive wound care and pain management
- Normalization of serum calcium and phosphate levels (calcium-phosphate product <55 mg^2/dL^2) via non-calcium–based phosphate binders (sevelamer and lanthanum carbonate)
- Normalization of PTH levels (cinacalcet or parathyroidectomy)

Second-Line Treatments

- Intravenous sodium thiosulfate (i.e., 25 g IV over 30 to 60 min three times weekly)
- Hyperbaric oxygen therapy
- Low dose tissue plasminogen activator

Suggested Readings

Arseculeratne G, Evans AT, Morley SM. Calciphylaxis—a topical overview. *J Eur Acad Dermatol Venereol.* 2006 May;20(5):493–502.

Bronson N, Menon R, Butler J, et al. Parathyroidectomy, excision and skin grafting with topical negative pressure for calciphylactic ulcers. *J Wound Care.* 2007 Jul;16(7):295–297.

Guldbakke KK, Khachemoune A. Calciphylaxis. *Int J Dermatol.* 2007 Mar;46(3):231–238.

Hayden MR, Goldsmith D, Sowers JR, et al. Calciphylaxis: Calcific uremic arteriolopathy and the emerging role of sodium thiosulfate. *Int Urol Nephrol.* 2008;40(2):443–451.

Llach F. The evolving pattern of calciphylaxis: Therapeutic considerations. *Nephrol Dial Transplant.* 2001 Mar;16(3):448–451.

Polizzotto MN, Bryan T, Ashby MA, et al. Symptomatic management of calciphylaxis: A case series and review of the literature. *J Pain Symptom Manage.* 2006 Aug;32(2):186–190.

Raymond CB, Wazny LD. Sodium thiosulfate, bisphosphonates, and cinacalcet for treatment of calciphylaxis. *Am J Health Syst Pharm.* 2008 Aug;65(15):1419–1429.

Weenig RH, Sewell LD, Davis MD, et al. Calciphylaxis: Natural history, risk factor analysis, and outcome. *J Am Acad Dermatol.* 2007 Apr;56(4):569–579.

Chondrodermatitis Nodularis Helicis

■■ Diagnosis Synopsis

Chondrodermatitis nodularis helicis (chondrodermatitis nodularis chronica helicis et antihelicis) is a benign, common inflammatory condition of the helical or antihelical cartilage and overlying skin with an exquisitely tender, small erythematous nodule or nodules. Patients preferentially sleep on the side of affected ear and cannot avoid doing so. Phone usage on the affected side is common. Repeated trauma, pressure, and subsequent ischemic necrosis of the affected cartilage and overlying dermis are felt to promote this condition. Cold, radiation therapy, and actinic damage may be exacerbating factors. It is more common in middle-aged to elderly, fair-skinned men. In men, the lesion favors the helix, whereas in women, the antihelix is more commonly affected. There have been no reports of malignant degeneration.

◉ Look For

A skin-colored or erythematous, firm, and exquisitely tender nodule, approximately 2 to 4 mm in diameter, located at the superior helical rim (Figs. 4-656 and 4-657) or antihelix (Figs. 4-658 and 4-659) of the ear. Sometimes there will be a small amount of scale or crusting at the center of the lesion (Figs. 4-657 and 4-659).

●● Diagnostic Pearls

- The tenderness and pain from these small, clinically unimpressive nodules is significant. Other causes of nodules at the helical rim, such as a squamous cell carcinoma, typically lack such significant pain.
- The patient's skin may exhibit evidence of sun damage.
- The development of the lesion on the antihelix is more common in women. Rarely, the condition occurs bilaterally.

?? Differential Diagnosis and Pitfalls

- Squamous cell carcinoma
- Actinic keratosis
- Basal cell carcinoma
- Amelanotic melanoma
- Picker's nodule
- Foreign body reaction
- Keratoacanthoma
- Gout
- Cutaneous horn
- Verrucae
- Calcinosis cutis

✓ Best Tests

- This diagnosis can often be made clinically. Skin biopsy will confirm the diagnosis and rule out malignancy if there is doubt. Histologically, acanthosis, hyperkeratosis, parakeratosis, hypergranulosis, and central ulceration are present with underlying degenerated collagen and fibrosis that may extend down to perichondrium.
- A skin biopsy can also have a therapeutic effect by the removal of affected cartilage and overlying lesion.

▲▲ Management Pearls

- Injection of 0.1 to 0.2 cc of triamcinolone (5 mg/cc) into the nodule can decrease inflammation and pain at the site.
- Skin biopsy can be both diagnostically and therapeutically beneficial for the patient.

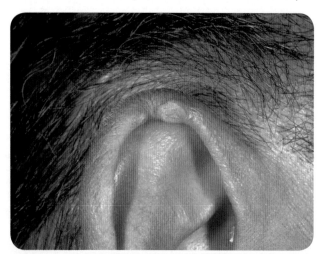

Figure 4-656 A painful papule or small ulceration on the helix is characteristic of chondrodermatitis nodularis helicis.

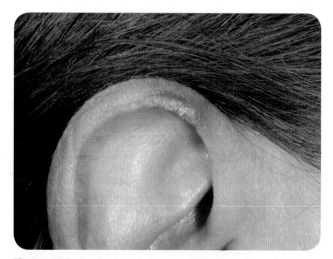

Figure 4-657 Scale/crust along the helix may obscure the ulceration of chondrodermatitis nodularis helicis.

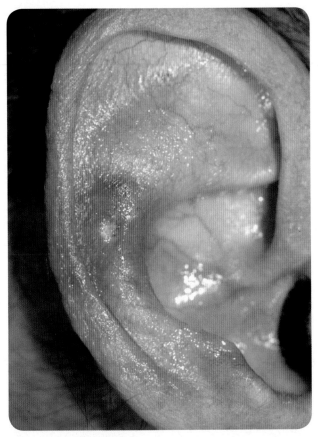

Figure 4-658 Clean-bordered ulcerations in chondrodermatitis nodularis helicis still require biopsy to exclude malignancy.

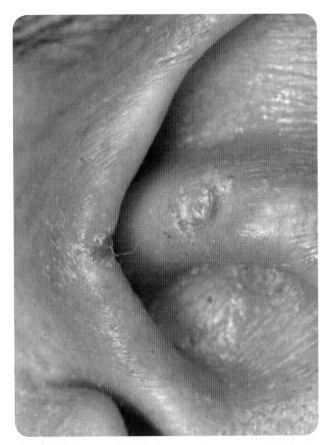

Figure 4-659 The ulcerations of chondrodermatitis nodularis helicis may be on the antihelix.

- Encourage the patient to sleep on the unaffected ear. Make sure that the patient protects the ear from trauma by taping a cotton ball just below the nodule or surrounding the ear in a foam protector. Such a pressure-relieving prosthesis can be fashioned by cutting a hole in a sponge. Specialized donut pillows are also commercially available.

Therapy

Pain and/or sleep disturbance are the only indications for treatment.

Consider intralesional triamcinolone as above. Clobetasol propionate cream twice daily to the area for 2 to 4 weeks may be used instead of intralesional triamcinolone.

Options for surgical treatment include removal by shave, punch, or elliptical excision if the lesion is small. Cryosurgery, curettage, and carbon dioxide laser ablation have also been used. The removal of affected cartilage without overlying skin often provides for a cure with a good cosmetic result.

Suggested Readings

James WD, Berger TG, Elston DM. Dermal and subcutaneous tumors. In: James WD, Berger TG, Elston DM, Odom RB, eds. *Andrews' Diseases of the Skin: Clinical Dermatology.* 10th Ed. Philadelphia, PA: Saunders Elsevier; 2006:610.

Long D, Maloney ME. Surgical pearl: Surgical planning in the treatment of chondrodermatitis nodularis chronica helicis of the antihelix. *J Am Acad Dermatol.* 1996 Nov;35(5 Pt 1):761–762.

Moncrieff M, Sassoon EM. Effective treatment of chondrodermatitis nodularis chronica helicis using a conservative approach. *Br J Dermatol.* 2004 May;150(5):892–894.

Sanu A, Koppana R, Snow DG. Management of chondrodermatitis nodularis chronica helicis using a 'doughnut pillow'. *J Laryngol Otol.* 2007 Nov;121(11):1096–1098.

Smith ML. Environmental and sports-related skin diseases. Borradori L, Bernard P. Pemphigoid Group. In: Bolognia JL, Jorizzo JL, Rapini RP, eds. *Dermatology.* 2nd Ed. St. Louis, MO: Mosby; 2008:1368–1369.

Taylor MB. Chondrodermatitis nodularis chronica helicis. Successful treatment with the carbon dioxide laser. *J Dermatol Surg Oncol.* 1991 Nov;17(11):862–864.

Thompson LD. Chondrodermatitis nodularis helicis. *Ear Nose Throat J.* 2007 Dec;86(12):734–735.

Diagnosis Synopsis

Corns (clavi) are keratinous thickenings of the skin of the toes that are caused by repeated friction or pressure to the area. The base of the corn is seen on the surface of the skin while the apex points inward, causing discomfort. Corns are classified as either hard or soft, depending upon their location and appearance. Hard corns typically affect the tops of the toes and are composed of a dense core that presses on sensory nerves, causing extreme pain. Soft corns occur between the toes and are continuously softened by sweat. They are macerated and white in appearance.

Factors that can lead to and exacerbate corns include ill-fitting shoes, not wearing shoes, the bunching up of socks, bony prominences in the feet or other faulty foot mechanics, and repetitive physical activities that stress the skin.

Immunocompromised Patient Considerations

Secondary infection of corns may occur, particularly in diabetic patients or patients who are otherwise immunosuppressed.

Look For

Well-circumscribed thickenings and conical, macerated papules between the toes (soft corns) (Fig. 4-660). Hard corns typically affect the tops of the toes or the side of the fifth toe and appear like callouses (Figs. 4-661–4-663). They can also appear on the top of the foot and even on the sole, basically anywhere friction occurs. They are dry and often have a waxy or transparent appearance.

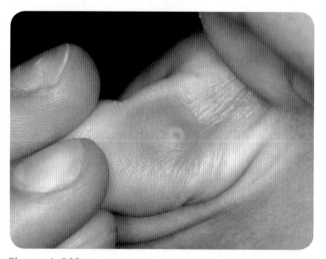

Figure 4-660 Corn between two toes. There is no hemorrhagic puncta suggesting a wart.

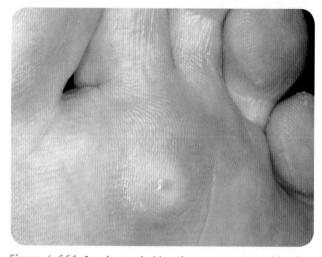

Figure 4-661 Corn in a typical location over a metatarsal head.

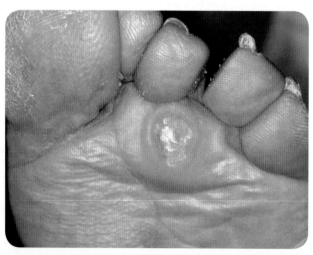

Figure 4-662 Corn over metatarsal head with irregular thickened callus.

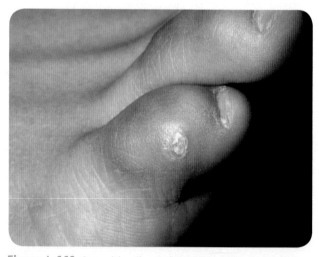

Figure 4-663 Corn with callus on lateral toe surface.

Diagnostic Pearls

The small, dark, and hemorrhagic foci seen in warts are absent in corns.

Differential Diagnosis and Pitfalls

Soft corns may be mistaken for tinea pedis or psoriasis.

Hard Corns may be Mistaken for the Following

- Warts
- Calluses—lack the dense core found in corns
- Porokeratosis plantaris discreta
- Eccrine poromas
- Foreign body reaction
- Palmoplantar keratoderma

Best Tests

- This is a clinical diagnosis based on morphology, symptoms, and location.
- Plain films of the feet in a weight-bearing position may help identify bony protuberances.

Management Pearls

- Make sure that shoes fit properly. There should be plenty of room in the toe box. Orthotic insoles may be necessary. Special corn pads are commercially available to redistribute the pressure over bony prominences. For interdigital soft corns, the web space can be padded with spacers specifically designed for this purpose.
- Patients with recurrent or recalcitrant corns may require referral to a podiatrist or orthopedic surgeon for the surgical correction of bony abnormalities.

Therapy

Instruct the patient in conservative measures, such as attention to foot hygiene, padding, and properly fitting footwear, as above.

Pare down the corn with a no. 15 blade, and remove the central core of the lesion. Alternatively, the patient can soak corns in warm water and file down with an emery board or pumice stone. Over-the-counter salicylic acid creams or lotions applied daily for 4 to 6 weeks can be effective.

Suggested Readings

Day RD, Reyzelman AM, Harkless LB. Evaluation and management of the interdigital corn: A literature review. *Clin Podiatr Med Surg.* 1996 Apr;13(2):201–206.

Freeman DB. Corns and calluses resulting from mechanical hyperkeratosis. *Am Fam Physician.* 2002 Jun;65(11):2277–2280.

Richards RN. Calluses, corns, and shoes. *Semin Dermatol.* 1991 Jun;10(2):112–114.

Singh D, Bentley G, Trevino SG. Callosities, corns, and calluses. *BMJ.* 1996 Jun;312(7043):1403–1406.

Cyst, Epidermoid (Sebaceous Cyst)

Diagnosis Synopsis

An epidermoid cyst, also known as an epidermal inclusion cyst, is a semisolid cyst. The cyst wall is stratified squamous epithelium, and the contents consist of macerated keratin and lipid-rich debris. The epidermoid cyst is a common lesion that can arise on the face, trunk, extremities, in the mouth, or on the genitals at any age. They are more common in men. Several etiologic factors have been implicated in the formation of epidermoid cysts, including traumatic or iatrogenic implantation of epidermal elements, sequestration of epidermal rests, occlusion of the eccrine duct or pilosebaceous unit, and human papillomavirus infection. Epidermoid cysts are a feature of several hereditary syndromes, such as Gardner syndrome, pachyonychia congenita, and the basal cell nevus syndrome. It is rare to see an epidermoid cyst in a prepubertal patient; in such cases, other diagnoses should be carefully considered.

Epidermoid cysts are benign and usually asymptomatic, but they may be painful if ruptured or infected. Rarely, malignancies such as basal cell carcinoma, squamous cell carcinoma, and mycosis fungoides have developed within these cysts.

Look For

A dome-shaped, firm, skin-colored nodule that is freely movable on palpation and sometimes has a small, dilated punctum (Figs. 4-664–4-667). Occasionally, a thick, cheesy material with a foul odor can be expressed. The cyst can be well defined or irregular due to prior rupture, scarring, and regrowth.

They can be located almost anywhere but are common on the face, neck, scalp, or trunk.

Dark Skin Considerations

The incidence is slightly higher in blacks than whites. In darker skin types, there may be a pigmented cyst lining.

Diagnostic Pearls

- Careful examination will frequently show a pore-like opening (also known as a central punctum). The lesion usually has a consistency a little firmer than the adult eyeball.
- Sudden pain or swelling may be related to bleeding, infection, or the rupture of the cyst contents into the surrounding tissue. The contents of the cyst, when exposed to air, have a foul-smelling odor.
- The presence of multiple epidermoid cysts and a family history of the same should lead to the consideration of a heritable condition such as Gardner syndrome, which is associated with GI polyps and malignancy.

?? Differential Diagnosis and Pitfalls

- Eruptive vellus hair cyst
- Lipoma
- Pilar cysts—most commonly located on the scalp and usually has a more firm consistency on palpation
- Pilomatrixoma
- Calcinosis cutis
- Steatocystoma
- Trichilemmal cyst
- Rheumatoid nodule
- Dermoid cyst

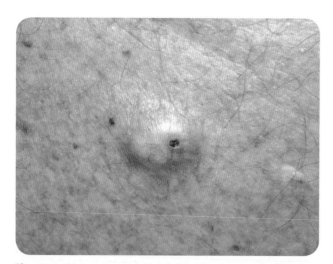

Figure 4-664 Prominent central pore in an epidermoid cyst.

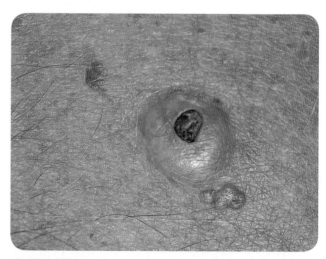

Figure 4-665 Epidermoid cyst with darkly pigmented keratin comprising most of the cyst.

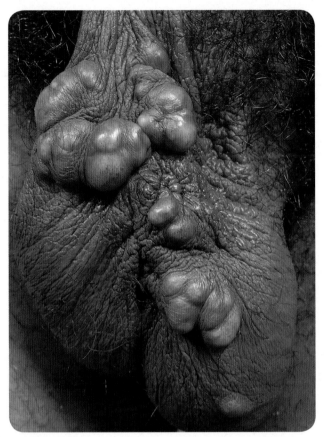

Figure 4-666 Multiple epidermoid cysts on the scrotum are not uncommon.

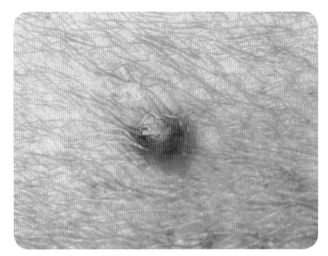

Figure 4-667 Inflamed epidermoid cyst. When inflamed, an epidermoid cyst may be mistaken for an abscess.

- Branchial cleft cyst or thyroglossal duct cyst
- Cutaneous metastatic malignancy

✓ Best Tests

The diagnosis can usually be made clinically. With pressure or a small incision, yellow, cheesy material can be expressed from the cyst. Skin biopsy can confirm the diagnosis by demonstrating characteristic histopathology but is usually not necessary. Ultrasound and MRI are both useful techniques but are usually not necessary. Obtain cultures and sensitivities, if possible, from any cysts suspected of being infected.

▲▲▲ Management Pearls

- Incision and drainage can provide immediate reduction in the cyst, but without removing the epidermal lining, the cyst will refill with layers of soft keratin. Using a punch biopsy to create a small skin opening and then using a curette to remove the cyst wall is sometimes effective and can reduce the incision size. Alternatively, the entire cyst (along with the wall) can be excised surgically. If the cyst wall is not completely removed, the cyst will likely regrow.

- If there is any concern for associated malignancy (e.g., rapid growth and ulceration), remove the cyst entirely, and send the specimen for pathologic analysis.

Therapy

Asymptomatic lesions require no treatment.

Symptomatic cysts can be excised in an elliptical fashion or, as described above, a punch biopsy can be used to create a small skin opening followed by curettage to remove the entire cyst wall. Incision and drainage is used for only temporary relief.

An infected cyst should be treated with systemic antibiotics prior to surgical intervention. The choice of antibiotic should be tailored to the suspected organism.

For methicillin-sensitive *Staphylococcus aureus* infection, a first generation cephalosporin can be given:

- Cephalexin 500 mg p.o. four times daily for 10 to 14 days

For methicillin-resistant *S. aureus,* the following medication is prescribed:

- Doxycycline 100 mg twice daily for 10 to 14 days
- Trimethoprim-sulfamethoxazole 1 to 2 double strength tabs p.o. twice daily

Inflamed cysts that are not infected may respond to intralesional triamcinolone, but incision and drainage is preferred to remove the "foreign body" (keratinous debris) causing the inflammatory reaction.

Suggested Readings

James WD, Berger TG, Elston DM. Nevi, neoplasms, and cysts. In: James WD, Berger TG, Elston DM, Odom RB, eds. *Andrews' Diseases of the Skin: Clinical Dermatology*. 10th Ed. Philadelphia, PA: Saunders Elsevier; 2006:676.

Khorsandi M, Lobby N, Harkaway RC, et al. Testicular cysts: Management and literature review. *J Am Osteopath Assoc*. 1999 Oct;99(10):537–538.

Mehrabi D, Leonhardt JM, Brodell RT. Removal of keratinous and pilar cysts with the punch incision technique: Analysis of surgical outcomes. *Dermatol Surg*. 2002 Aug;28(8):673–677.

Seabury, S.M. Cysts. In: Bolognia JL, Jorizzo JL, Rapini RP, eds. *Dermatology*. 2nd Ed. St. Louis, MO: Mosby; 2008:1681–1682.

Smoot EC. Removal of large inclusion cysts with minimal incisional scars. *Plast Reconstr Surg*. 2007 Apr;119(4):1395.

Wiesenthal JD, Ettler H, Razvi H. Testicular epidermoid cyst: A case report and review of the clinicopathologic features. *Can J Urol*. 2004 Feb;11(1):2133–2135.

Dermatofibroma

Diagnosis Synopsis

Dermatofibromas, or histiocytomas, are common, benign skin neoplasms composed of collagen, macrophages (histiocytes), capillaries, and fibroblasts. The etiology and pathogenesis are unknown, though some may arise at sites of trauma or insect bites. They are firm, skin-colored or slightly pigmented papules or nodules. They may be tender or pruritic, and they often persist for life. They are most common on the legs of women and usually appear in young adulthood. They may heal as depressed scars after several years.

Dermatofibromas are often solitary, though any individual may have more than one.

Look For

Firm, 0.5 to 2 cm papules or nodules that may be flesh-colored, tan, pink, yellowish, blue, brown, red, or black (Figs. 4-668–4-670). They are typically—but not exclusively—round or ovoid with a well-defined border. They are often found on the extremities, especially the legs. Because the epidermis is tethered to the underlying fibrotic component, the overlying skin does not slide over the underlying nodule.

Dark Skin Considerations

In darker-skinned individuals, the papules or nodules appear darker than on lightly pigmented skin and are still more frequent on the legs (Fig. 4-671).

Diagnostic Pearls

By squeezing laterally on these papules or nodules, the skin will pucker inward, creating a small dimple—the so-called "dimple sign" or "Fitzpatrick sign"—and confirming the diagnosis. An uncommon variant may have a targetoid appearance with a pale center and pigmented rim.

Differential Diagnosis and Pitfalls

- Dermatofibrosarcoma protuberans (DFSP) is a locally invasive malignant neoplasm that can begin as a dermatofibroma-size lesion. DFSP favors the trunk and progressively increases in size, while dermatofibromas do not substantially increase in size and favor the extremities.
- Melanocytic nevus
- Blue nevus
- Dysplastic nevus
- Keratoacanthoma
- Prurigo nodularis
- Melanoma
- Basal cell carcinoma
- Squamous cell carcinoma
- Spitz nevus
- Keloid or hypertrophic scar
- Fibroxanthoma
- Kaposi sarcoma
- Mastocytosis
- Neurilemmoma (schwannoma)
- Foreign body granuloma
- Pilomatrixoma
- Seborrheic keratosis

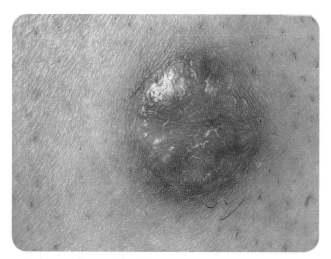

Figure 4-668 Dermatofibromas have a distinct border and often have mottled pigmentation.

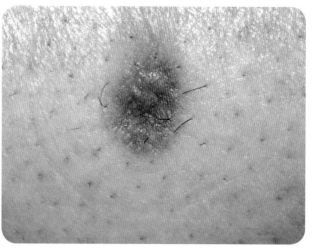

Figure 4-669 Dermatofibromas become depressed with time (often years).

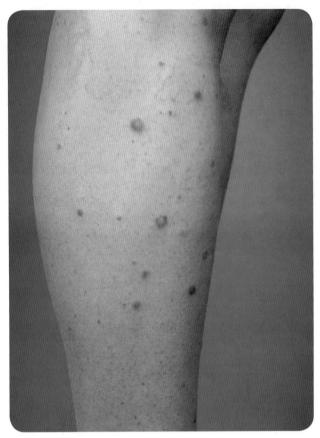

Figure 4-670 Multiple dermatofibromas are sometimes associated with connective tissue diseases.

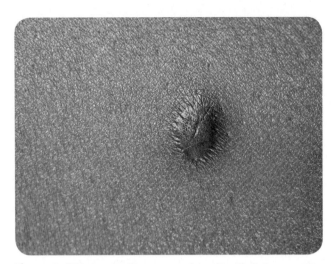

Figure 4-671 Dermatofibromas may be uniformly dark, suggesting a melanocytic malignancy.

- Patients who present with a diagnostic concern about a dermatofibroma. The diagnosis is overwhelmingly made on clinical grounds, in which case lesions can be identified as benign, and no therapy is required.
- Patients who present with symptomatic (e.g., tenderness, pruritus, or irritation with shaving) lesions or cosmetic concerns. Symptomatic, protruding dermatofibromas can be reduced in size by liquid nitrogen therapy or intralesional corticosteroids. Excision should be presented as an undesirable option because of the risk of recurrence or the probability that the resulting scar would be worse than the original lesion.

✓ Best Tests

- Clinical examination is the usual diagnostic method. In the unusual case in which the diagnosis is in question, an excisional biopsy will remove the lesion and confirm the diagnosis. However, recurrence is common, and, thus, the use of topical or intralesional steroids is often necessary to reduce the chance of regrowth. Shave biopsy can also confirm the diagnosis, but lesions are likely to recur.
- Dermatoscopy may be a useful tool for differentiating dermatofibromas from other pigmented lesions.

▲▲ Management Pearls

Patients with one or more dermatofibromas can be divided into one of the three categories, and management should be planned accordingly:

- Unconcerned patients with a dermatofibroma found incidentally on examination. Lesions can be identified as benign, and no therapy is required.

Therapy

No treatment is needed unless the lesion(s) are symptomatic and/or cosmetically unacceptable.

Intralesional corticosteroids (10 to 20 mg/cc of triamcinolone acetonide) achieve variable results. Cryotherapy with liquid nitrogen is a useful option that may result in flattening of lesions with lightening of pigmentation and lessening of symptoms. Freezing is performed for 20 to 30 s with a 2 mm margin and may be repeated at an interval of 4 to 8 weeks. As this is a longer freezing time than is used for other types of lesions, nonsteroidal anti-inflammatory drugs (NSAIDs) and ultrapotent topical steroids (clobetasol ointment) may be used to mitigate discomfort in the few days after treatment.

Excision can be performed, but due to the high incidence of recurrence, the use of topical or intralesional steroids post-excision is often necessary. Complete excision, including an underlying area of subcutaneous fat, gives the best chance of cure, as recurrences are more likely with cryosurgery or a superficial shave biopsy.

Suggested Readings

Andrews MD. Cryosurgery for common skin conditions. *Am Fam Physician.* 2004 May;69(10):2365–2372.

Fitzpatrick TB, Gilchrest BA. Dimple sign to differentiate benign from malignant pigmented cutaneous lesions. *N Engl J Med.* 1977 Jun;296(26):1518.

Fuciarelli K, Cohen PR. Sebaceous hyperplasia: A clue to the diagnosis of dermatofibroma. *J Am Acad Dermatol.* 2001 Jan;44(1):94–95.

Harting M, Hicks MJ, Levy ML. Dermal hypertrophies. In: Fitzpatrick TB, Wolff K, eds. *Fitzpatrick's Dermatology in General Medicine.* 7th Ed. New York, NY: McGraw-Hill; 2008:556–557.

Kamino H, Meehan SA, Pui J. Fibrous and fibrohistiocytic proliferations of the skin and tendons. In: Bolognia JL, Jorizzo JL, Rapini RP, eds. *Dermatology.* 2nd Ed. St. Louis, MO: Mosby; 2008:1815–1817.

Lanigan SW, Robinson TW. Cryotherapy for dermatofibromas. *Clin Exp Dermatol.* 1987 Mar;12(2):121–123.

Zaballos P, Puig S, Llambrich A, et al. Dermoscopy of dermatofibromas: A prospective morphological study of 412 cases. *Arch Dermatol.* 2008 Jan;144(1):75–83.

Zaccaria E, Rebora A, Rongioletti F. Multiple eruptive dermatofibromas and immunosuppression: Report of two cases and review of the literature. *Int J Dermatol.* 2008 Jul;47(7):723–727.

Zelger B, Zelger BG, Burgdorf WH. Dermatofibroma-a critical evaluation. *Int J Surg Pathol.* 2004 Oct;12(4):333–344.

Gout

Diagnosis Synopsis

Gout is the systemic deposition of monosodium urate crystals in tissues due to hyperuricemia. Elevated uric acid levels can be caused by the overproduction of uric acid from purine catabolism or insufficient excretion by the kidneys. The deposition of urate crystals in tissues leads to inflammation and subsequent tissue damage. Men aged 40 to 50 are most commonly affected. Other risk factors include renal insufficiency, obesity, increased alcohol consumption, medications (e.g., diuretics), lymphomas, leukemias, tumor lysis syndrome, and hemolysis.

The most common sites involved are the skin and joints. Gout can present in an acute and chronic form: acute gouty arthritis or chronic tophaceous gout, respectively. The acute form presents as a painful, swollen, warm, tender, and erythematous joint. Most common joints include the first metatarsophalangeal joint, the ankle, foot, and knee. The majority of attacks involve one joint. Chronic tophaceous gout presents most commonly on the joints or helix of the ear. Smooth or multilobulated nodules can ulcerate, leading to the extrusion of a chalk-like substance.

Look For

Acute gout often presents with a single joint that is hot, erythematous, tender, and occasionally edematous (Figs. 4-672–4-674). The most commonly affected joints are the great toe, ankle, wrist, and knee.

The nodules of gout vary in size and are yellow or cream in color (Fig. 4-675). It is common to have nodules that break down, heal, and then develop again. These deposits are mostly found on the rims of the ears (helix and antihelix), the distal toe and finger joints, the Achilles tendon, or the olecranon or prepatellar bursae.

Diagnostic Pearls

- There is a male preponderance of the disease. Diagnosing tophi in women is rare.
- The most common site of a first attack of acute gout is the great toe (podagra).

Differential Diagnosis and Pitfalls

Acute Gouty Arthritis

- Pseudogout
- Septic arthritis
- Psoriatic arthritis
- Reactive arthritis
- Osteoarthritis
- Cellulitis

Chronic Tophaceous Gout

- Rheumatoid nodules
- Calcinosis cutis
- Xanthomas
- Chondrodermatitis nodularis helices
- Squamous cell carcinoma

Best Tests

- Biopsy or aspirate with polarizing microscopy—Finding the characteristic needle-shaped negatively birefringent crystals of monosodium urate in the joint fluid confirms the diagnosis.

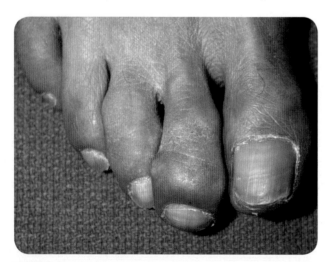

Figure 4-672 Gout is often a red nodule with white-to-yellow smaller nodules within it.

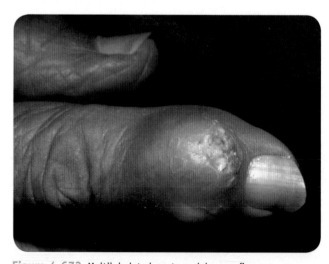

Figure 4-673 Multilobulated gouty nodule on a finger.

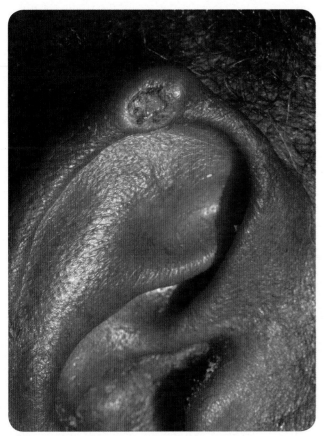

Figure 4-674 Ulcerated gouty nodule on helix that may be confused with chondrodermatitis nodularis helicis.

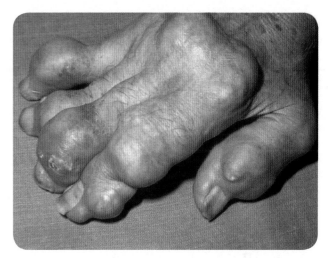

Figure 4-675 Multiple gouty nodules with marked joint deformity.

- Plain radiographs of the affected joint(s).
- Elevated serum uric acid level—Note that this test is not particularly sensitive or specific for the diagnosis of gout.
- WBC (joint fluid and blood) and erythrocyte sedimentation rate (ESR) are usually elevated during acute attacks.

▲▲ Management Pearls

- Patients with gout should avoid foods high in purines such as anchovies, organ meat, asparagus, oatmeal, cocoa, mushrooms, and spinach. Alcohol consumption should be limited to two drinks per day.
- As there are many causes of mild elevations in the serum uric acid, biopsy of presumptive lesions is necessary to avoid missing an infiltrative disease or a malignancy.

Therapy

Acute Attacks
- Rest and elevate affected joint, if possible.
- Nonsteroidal anti-inflammatory drugs (NSAIDs)—Ibuprofen (preferred) 800 mg p.o. three times daily for

5 days, indomethacin 50 mg p.o. four times daily for 5 days, or another NSAID at maximum dose. Doses must be lowered in cases of renal insufficiency, and NSAIDs are contraindicated with known peptic ulcer disease.
- Colchicine—0.6 to 1.2 mg p.o. initial dose, then 0.6 mg p.o. every 1 to 2 h until attack improves or gastrointestinal symptoms develop. Maximum total dose equals 4 to 6 mg.
- Steroids—Reserve for patients in whom NSAIDs or colchicine may be contraindicated or ineffective. Triamcinolone acetonide 60 mg IM or prednisone 20 to 40 mg p.o./IM daily.
- Intraarticular steroids, such as triamcinolone hexacetonide, may be used to treat a single inflamed joint.

Chronic Rx
The main indication for long-term, prophylactic treatment is recurrent attacks (i.e., three or more per year). Goal serum urate less than or equal to 6 mg/dL.

- Colchicine—0.6 to 1.2 mg p.o. daily for 1 to 2 weeks prior to initiating hypouricemic therapy; continue for several months after hypouricemic therapy has begun. Some patients will require long-term colchicine in addition to hypouricemics.
- Allopurinol—For overproducers of uric acid, 300 to 900 mg p.o. daily.
- Probenecid—For persons with decreased excretion of uric acid, 0.5 to 1 g p.o. twice daily.
- A 24-h urine collection is often useful in determining which hypouricemic agent is indicated.

Rarely, surgical intervention is required secondary to joint destruction.

Suggested Readings

Chen LX, Schumacher HR. Gout: Can we create an evidence-based systematic approach to diagnosis and management? *Best Pract Res Clin Rheumatol.* 2006 Aug;20(4):673–684.

Fitzgerald BT, Setty A, Mudgal CS. Gout affecting the hand and wrist. *J Am Acad Orthop Surg.* 2007 Oct;15(10):625–635.

Fox R. Management of recurrent gout. *BMJ.* 2008 Feb;336(7639):329.

Janssens HJ, Lucassen PL, Van de Laar FA, et al. Systemic corticosteroids for acute gout. *Cochrane Database Syst Rev.* 2008 Apr;(2):CD005521.

Jordan KM, Cameron JS, Snaith M, et al.; British Society for Rheumatology and British Health Professionals in Rheumatology Standards, Guidelines and Audit Working Group (SGAWG). British Society for Rheumatology and British Health Professionals in Rheumatology guideline for the management of gout. *Rheumatology (Oxford).* 2007 Aug;46(8):1372–1374.

Pascual E, Sivera F. Therapeutic advances in gout. *Curr Opin Rheumatol.* 2007 Mar;19(2):122–127.

Taylor WJ, Schumacher HR Jr, Singh JA, et al. Assessment of outcome in clinical trials of gout—a review of current measures. *Rheumatology (Oxford).* 2007 Dec;46(12):1751–1756.

Underwood M. Diagnosis and management of gout. *BMJ.* 2006 Jun;332(7553):1315–1319.

Yosipovitch G, DeVore A, Dawn A. Obesity and the skin: Skin physiology and skin manifestations of obesity. *J Am Acad Dermatol.* 2007 Jun;56(6):901–916; quiz 917–920.

Hidradenitis Suppurativa

Diagnosis Synopsis

Hidradenitis suppurativa is a destructive, chronic inflammatory disorder of the terminal follicular epithelium in apocrine gland–bearing regions of the body. Previously, this disease was thought to be due to bacterial infection, but it has now become clear that it is a noninfectious acneiform disease. It is believed that follicular occlusion leads to trapping of follicular contents, rupture, and inflammation of the dermis, with bacterial superinfection in some cases. Hidradenitis suppurativa is more common in women and blacks.

The nodules of hidradenitis suppurativa are seen most commonly on the buttocks, breasts, and in the groin and axillae. Usually, the onset of the disease occurs soon after puberty, and patients typically report recurring "boils." Shaving, depilation, deodorants, and mechanical irritation can worsen this condition, but irritation of the skin is usually not a major factor. Obesity and cigarette smoking are associated with hidradenitis suppurativa. Symptoms may include arthralgias and local pain and tenderness during a flare-up.

Interestingly, hidradenitis suppurativa shares similar clinical features (severe inflammation, occlusion of the follicle, and scarring) with dissecting cellulitis of the scalp and acne conglobata. Collectively, these three conditions are referred to as the follicular occlusion triad, and more than one may occur in a given patient. Some consider the pilonidal sinus (pilonidal cyst) to be an additional member of this group.

With a prevalence of up to 1% in some population-based studies, hidradenitis suppurativa is a common disease.

Look For

Firm, tender, erythematous nodules and often extensive scars and sinus tracking under the surface of the skin

(Figs. 4-676–4-678). These sinus tracts may drain pus, which is often malodorous.

The lesions are seen mostly on the groin, axillae, buttocks, and breasts. The disease is rarely seen on the arms or legs. The involvement of the scalp is usually referred to as dissecting cellulitis, and on the trunk it is considered as acne conglobata. Sinuses may involve the rectum and anus, and, in severe cases, vaginal and urethral fistulas can develop. Lesions heal with hypertrophic scarring (Fig. 4-679).

Diagnostic Pearls

- Double comedones on a single lesion (similar to the acne conglobata complex) are very suggestive of this diagnosis.
- Only half of bacterial cultures will demonstrate pathogens.
- Involvement of the axillae is more common in women, and involvement of the anogenital region is more common in men. It is most common in young women, and premenstrual flares are not uncommon.

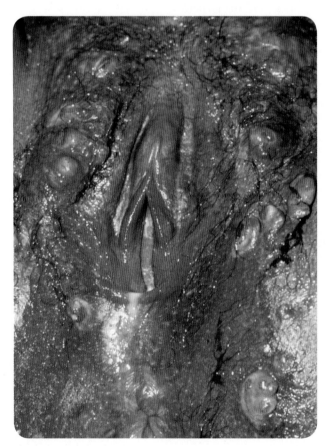

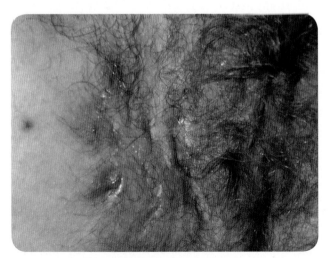

Figure 4-676 Sinus tracts and inflammatory cysts in the groin due to hidradenitis suppurativa.

Figure 4-677 Multiple vulval cysts and sinuses due to hidradenitis suppurativa.

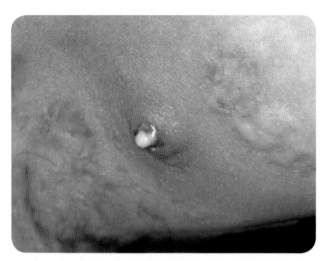

Figure 4-678 Inflamed axilla in hidradenitis suppurativa.

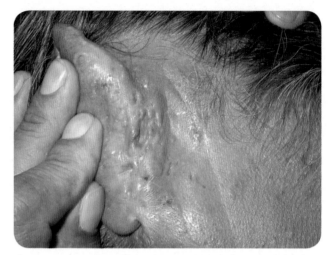

Figure 4-679 Scarring from retroauricular hidradenitis suppurativa.

?? Differential Diagnosis and Pitfalls

- Epidermoid cysts
- Bartholin gland abscess
- Crohn disease (perianal)
- Granuloma inguinale
- Tuberculosis
- Actinomycosis
- Lymphogranuloma venereum
- Abscess(es), including recurrent *Staphylococcus aureus* infection
- Pilonidal sinus (cysts)
- Candidiasis
- Folliculitis/furunculosis
- Tularemia
- Cat scratch disease

✓ Best Tests

- The diagnosis can often be made on clinical grounds.
- Gram stain, culture, and sensitivity can be performed on any pus/exudate as superinfection may occur.
- When in doubt, skin biopsy may aid in making the diagnosis.

▲▲ Management Pearls

- Advise patients that treatment can be difficult, but, with limited disease, conservative measures can be effective.
- Surgical excision is often the ideal treatment for extensive, recurrent disease. Very wide unroofing and debridement of individual sinus tracts, allowing for healing by secondary intention, is best. Incision and drainage may offer temporary relief from individual lesions but is generally avoided because cysts will simply re-form. When severe, refer to a dermatologist or surgeon who has special training in treating this disease.
- Instruct patients to avoid tight-fitting clothing and excessive friction to the involved areas. Encourage weight loss in the obese and smoking cessation in cigarette smokers.
- Squamous cell carcinoma may develop in scars after many years.
- Because of the severity of the disease and the foul odor of the drainage, social isolation and/or depression is commonly seen. Attention should be given to pain management and social factors.

Therapy

First-line treatments are antibiotics and surgery:

- Consider oral tetracycline (500 mg twice daily) or minocycline (100 mg twice daily) or doxycycline (100 mg twice daily) for months.
- Topical clindamycin 2% solution applied twice daily to affected areas may help with early lesions or between flares.

Surgical techniques include the excision of affected tissues and exteriorization of sinus tracts. Simple incision and drainage of large cysts may be performed with the recognition that the rate of recurrence is extremely high.

Intralesional triamcinolone to active cysts and nodules (triamcinolone 3 to 10 mg/cc), and hormonal therapy (in women only) with cyproterone acetate (50 mg days 5 to 14 of menstrual cycle), and ethinylestradiol (50 mcg of ethinylestradiol from days 5 to 25) can be considered as second-line therapies. Finasteride 5 mg per day for 3 months may benefit some patients of both sexes. Oral contraceptives may also have efficacy in women.

Isotretinoin 1 mg/kg daily has been beneficial in some patients as has acitretin 25 mg twice daily. Systemic anti-inflammatory agents, such as corticosteroids and cyclosporine, are occasionally used to palliate symptoms. Dapsone at daily doses from 25 to 150 mg has been proven effective in a small series of patients. Biologic agents, such as the anti-TNF drugs infliximab and etanercept are of questionable value in treating hidradenitis suppurativa. Additional studies are required to determine their efficacy.

Other techniques with some reported success include carbon dioxide laser ablation and liposuction.

Suggested empiric antibiotics for the treatment of super-infections include oral clindamycin (300 mg twice daily) or dicloxacillin (500 mg three times daily). Metronidazole is commonly used to treat anaerobic superinfections, but there is little evidence base to support this.

Attention to psychosocial ramifications of this disease is crucial. Depression is not uncommon, and patient suffering likely exceeds that of most common chronic skin diseases.

Suggested Readings

Giamarellos-Bourboulis EJ, Pelekanou E, Antonopoulou A, et al. An open-label phase II study of the safety and efficacy of etanercept for the therapy of hidradenitis suppurativa. *Br J Dermatol.* 2008 Mar;158(3):567–572.

Jemec GB. Medical treatment of hidradenitis suppurativa. *Expert Opin Pharmacother.* 2004 Aug;5(8):1767–1770.

Jemec GB, Wendelboe P. Topical clindamycin versus systemic tetracycline in the treatment of hidradenitis suppurativa. *J Am Acad Dermatol.* 1998 Dec;39(6):971–974.

Kraft JN, Searles GE. Hidradenitis suppurativa in 64 female patients: Retrospective study comparing oral antibiotics and antiandrogen therapy. *J Cutan Med Surg.* 2007 Jul–Aug;11(4):125–131.

Kurzen H, Jung EG, Hartschuh W, et al. Forms of epithelial differentiation of draining sinus in acne inversa (hidradenitis suppurativa). *Br J Dermatol.* 1999 Aug;141(2):231–239.

Lapins J, Marcusson JA, Emtestam L. Surgical treatment of chronic hidradenitis suppurativa: CO_2 laser stripping-secondary intention technique. *Br J Dermatol.* 1994 Oct;131(4):551–556.

Lee RA, Yoon A, Kist J. Hidradenitis suppurativa: An update. *Adv Dermatol.* 2007;23:289–306.

Mekkes JR, Bos JD. Long-term efficacy of a single course of infliximab in hidradenitis suppurativa. *Br J Dermatol.* 2008 Feb;158(2):370–374.

Mitchell KM, Beck DE. Hidradenitis suppurativa. *Surg Clin North Am.* 2002 Dec;82(6):1187–1197.

Revuz J. Medical treatments of hidradenitis suppurativa: A new paradigm. *Dermatology.* 2007;215(2):95–96.

Revuz JE, Canoui-Poitrine F, Wolkenstein P, et al. Prevalence and factors associated with hidradenitis suppurativa: Results from two case-control studies. *J Am Acad Dermatol.* 2008 Oct;59(4):596–601.

Wolkenstein P, Loundou A, Barrau K, et al.; Quality of Life Group of the French Society of Dermatology. Quality of life impairment in hidradenitis suppurativa: A study of 61 cases. *J Am Acad Dermatol.* 2007 Apr;56(4):621–623.

◼◼ Diagnosis Synopsis

Kaposi sarcoma (KS) is a malignancy of vascular endothelial cells that are infected with human herpesvirus type 8 (HHV-8). KS presents with violaceous nodules or plaques that may occur anywhere on the body. There are four different variants of KS, which include the AIDS-associated KS, and the three non-AIDS–associated KS variants (classic KS, African endemic KS, and KS in iatrogenically immunosuppressed patients). All four types can be linked to infection with HHV-8.

AIDS-Associated KS

In the United States, the AIDS-associated epidemic form of KS is seen primarily in men who have sex with men and African or Caribbean women. Patients with AIDS-associated KS often have concomitant widespread visceral KS and are at risk for hemorrhage from gastrointestinal lesions, cardiac tamponade, and pulmonary obstruction. AIDS-associated KS most commonly affects patients with CD4 counts less than 500 cells per cubic millimeter. The introduction of highly active antiretroviral therapy (HAART) has prolonged the average survival of patients with AIDS-associated KS and can often lead to complete resolution of lesions.

Non-AIDS–Associated KS

Classic (Traditional) KS

Classic KS is seen almost exclusively in people of Mediterranean and Ashkenazi Jewish descent. Older literature describes a higher male-to-female incidence of approximately 12:1. However, more recent studies suggest that the gender gap may not be so significant. Age of onset is typically between 50 and 70 years. Classic KS most commonly runs an indolent course for 10 to 15 years or more with slow enlargement of tumors and the gradual development of additional lesions. Eventually, systemic lesions can develop along the gastrointestinal tract, in lymph nodes, and in other organs. These visceral tumors are usually asymptomatic.

African Endemic KS

African endemic KS has 4 subgroups that include florid, nodular, lymphadenopathic, and infiltrative. Most pediatric cases are lymphadenopathic and rapidly disseminate, with a high mortality. This aggressive endemic form of KS exists in equatorial Africa and is unrelated to AIDS. Areas of highest prevalence include Uganda, the Democratic Republic of the Congo, Zambia, and the Republic of the Congo (Brazzaville). Systemic lesions are particularly prevalent in this form.

Immunocompromised Patient Considerations

Iatrogenic KS

Iatrogenic KS is the result of long-term systemic immunosuppression and is common in transplant recipients, especially renal transplant. It may resolve when immunosuppressive medications are discontinued.

◉ Look For

AIDS-Associated KS

Deep red, brown, or purple macules, plaques, and nodules (Figs. 4-680 and 4-681). Large tumors may be present.

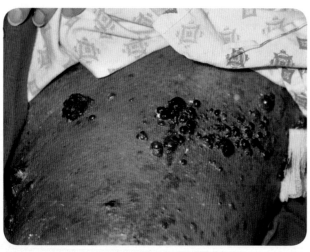

Figure 4-680 AIDS-associated KS with multiple purpuric and hemorrhagic nodules.

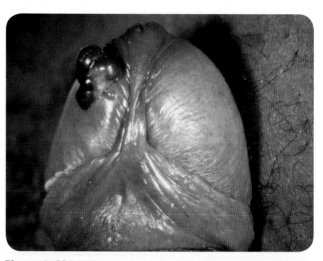

Figure 4-681 AIDS-associated KS with multiple purpuric and hemorrhagic nodules on the glans penis.

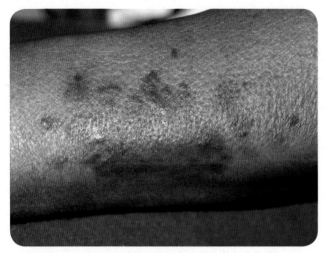

Figure 4-682 KS with purple papules and nodules on the leg.

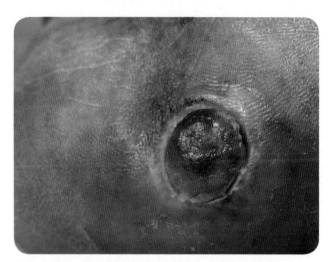

Figure 4-683 KS including an ulcerating lesion on the sole.

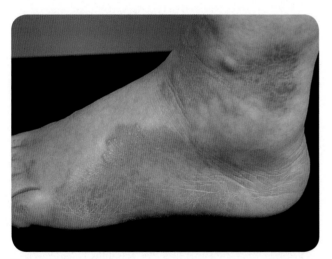

Figure 4-684 KS in its early stages may be a persistent red plaque on a lower leg.

KS may present anywhere on the body but is seen more frequently on the trunk, extremities, and face. Hard palate plaques are also common. Koebnerization (lesions occurring in areas of trauma) occasionally takes place.

Non-AIDS–Associated KS

Red, purple, or bluish-black patches that slowly progress into plaques/nodules (Figs. 4-682 and 4-683). The disease is often limited to the lower extremities, especially involving the ankles and feet (Fig. 4-684). Venous stasis and lymphedema of the involved lower extremity are frequently seen. Late lesions may appear verrucous. Oral and other mucosal tumors may occur.

Dark Skin Considerations

In darker skin, lesions will appear violaceous, hyperpigmented, brown, or black. The violaceous hue may be less conspicuous in darker skin.

Diagnostic Pearls

AIDS-Associated KS

AIDS-associated KS lesions can be distributed in many areas of the body, but the presence of palatal lesions may aid in diagnosis. Any purple plaque in an HIV-infected patient should raise suspicion of KS.

Non-AIDS–Associated KS

Classic KS favors the lower extremities. Lesions start distally, usually on the feet.

?? Differential Diagnosis and Pitfalls

- Bacillary angiomatosis is an infectious vascular process in AIDS patients, but lesions tend to be painful.
- Single lesions with rapid onset are consistent with a pyogenic granuloma.
- Dermatofibromas are tan brown, flat-topped solitary papules.
- Dermatofibroma sarcoma protuberans presents as a solitary brown to purple firm plaque.

507

- Hemangiomas tend to be bright red dome-shaped papules, but they can be darker purple or black when thrombosed.
- Kaposiform hemangioendotheliomas and spindle cell hemangiomas may clinically appear similar; a biopsy is often useful.
- Angiokeratomas often present with clustered purple, smooth dome-shaped papules.
- Lichen simplex chronicus is marked with lichenified pruritic skin.
- Prurigo nodularis typically has hyperpigmented, excoriated, and pruritic nodules.
- Metastatic carcinoma or melanoma can be distinguished via biopsy.
- Pigmented basal cell carcinoma can be seen more commonly in darker skin.
- Blue rubber bleb nevus syndrome is usually diagnosed at birth with the presence of blue vascular papules.
- Tufted angiomas are usually detected at an early age.
- Cavernous hemangiomas are detected at an early age and tend to be quite large.
- Arteriovenous malformation
- Hypertrophic lichen planus is marked with pruritic, purple papules and plaques, commonly over the anterior shins.
- Lymphoma can be distinguished via biopsy.
- Angiosarcoma may clinically resemble KS but usually presents on the head and neck.
- A large junctional nevus or port-wine stain may resemble early KS.
- Sarcoid can present with violaceous plaques; a biopsy is useful when in doubt.
- Acroangiodermatitis and chronic stasis dermatitis may also clinically resemble late stage KS.

✓ Best Tests

- Skin biopsy is diagnostic. Immunohistochemical staining or PCR for HHV-8 is confirmatory.
- Additional studies may be warranted to ascertain the extent of disease, including but not limited to CT scans, plain films, CBC, and fecal occult blood testing.
- Consider HIV testing if the patient's HIV status is unknown.

▲▲ Management Pearls

AIDS-Associated KS

The treatment of advanced AIDS-associated KS often necessitates a multidisciplinary approach. An infectious disease/HIV specialist should be involved in the treatment of HIV and opportunistic infections. Medical or radiation oncologists may be needed to administer systemic chemotherapy or radiation therapy, respectively.

Non-AIDS–Associated KS

The treatment of non-AIDS–associated KS is considered largely palliative. In elderly patients or those with multiple comorbidities and limited disease, the risks and benefits of pursuing aggressive treatment should be weighed carefully. However, the treatment of advanced non-AIDS–associated KS also necessitates a multidisciplinary approach.

Immunocompromised Patient Considerations

For iatrogenic KS, reduction or cessation of immunosuppressive medications may be sufficient for the resolution of KS and should be attempted first, when possible, before moving on to other forms of therapy. Changing cyclosporine to sirolimus has also led to resolution in many patients.

Therapy

AIDS-Associated KS

- HAART therapy results in a dramatic reduction of KS lesions and incidence. This benefit may be enhanced by the addition of pegylated liposomal doxorubicin.
- Etoposide has been used with greater than 75% response rate for AIDS-associated KS.
- Angiogenesis inhibitors (thalidomide, COL-3, bevacizumab [anti-VEGF], and TNP-470) have also shown promise.
- Drugs that target HHV-8 are currently being developed.

Solitary Lesions in Both AIDS- and Non-AIDS–Associated KS

- Superficial and small lesions can be treated with liquid nitrogen (5 to 10 s with three cycles) sufficient to cause ulceration. The resultant scar is thought to replace the KS lesion.
- Intralesional bleomycin (1.5 mg).
- Intralesional interferon alpha (3 to 5 MU three times per week).
- Intralesional vinblastine (0.1 mg).
- Radiotherapy with extended field radiation, electron beam, or cobalt therapy.
- Panretin gel (alitretinoin 0.1%) applied to the lesion(s) twice daily; cost may be prohibitive.
- Excision of solitary lesions; however, they can locally recur.

Widespread Skin Disease for AIDS- and Non-AIDS–Associated KS

- Radiation therapy can be effective in controlling widespread disease.
- Chemotherapy options include weekly intravenous vinblastine (4 to 6 mg) or vinblastine alternating with vincristine (2 mg IV) on a weekly basis. Combination regimens include doxorubicin, bleomycin, and vincristine. Liposomal preparations of anthracyclines are also being used in hopes of minimizing side effects of therapy.
- Interferon alpha can also be used as systemic therapy for KS. It is administered IV or with daily subcutaneous injections to a dose of 30 MU daily.

Suggested Readings

Aldenhoven M, Barlo NP, Sanders CJ. Therapeutic strategies for epidemic Kaposi's sarcoma. *Int J STD AIDS*. 2006 Sep;17(9):571–578.

Chor PJ, Santa Cruz DJ. Kaposi's sarcoma. A clinicopathologic review and differential diagnosis. *J Cutan Pathol*. 1992 Feb;19(1):6–20.

Cooley T, Henry D, Tonda M, et al. A randomized, double-blind study of pegylated liposomal doxorubicin for the treatment of AIDS-related Kaposi's sarcoma. *Oncologist*. 2007 Jan;12(1):114–123.

Dezube BJ. New therapies for the treatment of AIDS-related Kaposi sarcoma. *Curr Opin Oncol*. 2000 Sep;12(5):445–449.

Di Lorenzo G, Konstantinopoulos PA, Pantanowitz L, et al. Management of AIDS-related Kaposi's sarcoma. *Lancet Oncol*. 2007 Feb;8(2):167–176.

Gill PS, Wernz J, Scadden DT, et al. Randomized phase III trial of liposomal daunorubicin versus doxorubicin, bleomycin, and vincristine in AIDS-related Kaposi's sarcoma. *J Clin Oncol*. 1996 Aug;14(8):2353–2364.

Gottlieb JJ, Washenik K, Chachoua A, et al. Treatment of classic Kaposi's sarcoma with liposomal encapsulated doxorubicin. *Lancet*. 1997 Nov; 350(9088):1363–1364.

Hengge UR, Ruzicka T, Tyring SK, et al. Update on Kaposi's sarcoma and other HHV8 associated diseases. Part 1: Epidemiology, environmental predispositions, clinical manifestations, and therapy. *Lancet Infect Dis*. 2002 May;2(5):281–292.

Iscovich J, Boffetta P, Franceschi S, et al. Classic kaposi sarcoma: Epidemiology and risk factors. *Cancer*. 2000 Feb;88(3):500–517.

North PE, Kincannon J. Vascular neoplasms and neoplastic-like proliferations. In: Bolognia JL, Jorizzo JL, Rapini RP, eds. *Dermatology*. 2nd Ed. St. Louis, MO: Mosby; 2008:1785–1788.

Schwartz RA, Micali G, Nasca MR, Scuderi L. Kaposi sarcoma: A continuing conundrum. *J Am Acad Dermatol*. 2008 Aug;59(2):179–206; quiz 207–208.

Tappero JW, Conant MA, Wolfe SF, et al. Kaposi's sarcoma. Epidemiology, pathogenesis, histology, clinical spectrum, staging criteria and therapy. *J Am Acad Dermatol*. 1993 Mar;28(3):371–395.

Walmsley S, Northfelt DW, Melosky B, et al. Treatment of AIDS-related cutaneous Kaposi's sarcoma with topical alitretinoin (9-cis-retinoic acid) gel. Panretin Gel North American Study Group. *J Acquir Immune Defic Syndr*. 1999 Nov;22(3):235–246.

Diagnosis Synopsis

Keloids are dense, fibrous tissue nodules, typically found at areas of previously traumatized skin (burns, lacerations, and incision scars), or arising spontaneously on normal skin. Lesions may be single or multiple. Over weeks to months, these large nodules can become painful, tender, pruritic, and grow to become very large (up to 30 cm). They can cause chronic discomfort, be disfiguring, and restrict normal tissue motion. Keloids are most frequent in blacks and those of Mediterranean ancestry, but they can appear in any ethnicity. There is likely a genetic basis for the tendency to develop keloids. Spontaneous keloid formation is observed in the two extremely rare syndromes: Rubinstein-Taybi syndrome and Goeminne syndrome.

A distinction should be made between a keloid and a hypertrophic scar. All trauma that involves the dermis will heal with a scar; however, in certain individuals, the scar is much larger and thicker than what is considered normal. These lesions are termed hypertrophic scars. In contrast to keloids, hypertrophic scars are always preceded by trauma and always confined to the margin of the wound. Also, hypertrophic scars appear immediately after trauma and show a tendency to gradually regress, whereas keloids can be delayed in appearance and are thought to very rarely spontaneously resolve.

Immunocompromised Patient Considerations

A form of Kaposi sarcoma clinically resembling keloids (termed keloidal Kaposi sarcoma) has been reported in HIV-infected patients.

Look For

Keloids usually appear smooth and shiny. They can be red, hyperpigmented, or skin-colored, have regular or irregularly shaped ridges (Figs. 4-685–4-688), and are usually firm to the touch. They develop projections that extend beyond the area of original trauma. The growths can mostly be found on the neck, ears, extremities, and upper trunk, especially the chest. Keloids are rarely found on the central face, eyelids, and genitals.

Dark Skin Considerations

Darker skin types have significantly higher tendency to form keloids, with an incidence as high as 16% in black Africans.

Diagnostic Pearls

Keloids very rarely involute and are not confined to the margins of trauma.

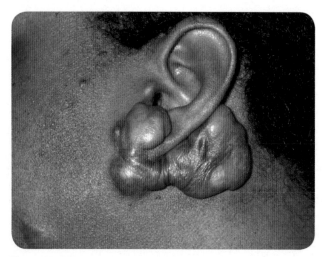

Figure 4-685 Keloid after ear piercing.

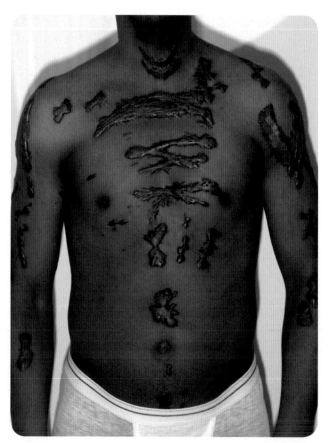

Figure 4-686 Multiple keloids, mostly spontaneous in origin.

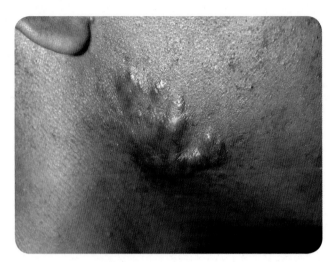

Figure 4-687 Keloidal acne scarring.

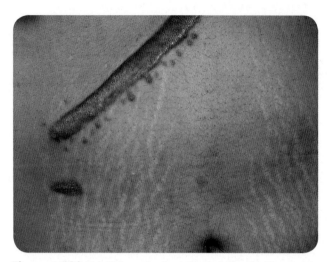

Figure 4-688 Keloidal scarring in a skin incision with tiny papular keloids in the sites of sutures.

?? Differential Diagnosis and Pitfalls

- Hypertrophic scars—see above
- Sarcoidosis—can localize in scars and form nodules clinically similar to keloids
- Foreign body reaction—should be associated with a history of trauma to the site
- Lobomycosis (keloidal blastomycosis)—infection with *Lacazia loboi*
- Dermatofibroma
- Dermatofibrosarcoma protuberans
- Xanthoma disseminatum (sclerotic form)
- Scleroderma
- Morphea
- Carcinoma en cuirasse

Immunocompromised Patient Differential Diagnosis

Keloidal Kaposi sarcoma

✓ Best Tests

The diagnosis is often made using history and appearance. If there is doubt, a biopsy will confirm the clinical diagnosis.

▲▲ Management Pearls

The surgical excision of keloids is inevitably fraught with the possibility of the keloid recurring in larger size than before the excision. Surgical excision is advised only if there is a post-op plan that includes regular follow-up for adjunctive therapy such as intralesional corticosteroids (5 to 20 mg/cc), pressure bandages, and/or silicone sheeting.

Therapy

Keloids are extremely difficult to treat.

Prevention and patient education are very important. Surgical wounds should parallel skin creases as much as possible, and wounds should be closed with minimal tension. Avoid making incisions overlying joints. Elective cosmetic surgery should be avoided in patients who are known keloid formers. The use of buried sutures and the application of pressure dressings and garments immediately postoperatively may reduce the likelihood of keloid formation.

- There has been some success in treating small earlobe keloids with pressure "clip-on" earrings.
- Some keloids and hypertrophic scars respond to topically applied silicone sheeting.
- Erythematous and inflamed keloids often respond to intralesional triamcinolone (10 to 40 mg/kg), depending on the density of the keloid tissue and the ability to infiltrate the medication. Use small quantities of high concentration triamcinolone (>20 mg/cc) to avoid skin atrophy.

Other therapies include
- Intralesional interferon, alpha, and gamma: 0.01 to 0.1 m three times per week
- Cryosurgery plus intralesional steroids
- Surgery plus local radiation therapy
- Laser therapy: argon, CO_2, Nd:YAG, or pulsed-dye laser to actively expanding lesions
- Imiquimod or intralesional verapamil post-excision
- Intralesional 5-FU

Suggested Readings

Boutli-Kasapidou F, Tsakiri A, Anagnostou E, et al. Hypertrophic and keloidal scars: An approach to polytherapy. *Int J Dermatol.* 2005 Apr;44(4):324–327.

Brown JJ, Ollier W, Arscott G, et al. Genetic susceptibility to keloid scarring: SMAD gene SNP frequencies in Afro-Caribbeans. *Exp Dermatol.* 2008 Jul;17(7):610–613.

Leventhal D, Furr M, Reiter D. Treatment of keloids and hypertrophic scars: A meta-analysis and review of the literature. *Arch Facial Plast Surg.* 2006 Nov–Dec;8(6):362–368.

O'Brien L, Pandit A. Silicon gel sheeting for preventing and treating hypertrophic and keloid scars. *Cochrane Database Syst Rev.* 2006 Jan;(1):CD003826.

Ragoowansi R, Cornes PG, Moss AL, et al. Treatment of keloids by surgical excision and immediate postoperative single-fraction radiotherapy. *Plast Reconstr Surg.* 2003 May;111(6):1853–1859.

Shaffer JJ, Taylor SC, Cook-Bolden F. Keloidal scars: A review with a critical look at therapeutic options. *J Am Acad Dermatol.* 2002 Feb;46(2 Suppl. Understanding):S63–S97.

Keratoacanthoma

Diagnosis Synopsis

A keratoacanthoma is a neoplasm considered by many to be a low-grade squamous cell carcinoma. It is a rapidly growing, well-differentiated neoplasm of squamous epithelium. It assumes a distinct crater-shaped appearance and usually occurs as a solitary lesion on the sun-exposed skin of the middle-aged and elderly. Men are more commonly affected than women, and fair-skinned individuals are at greater risk than those with dark skin.

In contrast to squamous cell carcinomas, keratoacanthomas appear and grow rapidly over the course of a few weeks to a month. If left untreated, most keratoacanthomas spontaneously involute and resolve within 6 months, leaving an atrophic scar.

Most keratoacanthomas are painless. Patients occasionally complain of pruritus within the lesion. They may cause mechanical or cosmetic deformity depending on the site of involvement. Most will cause only local destruction, but there are few that behave more aggressively. These are considered invasive variants. Metastases to draining lymph nodes, while seldom, have been reported.

Risk factors include sun exposure and immunosuppression. Skin injury may also be a predisposing factor, as there are many reports of keratoacanthomas developing in sites of previous trauma, in surgical scars, after laser resurfacing, and following radiation therapy.

In rare cases, multiple keratoacanthomas develop as part of a syndrome. The Ferguson-Smith syndrome is an autosomal dominant inherited disease characterized by multiple self-healing keratoacanthomas that affect young men in their third decade of life. Lesions occur within one localized area. The face, trunk, or penis is usually involved, and pruritus is a common feature. Each lesion clinically resembles a solitary keratoacanthoma. In eruptive keratoacanthomas of Grzybowski, hundreds of lesions occur in a generalized distribution and may involve mucous membranes. Keratoacanthomas may occur within the Muir-Torre syndrome along with sebaceous neoplasms and adenomatous colon carcinoma or other low-grade internal malignancies. Other familial syndromes have also been described.

Immunocompromised Patient Considerations

It is thought that the immune system plays a role in the spontaneous regression of keratoacanthomas. Patients on immunosuppressants (e.g., immunosuppression after solid organ transplantation) have increased numbers of more persistent and more chronic keratoacanthomas.

Look For

A solitary dome-shaped, skin-colored nodule with a central keratin-filled plug (Figs. 4-689 and 4-690). It is sharply demarcated from the surrounding skin and may have telangiectasias within the lesion. They range in size from 1 to 2 cm. The most common locations include the central face, dorsal hands, and arms. In women, the distal legs are also frequently involved. Multiple keratoacanthomas are not uncommon (Figs. 4-691 and 4-692).

Some rare variants include

- Keratoacanthoma centrifugum marginatum, which expands peripherally while involuting centrally. The most common site is the pretibial shin.
- Giant keratoacanthomas are greater than 2 cm in diameter and usually involve the nose or eyelids.

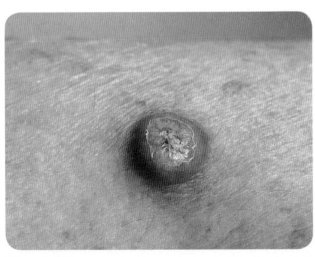

Figure 4-689 Average-sized keratoacanthoma with central keratotic core arising on sun-damaged skin.

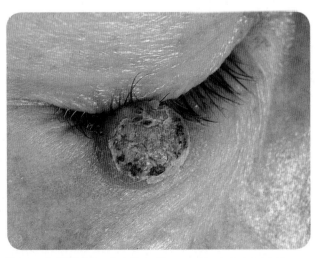

Figure 4-690 Large keratoacanthoma with central keratotic core arising on the eyelid.

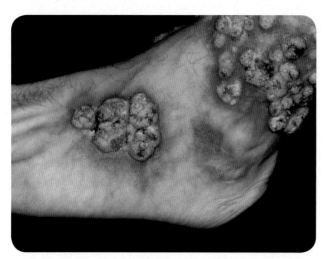

Figure 4-691 Multiple grouped keratoacanthomas on the lower legs.

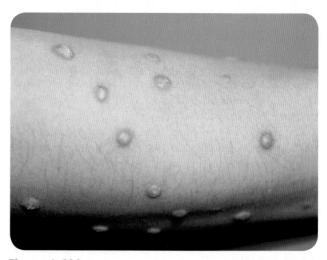

Figure 4-692 Multiple eruptive keratoacanthomas presenting as flesh-colored papules.

- Subungual keratoacanthomas are tender and result in nail dystrophy. These may also cause terminal phalanx destruction.

Diagnostic Pearls

Typical lesions of keratoacanthoma have a very distinct cup- or crater-shaped appearance. Patients will describe a very rapid growth (usually 2 to 6 weeks), which helps the clinician to distinguish it from squamous cell carcinoma or basal cell carcinoma.

?? Differential Diagnosis and Pitfalls

- Basal cell carcinoma
- Squamous cell carcinoma
- Merkel cell carcinoma
- Metastatic carcinoma
- Molluscum contagiosum
- Verruca vulgaris
- Actinic keratosis/cutaneous horn
- Prurigo nodularis
- Sporotrichosis

✓ Best Tests

Diagnosis should be based on biopsy to accurately differentiate keratoacanthoma from a malignancy.

▲▲ Management Pearls

Keratoacanthomas may regress spontaneously if left untreated; however, they may induce significant local destruction and psychological distress to the patient. Additionally, rare invasive variants have been documented, and it is clinically impossible to distinguish which lesions will behave in this fashion. There are reports of metastasis to regional lymph nodes. Therefore, treatment is recommended in order to speed resolution, prevent local destruction and metastasis, and improve cosmetic outcome.

Therapy

Complete excision is the recommended treatment of choice. Mohs surgery should be considered for tissue sparing and margin control. Electrodesiccation and curettage may be used for smaller tumors if the site is not of cosmetic concern. The argon laser, topical imiquimod, or 5-fluorouracil can also be tried on small lesions. Radiation therapy is efficacious with good cosmetic outcome for poor surgical candidates.

Medical management has been reported to be efficacious in small trials including intralesional 5-fluorouracil, methotrexate, interferon 2-alpha, and bleomycin. The disadvantage of this modality is the lack of a definitive diagnosis, as no specimen is sent for histopathology.

Multiple keratoacanthomas within syndromes have been successfully treated with oral isotretinoin with surgery used adjunctively for refractive lesions.

Suggested Readings

Bhatia N. Imiquimod as a possible treatment for keratoacanthoma. *J Drugs Dermatol.* 2004 Jan–Feb;3(1):71–74.

Dendorfer M, Oppel T, Wollenberg A, et al. Topical treatment with imiquimod may induce regression of facial keratoacanthoma. *Eur J Dermatol.* 2003 Jan–Feb;13(1):80–82.

Divers AK, Correale D, Lee JB. Keratoacanthoma centrifugum marginatum: A diagnostic and therapeutic challenge. *Cutis*. 2004 Apr;73(4):257–262.

Donahue B, Cooper JS, Rush S. Treatment of aggressive keratoacanthomas by radiotherapy. *J Am Acad Dermatol*. 1990 Sep;23(3 Pt 1):489–493.

Karaa A, Khachemoune A. Keratoacanthoma: A tumor in search of a classification. *Int J Dermatol*. 2007 Jul;46(7):671–678.

Kossard S, Tan KB, Choy C. Keratoacanthoma and infundibulocystic squamous cell carcinoma. *Am J Dermatopathol*. 2008 Apr;30(2):127–134.

Street ML, White JW, Gibson LE. Multiple keratoacanthomas treated with oral retinoids. *J Am Acad Dermatol*. 1990 Nov;23(5 Pt 1):862–866.

Lipoma

Diagnosis Synopsis

Lipomas are benign tumors of mature fat cells. They are the most common soft tissue tumor.

Clinically, lipomas present as soft, rubbery, freely mobile subcutaneous masses without overlying skin change. They are most often solitary but can be multiple. They can occur anywhere on the body where fat is found, with the highest predilection for the neck, trunk, extremities, and buttocks. They can be quite small (1 to 2 mm) to quite large (>10 cm) and occasionally are multilobular. They are usually asymptomatic; however, large tumors that compress nerves or limit normal tissue movement can cause discomfort and pain. Tumors with a vascular component (angiolipomas) also tend to be painful. They grow slowly to a stable size and do not spontaneously regress. Solitary lipomas are slightly more common in women, whereas multiple lipomas are more often seen in men. They may become more noticeable with weight gain but usually do not shrink with weight loss. An increased incidence is associated with diabetes, obesity, and hypercholesterolemia.

Multiple lipomas are associated with several rare syndromes:

- Diffuse lipomatosis—characterized by the infiltration of nonencapsulated fat into multiple tissues including muscle, skin, fascia, and bone. This entity can be seen in association with tuberous sclerosus.
- Familial multiple lipomatosis—characterized by multiple encapsulated lipomas in several family members.
- Proteus syndrome—characterized by multiple hamartomas (including lipomas) and disproportionate overgrowth of multiple tissues.
- Hemihyperplasia/multiple lipomatosis syndrome—characterized by multiple lipomas, asymmetric tissue overgrowth, capillary malformations, and accentuation of plantar skin creases.
- Benign symmetric lipomatosis (Madelung disease)—characterized by symmetric fat deposits around and above the shoulders associated with alcoholism.
- Adiposis dolorosa (Dercum disease)—characterized by multiple painful lipomas in postmenopausal women associated with weakness and depression.
- Gardner syndrome—characterized by multiple lipomas, colon polyposis, odontomas, epidermoid cysts, osteomas, leiomyomas, desmoid fibromatosis, and hypertrophy of the retinal pigment epithelium.
- Bannayan-Riley-Ruvalcaba syndrome—characterized by multiple lipomas, macrocephaly, intestinal polyposis, lentigines of the penis, and hemangiomas.

Immunocompromised Patient Considerations

Lipomas in the pubic area are commonly seen in HIV-infected patients with lipodystrophy.

Look For

Solitary or multiple soft tumors with no overlying color change that may grow to great size or stay limited to less than 2 to 2.5 cm (Figs. 4-693–4-696). The tumors have a soft and fluctuant feel and are often lobulated. They are freely movable.

Lipomas most commonly occur on the neck, shoulders, back, arms, and thighs.

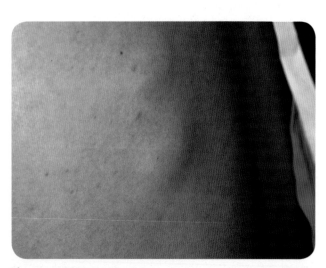

Figure 4-693 Lipomas may be single or multiple lesions in the dermis that are soft and freely movable.

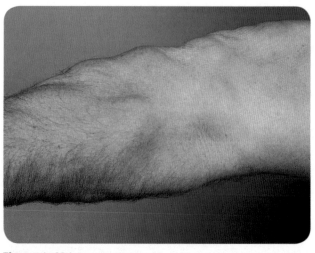

Figure 4-694 Multiple lipomas are not uncommon, and some are better felt than seen.

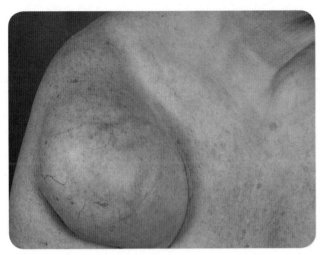

Figure 4-695 Huge lipomas with dilated surface vessels sometimes occur.

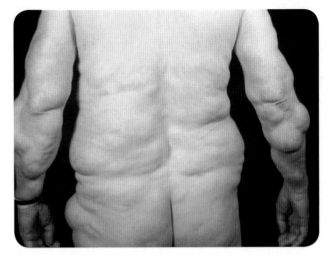

Figure 4-696 When multiple symmetrical lipomas are present, they may be painful (Dercum disease). Lesions—in this case—were not painful.

Diagnostic Pearls

- Lipomas are usually not tender; angiolipomas are tender and may have a faint overlying erythema.
- Malignant lesions tend to be tethered to the overlying skin and are, therefore, less mobile.

?? Differential Diagnosis and Pitfalls

- There is no overlying skin change, nor are there ostia or dilated pores as would be seen in an epidermoid cyst.
- Cysts are usually firmer and more superficial.
- Metastatic malignancy is usually much firmer to the touch.
- Liposarcoma
- Teratoma
- Angiomyolipomas
- Hibernomas (brown fat)
- Abscess—one would expect to see accompanying erythema and induration.
- Blue rubber bleb nevus syndrome
- Leiomyoma
- Dermatofibroma
- Glomus tumor

✓ Best Tests

- This diagnosis can often be made on clinical grounds. If the diagnosis is in doubt or there is concern for malignancy, perform a biopsy.
- A CT scan can help distinguish a lipoma from a liposarcoma.

▲▲ Management Pearls

Often, a lipoma can be fully excised through a small skin opening utilizing a "squeeze" technique. A 6 mm punch or stab incision can be made over the lipoma and then, through a combination of manual expression and curettage, the entire lipoma can be removed through the small opening.

Therapy

Lipomas do not have to be treated, but if they are progressively enlarging, excise them when they are small. Use the squeeze technique as above or make a small elliptical incision overlying the lipoma. Make sure to excise the tumor and its fibrous capsule fully to prevent recurrence.

Liposuction has also been used for the treatment of larger lesions. The advantage of liposuction is smaller incisions with less subsequent scarring.

Intralesional corticosteroids are sometimes employed to shrink smaller lipomas.

Suggested Readings

Brenn T. Neoplasms of subcutaneous fat. In: Fitzpatrick TB, Wolff K, eds. *Fitzpatrick's Dermatology in General Medicine*. 7th Ed. New York, NY: McGraw-Hill; 2008:1190–1194.

Dalal KM, Antonescu CR, Singer S. Diagnosis and management of lipomatous tumors. *J Surg Oncol*. 2008 Mar;97(4):298–313.

Furlong MA, Fanburg-Smith JC, Childers EL. Lipoma of the oral and maxillofacial region: Site and subclassification of 125 cases. *Oral Surg Oral Med Oral Pathol Oral Radiol Endod*. 2004 Oct;98(4):441–450.

Guaraldi G, Orlando G, Squillace N, et al. Prevalence of and risk factors for pubic lipoma development in HIV-infected persons. *J Acquir Immune Defic Syndr*. 2007 May;45(1):72–76.

Keskin G, Ustundag E, Ercin C. Multiple infiltrating lipomas of the tongue. *J Laryngol Otol*. 2002 May;116(5):395–397.

Kindblom LG, Angervall L, Stener B, et al. Intermuscular and intramuscular lipomas and hibernomas. A clinical, roentgenologic, histologic, and prognostic study of 46 cases. *Cancer*. 1974 Mar;33(3):754–762.

Mentzel T. Cutaneous lipomatous neoplasms. *Semin Diagn Pathol*. 2001 Nov;18(4):250–257.

Pinski KS, Roenigk HH. Liposuction of lipomas. *Dermatol Clin*. 1990 Jul;8(3): 483–492.

Silistreli OK, Durmuş EU, Ulusal BG, et al. What should be the treatment modality in giant cutaneous lipomas? Review of the literature and report of 4 cases. *Br J Plast Surg*. 2005 Apr;58(3):394–398.

Paget Disease, Extramammary

■ Diagnosis Synopsis

Extramammary Paget disease is a rare neoplastic condition of apocrine gland–bearing skin, which may be associated with internal malignancy. It is clinically and histologically similar to Paget disease of the nipple, appearing as pruritic, erythematous, scaling plaques, but the location is usually genital or perianal skin. It is more common in middle-aged to elderly white women. Extramammary Paget disease often goes undiagnosed because, clinically, it can appear similar to chronic dermatitis.

Approximately a quarter of cases are associated with an underlying neoplasm, usually adnexal apocrine carcinoma, but cases of carcinoma of the prostate, urethra, cervix, vagina, endometrium, bladder, and Bartholin glands have been described. Perianal disease is more frequently associated with an underlying carcinoma of the rectum. In light of these associations, a thorough investigation for an underlying carcinoma should accompany every confirmed diagnosis. The treatment of the condition is by surgical removal; however, recurrence is common.

◉ Look For

Dry or macerated, red (white if lichenified appearing), scaly plaques, sometimes with a verrucous surface (Figs. 4-697–4-700). Plaques are most frequently located in the perineum or genital region. There may be secondary crusting or erosion.

Less common locations include the umbilicus, cheeks, eyelids, and external auditory canal.

Pruritus is the most common symptom and may lead to excoriation and lichenification.

●● Diagnostic Pearls

- Scaly dermatic plaques, especially on the groin, that do not resolve with conventional therapies should be biopsied to exclude this diagnosis.
- Erythema of the involved area in an "underpants pattern" usually suggests dermal metastases.

?? Differential Diagnosis and Pitfalls

- Contact dermatitis
- Seborrheic dermatitis
- Psoriasis
- Lichen simplex chronicus
- Bowen disease
- Basal cell carcinoma
- Candidiasis
- Tinea cruris
- Intertrigo

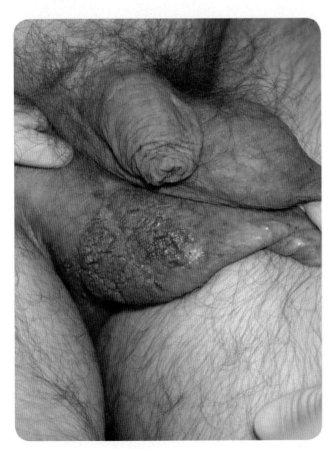

Figure 4-697 A large verrucous and eroded plaque on the scrotum is often mistaken for dermatitis when it has this type of presentation, as in this case extramammary Paget disease.

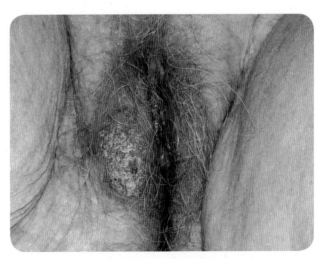

Figure 4-698 A vulvar hyperkeratotic erythematous plaque is very suggestive of Paget disease and requires a biopsy.

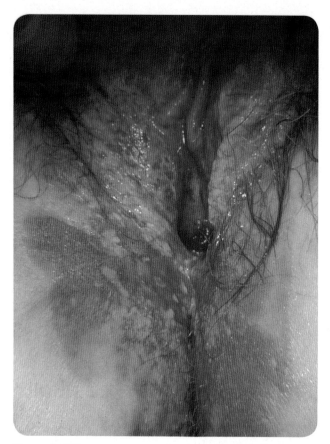

Figure 4-699 Sharply bordered, eroded plaque was extramammary Paget disease.

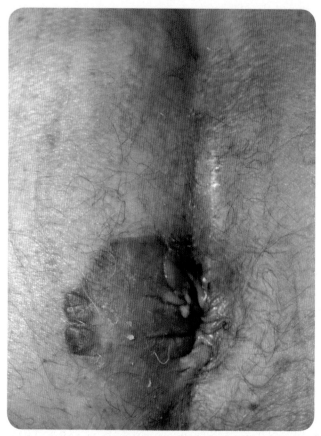

Figure 4-700 Sharply bordered, hyperpigmented plaque of extramammary Paget disease perianally and on the buttocks.

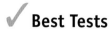

Best Tests

The diagnosis is confirmed by skin biopsy. Clinical suspicion is often elevated by a lack of response to standard topical corticosteroid regimens for presumed eczematous dermatitis.

Patients should undergo cancer screening including the following:

- Complete skin examination including lymph node exam
- Rectal exam with fecal occult blood test
- Urinalysis
- Pap smear
- Prostate-specific antigen
- Carcinoembryonic antigen
- Colonoscopy
- Possible investigations: colposcopy, urethrocystoscopy, ultrasound or CT/MRI, and esophagogastroduodenoscopy

Management Pearls

- A multidisciplinary team is often needed, including a medical oncologist. Depending on the specific location, consultation with a gynecologist, urologist, or colorectal surgeon may be needed. Consultation with a gastroenterologist may be needed to perform screening examinations.
- Patients will require frequent follow-up to assess for possible recurrence.

Therapy

Wide local excision of the entire lesion is essential. Lymph node dissection may be indicated as well. Because the lesion is often multifocal, Mohs micrographic surgery is considered optimal. Several techniques have been used to help delineate the extent of disease prior to surgery, including topical 5-fluorouracil and topical d-aminolevulinic acid with a Wood lamp.

Radiation and/or chemotherapy (mitomycin C, etoposide, cisplatin, and 5-FU) may be helpful as an adjuvant to surgery.

Imiquimod 5% cream is a useful patient-applied alternative or adjuvant in the treatment of extramammary Paget disease.

Recurrence is common, even with Mohs surgery.

Suggested Readings

Cohen Pr, Schulze KE, Tschen, JA. et al. Treatment of extramammary Paget disease with topical imiquimod cream: Case report and literature review. *South Med J.* 2006 April;99(4):396–402.

Hendi A, Brodland DG, Zitelli JA. Extramammary Paget's disease: Surgical treatment with Mohs micrographic surgery. *J Am Acad Dermatol.* 2004 Nov;51(5):767–773.

Kanitakis J. Mammary and extramammary Paget's disease. *J Eur Acad Dermatol Venereol.* 2007 May;21(5):581–590.

Mirer E, El Sayed F, Ammoury A, et al. Treatment of mammary and extramammary Paget's skin disease with topical imiquimod. *J Dermatolog Treat.* 2006;17(3):167–171.

Neuhaus IM, Grekin RC. Mammary and extramammary Paget disease. In: Fitzpatrick TB, Wolff K, eds. *Fitzpatrick's Dermatology in General Medicine.* 7th Ed. New York, NY: McGraw-Hill; 2008:1094–1096.

Shepherd V, Davidson EJ, Davies-Humphreys J. Extramammary Paget's disease. *BJOG.* 2005 Mar;112(3):273–279.

Ye JN, Rhew DC, Yip F, Edelstein L. Extramammary Paget's disease resistant to surgery and imiquimod monotherapy but responsive to imiquimod combination topical chemotherapy with 5-fluorouracil and retinoic acid: A case report. *Cutis.* 2006 Apr;77(4):245–250.

Zampogna JC, Flowers FP, Roth WI, et al. Treatment of primary limited cutaneous extramammary Paget's disease with topical imiquimod monotherapy: Two case reports. *J Am Acad Dermatol.* 2002 Oct;47(4 Suppl.):S229–S235.

Pseudolymphoma

Diagnosis Synopsis

Pseudolymphoma (cutaneous lymphoid hyperplasia) is a benign inflammatory response that histologically and often clinically mimics cutaneous lymphoma. Both T-cell and B-cell forms occur. Pseudolymphoma is characterized by dense lymphoid infiltrates of the skin, which may be focal or diffuse. Triggers include insect bites or stings, which cause local reactions, or anticonvulsant drugs, which can cause widespread eruptions. Other causes include a broad range of non-anticonvulsant drugs, tattoo dyes, trauma, vaccinations, jewelry, folliculitis, and infections such as varicella, molluscum contagiosum, HIV, and Lyme disease. Medication-related reactions may include fever, lymphadenopathy, and an erythematous skin eruption. Malaise, arthralgia, hepatosplenomegaly, eosinophilia, and abnormal liver function tests can also be present. Pseudolymphoma appears to be more common in young adult women. Very rarely, cases of pseudolymphoma evolving into lymphoma have occurred.

Look For

The typical lesion is a pruritic, smooth-surfaced papule, nodule, or plaque on the head or neck (Figs. 4-701–4-704).

Lesions are usually solitary and range from 0.5 to 3.0 cm in diameter.

Pseudolymphoma may also present as widespread dermal papules with or without scale. Lesions are often red to violaceous, but they may be skin colored.

Other sites of predilection are the chest and upper extremities.

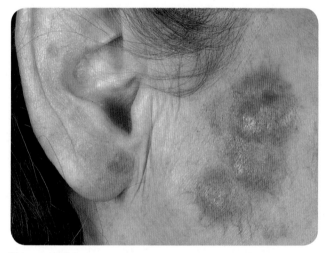

Figure 4-702 A red plaque on the face and a nodule on the ear were pseudolymphomas.

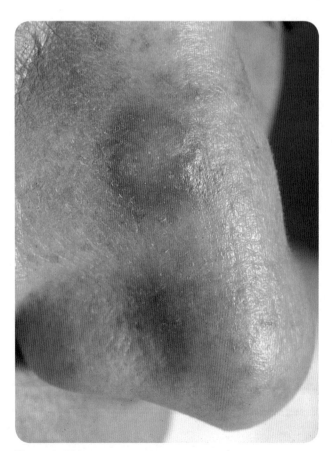

Figure 4-701 A discrete, red plaque was a pseudolymphoma.

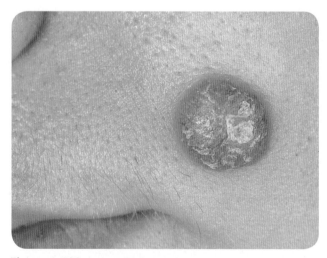

Figure 4-703 A well-demarcated facial plaque was a pseudolymphoma.

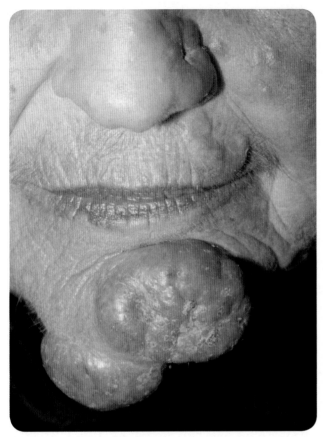

Figure 4-704 Clinically, this large nodule would be thought to be malignant but was a pseudolymphoma.

Diagnostic Pearls

- In pseudolymphoma, there is no atrophy of the skin, which distinguishes it from long-term lupus.
- The lesions of pseudolymphoma infrequently occur below the waist.

?? Differential Diagnosis and Pitfalls

- Insect bite—can be multiple
- B-cell lymphoma
- Mycosis fungoides—can be patches or plaques
- Nodular scabies—extremely pruritic
- Lymphomatoid papulosis—some of the papules are crusted with necrotic centers
- Lymphomatoid granulomatosis
- Actinic reticuloid
- Follicular mucinosis
- Lupus erythematosus
- Syphilis
- Sweet syndrome

✓ Best Tests

- Skin biopsy with immunophenotyping of the infiltrate. A highly sensitive technique, such as gene rearrangements, may be used to determine the presence of monoclonal receptor populations.
- No single laboratory test distinguishes cutaneous lymphoma from pseudolymphoma; clinicopathologic correlation is often required.

▲▲ Management Pearls

Patients should have close follow-up to rule out lymphoma.

Therapy

Remove the inciting agent, if it is known. Removal is often sufficient for disease resolution. Stopping anticonvulsants typically results in symptom resolution within 3 to 4 weeks.

Topical Corticosteroids
- Hydrocortisone valerate 0.2% applied twice daily until resolution
- Betamethasone 0.05% cream or ointment applied twice daily for up to 2 weeks
- Clobetasol applied twice daily for up to 2 weeks
- Fluocinonide cream or ointment 0.05% applied twice daily for up to 2 weeks

Other treatment modalities include simple surgical excision for solitary lesions, cryotherapy, photodynamic therapy, or local radiation. Topical tacrolimus, intralesional corticosteroids, and intralesional interferon alpha-2B have also been reported as useful approaches to treating pseudolymphoma.

Suggested Readings

Albrecht J, Fine LA, Piette W. Drug-associated lymphoma and pseudolymphoma: Recognition and management. *Dermatol Clin.* 2007 Apr;25(2):233–244, vii.

Cerroni L, Kerl H. Diagnostic immunohistology: Cutaneous lymphomas and pseudolymphomas. *Semin Cutan Med Surg.* 1999 Mar;18(1):64–70.

Dionyssopoulos A, Mandekou-Lefaki I, Delli FS, et al. T- and B-cutaneous pseudolymphomas treated by surgical excision and immediate reconstruction. *Dermatol Surg.* 2006 Dec;32(12):1526–1529.

Lee MW, Lee DK, Choi JH, et al. Clinicopathologic study of cutaneous pseudolymphomas. *J Dermatol.* 2005 Jul;32(7):594–601.

Maubec E, Pinquier L, Viguier M, et al. Vaccination-induced cutaneous pseudolymphoma. *J Am Acad Dermatol.* 2005 Apr;52(4):623–629.

Mikasa K, Watanabe D, Kondo C, et al. Topical 5-aminolevulinic acid-based photodynamic therapy for the treatment of a patient with cutaneous pseudolymphoma. *J Am Acad Dermatol*. 2005 Nov;53(5):911–912.

Moreno-Ramírez D, García-Escudero A, Ríos-Martín JJ, et al. Cutaneous pseudolymphoma in association with molluscum contagiosum in an elderly patient. *J Cutan Pathol*. 2003 Aug;30(7):473–475.

Ploysangam T, Breneman DL, Mutasim DF. Cutaneous pseudolymphomas. *J Am Acad Dermatol*. 1998 Jun;38(6 Pt 1):877–895; quiz 896–897.

Rijlaarsdam JU, Willemze R. Cutaneous pseudolymphomas: Classification and differential diagnosis. *Semin Dermatol*. 1994 Sep;13(3):187–196.

Schreiber MM, McGregor JG. Pseudolymphoma syndrome. A sensitivity to anticonvulsant drugs. *Arch Dermatol*. 1968 Mar;97(3):297–300.

Tomar S, Stoll HL, Grassi MA, et al. Treatment of cutaneous pseudolymphoma with interferon alpha-2b. *J Am Acad Dermatol*. 2009 Jan;60(1):172–174.

Rheumatoid Nodule

◼◼ Diagnosis Synopsis

Rheumatoid nodules occur as the most common cutaneous manifestation of rheumatoid arthritis. The characteristic rheumatoid nodule occurs in 20% of patients with rheumatoid arthritis and may be an indication of a more severe form of the disease. The etiology of rheumatoid nodules remains unclear, but both vascular and external trauma, combined with pooling of rheumatoid immune complexes, likely lead to the formation of the nodule. Rheumatoid nodules may also occur within internal organs such as the heart, lungs, and muscle. Visceral nodules may clinically mimic infection, malignancy, or other inflammatory processes such as Wegener granulomatosis. Very rarely, nodules occur in the sclera, causing it to atrophy and perforate.

These patients will have a moderate to high titer of rheumatoid factor. Sometimes, however, patients with mild rheumatoid arthritis may also develop nodules, as may patients who have rheumatoid disease without joint involvement. Nodules can also precede the onset of arthritis by a number of years.

Nodules on pressure areas, such as the sacrum, have a tendency to ulcerate. Subsequent secondary infection can lead to septicemia and septic arthritis. More complications of nodule formation are pain, reduced joint mobility, and neuropathy.

Nodules are composed of fibrous tissue with areas of fibrinoid necrosis, typically with palisaded granulomas in the deep dermis and subcutis. Nodules may stay the same size or grow larger. They may persist indefinitely or resolve spontaneously. Neuropathy and fistula formation are also known to occur.

Rheumatoid Nodulosis

This is a variant of rheumatoid disease in which nodules appear in the absence of synovitis. These nodules tend to be smaller than rheumatoid nodules and occur mostly on the hands and feet. After a number of years, rheumatoid nodulosis may convert to rheumatoid disease in which the joints are affected. The initiation of methotrexate therapy is a known trigger of nodulosis, especially on the hands.

Benign Rheumatoid Nodules

Nodules may sometimes be present in healthy young children in the absence of rheumatoid disease. The location of these nodules is different from those of typical rheumatoid nodules in that these occur mainly on the pretibial areas, feet, and scalp.

Immunocompromised Patient Considerations

Superinfection of rheumatoid nodules is a rare complication of immunosuppressive therapy for rheumatoid arthritis.

Various stages of HIV infection can lead to both improvement and worsening of the symptoms of rheumatoid arthritis, including nodules. Massive pulmonary rheumatoid nodules in an HIV-infected patient have been described.

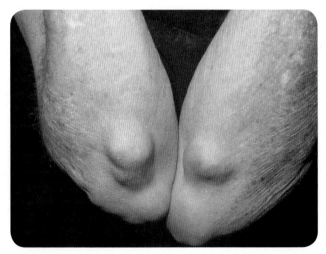

Figure 4-705 Typical location of rheumatoid nodules on the extensor surface of the elbows.

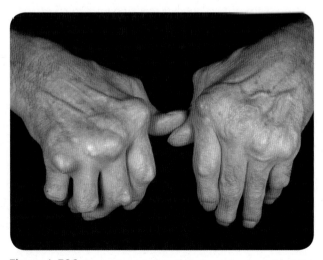

Figure 4-706 The extensor surface of the hands is a typical location for rheumatoid nodules.

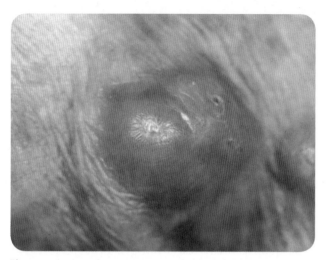

Figure 4-707 Rheumatoid nodules may have the "apple jelly" color of granulomatous inflammation.

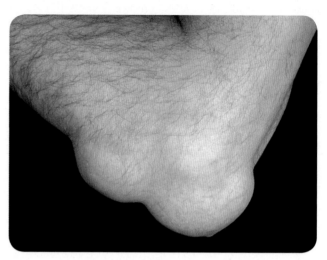

Figure 4-708 Nodules in the olecranon region may not seem inflammatory and have to be distinguished from gouty tophi.

Look For

Rheumatoid nodules are firm, skin-colored subcutaneous nodules (Figs. 4-705–4-708). They are semimobile and usually painless on palpation. Nodules are mostly located on the extensor surfaces and over pressure areas such as the sacrum. Nodules occur most commonly in periarticular locations and are most frequently seen on the ulnar border of the forearm. Other less common locations are the dorsa of the hands, on the knees and ears, along Achilles tendons, and across the scapulae. The size of the nodules varies, and they may reach 5 cm or more in diameter.

Look for ulceration of the nodule, as this may lead to septicemia or septic arthritis.

Diagnostic Pearls

The presence of firm subcutaneous nodules in an extensor distribution in a patient with existing rheumatoid arthritis is highly suggestive of the diagnosis of rheumatoid nodules.

?? Differential Diagnosis and Pitfalls

- Subcutaneous granuloma annulare
- Gout
- Pseudogout
- Xanthoma (reveal foam cells on histology)
- Foreign body reaction
- Calcinosis cutis
- Myxoid cyst
- Dermatomyositis

- Papulonecrotic tuberculid (tuberculin test will show a positive reaction, and associated signs of pulmonary or extra pulmonary disease will be present)
- Necrobiosis lipoidica diabeticorum
- Lipoma
- Sarcoidosis
- Lymphadenopathy
- Mycobacterial infection (*Mycobacterium marinum*)
- Deep fungal infection
- Churg-Strauss granuloma
- Erythema elevatum diutinum

Visceral Nodules

- Granulomatous infectious processes
- Wegener granulomatosis
- Malignancy

✓ Best Tests

Rheumatoid factor is usually high in patients with rheumatoid nodules.

▲▲ Management Pearls

- Nodules that are present over areas of repetitive trauma tend to recur in a very short time after being surgically removed.
- As rheumatoid nodules are predictors of severe or advanced arthritis, their presence indicates that more aggressive management of the underlying disease is required.

Therapy

As rheumatoid nodules are usually asymptomatic, treatment is generally requested for cosmetic purposes. Nodules that need to be treated are those that are exposed to constant trauma or those that are on weight-bearing prominences. If these nodules are not treated, complications may develop.

Treatment

- Surgical excision.
- Injecting corticosteroid directly into the nodule can also be tried and sometimes reduces its size.
- The underlying rheumatoid arthritis should also be managed aggressively, if not already done so.

Suggested Readings

Arnold C. The management of rheumatoid nodules. *Am J Orthop.* 1996 Oct;25(10):706–708.

Baan H, Haagsma CJ, van de Laar MA. Corticosteroid injections reduce size of rheumatoid nodules. *Clin Rheumatol.* 2006 Feb;25(1):21–23.

García-Patos V. Rheumatoid nodule. *Semin Cutan Med Surg.* 2007 Jun;26(2):100–107.

Highton J, Hessian PA, Stamp L. The Rheumatoid nodule: peripheral or central to rheumatoid arthritis? *Rheumatology (Oxford).* 2007 Sep;46(9):1385–7.

McGrath MH, Fleischer A. The subcutaneous rheumatoid nodule. *Hand Clin.* 1989 May;5(2):127–135.

Mine T, Tanaka H, Taguchi T, et al. A giant rheumatoid nodule. *Clin Rheumatol.* 2004 Oct;23(5):467–469.

Rencic A, Nousari CH. Other rheumatologic diseases. In: Bolognia J, Jorizzo JL, Rapini RP, eds. *Dermatology.* 2nd Ed. St. Louis, MO: Mosby; 2008:605–606.

Sander O, Scherer A. Mimicry of a rheumatoid nodule by tophaceous pseudogout at the elbow. *J Rheumatol.* 2008 Jul;35(7):1419.

Winne L, Praet M, Brusselle G, et al. Bilateral spontaneous pneumothorax in a patient with pulmonary rheumatoid nodules, secondary infected by Aspergillus. *Clin Rheumatol.* 2007 Jul;26(7):1180–1182.

Ziff M. The rheumatoid nodule. *Arthritis Rheum.* 1990 Jun;33(6):761–767.

Squamous Cell Carcinoma (SCC)

▪▪ Diagnosis Synopsis

Squamous cell carcinoma (SCC) is a malignancy of cutaneous epithelial cells occurring most frequently on sun-exposed areas of the skin, particularly the face and dorsal hands. Actinic keratoses may be a precursor lesion. The clinical presentation is highly variable among different demographic groups and tumor subtypes. SCC can involve the oral mucosa and lip and, when it does, it carries a much greater risk of metastases. Risk factors for the development of SCC include chronic sun exposure, fair skin and blue eyes, family history of skin cancer, scarring processes (chronic ulcers, burns, hidradenitis), ionizing radiation, immunosuppression, certain subtypes of human papillomavirus (HPV), and chemical carcinogens. Several genetic syndromes are associated with an increased risk of SCC as well. These include xeroderma pigmentosum, oculocutaneous albinism, epidermodysplasia verruciformis, epidermolysis bullosa, and KID syndrome (keratitis-ichthyosis-deafness).

Squamous cell carcinoma in situ (SCCIS) is confined to the epidermis and includes other specific clinical entities such as Bowen disease and erythroplasia of Queyrat (on the male genitalia). As in invasive disease, SCCIS is more frequent and more aggressive in immunosuppressed individuals.

Dark Skin Considerations

Although the yearly incidence of SCC is 3.4 per 100,000 among blacks, or about 80 times less than the rate observed among whites, it is the most commonly seen skin cancer in blacks. Unlike in whites, most SCC in blacks occurs on non–sun-exposed skin and is not as strongly associated with preexisting actinic keratoses. Blacks with SCC have a higher mortality rate, which may reflect later diagnosis and/or the more aggressive nature of the disease. SCC occurring on covered skin has a higher metastatic potential. Whether SCC is inherently more aggressive in blacks is not known. However, it may occur in chronic sun-exposed lesions of discoid lupus erythematosus and in keloids and chronic hidradenitis suppurativa lesions.

◉ Look For

The majority of SCC lesions appear on chronically sun-damaged skin of the head, neck, forearms, and dorsal hands. The clinical presentation may be variable. SCC often presents as an erythematous, hyperkeratotic papule or nodule that may ulcerate, but it may also be skin colored and/or smooth (Figs. 4-709–4-714). Over time, the tumor often develops a depressed center, and the growth becomes fixed

Immunocompromised Patient Considerations

SCC tends to be much more frequent and aggressive in the immunocompromised patient. These malignant tumors are prevalent in organ transplant recipients and those with HIV/AIDS. Patients with AIDS have a three to five times increased risk of SCC; even with antiretroviral therapy, the risk in HIV-infected patients is still 1.5–2 times that of the general population. Risk for SCC directly correlates to the length and degree of the immunosuppressive regimen. Azathioprine and cyclosporine use appears to present higher risk than other immunosuppressive agents. Other risk factors for developing SCC include increased lifetime UV exposure, increased age, a light skin type, blue eyes, personal or family history of skin cancer or actinic keratoses, and prior HPV infection. Heart transplant patients are at greatest risk, followed by renal patients, and finally liver transplant recipients. In one prospective study, the annual incidence of SCC in renal transplant patients was 3.5%, with increasing incidence and with longer duration of immunosuppression.

Penile or anal SCC is seen more frequently in patients with HIV/AIDS. The risk of anal SCC is at least two-fold greater in HIV-infected individuals. These tumors often develop within longstanding condyloma acuminata. Mucosal papillary tumors or flat lesions are seen, and symptoms may include pain, itching, burning, and/or bleeding. Over time, the lesions slowly progress into a tumorous mass or slowly infiltrate into deeper tissue.

In the HIV-infected patient, one must consider the possibility of anal intraepithelial neoplasia (AIN), which is a corollary to cervical intraepithelial neoplasia. HIV-infected patients should undergo routine screening for possible AIN and anal SCC.

to the underlying structures. New masses appearing within scars or chronic ulcers should be considered highly suspicious for SCC.

Verrucous carcinoma is a rare, well-differentiated variety of SCC that presents as a glassy or shiny nodular growth. Oral, anogenital, foot, and subungual variants exist.

Dark Skin Considerations

Patients of darker skin types may present with a pigmented variant of SCC. In blacks, the lesions may be erythematous with varying degrees of scale and crust, and they may be mistaken for psoriasis, eczema, infection, or trauma.

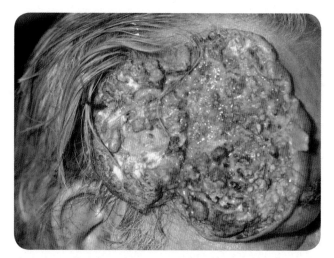

Figure 4-709 Giant ulcerating SCC of the forehead. The rolled border may be clinically confused with a basal cell carcinoma.

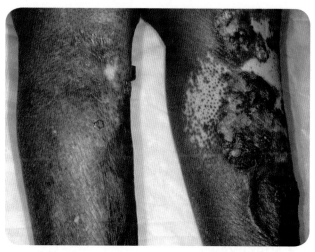

Figure 4-710 SCC can occur in the atrophic plaques secondary to burns (Marjolin ulcer).

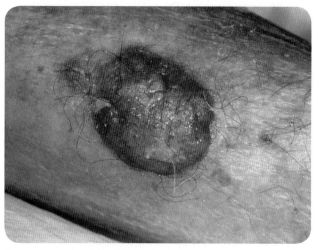

Figure 4-711 Red nodule with glistening epithelial surface that was a SCC on biopsy.

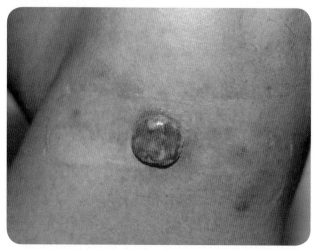

Figure 4-712 Merkel cell carcinomas arise on sun-exposed skin and clinically resemble a nodular SCC.

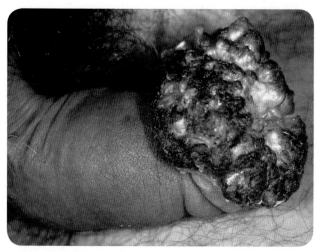

Figure 4-713 SCC of the penis is often a sequela of HPV-16 or HPV-18 infection.

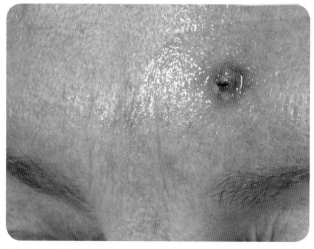

Figure 4-714 Irregular ulceration on the forehead with some scaling is one presentation of SCC.

Immunocompromised Patient Considerations

In the immunocompromised patient, an SCC can occur anywhere on the body, including the oral, anal, cervical mucosa, and male genitals. In the fair-skinned transplant patient, SCCs typically arise as scaly or warty papules in an area of prior sun damage. Thick, scaly, crusted papules can quickly evolve into nodules and even tumors. Some plaques will ulcerate and bleed. Multiple primary lesions are frequently present in this population.

 ## Diagnostic Pearls

The skin of patients with SCC will often display other evidence of sun exposure (e.g., solar elastosis, actinic keratoses, and solar lentigines).

Dark Skin Considerations

Predisposing factors that are important in the development of SCC in blacks include old burn scars, chronic cutaneous ulcers or inflammation, previous sites of irradiation, chronic lymphedema, stasis, albinism, and chronic discoid lupus erythematosus.

Immunocompromised Patient Considerations

In the immunocompromised, such as transplant patients, keep a high index of suspicion when looking at any warty or scaly solitary lesion. With a persistent nonhealing lesion, one must always consider SCC.

?? Differential Diagnosis and Pitfalls

- Actinic keratosis
- Bowen disease
- Basal cell carcinoma
- Verruca vulgaris
- Keratoacanthoma
- Eccrine poroma
- Pyogenic granuloma
- Amelanotic melanoma
- Deep fungal infection
- Nummular eczema
- Atypical fibroxanthoma
- Cutaneous neuroendocrine carcinoma

- Irritated seborrheic keratosis
- Chronic draining or ulcerative lesions
- Hypertrophic discoid lupus erythematosus
- Hypertrophic lichen planus
- Prurigo nodularis

 ## Best Tests

- A thorough history and physical exam is the most effective means of detection. Biopsy of the lesion will demonstrate characteristic histopathology.
- Palpate for regional lymphadenopathy, and perform a complete skin examination in any patient with a suspicious lesion.
- Depending on the clinical scenario, imaging such as a CT scan may prove helpful in a staging workup.

▲▲ Management Pearls

SCC of the head and neck, including the oral mucosa, has a higher likelihood of metastasis. Refer these patients to a specialist.

Immunocompromised Patient Considerations

SCC in the immunocompromised patient has a high propensity for metastasis. Refer these patients to a specialist if the tumor is not easily excised or there are multiple lesions. In the transplant patient with widespread multiple SCCs and precancerous actinic keratoses, consider using an oral retinoid for chemoprophylaxis.

Therapy

Both Mohs micrographic surgery and standard surgical excision with 3 to 4 mm margins are first-line treatments. In high-risk SCC in which Mohs surgery is not performed, 6 mm margins are typically required. In cases of known or suspected nodal metastases, sentinel or formal lymph node dissection is often indicated.

For patients who are not surgical candidates, a number of therapeutic modalities are available. For superficial SCCs, electrodesiccation and curettage (times 3) with margins of 3 to 4 mm may be used. Radiation therapy is another reasonable alternative for poor surgical candidates.

Several treatments may be tried as second- or third-line options, particularly in patients who are not amenable to surgery or those with an extensive burden of disease. These include

- Topical imiquimod
- Topical or intralesional 5-fluorouracil
- Electrochemotherapy with intralesional bleomycin
- Intralesional interferon alpha
- Photodynamic therapy

Immunocompromised Patient Considerations

Complete, timely excision of the lesion is indicated. Staging is essential to select the most appropriate surgical approach and the necessity for node dissection. Mohs surgery is the most appropriate treatment for almost all lesions except for smaller and superficial SCC lesions that can be excised easily. Wide local excision is suggested for scrotal SCC. Partial and total penectomy are last resort options.

Suggested Readings

Alam M, Ratner D. Cutaneous squamous-cell carcinoma. *N Engl J Med.* 2001 Mar;344(13):975–983.

Drake LA, Dinehart SM, Goltz RW, et al. Guidelines of care for Mohs micrographic surgery. American Academy of Dermatology. *J Am Acad Dermatol.* 1995 Aug;33(2 Pt 1):271–278.

Drake AL, Walling HW. Variations in presentation of squamous cell carcinoma in situ (Bowen's disease) in immunocompromised patients. *J Am Acad Dermatol.* 2008 Jul;59(1):68–71.

Grossman DG, Leffell DJ. Squamous cell carcinoma. In: Fitzpatrick TB, Wolff K, eds. *Fitzpatrick's Dermatology in General Medicine.* 7th Ed. New York, NY: McGraw-Hill; 2008:1028–1036.

Hashi N, Shirato H, Omatsu T, et al. The role of radiotherapy in treating squamous cell carcinoma of the external auditory canal, especially in early stages of disease. *Radiother Oncol.* 2000 Aug;56(2):221–225.

Miller SJ, Alam M, Andersen J, et al.; National Comprehensive Cancer Network. Basal cell and squamous cell skin cancers. *J Natl Compr Canc Netw.* 2007 May;5(5):506–529.

Pivot X, Felip E; ESMO Guidelines Working Group. Squamous cell carcinoma of the head and neck: ESMO clinical Recommendations for diagnosis, treatment and follow-up. *Ann Oncol.* 2008 May;19(Suppl. 2):ii79–ii80.

Rigel DS, Cockerell CJ, Carucci J, et al. Actinic keratosis, basal cell carcinoma, and squamous cell carcinoma. In: Bolognia J, Jorizzo JL, Rapini RP, eds. *Dermatology.* 2nd Ed. St. Louis, MO: Mosby; 2008:1645–1651.

Smeets NW, Kuijpers DI, Nelemans P, et al. Mohs' micrographic surgery for treatment of basal cell carcinoma of the face—results of a retrospective study and review of the literature. *Br J Dermatol.* 2004 Jul;151(1):141–147.

Stasko T, Brown MD, Carucci JA, et al.; International Transplant-Skin Cancer Collaborative, European Skin Care in Organ Transplant Patients Network. Guidelines for the management of squamous cell carcinoma in organ transplant recipients. *Dermatol Surg.* 2004 Apr; 30(4 Pt 2):642–650.

Tillman DK, Carroll MT. Topical imiquimod therapy for basal and squamous cell carcinomas: A clinical experience. *Cutis.* 2007 Mar;79(3):241–248.

Acne Keloidalis Nuchae

■■ Diagnosis Synopsis

Acne keloidalis nuchae (AKN), or folliculitis keloidalis, is a chronic inflammatory disease in which keloid-like papules, plaques, and pustules occur at the nape of the neck and on the occipital scalp. Inflammation of the hair follicle and fibrosis of the tissue typically result in scarring. The condition is often painful and disfiguring. The etiology is idiopathic, although a number of causes have been suggested, including friction from shirt collars, football or military helmets, trauma from shaving or short haircuts, chronic bacterial infection, or an autoimmune process. Some believe that AKN is a form of scarring alopecia. Furthermore, the term "acne keloidalis" is a misnomer, as keloids at other locations or a family history of keloids are not features of the disease. The overwhelming majority of patients with AKN are young adult black or Hispanic men. AKN is rare in prepubertal children.

◉ Look For

AKN starts as follicular papules and pustules (often eroded or excoriated) on the superior back, nape of the neck, and the occipital scalp (Figs. 4-715–4-718). The papules and pustules may coalesce as they partially heal to form keloid-like, firm plaques. Scarring alopecia and subcutaneous abscesses with draining sinuses may be present.

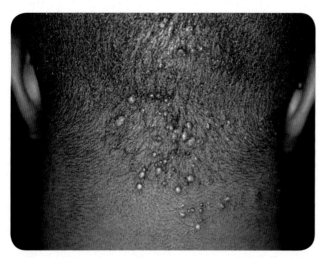

Figure 4-715 Mildest forms of AKN often have multiple discrete shiny papules.

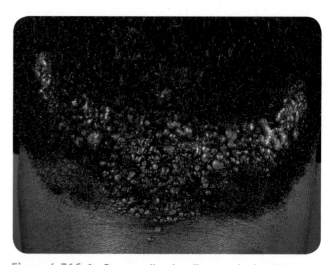

Figure 4-716 Confluent small and medium papules in AKN.

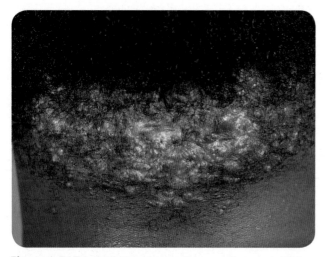

Figure 4-717 Inflammation and erosions are often seen in AKN.

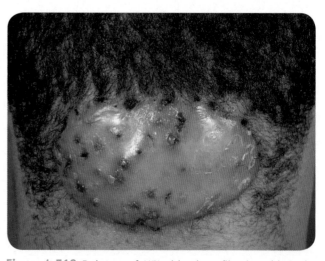

Figure 4-718 End stage of AKN with a large fibrotic and hypopigmented mass.

Dark Skin Considerations

This condition mostly commonly affects dark-skinned males, especially those with coarse, curly hair.

Diagnostic Pearls

Comedones (such as in cases of acne) are not present. Early lesions have a follicular distribution. Patients frequently have a history of sports helmet use or occupational headgear that presses on the affected sites.

?? Differential Diagnosis and Pitfalls

- Sarcoidosis can present with keloid-like papules in this area.
- Tinea capitis/kerion is a dermatophyte infection commonly seen in children.
- Folliculitis may affect other hair-bearing areas of the body.
- Dissecting cellulitis of the scalp frequently involves the vertex in addition to the occiput.
- Hidradenitis suppurativa—Usually located in axillary, inguinal, or anogenital areas.
- Acne vulgaris—Look for comedones.
- Keloids
- Nevus sebaceous
- Pseudofolliculitis barbae

✓ Best Tests

- The diagnosis may be made clinically, as the presence of papules, pustules, and scar formation at the occiput of a black male is virtually pathognomonic, but a definitive diagnosis can only be made by deep biopsy (below the level of the follicular bulbs and scar tissue). Proceed with biopsy if the presentation is atypical.
- Obtain a bacterial culture with sensitivities from any pustular or draining lesions. This will help identify infected lesions and exclude other diagnoses (e.g., *Staphylococcus aureus* folliculitis).

▲▲ Management Pearls

If excising lesions and closing the defect primarily, always follow surgery with regular (every 3 to 4 weeks) intralesional triamcinolone injections and a silastic pressure dressing to the site. Concerns over keloidal scarring should not prohibit obtaining a biopsy.

Therapy

Discourage skin picking, wearing shirts with tight collars, and close hair cutting/shaving. Athletes who frequently wear helmets should ensure that they fit properly.

Topical Therapies
Clindamycin 1% applied twice daily to pustular, crusted, or draining lesions. If there is no improvement with topical antimicrobials, consider systemic therapy (see below). A combination of tretinoin and a class 2 or 3 topical steroid may improve symptoms and flatten lesions.

High-potency topical corticosteroids (class 2)

- Fluocinonide cream, ointment—apply twice daily (15, 30, 60, 120 g)
- Desoximetasone cream, ointment—apply twice daily (15, 60, 120 g)
- Halcinonide cream, ointment—apply twice daily (15, 60, 240 g)
- Amcinonide ointment—apply twice daily (15, 30, 60 g)

Mid-potency topical corticosteroids (classes 3 and 4)

- Triamcinolone cream, ointment—apply twice daily (15, 30, 60, 120, 240 g)
- Mometasone cream, ointment—apply twice daily (15, 45 g)
- Fluocinolone ointment, cream—apply twice daily (15, 30, 60 g)

Intralesional triamcinolone acetonide (10 to 40 mg/mL) is another alternative. Patients should be warned that the injected areas may become hypopigmented.

Systemic Therapies
- Antibiotics—Erythromycin 333 mg three times daily, minocycline 100 mg twice daily, or tetracycline 500 to 1,000 mg twice daily are possibilities
- Isotretinoin has resulted in dramatic improvement in one case report

Surgical Treatments
- Laser therapy—Carbon dioxide or Nd:YAG laser treatments have been successful for a few patients. Follow up with intralesional triamcinolone injections every 2 to 3 weeks.
- Excision—Numerous methods have been described. Elliptical excision with primary closure works well for smaller lesions. Excision should extend to the deep fat or fascia below the hair follicles. Larger lesions should be excised in stages or permitted to heal by secondary intention.

Suggested Readings

Adegbidi H, Atadokpede F, do Ango-Padonou F, et al. Keloid acne of the neck: Epidemiological studies over 10 years. *Int J Dermatol.* 2005 Oct;44(Suppl. 1):49–50.

Gloster HM. The surgical management of extensive cases of acne keloidalis nuchae. *Arch Dermatol.* 2000 Nov;136(11):1376–1379.

Kantor GR, Ratz JL, Wheeland RG. Treatment of acne keloidalis nuchae with carbon dioxide laser. *J Am Acad Dermatol.* 1986 Feb;14(2 Pt 1):263–267.

Kelly AP. Pseudofolliculitis barbae and acne keloidalis nuchae. *Dermatol Clin.* 2003 Oct;21(4):645–653.

Knable AL, Hanke CW, Gonin R. Prevalence of acne keloidalis nuchae in football players. *J Am Acad Dermatol.* 1997 Oct;37(4):570–574.

McMichael A, Guzman Sanchez D, Kelly P. Folliculitis and the Follicular Occlusion Tetrad. In: Bolognia JL, Jorizzo JL, Rapini RP, eds. *Dermatology.* 2nd Ed. St. Louis, MO: Mosby; 2008:526–527.

Quarles FN, Brody H, Badreshia S, et al. Acne keloidalis nuchae. *Dermatol Ther.* 2007 May–Jun;20(3):128–132.

Alopecia Areata

⬛ Diagnosis Synopsis

Alopecia areata is a T-lymphocyte–mediated autoimmune disease of the hair follicle resulting in nonscarring hair loss. Most cases are limited to one or two small patches of alopecia, but in severe cases all the hair on the scalp is lost (alopecia totalis) or all body hair is lost (alopecia universalis). Hair in most patients will spontaneously regrow, though recurrences are common. Alopecia areata is seen equally in both sexes and in patients of all ages and ethnicities. It may be seasonal. There is an increased incidence of alopecia areata in patients with Down syndrome, lichen planus, and other autoimmune diseases such as vitiligo, lupus erythematosus, rheumatoid arthritis, pernicious anemia, or thyroid disease. The most frequent association is with thyroid disease. Patients with alopecia areata are also more likely to have atopy, and its

presence is felt to be a poor prognostic indicator for alopecia areata. The condition is treatable but cannot be cured.

◉ Look For

The course of alopecia areata is unpredictable, with wide variation in duration and extent of disease occurring from patient to patient. Also look for round, patchy areas of nonscarring hair loss (Figs. 4-719 and 4-720). Although it usually affects the scalp, the condition can also target the eyebrows (Fig. 4-721), eyelashes, beard (Fig. 4-722), and other body sites. Additionally, pitting and ridging of the fingernails can occur with this disease. Hairs that grow back are often hypopigmented, temporarily or permanently. This hypopigmentation is not seen in other forms of alopecia.

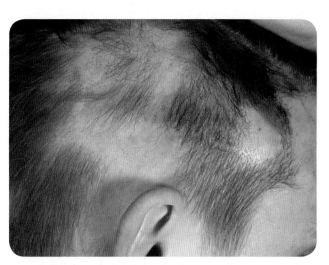

Figure 4-719 Multiple regions of alopecia areata of the scalp.

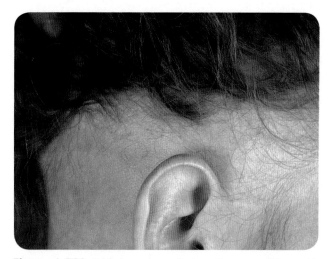

Figure 4-720 Ophiasis pattern of alopecia areata with a wide peripheral rim of baldness.

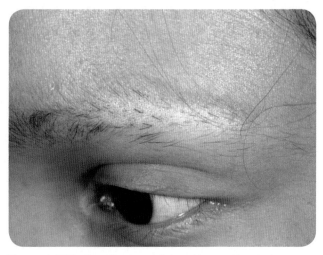

Figure 4-721 Alopecia areata of the eyebrow and eyelashes.

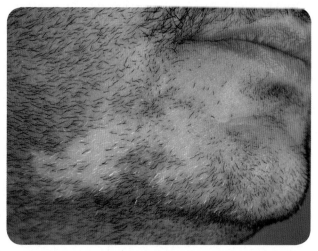

Figure 4-722 Alopecia areata of the beard with associated hypopigmentation (poliosis) of regrowing hairs.

Often when there is a regrowth after diffuse loss, a patch of alopecia also along the inferior hairline from ear to ear remains, and this is temporal ophiasis pattern.

Diagnostic Pearls

- Scalp burning with or without slight erythema (peach colored) can accompany the lesions. Exclamation point hairs with a tapering base and a ragged proximal portion are diagnostic of the disease. They are frequently at the border of the lesions and can be seen with the aid of a magnifying glass. The ragged end is easily seen under the microscope.
- A positive pull test from the periphery of a patch of hair loss indicates that the disease is active and additional hair loss can be expected.

Dark Skin Considerations

In blacks, traction alopecia often resembles ophiasis, a form of alopecia areata where the hair loss occurs at the hairline. The ragged end is easily seen microscopically.

Differential Diagnosis and Pitfalls

- Trichotillomania, from the twisting and pulling of hair, may mimic alopecia areata. Hairs are broken off at varying lengths.
- Telogen effluvium from nutritional, hormonal, and drug etiologies can lead to large clumps of hair coming out in a similar fashion to alopecia areata. The loss is diffuse, not localized.
- Tinea capitis
- Syphilis
- Loose anagen syndrome
- Androgenetic alopecia
- Pseudopelade of Brocq/scarring alopecia

✓ Best Tests

- This diagnosis can usually be made clinically.
- Scalp biopsy is diagnostic in equivocal cases.
- If the clinical situation warrants, tests for associated conditions may be fruitful:
  - ANA, rheumatoid factor
  - Thyroid function tests
  - Serum vitamin B_{12}

Dark Skin Considerations

In a black patient, a fungal culture is an effective way of establishing or excluding tinea capitis.

▲▲ Management Pearls

- It is important to help the patient understand the unpredictable nature of the disease and that there is often a chance of some regrowth. The condition is benign, and, therefore, treatment is optional.
- Wigs, hats, caps, and scarves are important options for some patients.

Therapy

Counsel carefully before attempting treatment, which is often unsuccessful. Patients with limited areas of loss in regions of no cosmetic importance are often best left untreated because spontaneous regrowth often occurs within a year. Treatments may stimulate hair growth, but there is no evince that the natural course of disease is altered.

Very limited mild alopecia areata and children with alopecia areata are often treated with topical mid-high potency steroids. A common side effect is atrophy. Greater extent of disease (totalis and universalis) confers a worse prognosis.

Mild to moderate alopecia areata (<25% involvement) can be treated with intralesional corticosteroids to speed regrowth: triamcinolone acetonide aqueous suspension (5 to 10 mg/mL) injected just beneath the dermis in per 0.1 mL injection (maximum 1 to 2 mL per monthly visit). Repeat at 4 to 6 week intervals. Adverse effects including pain during injection and atrophy are generally temporary.

Topical immunotherapy with diphencyprone to induce a contact dermatitis is another alternative. A 2% lotion is applied initially to a small area of alopecia to incite an allergic contact reaction. Subsequent weekly applications to larger areas of alopecia should be at more dilute concentrations (0.001% to 0.1%) that maintain a tolerable level of pruritus and erythema.

Topical steroids (clobetasol propionate gel or solution twice daily and/or with occlusion nightly) and anthralin cream 1.0% applied for 10 to 20 min daily to the area and approximately 1 cm beyond the border (wash off with shampoo) are other approved therapies. Anthralin is messy and stains fabrics and often stains skin.

For extensive disease, consider psoralen plus UVA (PUVA) or topical steroids plus minoxidil (each applied twice daily). The efficacy of each is debated. Systemic corticosteroids may offer short-term help, but they have no long-term benefit and should be considered cautiously.

Suggested Readings

Ajith C, Gupta S, Kanwar AJ. Efficacy and safety of the topical sensitizer squaric acid dibutyl ester in Alopecia areata and factors influencing the outcome. *J Drugs Dermatol*. 2006 Mar;5(3):262–266.

Delamere FM, Sladden MM, Dobbins HM, et al. Interventions for alopecia areata. *Cochrane Database Syst Rev*. 2008 Apr;(2):CD004413.

Joly P. The use of methotrexate alone or in combination with low doses of oral corticosteroids in the treatment of alopecia totalis or universalis. *J Am Acad Dermatol*. 2006 Oct;55(4):632–636.

Olsen E, Hordinsky M, McDonald-Hull S, et al. Alopecia areata investigational assessment guidelines. National Alopecia Areata Foundation. *J Am Acad Dermatol*. 1999 Feb;40(2 Pt 1):242–246.

Paus R, Olsen EA, Messenger AG. Hair growth disorders. In: Fitzpatrick TB, Wolff K, eds. *Fitzpatrick's Dermatology in General Medicine*. 7th Ed. New York, NY: McGraw-Hill; 2008:762–765.

Price VH. Treatment of hair loss. *N Engl J Med*. 1999 Sep;341(13):964–973.

Wasserman D, Guzman-Sanchez DA, Scott K, et al. Alopecia areata. *Int J Dermatol*. 2007 Feb;46(2):121–131.

■ Diagnosis Synopsis

Female pattern hair loss (FPHL) is frequently referred to as androgenetic alopecia. It is most commonly noticed after menopause, although it may begin any time after puberty. The incidence of androgenetic alopecia in women is thought to be less than that in males, although some argue that differences in expression only make it seem that this is the case. Both frequency and severity increase with age.

Hereditary transmission of FPHL is consistent with a polygenic trait where many genes are involved in its susceptibility. In susceptible hair follicles, dihydrotestosterone (DHT) binds to the androgen receptor, and the hormone-receptor complex activates the genes responsible for the gradual transformation of large terminal follicles to miniaturized follicles. The role of DHT is less certain in pattern hair loss in women compared with men. In contrast to men, female pattern alopecia usually presents as diffuse thinning of the central portion of the scalp with sparing of the frontal hairline. Hair thinning is often more evident in the frontal portion of the scalp resulting in "Christmas tree pattern" thinning of the central part.

◉ Look For

Diffuse thinning of the crown and widening of the midline part with retention of the frontal hairline (Fig. 4-723–4-725). Bitemporal recession is not typical.

Hairs themselves undergo a transition from thick, pigmented terminal hairs to shorter, indeterminate hairs to wispy, nonpigmented vellus hairs.

Follicles are intact without the evidence of scarring.

●● Diagnostic Pearls

- Women rarely develop a male pattern (bitemporal recession/vertex thinning) of hair loss; if this is present, further clinical and laboratory evaluation is warranted to rule out a virilizing tumor.
- Young women with pronounced FPHL or other features of hyperandrogenism (hirsutism, acne, and irregular menses) should be evaluated for an underlying functional endocrine disorder such as polycystic ovary syndrome or late-onset congenital adrenal hyperplasia.
- Increased hair shedding is generally not a prominent feature, although a subset of women present with FPHL that is unmasked by an episode of telogen effluvium.
- Concomitant seborrheic dermatitis is often present, confusing the diagnosis with an inflammatory process because of the natural tendency to minimize normal grooming practices such as frequent hair washing.

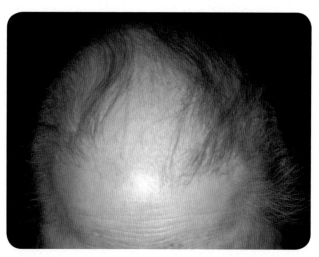

Figure 4-723 Very extensive female pattern alopecia.

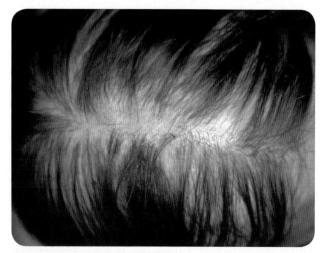

Figure 4-724 Female pattern alopecia with a wide central part and diffuse thinning.

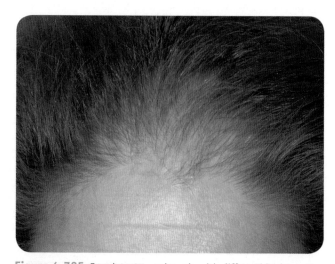

Figure 4-725 Female pattern alopecia with diffuse thinning.

?? Differential Diagnosis and Pitfalls

- Telogen effluvium—anemia, thyroid disease, medications, and major illness
- Anagen effluvium—toxins and chemotherapy
- Alopecia areata
- Traumatic—traction alopecia or trichotillomania
- Alopecia associated with virilizing disorders
- Scarring alopecia secondary to infections, radiation, auto-immune disease, burns, infiltrating metastatic carcinomas, or sarcoidosis

✓ Best Tests

This is usually a clinical diagnosis. The hair-pull test may be helpful. Grasp approximately 15 to 20 hairs between the thumb and the index finger, and pull gently but firmly; three or fewer lost hairs indicate normal shedding.

The decision to pursue further testing should be based on history and physical exam, but the following may be helpful in making the diagnosis:

- Biopsy—may help rule out underlying inflammatory disorders
- Androgen profile (testosterone- free/total, DHEA, etc.)— if features of hyperandrogenism present
- Iron studies
- Treatment of iron deficiency (decreased ferritin level) may enhance the efficacy of other hair loss treatments
- Thyroid function tests
- VDRL
- ANA

▲▲ Management Pearls

- Standardized scalp photography every 6 to 12 months is helpful in tracking treatment progress and/or disease progression.

- Patients with alopecia require scalp protection from UV radiation.
- Finasteride, spironolactone, and cyproterone can result in the feminization of a male fetus if used in women of childbearing potential.

Therapy

Hair pieces and other methods of camouflage should be offered as treatment alternatives and adjuncts.

Medical Treatments
- Topical minoxidil 2%—1 mL twice daily (only FDA-approved drug for women with FPHL)
- Topical minoxidil 5%—1 mL twice daily is often used off-label
- Spironolactone 200 mg daily
- Cyproterone acetate

Surgery
Scalp reduction, flaps, and hair transplant (micrografting)

Reassure patient that normal hair grooming practices, including washing, perming, coloring, etc., are not harmful because FPHL is not a primary hair shaft disorder associated with increased fragility.

Suggested Readings

Dinh QQ, Sinclair R. Female pattern hair loss: current treatment concepts. *Clin Interv Aging.* 2007;2(2):189–199.

Norwood OT. Incidence of female androgenetic alopecia (female pattern alopecia). *Dermatol Surg.* 2001 Jan;27(1):53–54.

Olsen EA, Messenger AG, Shapiro J, et al. Evaluation and treatment of male and female pattern hair loss. *J Am Acad Dermatol.* 2005 Feb;52(2): 301–311.

Price VH. Treatment of hair loss. *N Engl J Med.* 1999 Sep;341(13):964–973.

Trost LB, Bergfeld WF, Calogeras E. The diagnosis and treatment of iron deficiency and its potential relationship to hair loss. *J Am Acad Dermatol.* 2006 May;54(5):824–844.

■■ Diagnosis Synopsis

Male pattern alopecia (MPA), or androgenetic alopecia, refers to the common patterned balding affecting many men (although androgenetic alopecia may affect women as well). There is the gradual conversion of terminal hairs into indeterminate and finally vellus hairs. The condition may profoundly affect self-esteem and impair psychosocial functioning for some men, and an association between early onset MPA and coronary artery disease has been shown. The hair loss has a strong genetic basis. The incidence is highest in white men, followed by Asians and black men. The onset is usually prior to age 40.

⦿ Look For

Hair loss can begin at the anterior hairline with bitemporal recession and move posteriorly (Fig. 4-726), or it can present with thinning at the vertex of the scalp (Figs. 4-727 and 4-728). Carefully examine with a magnifying glass to see the progressive miniaturization of hair in areas of alopecia. Follicles are intact.

Dark Skin Considerations

Black men have a lower incidence of MPA and, in addition, tend to have more frontal baldness.

●● Diagnostic Pearls

May be precipitated or hastened by other forms of hair loss such as chemotherapy-induced hair loss (anagen effluvium) or telogen effluvium.

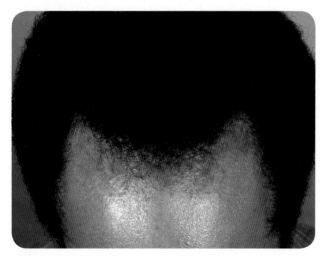

Figure 4-726 Frontal regression in MPA.

?? Differential Diagnosis and Pitfalls

- Other causes of nonscarring alopecia should be considered if the hair loss does not fit the typical frontal/temporal or vertex pattern of hair loss.
- Alopecia areata
- Drug-related alopecia
- Telogen effluvium
- Anagen effluvium
- Tinea capitis
- Trichotillomania

✓ Best Tests

This is a clinical diagnosis most easily confirmed by the specific pattern of hair loss. Take a family history.

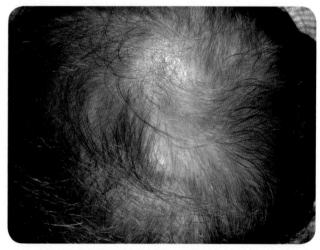

Figure 4-727 Moderate vertex balding in androgenetic alopecia. Note smaller diameter hairs with area of alopecia.

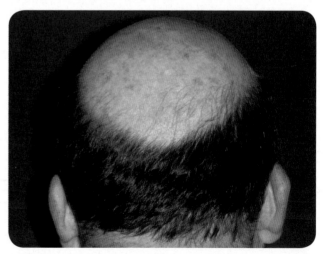

Figure 4-728 Severe vertex balding in androgenetic alopecia. Red papules are actinic keratoses that are a common complication of alopecia and sun exposure in lightly pigmented men.

▲▲▲ Management Pearls

- Patient should be advised that the hair loss is nonscarring, so there is a population of cells that can grow and enlarge the hair. The only clinically proven pharmacologic methods to prevent loss are minoxidil (Rogaine) or finasteride (Propecia). If these treatments are discontinued, the extent of loss will rapidly progress to where it would have been had treatment not been initiated.
- Individuals with hair loss should take measures to protect their scalp from UV radiation with sunscreens, hats, or hairpieces.

Therapy

Hairpieces and certain hair weaving techniques are an alternative to medical or surgical intervention.

Topical Therapy
Minoxidil 5% or 2% solution—1 mL applied to the affected area twice daily

Systemic Therapy
Finasteride—1 mg daily; note: finasteride should not be administered to women

Scalp reduction or hair transplantation surgeries are effective but expensive surgical procedures that should be performed by a qualified dermatologic surgeon or plastic surgeon.

Dark Skin Considerations

Black men usually prefer the oily 5% minoxidil over the 2% minoxidil, which has an alcohol base.

Suggested Readings

Lotufo PA, Chae CU, Ajani UA, et al. Male pattern baldness and coronary heart disease: The Physicians' Health Study. *Arch Intern Med*. 2000 Jan;160(2):165–171.

Olsen EA, Dunlap FE, Funicella T, et al. A randomized clinical trial of 5% topical minoxidil versus 2% topical minoxidil and placebo in the treatment of androgenetic alopecia in men. *J Am Acad Dermatol*. 2002 Sep;47(3):377–385.

Olsen EA, Messenger AG, Shapiro J, et al. Evaluation and treatment of male and female pattern hair loss. *J Am Acad Dermatol*. 2005 Feb;52(2): 301–311.

Price VH. Treatment of hair loss. *N Engl J Med*. 1999 Sep;341(13):964–973.

Sinclair R. Male pattern androgenetic alopecia. *BMJ*. 1998 Sep;317(7162): 865–869.

Stough D, Stenn K, Haber R, et al. Psychological effect, pathophysiology, and management of androgenetic alopecia in men. *Mayo Clin Proc*. 2005 Oct;80(10):1316–1322.

Diagnosis Synopsis

Nevus sebaceous (of Jadassohn) is a common hamartomatous malformation that is usually present at birth or develops in early childhood. Its presence may be subtle and not be noted until later childhood or adolescence, when it thickens due to hormonal influence. It consists of a yellow to orange oval or linear verrucous plaque, most often on the scalp or, more rarely, the forehead and neck. Most lesions are sporadic. There is no predilection for either sex or any ethnicity. Removal, if not cosmetically a problem, is recommended before adulthood due to the small risk of a malignancy developing within the lesion during adulthood. In the past, the risk of development of basal cell carcinoma within lesions was approximated at 10%, though this is now considered to be an overestimation. Other benign adnexal neoplasms, including trichoblastoma and syringocystadenoma papilliferum, occur more frequently within the lesion. In very rare cases, sebaceous or apocrine carcinomas can occur within nevus sebaceous.

A small number of patients with this lesion will have nevus sebaceous syndrome, which is analogous to epidermal nevus syndrome. They may manifest neurologic, skeletal, or ocular abnormalities.

Look For

A solitary yellow-orange plaque, which thickens and darkens with age, typically in early adolescence at the onset of puberty (Figs. 4-729–4-732). It often has a rubbery, verrucous quality.

The lesion usually occurs on the scalp and is accompanied by alopecia. Less commonly, nevus sebaceous may also occur on the face, neck, trunk, and extremities.

Dark Skin Considerations

In blacks, the plaque can appear very dark and similar in appearance to a seborrheic keratosis.

Diagnostic Pearls

The lesion is often flat and slightly pink-to-yellow in the neonate, and there is an absence of hair in a round or oval configuration that suggests the lesion.

Differential Diagnosis and Pitfalls

- Basal cell carcinoma
- Epidermal nevus
- Aplasia cutis congenita
- Solitary mastocytoma
- Juvenile xanthogranuloma
- Nevus comedonicus
- Syringocystadenoma or other adnexal neoplasm

Best Tests

The diagnosis can often be made clinically. Perform a skin biopsy if there is doubt.

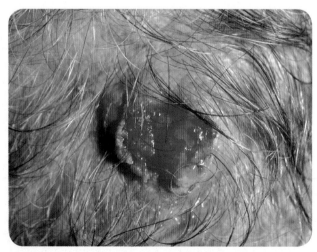

Figure 4-729 Tumors may develop in a nevus sebaceous with increasing age; most are basal cell carcinomas, and in this case, a syringocystadenoma papilliferum.

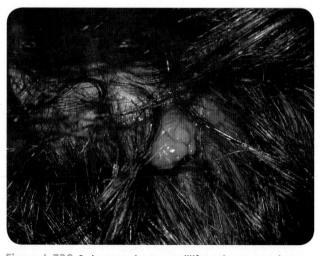

Figure 4-730 Syringocystadenoma papilliferum in a nevus sebaceous.

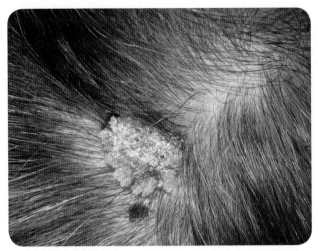

Figure 4-731 Verrucous plaque of a nevus sebaceous with a basal cell carcinoma on biopsy.

 ## Management Pearls

In the adult years, benign neoplasms or malignancy (basal cell or squamous cell carcinoma) can develop within a nevus sebaceous. Prophylactic excision of the entire lesion is usually recommended, if feasible. If not, careful observation for changes is needed. Subtotal treatments, such as shave excision or laser therapy, typically lead to recurrence.

Therapy

Surgical excision is the treatment of choice. Because the risk of malignant transformation is low, especially in children, removal can be delayed until adolescence with careful observation.

If surgery is contraindicated or undesired, the following techniques have been used to improve the appearance of the lesion, but continued observation is recommended:

- Curettage and cautery
- Laser resurfacing (carbon dioxide laser)
- Photodynamic therapy
- Cryotherapy

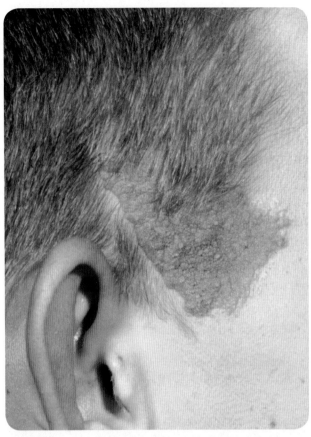

Figure 4-732 A nevus sebaceous persistent into adulthood can be mistaken for a seborrheic keratosis unless a careful history is obtained.

Suggested Readings

Cribier B, Scrivener Y, Grosshans E. Tumors arising in nevus sebaceous: A study of 596 cases. *J Am Acad Dermatol.* 2000 Feb;42(2 Pt 1):263–268.

McCalmont TH. Adnexal neoplasms. In: Bolognia J, Jorizzo JL, Rapini RP, eds. *Dermatology.* 2nd Ed. St. Louis, MO: Mosby; 2008:1695–1696.

Sugarman JL. Epidermal nevus syndromes. *Semin Cutan Med Surg.* 2007 Dec;26(4):221–230.

Terenzi V, Indrizzi E, Buonaccorsi S, et al. Nevus sebaceous of Jadassohn. *J Craniofac Surg.* 2006 Nov;17(6):1234–1239.

Diagnosis Synopsis

Telogen effluvium is one of many nonscarring alopecias. Normally, hair growth occurs in a cycle of growing hair (anagen phase) and then goes into a resting phase (telogen phase) and finally is shed. In telogen effluvium, a physiologic stressor causes many more hairs than normal to enter the resting phase, resulting in the key feature being diffuse hair shedding. Triggers include an episode of serious illness, high fevers, drugs, fad diets (usually low protein), childbirth, heavy blood loss, other significant physical or emotional stress, or thyroid disease. The interval between the inciting event or exposure and the shedding is generally a few months. Less commonly, a chronic form of telogen effluvium can last several years. Telogen effluvium itself is a benign and self-limited condition, although its presence may provide a clue to an underlying disease state.

Look For

Patients usually complain only that their hair is falling out at an increased rate (Figs. 4-733–4-736). Occasionally, there may be diffuse thinning without areas of total alopecia or a bitemporal prominence or thinning.

Diagnostic Pearls

Pull on a group of about 50 hairs, holding firmly with your fingers. Normally, just one to two hairs should come out from their "roots" (hair bulb). In telogen effluvium, many hairs should come out easily, and their roots will have an elongated hair bulb. The scalp should appear nonerythematous and be entirely unremarkable.

?? Differential Diagnosis and Pitfalls

- Androgenetic alopecia (pattern hair loss)
- Alopecia areata
- Trichotillomania
- Secondary syphilis
- Traction alopecia
- Anagen effluvium
- Tinea capitis (black dot disease)

✓ Best Tests

- Perform the hair-pull test as described in Diagnostic Pearls. Biopsy is usually not necessary. The decision to pursue further testing should be made on an individual basis.
- A drug history is essential. Potential drug culprits are numerous; thus, timing of initiation of new exposure is particularly important.
- Low iron stores, as measured with serum ferritin, are a common and easily correctable cause that is seen in patients who do not eat meat or women with heavy menstrual periods.

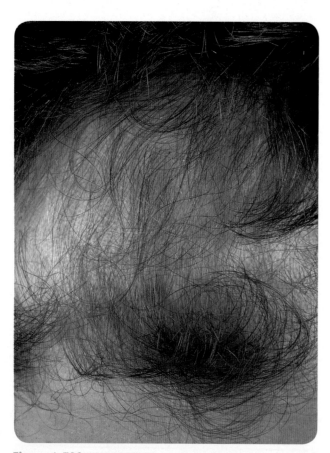

Figure 4-733 Telogen effluvium with no evidence of scaling; the hair loss is not uniform in telogen effluvium.

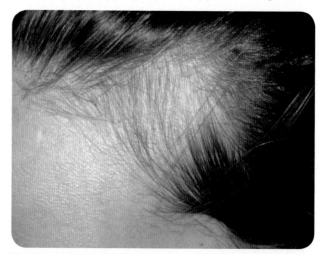

Figure 4-734 Diffuse thinning in telogen effluvium.

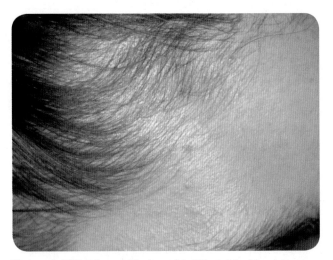

Figrue 4-735 Telogen effluvium with diffuse thinning.

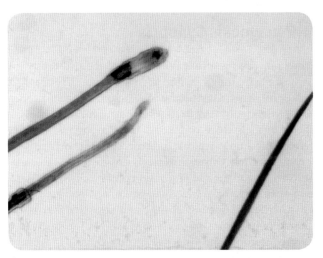

Figure 4-736 Methotrexate overdose with a dystrophic anagen hair (lower) and a telogen hair (upper).

- Consider thyroid function tests (e.g., TSH) in patients with other manifestations of thyroid disease.
- Systemic causes of telogen effluvium may occasionally be detected by further metabolic testing, including serum chemistries and liver enzymes.

▲▲ Management Pearls

- Give patients reassurance that hair will spontaneously regrow and will not progress to baldness. In a subset of patients, the episode of telogen effluvium may unmask or hasten androgenetic alopecia.
- If dietary factors are thought to play a role, consultation with a dietitian may be prudent.

Therapy

The condition is self-limited, and, usually, reassurance is the best therapy.

Patients who are significantly distressed by their hair loss and are motivated to pursue an active role in treatment may wish to try minoxidil (1 mL top twice daily). Of note, this treatment is only of theoretical (not proven) benefit in the treatment of telogen effluvium.

Suggested Readings

Harrison S, Sinclair R. Telogen effluvium. *Clin Exp Dermatol.* 2002 Jul;27(5):389–395.

Pilar Garc. Telogen effluvium associated with albendazole therapy. *Int J Dermatol.* 1990 Nov;29(9):669–670.

Rebora A. Telogen effluvium. *Dermatology.* 1997;195(3):209–212.

Sinclair R. Chronic telogen effluvium: a study of 5 patients over 7 years. *J Am Acad Dermatol.* 2005 Feb;52(2 Suppl. 1):12–16.

Tosti A, Pazzaglia M. Drug reactions affecting hair: diagnosis. *Dermatol Clin.* 2007 Apr;25(2):223–231, vii.

Trost LB, Bergfeld WF, Calogeras E. The diagnosis and treatment of iron deficiency and its potential relationship to hair loss. *J Am Acad Dermatol.* 2006 May;54(5):824–844.

■■ Diagnosis Synopsis

Onychomycosis is a fungal infection of the nail caused by dermatophyte fungi (tinea unguium), nondermatophyte molds, or yeasts. Onychomycosis is more frequent in men and is commonly associated with concurrent tinea pedis. It affects toenails more commonly than fingernails, and fingernail infection is typically preceded by or associated with toenail infection. Onychomycosis is classified into three patterns relating to the site of invasion of the nail: distal lateral subungual, superficial white, and proximal subungual.

Distal lateral subungual onychomycosis (DLSO) is the most common form of onychomycosis and begins with a fungal invasion of the distal nail (hyponychium). In Western countries, DLSO is mainly due to *Trichophyton rubrum*.

Superficial white onychomycosis (SWO) is due to fungal invasion of the superficial dorsal nail plate, typically caused by *T. rubrum* in HIV-infected patients and *T. mentagrophytes* in immunocompetent individuals.

Proximal subungual onychomycosis (PSO) is caused by invasion of the proximal nail fold. In the absence of paronychia, PSO is typically due to *T. rubrum*.

While *Candida* species are frequently cultured from nails, these species are not thought to be the primary pathogen. *Candida* is commonly associated with chronic paronychia and occasionally secondarily infects the nail plate. True nail invasion by *Candida* is seen almost exclusively in chronic mucocutaneous candidiasis.

Immunocompromised Patient Considerations

SWO and PSO have been reported to be more common in HIV infection and immunocompromised states.

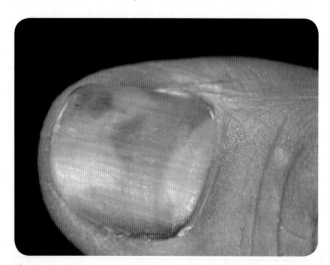

Figure 4-737 Onychomycosis secondary to *Candida*.

546

◉ Look For

Onychomycosis is marked by nail thickening, yellowish nail discoloration, onycholysis, and subungual debris (Figs. 4-737–4-740). If left untreated, nail infections can lead to total nail dystrophy.

Paronychia (erythema and swelling surrounding the nail plate) may be an associated finding.

In the setting of a dermatophyte infection, there frequently is concomitant tinea pedis, marked by scaly, erythematous plaques in the web spaces of the toes and on the soles or sides of the feet. There may also be concomitant tinea corporis or tinea capitis.

Immunocompromised Patient Considerations

Onychomycosis can serve as a nidus for infection in diabetic and immunocompromised patients, resulting in cellulitis. Treatment needs to be more aggressive in these patients.

●● Diagnostic Pearls

It is important to do a thorough skin exam, particularly of the feet and scalp, to rule out coexistent infection.

Immunocompromised Patient Considerations

Apparent SWO due to *T. rubrum* should raise concern for possible HIV/AIDS.

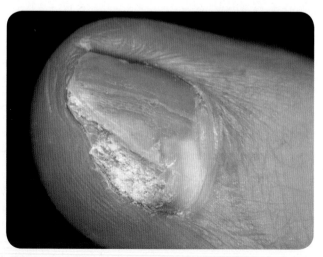

Figure 4-738 Lateral onychomycosis.

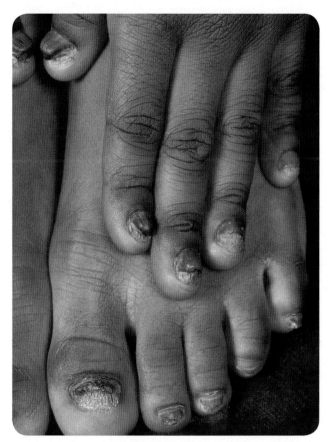

Figure 4-739 Round, irregular nail plates in onychomycosis.

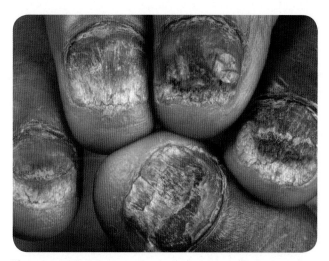

Figure 4-740 Onychomycosis with rough and thickened nail plates.

Immunocompromised Patient Differential Diagnosis

Chronic mucocutaneous candidiasis is characterized by chronic paronychia, nail dystrophy, and chronic mucocutaneous candidal infections.

✔ Best Tests

- A nail clipping sent in formalin for standard histopathology with a PAS stain is a very sensitive method of detection, though it cannot identify viable or specific pathogens and is somewhat costly.
- KOH preparation of nail scrapings is also a sensitive method for detecting nail infection, but it cannot identify the specific pathogen. It can rapidly be performed in the office.
- Fungal culture is also helpful and allows for identification of the specific pathogen but has a low sensitivity of only 50% to 70% and may show false-positive results due to contamination.

▲▲ Management Pearls

- Although 50% of nail dystrophies are due to onychomycosis, a patient should never be treated with systemic antifungal agents without confirmed infection based on direct microscopy, fungal culture, or histopathology. Systemic antifungal agents are costly and can have rare undesirable side effects and toxicities.
- If a patient has no complicating comorbidities or associated symptoms, it is important to consider conservative management strategies such as watchful waiting.

?? Differential Diagnosis and Pitfalls

- Psoriasis nail changes include nail pitting, "oil spot" yellow nail discoloration, and onycholysis.
- Lichen planus is characterized by red longitudinal ridging and grooves.
- Alopecia areata is classically characterized by red lunula and nail pitting.
- Chronic paronychia has associated changes in the nail fold and distal finger.
- Congenital nail dystrophy presents early and usually affects all nails.
- Trauma will elicit an associated history and commonly affects one nail.
- Median nail dystrophy
- Melanoma can present with Hutchinson sign (pigment in the proximal nail fold).
- Squamous cell carcinoma of the nail is commonly friable and bleeds easily.
- Subungual verruca vulgaris can result in dystrophic nails.
- Pseudomonas nail infection is usually associated with a greenish discoloration.

Immunocompromised Patient Considerations

Keep in mind potential drug interactions for HIV and immunocompromised patients. Achlorhydria, often seen in AIDS, may reduce drug absorption and needs to be factored into management.

Therapy

Oral antifungal treatments offer the best cure rates for onychomycosis.

First-Line Therapy

Terbinafine 250 mg p.o. for 12 weeks is the most effective treatment for onychomycosis. As a less expensive alternative regimen, pulse dosing of terbinafine can be used with only a slight decrease in efficacy (250 mg p.o. for 7 days, for 1 week per month for 3 months).

Alternative Therapies

- Itraconazole 200 mg p.o. for 12 weeks or pulse therapy using 200 mg p.o. twice daily for 1 week per month for 3 to 4 months
- Griseofulvin 1 to 2 g p.o. per day until nail changes resolve
- Fluconazole 150 to 200 mg p.o. for 9 months

Hepatotoxicity is associated with some oral antifungal agents. Baseline LFTs are useful prior to initiation of therapy.

Topical Therapy

Topical treatments are usually ineffective for the nails, although they may help to reduce or stabilize infection. Options include imidazole creams, urea gels or creams, and ciclopirox nail lacquer (more costly).

Nondermatophyte molds are often resistant to oral antifungal agents but may respond to topical therapy, especially after debridement.

Other Therapy

Mechanical debridement with total or partial surgical nail avulsion or chemical nail avulsion with topical 40% urea ointment under occlusion can be used as adjunctive therapy to either topical or oral antifungal agents.

Suggested Readings

Chang CH, Young-Xu Y, Kurth T, et al. The safety of oral antifungal treatments for superficial dermatophytosis and onychomycosis: A meta-analysis. *Am J Med.* 2007 Sep;120(9):791–798.

Elewski BE. Onychomycosis: Pathogenesis, diagnosis, and management. *Clin Microbiol Rev.* 1998 Jul;11(3):415–429.

Faergemann J, Baran R. Epidemiology, clinical presentation and diagnosis of onychomycosis. *Br J Dermatol.* 2003 Sep;149(Suppl. 65):1–4.

Gupta AK, Ryder JE, Lynch LE, et al. The use of terbinafine in the treatment of onychomycosis in adults and special populations: A review of the evidence. *J Drugs Dermatol.* 2005 May–Jun;4(3):302–308.

Krob AH, Fleischer AB, D'Agostino R, et al. Terbinafine is more effective than itraconazole in treating toenail onychomycosis: Results from a meta-analysis of randomized controlled trials. *J Cutan Med Surg.* 2003 Jul–Aug;7(4):306–311.

Piraccini BM, Tosti A. White superficial onychomycosis: epidemiological, clinical, and pathological study of 79 patients. *Arch Dermatol.* 2004 Jun;140(6):696–701.

Roberts DT, Taylor WD, Boyle J, British Association of Dermatologists. Guidelines for treatment of onychomycosis. *Br J Dermatol.* 2003 Mar;148(3):402–410.

Scher RK, Tavakkol A, Sigurgeirsson B, et al. Onychomycosis: Diagnosis and definition of cure. *J Am Acad Dermatol.* 2007 Jun;56(6):939–944.

Sobera JO, Elewski BE. Fungal diseases. In: Bolognia JL, Jorizzo JL, Rapini RP, eds. *Dermatology.* 2nd Ed. St. Louis, MO: Mosby; 2008:1144–1149.

Tosti A, Piraccini BA. Biology of nails and nail disorders. In: Fitzpatrick TB, Wolff K, eds. *Fitzpatrick's Dermatology in General Medicine.* 7th Ed. New York, NY: McGraw-Hill; 2008:778–794.

Diagnosis Synopsis

Acute paronychia is defined as the inflammation of a nail fold for fewer than 6 weeks. Pain, swelling, and redness are the cardinal symptoms, sometimes accompanied by abscess formation.

The anatomy surrounding a nail includes two lateral nail folds at the junction of the lateral nail plate and the skin of the distal phalanx and a proximal nail fold that includes the eponychium (or cuticle) sandwiched between the proximal aspect of the nail plate and the skin of the distal phalanx. Acute paronychia frequently arises from trauma to one of these structures, resulting in compromise of the physiologic barrier to entry of microorganisms. Examples of inciting trauma include foreign bodies, such as splinters; manipulations, such as manicures or pedicures; fingernail biting; finger sucking in children; or "hangnail" removal. Occasionally, acute paronychia arises as a painful exacerbation of chronic paronychia, which is now understood to be a localized form of chronic irritant/allergic dermatitis.

Certain drugs—including retinoids (isotretinoin, acitretin), methotrexate, antiretroviral protease inhibitors (indinavir and lamivudine), and epidermal growth factor receptor inhibitors (cetuximab, gefitinib, and lapatinib)—can cause paronychia, in some cases with associated periungual pyogenic granuloma.

Specific bacteria predominate in trauma-related acute paronychia. They include *Staphylococcus aureus*, *Streptococcus pyogenes*, and anaerobic bacteria derived from the oral flora. Other bacteria that have been reported as causes include

- *Pseudomonas*
- *Proteus*
- *Hendersonula*
- *Scytalidium*
- *Fusarium*
- *Prevotella*
- *Bartonella*

Patients with diabetes mellitus may be at increased risk of acute paronychia.

Look For

Periungual erythema, tenderness, and swelling that may be fluctuant or exude pus (Figs. 4-741–4-744).

Immunocompromised Patient Considerations

Drug-induced paronychias must be considered in patients with HIV/AIDS.

Diagnostic Pearls

- Acute paronychia presents within 6 weeks of onset of symptoms and often affects just one digit. Chronic paronychia may affect more than one digit, is present for more than 6 weeks after onset of symptoms, and is associated with irritant/allergen exposure, often of an occupational nature (e.g., dishwashing).
- The presence of nail plate changes suggests a chronic process.
- The digital pressure test: Having the patient appose the fingertip pad of the affected digit to a firm surface or the thumb will blanch the skin overlying an area that is involved by abscess. If blanching occurs, it is more likely

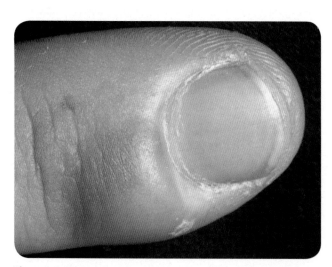

Figure 4-741 Acute paronychia 4 days after manipulation of a hangnail.

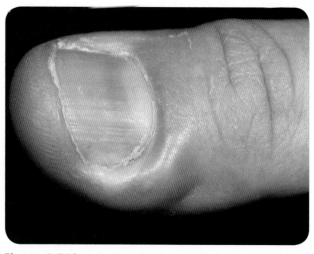

Figure 4-742 Acute bacterial paronychia of the posterior and lateral nail folds.

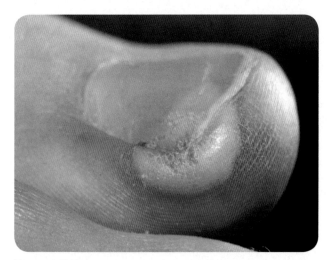

Figure 4-743 Acute bacterial paronychia laterally and subungually.

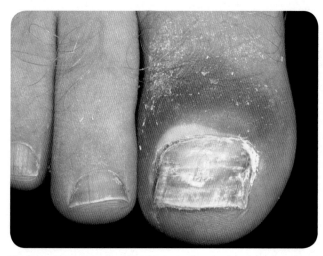

Figure 4-744 Acute bacterial paronychia after dermatophyte destruction of the nail plate.

overlying an abscess. This can help guide the decision to incise and drain.

?? Differential Diagnosis and Pitfalls

- Chronic paronychia—complicated by acute paronychia
- Trauma, including fracture of the distal phalanx—X-ray is indicated for a history of blunt trauma
- Herpetic whitlow—one or more vesicles near the nail with honeycomb appearance; painful
- Onychocryptosis (ingrown nail)
- Felon (purulent infection of the distal fingertip)
- Osteomyelitis
- Pemphigus vulgaris
- Pyogenic granuloma
- Pustular psoriasis
- Acrodermatitis continua of Hallopeau
- Reactive arthritis (previously referred to as Reiter disease)
- Digital mucinous cyst
- Onychomycosis
- Syphilitic chancre
- Acropustulosis continua

✓ Best Tests

- Culture for bacteria, including anaerobic bacterial culture.
- Culture for fungi.
- If lesion is vesicular and painful, consider viral culture, Tzanck smear, and/or direct fluorescent antibody testing for herpes simplex virus.

▲▲ Management Pearls

If purulent drainage or abscess is present, contact precautions for presumptive methicillin-resistant *S. aureus* (MRSA) should be followed until culture results confirm another organism. In recurrent cases, investigation into the precipitating factors or traumatic events may help prevent future occurrences.

Therapy

If no abscess is present, warm water soaks four times daily for 15 minutes or soaks in aluminum acetate (Burow solution) or diluted white vinegar may prove sufficient.

A topical antibacterial agent such as mupirocin, bacitracin/neomycin/polymyxin b sulfate, or gentamicin two or three times daily may be added in uncomplicated cases. Limited data support the concomitant use of a potent topical steroid such as betamethasone.

More extensive or recalcitrant cases may require oral antibiotics. Such drugs should have antistaphylococcal coverage as well as activity against anaerobes. The prevalence of MRSA should be considered in the choice of antibiotics.

- Clindamycin
- Doxycycline
- Trimethoprim-sulfamethoxazole

Drug-induced cases may improve with cessation or substitution of the causative agent. In the case of EGF-receptor antagonist-induced paronychia, drug substitution may be undesirable because these are typically used as cancer chemotherapeutics. In the case of cetuximab-induced paronychia, doxycycline 100 mg twice has shown efficacy.

Incision and drainage is indicated when abscess is present (i.e., with fluctuance or a positive digital pressure test). In most cases, a digital anesthetic block is used with one of the following approaches:

- Incise with a no. 11 or 15 blade angled away from the nail bed. Pack with plain gauze for 48 h, and then remove packing and commence soaks four times daily.
- Run a no. 11 blade parallel to the nail plate and under the cuticle. Turn the blade 90 degrees with the sharp side toward the nail to lift the cuticle from the nail plate and allow pus to drain.
- Lift the nail fold with a 21- or 23-gauge needle, and allow pus to drain. (Some describe using this approach without any anesthesia.)

Suggested Readings

Black JR. Paronychia. *Clin Podiatr Med Surg*. 1995 Apr;12(2):183–187.

Guly HR. Fractures of the terminal phalanx presenting as a paronychia. *Arch Emerg Med*. 1993 Dec;10(4):301–305.

Lawry M, Daniel CR III. Nonfungal infections and acute paronychia. In: Scher RK, Daniel CR. *Nails: Diagnosis, Therapy, Surgery*. 3rd Ed. Oxford: Elsevier Saunders; 2005:143–144.

Ogunlusi JD, Oginni LM, Ogunlusi OO. DAREJD simple technique of draining acute paronychia. *Tech Hand Up Extrem Surg*. 2005 Jun;9(2):120–121.

Rigopoulos D, Gregoriou S, Belyayeva Y, et al. Acute paronychia caused by lapatinib therapy. *Clin Exp Dermatol*. 2009 Jan;34(1):94–95.

Sander A, Frank B. Paronychia caused by Bartonella henselae. *Lancet*. 1997 Oct;350(9084):1078.

Shaw J, Body R. Best evidence topic report. Incision and drainage preferable to oral antibiotics in acute paronychial nail infection? *Emerg Med J*. 2005 Nov;22(11):813–814.

Sibel S, Macher A, Goosby E. Paronychia in patients receiving antiretroviral therapy for human immunodeficiency virus infection. *J Am Podiatr Med Assoc*. 2000 Feb;90(2):98–100.

Tosti A, Piraccini BM, D'Antuono A, et al. Paronychia associated with antiretroviral therapy. *Br J Dermatol*. 1999 Jun;140(6):1165–1168.

Turkmen A, Warner RM, Page RE. Digital pressure test for paronychia. *Br J Plast Surg*. 2004 Jan;57(1):93–94.

Wollina U. Acute paronychia: Comparative treatment with topical antibiotic alone or in combination with corticosteroid. *J Eur Acad Dermatol Venereol*. 2001 Jan;15(1):82–84.

Diagnosis Synopsis

Chronic paronychia is defined as inflammation of a nail fold (the skin surrounding the fingernails) lasting at least 6 weeks. Symptoms may include redness, swelling, and sometimes pain. There may be disruption or absence of the cuticle, and protracted cases may manifest with changes in the nail plate itself. Nail plate involvement signals damage to the nail matrix, which lies deep to and proximal to the proximal nail fold. Acute paronychia with marked tenderness, erythema, and even abscess formation may complicate chronic paronychia.

There is debate as to whether chronic paronychia is primarily an infectious or an inflammatory disease process; the emerging view is that chronic paronychia is a species of chronic irritant or allergic hand dermatitis. Evidence for this view includes (i) it is frequently associated with occupational exposures in dishwashers, bartenders, laundry workers, nurses, swimmers, fishmongers, and cooks; (ii) the frequent occurrence of disease in more than one digit; and (iii) a well-designed study that demonstrated the superiority of treatment with potent topical steroids over systemic antifungals. Women are more frequently affected than men.

Nevertheless, infectious pathogens do play a role in this disease. The chronic inflammatory process compromises the nail fold barrier to the entry of microorganisms. Superinfection with bacteria may result in acute paronychia developing in the context of chronic paronychia. Fungal colonization and/or infection, especially with *Candida albicans*, is common. In one study, *Candida* was cultured in over 90% of patients with chronic paronychia.

Certain drugs can cause paronychia (potentially either acute or chronic). These include retinoids (isotretinoin and acitretin), methotrexate, antiretroviral protease inhibitors (indinavir and lamivudine), and epidermal growth factor receptor inhibitors (cetuximab, gefitinib, and lapatinib). In some cases, drug-induced paronychia is associated with periungual pyogenic granulomas.

Diabetes mellitus is a risk factor for developing paronychia.

Look For

Erythema, edema, and tenderness of one or more nail folds, damage or absence of the cuticle, and pitting or Beau lines (transverse lines in the nail plate) (Figs. 4-745–4-748). Onycholysis (separation of the nail plate from the nail bed) is also observed.

Diagnostic Pearls

- Chronic paronychia may affect more than one digit, presents more than 6 weeks after onset of symptoms, and is associated with irritant/allergen exposure, often of an occupational nature (e.g., dishwashing).
- Nail changes strongly suggest a chronic process.
- Acute paronychia presents within 6 weeks of onset of symptoms and often affects just one digit. A history of trauma 2 to 5 days prior to onset of symptoms strongly suggests acute paronychia.

Differential Diagnosis and Pitfalls

- Acute paronychia—may complicate chronic paronychia
- Herpetic whitlow—one or more blisters near the nail with honeycomb appearance

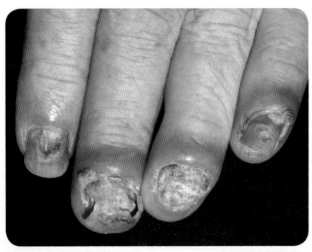

Figure 4-745 Chronic paronychia with swollen nail folds and destruction of nail plates.

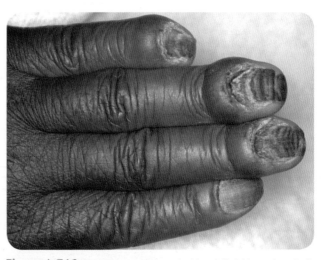

Figure 4-746 Massively swollen posterior nail folds and periodic ridging of the nail plate due to chronic *Candida* infection.

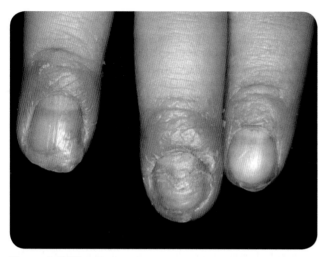

Figure 4-747 Different degrees of nail fold swelling and nail plate distortion on three adjacent nails.

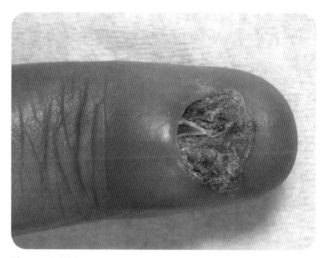

Figure 4-748 Chronic paronychia consistent with chronic infection with *Pseudomonas*.

- Onychocryptosis (ingrown nail)
- Felon
- Osteomyelitis
- Pemphigus vulgaris
- Pyogenic granuloma
- Pustular psoriasis
- Acrodermatitis continua of Hallopeau
- Reactive arthritis (previously referred to as Reiter disease)
- Digital mucous cyst—usually not inflamed
- Onychomycosis
- Squamous cell carcinoma or squamous cell carcinoma in situ (Bowen disease)
- Periungual verruca vulgaris—usually with verrucous surface and not inflamed
- Atypical mycobacterial infection—associated with cleaning fish tanks

✓ Best Tests

Typical cases do not require special testing.

Refractory cases or cases in which acute paronychia may be superimposed may require the following:

- Biopsy to rule out malignancy
- Culture for bacteria, including anaerobic bacterial culture
- Culture for fungi or nail clippings for PAS or methenamine silver staining or a KOH scraping for fungal forms
- Culture for atypical mycobacteria

▲▲ Management Pearls

- Chronic paronychia responds to avoidance of inciting factors. Dishwashers and others who cannot avoid exposures

should be urged to use rubber gloves with cotton liner inserts.
- Nail acrylics and artificial nail adhesives are sometimes implicated in chronic contact dermatitis or irritant dermatitis of the nail folds.

Therapy

In addition to the avoidance of inciting allergens/irritants, treatment includes

Ultra-potent topical steroids (first line):

- Clobetasol 0.05% ointment or cream—twice daily for 1 to 2 weeks
- Betamethasone dipropionate augmented cream or ointment—0.05% cream twice daily for 1 to 2 weeks

Topical antifungals may also be added until clinically resolved (often 4 weeks):

- Ciclopirox 0.8% liquid or 0.77% cream/lotion twice daily
- Clotrimazole 1% cream three times daily
- Econazole 1% cream three to four times daily
- Ketoconazole 2% cream once or twice daily
- Nystatin 100,000 U/g three times daily
- Terbinafine 1% cream twice daily
- Thymol 1% to 4% in alcohol three times daily

Intralesional corticosteroid injection (e.g., triamcinolone acetonide) may prove beneficial in cases that do not respond to initial topical therapy.

(Continued)

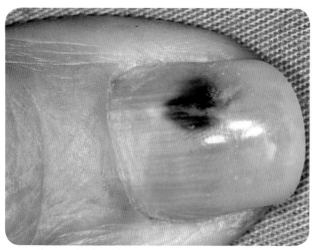

Figure 4-751 Colonization of the undersurface of an artificial nail with *Pseudomonas* sp.

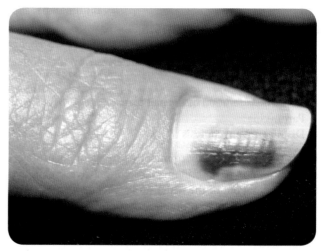

Figure 4-752 Infection between the nail plate and the nail bed with *Pseudomonas* sp.

▲▲ Management Pearls

- The most important method for preventing future infection is to protect the hands/nails from water by using vinyl gloves. Be sure the patient turns the gloves inside out after use to prevent the growth of the organism in the gloves.
- Other predisposing factors, such as trauma and underlying nail disease (psoriasis, etc.), should be minimized whenever possible. Nails should be kept clipped short.

Therapy

The best treatment is to trim the nail plate and to soak the fingers in 0.1% polymyxin B and 1% acetic acid solution (1:5 dilution of white vinegar) twice daily for 1-h periods. Topical solutions of fluoroquinolones or an aminoglycoside, such as tobramycin, are also effective. Treatment for 1 to 4 months with topical agents is typically required.

Ciprofloxacin 500 mg twice daily for 1 to 2 weeks.
Note: It will take several months for the discoloration to grow out with the nail plate.

Suggested Readings

Agger WA, Mardan A. Pseudomonas aeruginosa infections of intact skin. *Clin Infect Dis*. 1995 Feb;20(2):302–308.

Elewski BE. Bacterial infection in a patient with onychomycosis. *J Am Acad Dermatol*. 1997 Sep;37(3 Pt 1):493–494.

LeFeber WP, Golitz LE. Green foot. *Pediatr Dermatol*. 1984 Jul;2(1):38–40.

Mermel LA, McKay M, Dempsey J, et al. Pseudomonas surgical-site infections linked to a healthcare worker with onychomycosis. *Infect Control Hosp Epidemiol*. 2003 Oct;24(10):749–752.

Sakata S, Howard A. Pseudomonas chloronychia in a patient with nail psoriasis. *Med J Aust*. 2007 Apr;186(8):424.

Shellow WV, Koplon BS. Green striped nails: Chromonychia due to Pseudomonas aeruginosa. *Arch Dermatol*. 1968 Feb;97(2):149–153.

Swartz MN. Gram-negative coccal and bacillary infections. In: Fitzpatrick TB, Wolff K, eds. *Fitzpatrick's Dermatology in General Medicine*. 7th Ed. New York, NY: McGraw-Hill; 2008:1735–1739.

Winslow EH, Jacobson AF. Can a fashion statement harm the patient? Long and artificial nails may cause nosocomial infections. *Am J Nurs*. 2000 Sep;100(9):63–65.

▪ Diagnosis Synopsis

Angiokeratomas of the scrotum (Fordyce angiokeratoma) are benign, often asymptomatic, 2 to 5 mm, warty or smooth-topped, red to violaceous papules composed of dilated dermal capillaries. The pathophysiology is unknown, but it is speculated that they may be caused by increased venous pressure due to their occasional association with vascular conditions such as varicoceles. The lesions may bleed spontaneously or with slight trauma, which is distressing to patients.

As the name implies, the condition is more common in men. However, angiokeratomas may also be seen on the inner thighs, lower abdomen, and on the vulva in women.

Prevalence data indicate that the condition is more common in whites and the Japanese, and that incidence increases with advancing age.

◉ Look For

Dark red to purple papules that are 2 to 5 mm in diameter (Figs. 4-753–4-756). The color has occasionally been described as blue or black. Lesions are most often multiple. There may be a superficial wart-like appearance to some lesions.

The scrotum is the most common site, but lesions may also be seen on the inner thighs, lower abdomen, or the vulva of women.

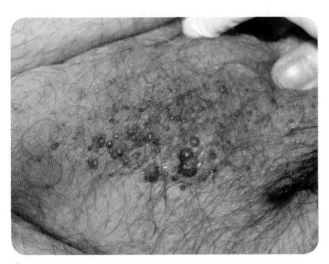

Figure 4-753 Angiokeratomas of scrotum may vary in size.

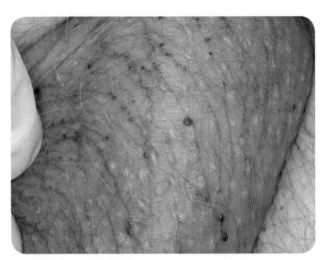

Figure 4-754 Angiokeratomas and Fordyce spots on the scrotum.

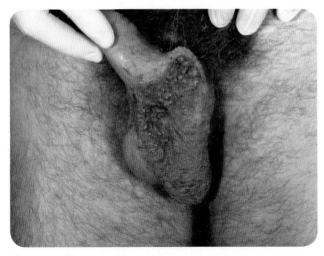

Figure 4-755 Plaque-like angiokeratomas on the scrotum.

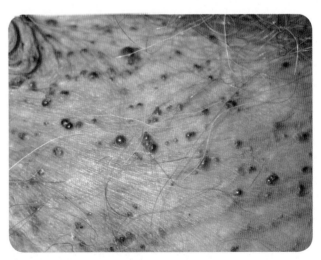

Figure 4-756 The color of scrotal angiokeratomas varies from red to deep purple, as in these lesions.

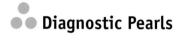

Diagnostic Pearls

- Fabry lesions are smaller and appear at an earlier age. Patients with Fabry disease may also report limb pain, history of renal or cardiac disease, and decreased sweating.
- Red scrotum occurs in half of the patients with angiokeratoma of the scrotum. The scrotum is not tender or edematous; it is red in color due to a background of telangiectasia. This asymptomatic redness may be the presenting factor for many patients.

?? Differential Diagnosis and Pitfalls

- Angiokeratoma corporis diffusum (Fabry disease)
- Hereditary hemorrhagic telangiectasia
- Condyloma acuminatum
- Melanoma
- Melanocytic nevi
- Cherry hemangiomas

✓ Best Tests

- Skin biopsy will confirm the clinical impression.
- Examination with a hand lens or dermatoscope may help to distinguish a vascular from a melanocytic lesion.

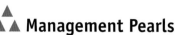

Management Pearls

Lesions do not have to be treated, but symptomatic, bleeding lesions can easily be treated by electrodesiccation.

Therapy

No treatment is necessary. If treatment is desired, however, cryotherapy, electrocautery, and laser therapy have all demonstrated success in clearing the lesions. Excision is impractical in cases where there are many lesions.

Lasers that have reportedly achieved success with single treatments include the 578-nm copper laser, the argon laser, and the 532-nm KTP laser.

Suggested Readings

Baker C, Kelly B. Other vascular disorders. In: Bolognia JL, Jorizzo JL, Rapini RP, eds. *Dermatology*. 2nd Ed. St. Louis, MO: Mosby; 2008:1623.

Lapidoth M, Ad-El D, David M, et al. Treatment of angiokeratoma of Fordyce with pulsed dye laser. *Dermatol Surg*. 2006 Sep;32(9):1147–1150.

Miller C, James WD. Angiokeratoma of Fordyce as a cause of red scrotum. *Cutis*. 2002 Jan;69(1):50–51.

Occella C, Bleidl D, Rampini P, et al. Argon laser treatment of cutaneous multiple angiokeratomas. *Dermatol Surg*. 1995 Feb;21(2):170–172.

Trickett R, Dowd H. Angiokeratoma of the scrotum: A case of scrotal bleeding. *Emerg Med J*. 2006 Oct;23(10):e57.

Balanitis, Nonspecific

Diagnosis Synopsis

Balanitis, or inflammation of the glans penis, can be triggered by a number of different infections and factors. The term *nonspecific balanitis* refers to those cases where an exact etiology for this penile inflammation cannot be found (a common occurrence). Patients may experience a burning sensation, itching, pain, or tenderness. Periurethral involvement may have associated pain with urination. Balanoposthitis refers to the inflammation of both the glans and of the foreskin in uncircumcised males.

Balanitis is common, affecting 11% of men presenting to urology clinics. Uncircumcised men with poor personal hygiene are most often affected.

Common infectious triggers include *Candida, Gardnerella vaginalis, Trichomonas vaginalis, Neisseria gonorrhoeae,* and *Streptococcus*. Smegma retention, trauma from intercourse, spermicides, and deodorants are other triggers. In older males, diabetes mellitus may be a factor. Other common causes are fixed drug eruption, malignancy, and allergic contact dermatitis (e.g., sensitization to an allergen within a condom). Complications include phimosis, fissuring, meatal stenosis, and involvement of the urethra requiring surgery.

Look For

Patients complain of pain, itch, penile discharge, inability to retract the foreskin, impotence, or difficulty in urinating. The glans penis and foreskin are red (Figs. 4-757–4-759) and, at times, may be studded with pustules or show erosions that may form ulcers. Swelling may be present and can cause the onset of phimosis or paraphimosis. Periurethral involvement may have associated pain with urination. A penile discharge may be present if infection is the cause. Look for possible meatal stenosis and bladder distention.

Diagnostic Pearls

Take an adequate sexual history, and rule out infections such as syphilis and gonorrhea.

Differential Diagnosis and Pitfalls

- If pustules are present, consider candidiasis, scabies, or psoriasis.
- Squamous cell carcinoma
- Extramammary Paget disease
- Drug eruption (including fixed drug eruption, which may be erosive)
- Zoon plasma cell balanitis
- Circinate balanitis (Reiter syndrome)

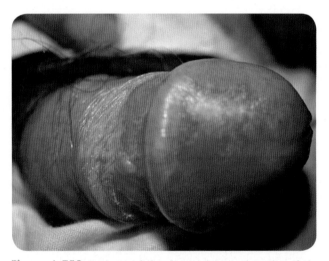

Figure 4-758 Erythema of the glans and mucosal portion of the shaft.

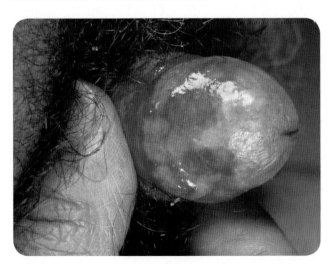

Figure 4-757 Poorly bordered erythema.

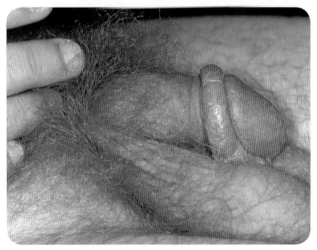

Figure 4-759 Redness and edema of the glans and corona in a patient with reactive arthritis.

559

- Contact dermatitis (e.g., exposure to skin cleansers, topical medications, condoms)
- Lichen sclerosus et atrophicus
- Lichen planus
- Pemphigus
- Syphilis
- Gonorrhea
- Genital herpes simplex virus

Immunocompromised Patient Differential Diagnosis

Syphilis should be high on the differential diagnosis list of any HIV-infected individual presenting with balanitis.

✓ Best Tests

- Take a thorough history
- Evaluate for diabetes
- Bacterial cultures and Gram stain test
- Fungal KOH preparation and fungal culture
- Tzanck smear and viral culture
- Serologic test for syphilis (VDRL, RPR)
- Patch testing if allergic contact dermatitis is suspected
- Biopsy in recalcitrant cases
- Consider ultrasound to detect urinary obstruction or urology referral

▲▲▲ Management Pearls

- Soap residues in the affected area are to be avoided by careful and copious rinsing with soap-free water.
- Close follow-up with these patients is mandatory. Biopsy should be performed in cases not responding to treatment to rule out malignancy.

Therapy

Treatment is specific to the causative agent. Often, non-specific balanitis must be treated empirically.

Temporary relief for nonspecific balanitis can be achieved with improved personal hygiene. Try daily foreskin retraction and cleansing with warm water. Vinegar and water soaks (one-half teaspoon of vinegar per 8 oz glass of water) or saline soaks are alternatives. Avoid any other cosmetic or lotion products.

If symptoms persist after 2 to 3 weeks, add application of low-to-medium–potency topical steroid only until

improved. An ointment base is usually better tolerated. Do not continue long-term topical corticosteroid use (i.e., more than 2 to 3 weeks).

Low-potency topical corticosteroids (*classes* 6 *and* 7)

- Prednicarbate cream, ointment—apply twice daily (15 g)
- Desonide cream, lotion—apply twice daily (25 g cream, 10, 30 mL ointment)
- Hydrocortisone 1% (many over-the-counter brands)—apply twice daily
- Hydrocortisone 2.5% cream, lotion—apply twice daily (1 oz tubes cream, 2 oz bottle lotion)

Mid-potency topical corticosteroids (*classes* 3 *to* 5)

Note: Do not use these for more than 3 to 4 days, as they easily induce atrophy in this region.

- Triamcinolone 0.1% cream, ointment—apply twice daily (15 g)
- Mometasone cream, ointment—apply twice daily (15 g)
- Fluocinolone ointment, cream—apply twice daily (15 g)
- Fluticasone cream—apply twice daily (15 g)

Topical tacrolimus 0.1% ointment applied twice daily is another option.

Further treatments that can be tried include

- Carbenoxolone gel
- 2.5% testosterone propionate ointment
- Intralesional corticosteroids
- High-potency topical corticosteroids (if lower potency formulations fail first) for very short periods (3 to 4 days)

Circumcision will cure balanoposthitis.

Immunocompromised Patient Considerations

If the causative agent is infectious, immunocompromised patients may need longer courses of appropriate systemic therapy.

Suggested Readings

Escala JM, Rickwood AM. Balanitis. *Br J Urol.* 1989 Feb;63(2):196–197.

Krueger H, Osborn L. Effects of hygiene among the uncircumcised. *J Fam Pract.* 1986 Apr;22(4):353–355.

Röchen M, Ghoreschi K. Morphea and lichen sclerosis. In: Bolognia JL, Jorizzo JL, Rapini RP, eds. *Dermatology.* 2nd Ed. St. Louis, MO: Mosby; 2008:1477–1478.

Diagnosis Synopsis

Candidiasis refers to a fungal infection caused by the yeast *Candida albicans*. Other species of *Candida* are occasionally causative. When in the male genital area, it might have been acquired through intercourse with an infected partner. It may also arise idiopathically. Predisposing factors include a history of diabetes mellitus, other forms of immunosuppression (including steroid use), obesity, preexisting intrinsic skin disease, or recent treatment with antibiotics.

Candidiasis presents clinically as small erythematous erosions and pustules with associated itching and burning. In its mildest form, the condition may be intermittent and transient. *Candida* most often infects warm, moist, occluded areas, and the proximal shaft of the penis, the scrotum, and the crural folds are frequently involved. Candidal balanitis is a fungal infection of the glans penis. It occurs more frequently in the uncircumcised male.

Immunocompromised Patient Considerations

It frequently occurs in diabetics, in the immunosuppressed, and after treatment with oral antibiotics.

Look For

Look for erythema of the shaft of the penis or glans, sometimes with erosions (Fig. 4-760). Candidiasis can involve the scrotum, presenting with erythema and edema (Fig. 4-761). Inguinal fold involvement tends to be macerated with satellite pustules (Fig. 4-762). Burning and pruritus are common symptoms.

Diagnostic Pearls

- Pustules, when seen, are usually subtle, fragile, and have a red halo.
- Inquire specifically about a history of diabetes mellitus, HIV, or other immune deficiency diseases. Take a thorough medication history, including any recent antibiotic usage or use of corticosteroids or other immunosuppressive agents.

Differential Diagnosis and Pitfalls

- Allergic or irritant contact dermatitis
- Psoriasis
- Lichen planus

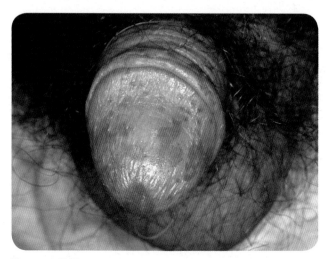

Figure 4-760 Candidiasis of the glans with red, somewhat eroded plaques.

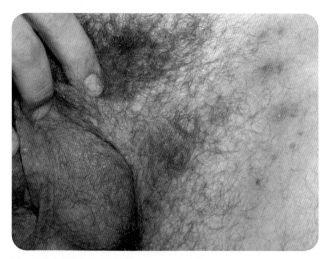

Figure 4-761 Candidiasis often involves the inguinal region, scrotum, and penis with very red papules and sometimes pustules.

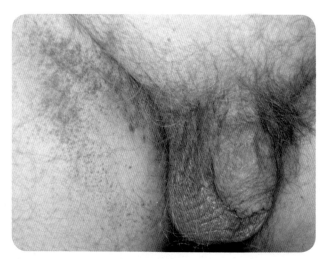

Figure 4-762 Penile edema and redness with scrotal and inguinal papules.

- Zoon balanitis (plasma cell balanitis)
- Nonspecific balanitis
- Reactive arthritis (formerly Reiter syndrome)
- Erythroplasia of Queyrat
- Herpes simplex virus
- Pemphigus vulgaris
- Lichen sclerosus

 Best Tests

A KOH preparation will show pseudo-hyphae and budding yeasts. Culture to allow the growth of yeast colonies.

 Management Pearls

- If lesions persist despite "adequate" therapy, consider reinfection from a sexual partner with *Candida* infection. Examine and treat the partner accordingly.
- In recurrent cases, consider screening for diabetes mellitus and HIV.
- It is possible for a candidate to develop a resistance to the drugs; therefore, a culture with sensitivity should be performed in persistent cases.

Therapy

Optimize the treatment of any underlying disease, such as diabetes.

Some antifungal agents come in powder form (miconazole powder), which are ideal for prevention.

Other Topical Therapies

- Spectazole cream—apply twice daily (15, 30, 85 g) for 10 days
- Miconazole cream—apply twice daily (15, 30, 85 g) for 10 days
- Clotrimazole cream—apply twice daily (15, 30, 45, 90 g) for 10 days
- Oral fluconazole (single dose of 100 to 200 mg) can be used for cases that are refractory to local therapy.

Immunocompromised Patient Considerations

Treat underlying disease or cause of immunosuppression.

Suggested Readings

Kyle AA, Dahl MV. Topical therapy for fungal infections. *Am J Clin Dermatol.* 2004;5(6):443–451.

Pappas PG, Rex JH, Sobel JD, et al; Infectious Diseases Society of America. Guidelines for treatment of candidiasis. *Clin Infect Dis.* 2004 Jan;38(2): 161–189.

Condyloma Acuminatum (Genital Wart)

■■ Diagnosis Synopsis

Condylomata acuminata, or genital warts, are caused by the human papillomavirus (HPV), a DNA virus that multiplies within the nuclei of infected epithelial cells. Approximately 90% of condylomata acuminata are related to HPV types 6 and 11. Genital warts are the most common sexually transmitted disease and should be considered in the differential diagnosis of patients presenting with genital papules.

The virus can remain latent in skin cells without any visible sign of infection. Subclinical infection is common and carries both infection and oncogenic potential. The highest prevalence rates occur in sexually active young adults, but do not discount this diagnosis in older individuals. Most lesions are asymptomatic, although pruritus and bleeding may occur. Recurrent disease is common.

Smoking, oral contraceptive use, multiple sexual partners, and early coital age are risk factors. HPV infection is more common and severe in patients with various immunologic deficiencies. HPV infection appears to be more common and more severe in immunocompromised patients. Warts are found in 5% to 30% of HIV-infected patients. Anogenital warts are more common in seropositive intravenous drug users.

The significant public health problem posed by genital HPV infection lies in the oncogenic potential of the virus. Subtypes 16, 18, 31, and many others predispose infected individuals to the development of squamous cell carcinoma (SCC) of the anogenital area.

Immunocompromised Patient Considerations

The treatment of genital warts in HIV-infected patients is often less effective than immunocompetent patients, necessitating combining medical and surgical procedures.

◉ Look For

Small 1 to 2 mm or larger white, gray, or skin-colored warty papules (Figs. 4-763–4-766) most commonly involving the penile glans and shaft in men and the vulvovaginal and cervical areas in woman. Sometimes there may be giant cauliflower-like lesions. In incompletely keratinized surfaces, like the vulva or under the foreskin, the papules will have a smoother surface (Fig. 4-767). Search carefully for

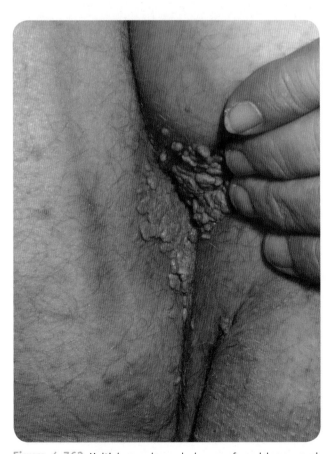

Figure 4-763 Multiple papules and plaques of condyloma acuminata in the perianal area.

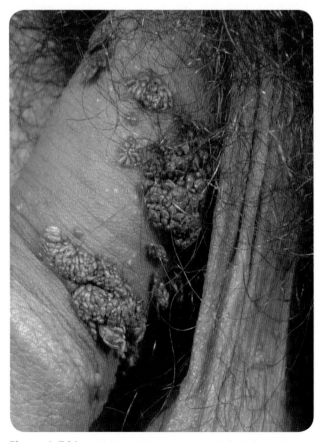

Figure 4-764 Multiple condylomata on the shaft of the penis.

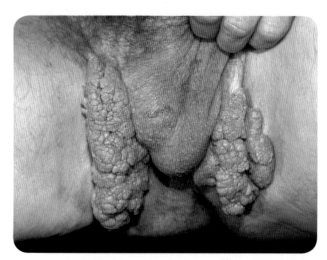

Figure 4-765 Giant condylomata bilaterally in both inguinal regions.

simultaneously involved multiple sites. Presence of external condylomata in both men and women warrants a thorough search for cervical and urethral lesions.

 Diagnostic Pearls

Recurrence rates and risk of oncogenic progression are highest among patients with immunologic deficiencies.

 Differential Diagnosis and Pitfalls

There are many verrucous-looking lesions of the genitals:

- Bowenoid papulosis
- SCC
- Psoriasis
- Condyloma latum (associated with syphilis)
- Seborrheic keratoses
- Lichen nitidus
- Pearly penile papules
- Sebaceous glands
- Acrochordons
- Lichen planus
- Nevocellular nevi
- Papillae
- Fordyce spots
- Molluscum contagiosum

 Best Tests

- As per the CDC, diagnosis of genital warts is made by visual inspection and may be confirmed by biopsy, although biopsy is needed only under certain circumstances (e.g., if the diagnosis is uncertain, the lesions do not respond

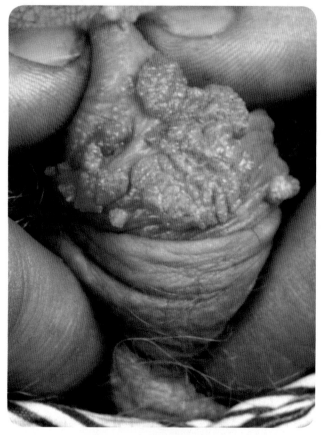

Figure 4-766 Extensive condylomata on the glans penis.

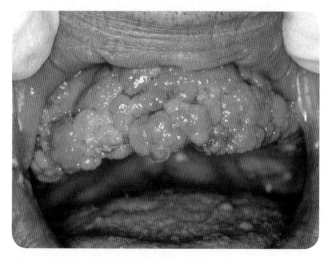

Figure 4-767 Large condylomata on the oral mucosa.

to standard therapy, the disease worsens during therapy, the patient is immunocompromised, or the warts are pigmented, indurated, fixed, bleeding, or ulcerated).

- The acetowhitening test involves the application of diluted acetic acid solution (3% to 5%) to genital tissue for 5 to 10 min before clinical examination. The solution whitens the warts, making it easier to visualize and focus treatment.

▲▲ Management Pearls

- The wart virus persists and is often present beyond the clinically visible borders of the lesions. This must be considered during destructive therapies. Lesions frequently recur, requiring vigilant surveillance.
- Other concomitant sexually transmitted diseases should be considered. Patients should be checked for immunodeficiency when there is severe involvement.
- Sexual partners of patients should be evaluated for disease, and female patients and partners should have regular Pap smears indefinitely.
- Patients should be advised that using condoms cannot completely protect them from HPV because vaginal or anal penetration does not need to occur to contract the virus.
- Consultations with specialists in gynecology, urology, or general or colorectal surgery may be needed.
- Gardasil (http://www.gardasil.com/) is a vaccine that protects against 4 strains of HPV (types 6, 11, 16, and 18), which cause 70% of cervical cancers and 90% of genital warts. In 2006, the FDA licensed this vaccine for use in girls/women ages 9 to 26.

Therapy

CDC-Recommended Regimens for External Genital Warts
Patient-Applied
Podofilox 0.5% solution or gel—Patients should apply podofilox solution with a cotton swab, or podofilox gel with a finger, to visible genital warts twice daily for 3 days, followed by 4 days of no therapy. This cycle may be repeated, as necessary, for up to four cycles.

OR

Imiquimod 5% cream—Patients should apply imiquimod cream once daily at bedtime, three times a week for up to 16 weeks.

Provider-Administered
Cryotherapy with liquid nitrogen or cryoprobe—Repeat applications every few weeks.

OR

Podophyllin resin 10% to 25% in a compound tincture of benzoin—A small amount should be applied to each wart and allowed to air-dry. The treatment can be repeated weekly, if necessary. Important guidelines should be followed to avoid the possibility of complications associated with systemic absorption and toxicity.

OR

Trichloroacetic acid (TCA) or bichloracetic acid (BCA) 80% to 90%—A small amount should be applied to only the warts and allowed to dry, at which time a white "frosting" develops. If an excess amount of acid is applied, the treated area should be powdered with talc, sodium bicarbonate (i.e., baking soda), or liquid soap preparations to remove unreacted acid. This treatment can be repeated weekly, if necessary.

OR

Surgical removal by scissor excision, shave excision, curettage, or electrosurgery.

CDC-Recommended Alternative Regimens
Intralesional interferon

OR

Laser surgery

CDC-Recommended Regimens for Cervical Warts
For women who have exophytic cervical warts, high-grade SIL must be excluded before treatment is initiated. The management of exophytic cervical warts should include consultation with a specialist.

CDC-Recommended Regimens for Vaginal Warts
Cryotherapy with liquid nitrogen—The use of a cryoprobe in the vagina is not recommended because of the risk for vaginal perforation and fistula formation.

OR

TCA or BCA 80% to 90% applied to warts—A small amount should be applied to only the warts and allowed to dry, at which time a white "frosting" develops. If an excess amount of acid is applied, the treated area should be powdered with talc, sodium bicarbonate, or liquid soap preparations to remove unreacted acid. This treatment can be repeated weekly, if necessary.

CDC-Recommended Regimens for Urethral Meatus Warts
Cryotherapy with liquid nitrogen

OR

Podophyllin 10% to 25% in compound tincture of benzoin—The treatment area must be dry before contact with normal mucosa. This treatment can be repeated weekly, if necessary.

Although data evaluating the use of podofilox and imiquimod for the treatment of distal meatal warts are limited, some specialists recommend their use in some patients.

(Continued)

CDC-Recommended Regimens for Anal Warts

Cryotherapy with liquid nitrogen

OR

TCA or BCA 80% to 90% applied to warts

OR

Surgical removal

Warts on the rectal mucosa should be managed in consultation with a specialist. Many persons with warts on the anal mucosa also have warts on the rectal mucosa, so persons with anal warts can benefit from an inspection of the rectal mucosa by digital examination or anoscopy.

Suggested Readings

Arican O, Guneri F, Bilgic K, et al. Topical imiquimod 5% cream in external anogenital warts: A randomized, double-blind, placebo-controlled study. *J Dermatol*. 2004 Aug;31(8):627–631.

Brodell LA, Mercurio MG, Brodell RT. The diagnosis and treatment of human papillomavirus-mediated genital lesions. *Cutis*. 2007 Apr; 79(4 Suppl.):5–10.

Centers for Disease Control and Prevention (CDC). Sexually transmitted diseases treatment guidelines, 2006. *MMWR Morb Mortal Wkly Rep*. 2006 Aug;59(RR1):1–94.

Centers for Disease Control and Prevention; Workowski KA, Berman SM. Sexually transmitted diseases treatment guidelines, 2006. *MMWR Recomm Rep*. 2006 Aug;55(RR-11):1–94.

Gotovtseva EP, Kapadia AS, Smolensky MH, et al. Optimal frequency of imiquimod (aldara) 5% cream for the treatment of external genital warts in immunocompetent adults: A meta-analysis. *Sex Transm Dis*. 2008 Apr;35(4):346–351.

Hagensee ME, Cameron JE, Leigh JE, et al. Human papillomavirus infection and disease in HIV-infected individuals. *Am J Med Sci*. 2004 Jul;328(1):57–63.

Huang CM. Human papillomavirus and vaccination. *Mayo Clin Proc*. 2008 Jun;83(6):701–706; quiz 706–707.

O'Mahony C. Genital warts: Current and future management options. *Am J Clin Dermatol*. 2005;6(4):239–243.

Partridge JM, Koutsky LA. Genital human papillomavirus infection in men. *Lancet Infect Dis*. 2006 Jan;6(1):21–31.

Reichman RC, Oakes D, Bonnez W, et al. Treatment of condyloma acuminatum with three different interferon-alpha preparations administered parenterally: A double-blind, placebo-controlled trial. *J Infect Dis*. 1990 Dec;162(6):1270–1276.

Scheinfeld N, Lehman DS. An evidence-based review of medical and surgical treatments of genital warts. *Dermatol Online J*. 2006;12(3):5.

Schöfer H. Evaluation of imiquimod for the therapy of external genital and anal warts in comparison with destructive therapies. *Br J Dermatol*. 2007 Dec;157 Suppl 2:52–55.

Sherrard J, Riddell L. Comparison of the effectiveness of commonly used clinic-based treatments for external genital warts. *Int J STD AIDS*. 2007 Jun;18(6):365–368.

Urman CO, Gottlieb AB. New viral vaccines for dermatologic disease. *J Am Acad Dermatol*. 2008 Mar;58(3):361–370.

Diagnosis Synopsis

Erythrasma is a common, chronic superficial bacterial infection of the skin caused by *Corynebacterium minutissimum*. It is characterized by distinct, superficial hyperpigmented or erythematous patches localized to intertriginous areas. A "disciform" variant (large disklike lesions) usually occurs outside of intertriginous areas, and it is associated with type 2 diabetes mellitus. Erythrasma may be acute or chronic. It may be pruritic.

The highest incidence is seen in regions of high humidity, especially in the tropics. Obesity, diabetes mellitus, immunosuppression, a history of atopy, and hyperhydrosis are risk factors. All age groups may be affected, but incidence increases with age.

Immunocompromised Patient Considerations

Although the overwhelming majority of *C. minutissimum* infections are localized to the superficial skin, deeper skin infections and extracutaneous disease have been reported. Cases of cutaneous granulomas and costochondral abscesses have been reported in HIV-infected individuals. Several cases of *C. minutissimum* bacteremia have been reported in patients with leukemia/lymphoma.

Look For

Brown, almost flat, minimally scaly plaques with fine scale on the webs of the toes, axillae, inframammary (beneath the breasts) folds, around the anus, and in the groin (Figs. 4-768

and 4-769). In the web spaces of the feet, macerated, white plaques can have a surrounding yellowish color.

Dark Skin Considerations

In black patients, the involved areas usually have an overlying fine, grayish scale.

Diagnostic Pearls

Plaques are usually sharply marginated. The lesions may be subtle but are almost always symmetrical. These are noninflammatory plaques with minimal, if any, erythema.

Immunocompromised Patient Considerations

The condition may be widespread in immunocompromised individuals.

Differential Diagnosis and Pitfalls

- Inverse psoriasis
- Seborrheic dermatitis
- Tinea corporis
- Tinea pedis
- Tinea versicolor
- Acanthosis nigricans
- Intertrigo
- Contact dermatitis
- Confluent and reticulated papillomatosis

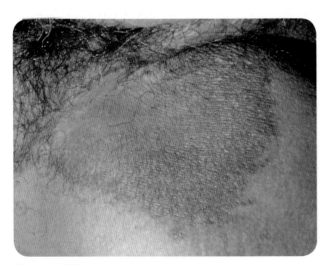

Figure 4-768 Plaque of erythrasma in the groin.

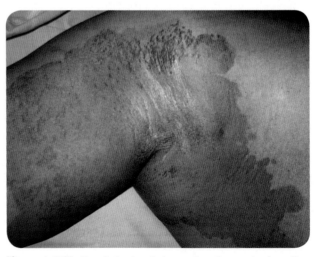

Figure 4-769 Sharply bordered plaque of erythrasma in the axilla.

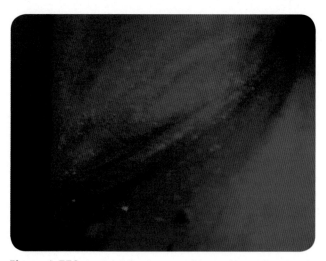

Figure 4-770 Coral-red fluorescence with Wood lamp shows erythrasma in the axilla.

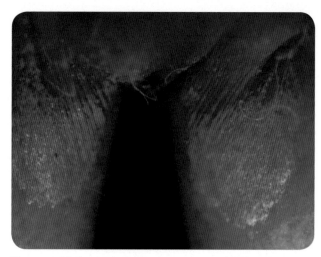

Figure 4-771 Coral-red fluorescence with Wood lamp shows erythrasma in the groin.

Immunocompromised Patient Differential Diagnosis

May present as granulomatous plaques in immunocompromised patients.

✓ Best Tests

- If a Wood lamp (UVA lamp) is available, the diagnosis is confirmed by coral red (pink-red) fluorescence due to the presence of coproporphyrin III produced by the organism (Figs. 4-770 and 4-771). Bathing may result in removing the superficially deposited fluorescing coproporphyrins and can result in a false-negative Wood light exam.
- KOH preparations of skin scrapings will often show chains of bacilli. Stain with methylene blue to facilitate identification.

▲▲ Management Pearls

Washing with an antibacterial soap may both treat active infections and prevent recurrences. Topical 10% to 20% aluminum chloride and 2% clindamycin may also be effective. Oral therapy (for recalcitrant cases) is with erythromycin (for 5 days).

Therapy

- Topical imidazole creams—Miconazole, clotrimazole, or econazole applied to affected areas twice daily for 2 weeks.
- Topical antibiotics—Topical erythromycin solution 2%, topical clindamycin solution 2%, or topical fusidic acid cream 2% applied twice daily for 2 weeks.
- Benzoic acid 6%, salicylic acid 3% (Whitfield ointment)—Apply twice daily for 4 weeks. May be irritating.
- Severe cases—Oral erythromycin, 250 mg four times daily for 2 weeks.

Suggested Readings

Dalal A, Likhi R. *Corynebacterium minutissimum* bacteremia and meningitis: A case report and review of literature. *J Infect*. 2008 Jan;56(1):77–79.

Hamann K, Thorn P. Systemic or local treatment of erythrasma? A comparison between erythromycin tablets and Fucidin cream in general practice. *Scand J Prim Health Care*. 1991 Mar;9(1):35–39.

Holdiness MR. Management of cutaneous erythrasma. *Drugs*. 2002;62(8): 1131–1141.

Tschen JA, Ramsdell WM. Disciform erythrasma. *Cutis*. 1983 May;31(5): 541–542, 547.

Washington JA, Wilson WR. Erythromycin: a microbial and clinical perspective after 30 years of clinical use (2). *Mayo Clin Proc*. 1985 Apr;60(4): 271–278.

Wharton JR, Wilson PL, Kincannon JM. Erythrasma treated with single-dose clarithromycin. *Arch Dermatol*. 1998 Jun;134(6):671–672.

Herpes Simplex Virus (HSV), Genital

■■ Diagnosis Synopsis

Genital herpes simplex virus is a sexually transmitted viral infection that is caused most commonly by herpes simplex virus type 2 (HSV-2) and less often by herpes simplex virus type 1 (HSV-1). This viral infection is spread from direct contact with active lesions (most common) or the asymptomatic shedding (less common) of infected individuals. The initial eruption usually develops within 5 to 7 days of inoculation and consists of grouped painful vesicles, pustules, and/or erosions on an erythematous base. In females, vulvar, vaginal, and perineal lesions are most common. In males, lesions most commonly occur on the glans penis or penile shaft. A prodrome of fever, malaise, and lymphadenopathy may precede the primary mucocutaneous eruption. In some individuals, primary infection can be severe and include symptoms of aseptic meningitis such as fever, headache, stiff neck, and photophobia. In women, there can be severe local symptoms of pain, dysuria, and vaginal discharge. It is important to note that even when asymptomatic a person sheds the virus and can, therefore, transmit the disease to another.

Mucocutaneous HSV infection is characterized by initial outbreaks (primary infection), periods of latency (regional sensory ganglia), and recurrent flares localized to the area of the initial outbreak (recurrent infection). Stress, ultraviolet light, fever, tissue damage, and immunosuppression have all been associated with triggering recurrent flares. Recurrent eruptions are usually less severe (fewer lesions and less painful), resolve within 1 week, and lack a prodromal phase. Patients with genital HSV have an average of four to seven recurrent outbreaks per year.

Females, the elderly, African American race, low socioeconomic status, early age of first intercourse, high number of sexual partners, and history of prior sexually transmitted disease all confer an increased risk of developing genital HSV.

Immunocompromised Patient Considerations

Immunocompromised patients generally have more severe disease. Recurrent outbreaks are more painful, more widespread, last longer, are poorly responsive to therapy, and have a higher risk of viremic dissemination. In addition, genital HSV infections in immunocompromised patients can have atypical presentations. Verrucous and exophytic nodules resembling condyloma acuminatum and verrucous carcinoma have been described. Infection with genital HSV confers an increased risk of acquiring and transmitting HIV.

◉ Look For

Grouped, umbilicated (with central depressions) vesicles and vesiculopustules or grouped erosions or small ulcers on an erythematous base (Figs. 4-772–4-775). Spreading lesions can be seen in the pubic area as well.

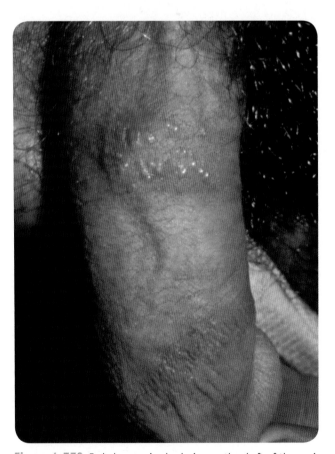

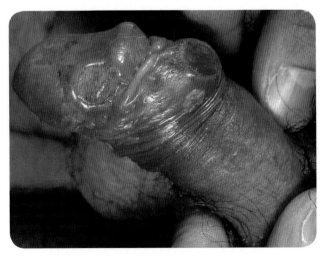

Figure 4-772 Multiple large herpetic ulcers on the penis.

Figure 4-773 Early herpes simplex lesion on the shaft of the penis with multiple grouped intact vesicles.

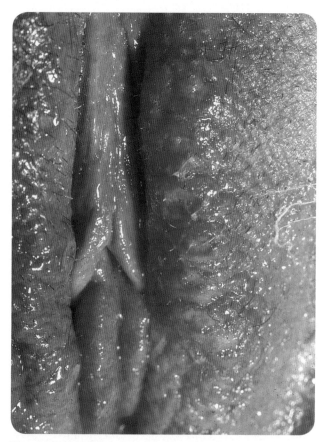

Figure 4-774 Vaginal labial herpetic infections.

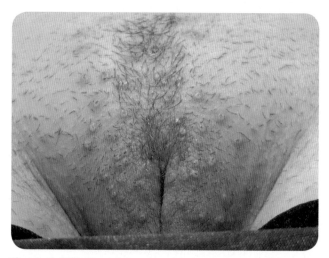

Figure 4-775 Mons pubis herpetic infection identified by umbilicated lesions.

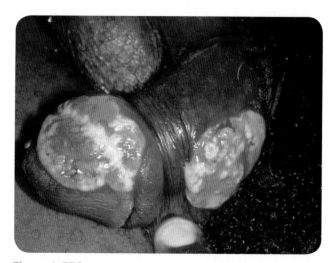

Figure 4-776 Herpes infection in an HIV-infected patient.

Immunocompromised Patient Considerations

Genital HSV can present as exophytic masses, verrucous nodules, or persistent ulcers in immunocompromised hosts (Fig. 4-776).

Diagnostic Pearls

- Vesicles are short-lived when they arise in the genital areas. Thus, grouped erosions are common.
- Lesions, especially erosions or ulcers, may be persistent in immunosuppressed patients.
- Patients may experience a burning sensation before the appearance of lesions.
- Consider this diagnosis for any recurrent eruption in the bathing trunk area.

?? Differential Diagnosis and Pitfalls

- Consider herpes zoster if the lesions seem to be unilateral or if the outbreak occurs in an older patient.
- Molluscum contagiosum lesions are usually not painful, are slow to evolve, and are rarely grouped.
- Fixed drug eruption
- Syphilis
- Lymphogranuloma venereum
- Chancroid
- Trauma
- *Candida*
- Pyoderma
- Erosive lichen planus

Immunocompromised Patient Differential Diagnosis

- Condyloma acuminatum
- Verrucous carcinoma

✓ Best Tests

- Immediate diagnosis to confirm acute herpetic infection, which includes varicella-zoster virus (VZV), can be made by demonstrating multinucleated giant cells on Tzanck prep.
- Direct fluorescence antigen (DFA) testing is a rapid (<24 h) and sensitive test for HSV-1, HSV-2, and VZV. This test is performed by vigorously scraping the base of a vesicle with a sterile cotton-tipped swab or 15 blade and smearing the cells onto a glass slide from a DFA kit. The slide is then fixed (usually contained in a kit) and sent for immunofluorescence analysis. Individual slides must be sent for each virus suspected. Slides can be stored at room temperature for 24 h after fixation, if needed.
- PCR-based clinical assays are rapid, highly sensitive tests for both HSV-1 and HSV-2 detection.
- Viral culture of skin lesions.

▲▲▲ Management Pearls

- Lesions normally resolve on their own within 5 to 10 days. Pain management is important, especially in the primary episode. Consider topical 5% lidocaine ointment and oral anti-inflammatories/analgesics.
- According to the CDC, antiviral chemotherapy offers clinical benefits to the majority of symptomatic patients and is the mainstay of management.
- Counseling regarding the natural history of genital herpes, sexual and perinatal transmission, and methods to reduce transmission is integral to clinical management. Additionally, the sex partners of patients who have genital HSV can benefit from evaluation and counseling. Symptomatic sex partners should be evaluated and treated in the same manner as patients who have genital lesions. Asymptomatic sex partners of patients who have genital HSV should be questioned concerning histories of genital lesions and offered type-specific serologic testing for HSV infection.

Precautions: Standard and Contact. (Isolate patient, wear gloves and a gown, limit patient transport, and avoid sharing patient-care equipment.)

Therapy

CDC-Recommended Regimens—First Clinical Episode

Systemic antiviral drugs can partially control the signs and symptoms of HSV episodes when used to first treat clinical and recurrent episodes or when used as daily suppressive therapy. However, these drugs neither eradicate latent virus nor affect the risk, frequency, or severity of recurrences after the drug is discontinued. Randomized trials have indicated that three antiviral medications provide clinical benefit for genital HSV: acyclovir, valacyclovir, and famciclovir.

Acyclovir 400 mg orally three times daily for 7 to 10 days

OR

Acyclovir 200 mg orally five times daily for 7 to 10 days

OR

Famciclovir 250 mg orally three times daily for 7 to 10 days

OR

Valacyclovir 1.0 g orally twice daily for 7 to 10 days

CDC-Recommended Regimens—Suppressive Therapy

Suppressive therapy reduces the frequency of genital HSV recurrences by 70% to 80% in patients who have frequent recurrences (i.e., six or more per year), and many patients report no symptomatic outbreaks. Treatment is also effective in patients with less frequent recurrences. Safety and efficacy have been documented among patients receiving daily therapy with acyclovir for as long as 6 years and with valacyclovir or famciclovir for 1 year. The quality of life is frequently improved in patients with frequent recurrences who receive suppressive therapy compared with episodic treatment.

Acyclovir 400 mg orally twice daily

OR

Famciclovir 250 mg orally twice daily

OR

Valacyclovir 500 mg orally once daily

OR

Valacyclovir 1.0 g orally once daily

(Continued)

CDC-Recommended Regimens—Episodic Therapy

Effective episodic treatment of recurrent HSV requires the initiation of therapy within 1 day of lesion onset or during the prodrome that precedes some outbreaks. The patient should be provided with a supply of the drug or a prescription for the medication with instructions to immediately initiate treatment when symptoms begin.

Acyclovir 400 mg orally three times daily for 5 days

OR

Acyclovir 800 mg orally twice daily for 5 days

OR

Acyclovir 800 mg orally three times daily for 2 days

OR

Famciclovir 125 mg orally twice daily for 5 days

OR

Famciclovir 1,000 mg orally twice daily for 1 day

OR

Famciclovir 1,500 mg orally once

OR

Valacyclovir 500 mg orally twice daily for 3 days

OR

Valacyclovir 1.0 g orally once daily for 5 days

CDC-Recommended Regimens—Suppressive Therapy in HIV-Infected Individuals

Acyclovir 400 to 800 mg orally two to three times daily

OR

Famciclovir 500 mg orally twice daily

OR

Valacyclovir 500 mg orally twice daily

CDC-Recommended Regimens—Episodic Therapy in HIV-Infected Individuals

Acyclovir 400 mg orally three times daily for 5 to 10 days

OR

Famciclovir 500 mg orally twice daily for 5 to 10 days

OR

Valacyclovir 1.0 g orally twice daily for 5 to 10 days

Acyclovir, valacyclovir, and famciclovir are safe for use in immunocompromised patients in the doses recommended for the treatment of genital HSV. For severe HSV disease, initiating therapy with acyclovir 5 to 10 mg/kg body weight IV every 8 h might be necessary.

Suggested Readings

ACOG Committee on Practice Bulletins—Gynecology. ACOG practice bulletin: Clinical management guidelines for obstetrician-gynecologists, no. 57, November 2004. Gynecologic herpes simplex virus infections. *Obstet Gynecol.* 2004 Nov;104(5 Pt 1):1111–1118.

Centers for Disease Control and Prevention; Workowski KA, Berman SM. Sexually transmitted diseases treatment guidelines, 2006. *MMWR Recomm Rep.* 2006 Aug;55(RR-11):1–94.

Corey L, Wald A, Patel R, et al; Valacyclovir HSV Transmission Study Group. Once-daily valacyclovir to reduce the risk of transmission of genital herpes. *N Engl J Med.* 2004 Jan;350(1):11–20.

Fatahzadeh M, Schwartz RA. Human herpes simplex virus infections: Epidemiology, pathogenesis, symptomatology, diagnosis, and management. *J Am Acad Dermatol.* 2007 Nov;57(5):737–763; quiz 764–766.

Fife KH, Warren TJ, Justus SE, et al; HS2100275 STUDY TEAM. An international, randomized, double-blind, placebo-controlled, study of valacyclovir for the suppression of herpes simplex virus type 2 genital herpes in newly diagnosed patients. *Sex Transm Dis.* 2008 Jul;35(7):668–673.

Gupta R, Warren T, Wald A. Genital herpes. *Lancet.* 2007 Dec;370(9605): 2127–2137.

Lebrun-Vignes B, Bouzamondo A, Dupuy A, et al. A meta-analysis to assess the efficacy of oral antiviral treatment to prevent genital herpes outbreaks. *J Am Acad Dermatol.* 2007 Aug;57(2):238–246.

Xu F, Sternberg MR, Kottiri BJ, et al. Trends in herpes simplex virus type 1 and type 2 seroprevalence in the United States. *JAMA.* 2006 Aug;296(8): 964–973.

Lichen Sclerosus

■■ Diagnosis Synopsis

Lichen sclerosus (lichen sclerosus et atrophicus) is a chronic dermatosis characterized by an initial short inflammatory phase followed by chronic scarring and skin atrophy. It is a disease primarily of anogenital skin in both males and females of all races.

Clinically, over 85% of lesions are found on anogenital skin. Anogenital lichen sclerosus usually presents as dry, tender, and severely pruritic white plaques with epidermal atrophy resembling scarring. Plaques can progress to cause functional impairment, most commonly phimosis in males and sclerosis of the vaginal introitus in females. It is more common in females, with two peaks in age distribution: (i) prepubertal children and (ii) postmenopausal women. It is one of the most common causes of chronic vulvar symptoms in adult females. The majority of cases of male genital lichen sclerosus occur in uncircumcised men.

Lichen sclerosus on nongenital skin is frequently asymptomatic; however, it can also be xerotic and pruritic. It most commonly presents as ivory-colored, atrophic, scar-like plaques with follicular accentuation on the neck, shoulders, back, and upper extremities. It also has a predilection for sites of previous trauma (Koebner phenomenon).

Lesions of lichen sclerosus should be treated. Squamous cell carcinoma can arise in genital lesions, and there may be complications related to genital scarring—including dyspareunia, urinary obstruction, ulceration, painful erection, and phimosis. Nongenital lesions may cause psychosocial distress secondary to cosmesis and chronic pruritus.

Currently, the etiology of lichen sclerosus is unknown.

◉ Look For

The lesions begin as flat, white plaques surrounded by a red-, purple-, or violet-colored border (Fig. 4-777). Over time, the lesions become sclerotic and atrophied and develop a shiny, porcelain appearance (Fig. 4-778). Telangiectasias and follicular plugs may be present in chronic lesions.

Extragenital lesions most commonly occur on the back and shoulders and often begin as white, polygonal papules that coalesce into plaques. Oral lichen sclerosus is rare. It presents as bluish white papules on the buccal mucosa that evolve into scar-like plaques or superficial erosions.

Female genital lesions may eventually obliterate the labia minora and narrow the introitus. An "hourglass" or "figure-of-eight" pattern may be seen surrounding the perivaginal and perianal areas (Fig. 4-779). When inflammation is severe, ulcerations/erosions and bullae can be seen.

Male genital lesions are often confined to the glans and prepuce. Often, the presenting lesion is a sclerotic band or ring at the edge of the prepuce (Fig. 4-780).

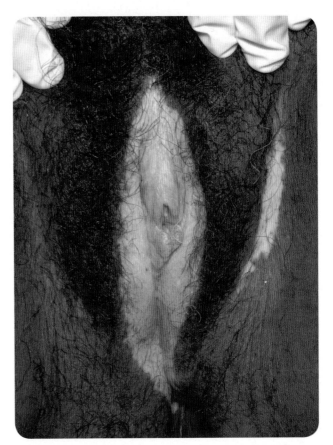

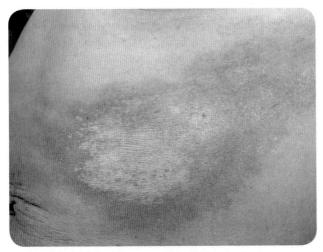

Figure 4-777 Lichen sclerosus can affect nongenital skin with white atrophic plaques that must be distinguished from morphea and a lichen sclerosus/morphea overlap syndrome.

Figure 4-778 Perivaginal hypopigmentation with atrophy and sclerosis.

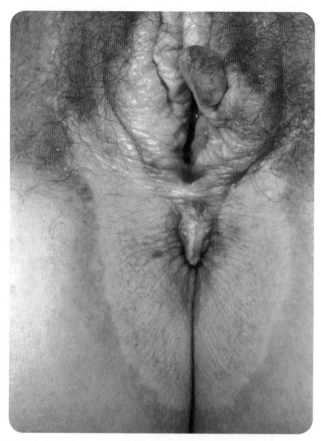

Figure 4-779 Hourglass hypopigmentation of the vulva with inflammation in lichen sclerosus.

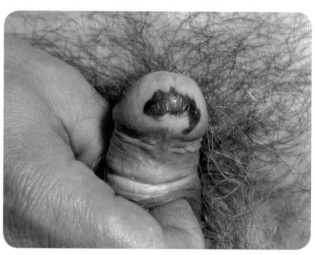

Figure 4-780 Balanitis xerotica obliterans in the male is analogous to lichen sclerosus. The glans in this case is white and sclerotic. Purpura occurs in lesions of the disorder in both sexes.

- Anetoderma
- Atrophoderma of Pasini and Pierini
- Extramammary Paget disease
- Lichen planus

✓ Best Tests

Skin biopsy will confirm the clinical suspicion.

▲▲ Management Pearls

- Seemingly paradoxical (one would not think using a strong corticosteroid on atrophic skin would be safe), high-potency (class 1) topical steroids are highly efficacious for this condition. See the patient frequently, and monitor for the correct use of the medication.
- Affected patients should be referred to a dermatologist and a gynecologist or urologist if the situation warrants (e.g., for management of genitourinary complications, biopsy of chronic ulcer or nodule to rule out squamous cell carcinoma). Uncircumcised males with lichen sclerosus may benefit from circumcision.

Therapy

Class 1 corticosteroids, such as clobetasol propionate 0.05% cream, applied daily or twice daily to the site until thickening and/or discomfort resolves is first-line therapy. In a limited number of studies, nearly all patients with vulvar disease achieved a response with 20% of responders achieving complete clearance.

●● Diagnostic Pearls

- When on the genitals, the lesions may have purpura, and caretakers of affected individuals must consider abuse.
- The Koebner phenomenon has been described in this condition, with lesions being found in surgical and burn scars and areas subject to trauma.

?? Differential Diagnosis and Pitfalls

There is often an overlap between lichen sclerosus and morphea (localized scleroderma); however, treatment remains the same.

Abuse should always be considered in individuals with scar-like lesions of the anogenital area.

- Scar
- Sclerosing basal cell carcinoma
- Chronic radiation dermatitis
- Vitiligo
- Tinea versicolor
- Idiopathic guttate hypomelanosis
- Bowen disease/erythroplasia of Queyrat

The use of long-term topical retinoids (tretinoin 0.025% applied five times weekly) has shown benefit in an open-label trial.

Topical immunomodulators (tacrolimus ointment 0.1% applied daily for 10 months) induced remission in all six patients in a case series. Pimecrolimus 1% cream twice daily for 3 months benefitted three of four patients in another series. Theoretically, there is the potential for an increased risk of malignancy with the chronic use of the calcineurin inhibitors. Because malignancies have been reported to develop within lesions of lichen sclerosus, calcineurin inhibitors are not used as chronic therapy by many dermatologists for this condition.

Oral retinoids (acitretin 20 to 30 mg daily for 16 weeks) provided benefit to some patients in a small clinical trial.

Various supportive measures may be needed:

- Stool softeners (i.e., docusate) when there is painful defecation
- Treatment of any postinflammatory pain syndromes (e.g., vulvodynia) with topical 5% lidocaine ointment
- Avoidance of local irritants and use of soap substitutes

- Education and/or counseling regarding impact on sexual functioning

Recent systematic review shows phototherapy to be an effective option for treating sclerotic skin diseases including lichen sclerosus. UVA-1 treatment can shorten the active phase of disease and prevent disease progression.

Suggested Readings

Hallel-Halevy D, Grunwald MH, Yerushalmi J, et al. Bullous lichen sclerosus et atrophicus. *J Am Acad Dermatol*. 1998 Sep;39(3):500–501.

Hengge UR, Krause W, Hofmann H, et al. Multicentre, phase II trial on the safety and efficacy of topical tacrolimus ointment for the treatment of lichen sclerosus. *Br J Dermatol*. 2006 Nov;155(5):1021–1028.

Kroft EB, Berkhof NJ, van de Kerkhof PC, et al. Ultraviolet A phototherapy for sclerotic skin diseases: A systematic review. *J Am Acad Dermatol*. 2008 Dec;59(6):1017–1030.

Neill SM, Tatnall FM, Cox NH; British Association of Dermatologists. Guidelines for the management of lichen sclerosus. *Br J Dermatol*. 2002 Oct;147(4):640–649.

Ridley CM. Lichen sclerosus et atrophicus. *Semin Dermatol*. 1989 Mar;8(1):54–63.

Tremaine RD, Miller RA. Lichen sclerosus et atrophicus. *Int J Dermatol*. 1989 Jan–Feb;28(1):10–16.

■ Diagnosis Synopsis

Pediculosis pubis (pubic lice, crabs) is a highly contagious sexually transmitted parasitic infestation with the pubic or crab louse, *Phthirus pubis*. Disease is most often spread from person to person by close physical contact, but it may occasionally be spread by fomites such as clothing or linens. Lice feed on human blood several times daily. The bites of the lice are usually painless, but patients often experience intense pruritus. The itching is the result of a reaction to the saliva and/or an anticoagulant injected into the skin by the louse as it feeds. The eggs (nits) are cemented to hair shafts with chitin and are difficult to remove. Lice hatch in approximately 6 to 10 days. Pubic lice are more common in sexually active individuals. In addition to the pubic hair, infestation may involve perianal skin, the axillae, and, rarely, the eyelashes, eyebrows, chest, or facial hair. Black patients may have scalp infestation. Treatment is aimed at eliminating lice via the use of medications and environmental control measures, including the treatment of all close contacts.

Immunocompromised Patient Considerations

Coexistent sexually transmitted infections, including HIV-AIDS, are more common in patients with pediculosis pubis versus the general population. In one study, a quarter of patients with HIV had a previous diagnosis of pubic lice. However, HIV seropositivity does not appear to affect the clinical course of pubic lice infections. Treatment regimens are typically the same as in seronegative patients.

◉ Look For

Lice and nits in the pubic hair (Fig. 4-781). They are also occasionally found on eyelashes, eyebrows, facial hair, body hair, or on the scalp. The lice are approximately 1 mm in diameter and may be tightly adherent to hair shafts (Figs. 4-782 and 4-783). They may be mistaken for crusts or hair casts when attached near the ostia, or openings, of hair follicles.

Inguinal lymph node swelling may be seen.

Erythematous macules or papules may appear at feeding sites after hours or days, and acute wheals may be seen as an immediate reaction. Erythema is often perifollicular. In patients with longstanding infection, *maculae ceruleae*, bluish-gray macules, may form at feeding sites.

Dark Skin Considerations

Black patients may have scalp infestation.

●● Diagnostic Pearls

- Itching is the main symptom.
- Nits fluoresce under a Wood light.

?? Differential Diagnosis and Pitfalls

- Trichorrhexis nodosa
- White piedra
- Peripilar hair casts may be mistaken for nits
- Bites from other insects
- Scabies

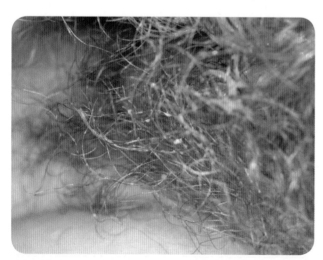

Figure 4-781 Multiple nits on pubic hairs suggestive of pubic lice infestation.

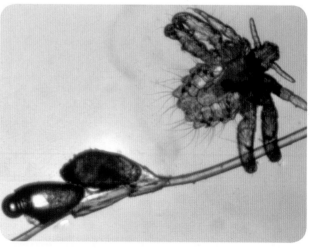

Figure 4-782 Pubic louse with nits on hair.

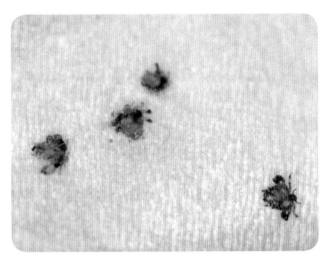

Figure 4-783 Pubic lice from infested skin.

- Impetigo
- Other causes of anogenital itch, including tinea cruris, contact dermatitis, and candidiasis

✓ Best Tests

Demonstration of the insect or the nit (from a hair visually or under the microscope) is diagnostic. A magnification glass or a Wood lamp may facilitate the diagnosis.

▲▲ Management Pearls

- The CDC recommends that sex partners within the previous month should be treated. Patients should avoid sexual contact with their sex partner(s) until patients and partners have been treated and reevaluated to rule out persistent disease. Patients should be evaluated and treated for other sexually transmitted diseases. Patients should be aware that condoms do not prevent transmission.
- All potential fomites should be discarded or laundered in hot water with drying on the highest heat. Dry cleaning may also be used. Items that are not easily washed can be sealed in air-tight plastic bags for 12 to 14 days. Soak combs and brushes in very hot water for a minimum of 5 min. Vacuum the carpets and furniture within the home.
- Shaving the involved area(s) may help eradicate the lice; however, this is not acceptable to many patients.

Precautions: Standard and Contact. (Isolate patient, wear gloves and a gown, limit patient transport, and avoid sharing patient-care equipment.)

Therapy

CDC-Recommended Regimens
Permethrin 1% cream rinse applied to affected areas and washed off after 10 min

OR

Pyrethrins with piperonyl butoxide applied to the affected area and washed off after 10 min. (Do not use in those with ragweed or turpentine allergy.)

CDC-Recommended Alternative Regimens
Malathion 0.5% lotion applied for 8 to 12 h and washed off

OR

Ivermectin 250 μg/kg repeated in 2 weeks

Use only aqueous preparations. For all topical preparations, rectal hair treatment is necessary to ensure complete eradication. Hairy individuals should treat their thighs, trunk, and axillary hair.

Infestation of the eyelashes can be treated with ophthalmic petroleum jelly applications twice daily for 2 weeks. Alternatively, nits and lice can be removed with forceps.

Treat any secondarily infected lesions with an appropriate topical or systemic antibiotic.

Additional Information from the CDC Website
Reported resistance to pediculicides has been increasing and is widespread. Malathion may be used when treatment failure is believed to have occurred because of resistance. The odor and long duration of application for Malathion make it a less attractive alternative than the recommended pediculicides. Ivermectin has been successfully used to treat lice but has only been evaluated in small studies.

Lindane is not recommended as first-line therapy because of toxicity. It should only be used as an alternative because of inability to tolerate other therapies or if other therapies have failed. Lindane toxicity, as indicated by seizure and aplastic anemia, has not been reported when treatment was limited to the recommended 4-min period. Permethrin has less potential for toxicity than lindane.

Immunocompromised Patient Considerations

CDC recommendations are the same for HIV-infected individuals and the general population.

Suggested Readings

Billstein SA, Mattaliano VJ. The "nuisance" sexually transmitted diseases: Molluscum contagiosum, scabies, and crab lice. *Med Clin North Am*. 1990 Nov;74(6):1487–1505.

Burkhart CG, Burkhart CN. Oral ivermectin for *Phthirus pubis*. *J Am Acad Dermatol*. 2004 Dec;51(6):1037; author reply 1037–1038.

Centers for Disease Control and Prevention; Workowski KA, Berman SM. Sexually transmitted diseases treatment guidelines, 2006. *MMWR Recomm Rep*. 2006 Aug;55(RR-11):1–94.

Elston DM. Drugs used in the treatment of pediculosis. *J Drugs Dermatol*. 2005 Mar-Apr;4(2):207–211.

Galiczynski EM, Elston DM. What's eating you? Pubic lice (Pthirus pubis). *Cutis*. 2008 Feb;81(2):109–114.

Ko CJ, Elston DM. Pediculosis. *J Am Acad Dermatol*. 2004 Jan;50(1):1–12; quiz 13–14.

Leone PA. Scabies and pediculosis pubis: An update of treatment regimens and general review. *Clin Infect Dis*. 2007 Apr;44(Suppl. 3):S153–S159.

Meinking DL, Burkhart CN, Burkhart CG, Elgart G. Infestations. In: Bolognia J, Jorizzo JL, Rapini RP, eds. *Dermatology*. 2nd Ed. St. Louis, MO: Mosby; 2008:1297–1298.

Diagnosis Synopsis

Syphilis is a sexually transmitted infection (STI) caused by the bacterium *Treponema pallidum* and is characterized by a chronic, intermittent, clinical course. It is transmitted from person to person via direct contact with a syphilis ulcer during vaginal, anal, or oral sex. Hence, the locations for syphilitic ulcers include the vagina, cervix, penis, anus, rectum, lips, and inside of the mouth. According to the Centers for Disease Control and Prevention (CDC), over 36,000 cases of syphilis were reported in the United States in 2006. Between 2005 and 2006, the number of primary and secondary syphilis cases increased by 11.8%. Sixty-four percent of syphilis cases were among men who have sex with men (MSM). An increased incidence of syphilis in the United States has been observed in black and Hispanic individuals, sex workers, individuals who sexually expose themselves to sex workers, and individuals with a history of other STIs and/or HIV.

The natural history of primary syphilis is as follows:

- Primary lesion develops 10 to 90 days (average of 3 weeks) after direct inoculation.
- Primary lesion is a painless, asymptomatic papule, followed by ulceration (chancre) and regional lymphadenopathy.
- Chancre lasts 3 to 6 weeks and heals spontaneously.
- All patients with primary syphilis will go on to develop secondary syphilis if left untreated.

Secondary syphilis usually appears 3 to 10 weeks after the primary chancre and is characterized by papulosquamous eruptions on the body and mucosal involvement in some cases. Tertiary syphilis may appear months to years after secondary syphilis resolves and can involve the CNS, heart, bones, and skin.

Immunocompromised Patient Considerations

Genital ulcers caused by syphilis increase the risk of HIV transmission due to epithelial barrier compromise and increased numbers of macrophages and T-lymphocytes with HIV-specific receptors.

Note that HIV infection can alter the clinical presentation of syphilis. HIV-associated manifestations include multiple chancres, atypical cutaneous eruptions, increased severity of organ involvement (such as hepatitis and glomerulonephritis), and rapidly developing arteritis and neurosyphilis. Neurosyphilis can occur at any stage of syphilis.

Look For

For primary syphilis, painless ulcer (chancre) in the vagina, cervix, penis, anus, rectum, lips, and inside of the mouth (Figs. 4-784–4-787). A characteristic lesion has a nonpurulent clean base with scanty serous exudate and an indurated, raised border. The primary chancre typically lasts 3 to 6 weeks. Unilateral regional lymphadenopathy is nontender and firm.

Diagnostic Pearls

A syphilis ulcer is a painless, solitary ulcer with a clean base and an indurated, smooth, firm border.

Differential Diagnosis and Pitfalls

All patients with a genital ulcer should have serologic testing for syphilis. The following differential will be focused on the chancre of primary syphilis.

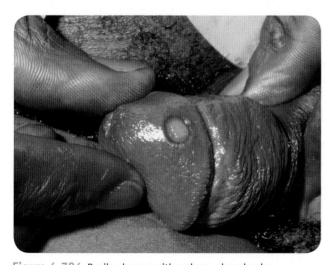

Figure 4-784 Penile chancre with a sharp, clean border.

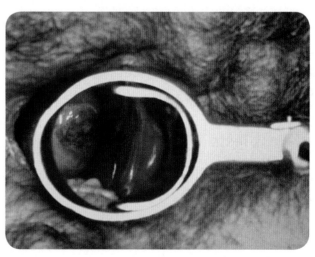

Figure 4-785 Primary syphilitic chancre on the cervix.

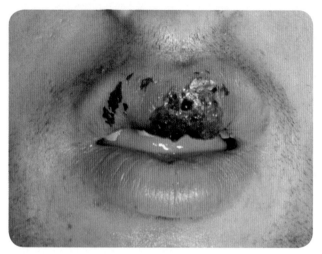

Figure 4-786 Chancre on the lip.

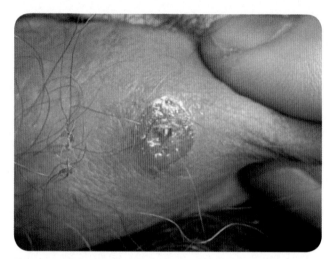

Figure 4-787 Primary chancres on the shaft of the penis.

Infectious

- Genital HSV—Look for multiple small vesicles on an erythematous base; usually painful; check direct fluorescence antigen , Tzanck smear, PCR, and viral culture.
- Chancroid (*Haemophilus ducreyi*)—Multiple nonindurated ulcers with irregular, ragged undermined edges, very painful; do Gram stain and culture on selective media for *H. ducreyi*.
- Lymphogranuloma venereum (LGV, *Chlamydia trachomatis* serovars L1–3)—Ulcers usually not observed but can have small, shallow, painless ulcer; do serologic testing for LGV.
- Granuloma inguinale (*Klebsiella granulomatis*)—Painless, extensive, and progressive; looks like granulation tissue; do tissue biopsy.

Noninfectious

- Fixed drug eruption—Red-brown papules or annular plaques that are commonly on the penis; can progress to bullae and erosions mimicking syphilis.
- Behçet disease—Do tissue biopsy if suspecting this diagnosis, and look for recurrent oral ulceration, recurrent genital ulceration, and ocular abnormalities.
- Ulcerative genital carcinoma—Do a tissue biopsy.
- Genital trauma
- Contact dermatitis

✓ Best Tests

The diagnosis of syphilis includes the following strategies:

- Direct visualization of the bacteria via dark field microscopy
- Direct detection of the bacterial DNA via PCR
- Serologic antibody tests (nonspecific and treponemal specific)

Non-treponemal Tests (Detection of Antibodies to Cardiolipin)

- Venereal Disease Research Laboratory
- Rapid plasma reagin (RPR or STS)
- Titers correlate with disease activity, and, therefore, it is useful in screening and monitoring treatment
- False positives due to pregnancy, lupus erythematosus, lymphoma, antiphospholipid syndrome, cirrhosis, vaccinations, drug abuse, and infectious diseases

Treponemal Specific Tests (To be Performed when Non-treponemal Test is Reactive)

- Microhemagglutination assay for *T. pallidum*
- Fluorescent treponemal antibody absorption (FTA-ABS) test
- Not reactive in early primary syphilis
- Will remain positive forever, so not useful for monitoring response to treatment
- False positives in HIV infection, autoimmune diseases, and additional bacteria from treponeme and spirochete families

Note that an early primary lesion (<1 to 2 weeks) must be evaluated by dark-field examination or direct immunofluorescent microscopy of the spirochete (recall that primary lesion occurs *prior* to hematogenous dissemination, so serology will be negative early on).

Do not perform a dark-field examination on oral lesions because nonpathogenic spirochetes are present in normal oral flora.

▲▲ Management Pearls

- All patients diagnosed with syphilis should be screened for HIV infection and retested 3 months later if the first HIV test is negative.

- Patients with neurologic or ophthalmic symptoms should have CSF analysis and ocular slit lamp examination performed.
- It is not necessary to perform CSF analysis if the patient does not demonstrate neurologic symptoms.
- Pregnancy—Note that no alternative exists for penicillin. If the patient has a history of penicillin allergy, she should undergo desensitization.
- Management of sex partners—Persons exposed to an infected sexual partner within 90 days preceding the diagnosis of primary, secondary, or early latent syphilis may also be infected, irrespective of serologic results; such persons should be treated presumptively.

Therapy

Current CDC guidelines:

- Penicillin G, IM or IV, for all stages of syphilis, remains the gold standard.
- Type of preparation, dosage, length of treatment depends on stage and clinical manifestations.

Primary and Secondary Syphilis
Adults:

- Benzathine penicillin G 2.4 MU IM, single dose

Pregnancy:

- Treatment during pregnancy is dictated by the penicillin schedule that is appropriate for the given stage of syphilis.
- Note that no alternative exists for penicillin. If the patient has a history of penicillin allergy, she should undergo desensitization.

Immunocompromised Patient Considerations

HIV-infected patients who contract early syphilis may be at an increased risk for neurologic complications and may have higher rates of treatment failure with currently recommended regimens. No treatment regimens for syphilis have been demonstrated to be more effective in preventing neurosyphilis in HIV-infected patients than in HIV-negative patients. Careful follow-up post-therapy intervention is essential.

Suggested Readings

Buchacz K, Klausner JD, Kerndt PR, et al. HIV incidence among men diagnosed with early syphilis in Atlanta, San Francisco, and Los Angeles, 2004 to 2005. *J Acquir Immune Defic Syndr.* 2008 Feb;47(2):234–240.

Centers for Disease Control and Prevention, Workowski KA, Berman SM. Sexually transmitted diseases treatment guidelines, 2006. *MMWR Recomm Rep.* 2006 Aug;55(RR-11):1–94.

Domantay-Apostol GP, Handog EB, Gabriel MT. Syphilis: The international challenge of the great imitator. *Dermatol Clin.* 2008 Apr;26(2):191–202, v.

Eccleston K, Collins L, Higgins SP. Primary syphilis. *Int J STD AIDS.* 2008 Mar;19(3):145–151.

Lautenschlager S. Cutaneous manifestations of syphilis: Recognition and management. *Am J Clin Dermatol.* 2006;7(5):291–304.

Lee V, Kinghorn G. Syphilis: An update. *Clin Med.* 2008 Jun;8(3):330–333.

Nandwani R, Fisher M, Medical Society for the Study of Venereal Diseases HIV Special Interest Group. Clinical standards for the screening and management of acquired syphilis in HIV-positive adults. *Int J STD AIDS.* 2006 Sep;17(9):588–593.

Park WB, Jang HC, Kim SH, et al. Effect of highly active antiretroviral therapy on incidence of early syphilis in HIV-infected patients. *Sex Transm Dis.* 2008 Mar;35(3):304–306.

Pialoux G, Vimont S, Moulignier A, et al. Effect of HIV infection on the course of syphilis. *AIDS Rev.* 2008 Apr–Jun;10(2):85–92.

Rolfs RT, Joesoef MR, Hendershot EF, et al. A randomized trial of enhanced therapy for early syphilis in patients with and without human immunodeficiency virus infection. The Syphilis and HIV Study Group. *N Engl J Med.* 1997 Jul;337(5):307–314.

Sanchez MR. Syphilis. In: Fitzpatrick TB, Wolff K, eds. *Fitzpatrick's Dermatology in General Medicine.* 7th Ed. New York, NY: McGraw-Hill; 2008:1955–1977.

Stevenson J, Heath M. Syphilis and HIV infection: An update. *Dermatol Clin.* 2006 Oct;24(4):497–507, vi.

Stoner BP. Current controversies in the management of adult syphilis. *Clin Infect Dis.* 2007 Apr;44(Suppl. 3):S130–S146.

Tinea Cruris

Diagnosis Synopsis

Tinea cruris (jock itch) is a superficial fungal infection of the skin most commonly caused by *Trichophyton rubrum* or other dermatophytes. Tinea cruris manifests as a symmetric erythematous rash in the inner thighs and the crural folds. It rarely spreads to the penis, but if it does, it will be found only at the base of the penis. It is often spread to the groin from fungal infection of the feet (tinea pedis).

Tinea cruris is usually associated with pruritus and is more common in postpubertal males. People at higher risk include those who have diabetes mellitus, are obese, recently visited a tropical climate, wear tight-fitting or wet clothes (including bathing suits) for extended periods, share clothing with others, or participate in sports.

Immunocompromised Patient Considerations

In the immunocompromised patient, pruritus may be absent. There is an increased risk of all dermatophyte infections (tinea pedis, cruris, corporis, faciale, as well as Majocchi granuloma) in the immunocompromised patient.

Look For

Look for annular, red, scaly plaques extending from the inguinal creases, down the medial thigh, and all around the pubic area and buttocks (Figs. 4-788–4-791). The plaques usually have a sharply demarcated edge and a central clearing. Plaques are described as having an active border,

meaning that the advancing edge of the plaque has prominent scale containing fungal hyphae. The central clearing of the elevated patches or plaques leads to the appearance of annular lesions and, thus, the description "ringworm" (a misnomer). The area affected may be moist and exudative in acute infections and dry in chronic infections.

Dark Skin Considerations

Chronic infections may result in either hyperpigmentation or hypopigmentation, even after resolution.

Immunocompromised Patient Considerations

In the immunocompromised patient, infection can be quite extensive. Tinea cruris may extend well beyond the typical crural or intragluteal distribution to involve the trunk or lower extremities. Plaques may show only well-demarcated hyperkeratosis as opposed to the typical annular pattern.

Diagnostic Pearls

In fungal lesions that have been treated with topical steroids, the redness can be absent, and minimal scaling may be present while the lesion is loaded with fungi. If the scraping is negative in a lesion that has not been treated, the lesion is probably *not* fungal in etiology.

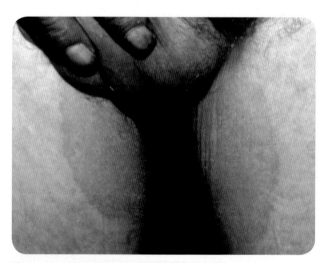

Figure 4-788 Bilateral, well-demarcated, hyperpigmented plaques are common in tinea cruris.

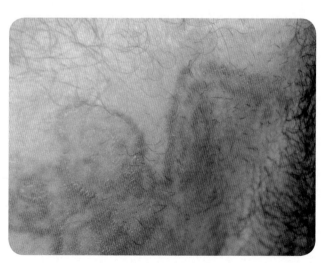

Figure 4-789 A red plaque with a polycyclic border is characteristic of tinea cruris.

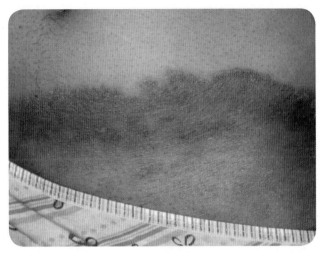

Figure 4-790 Tinea cruris with a polycyclic border and hyperpigmentation extending to the lower abdomen.

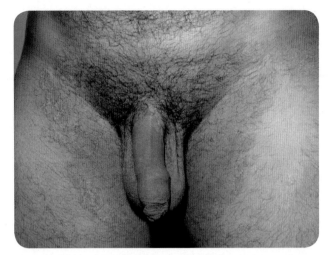

Figure 4-791 In this case of tinea cruris due to *T. rubrum*, there is sparing of the penis and scrotum, which is common with dermatophyte infections.

?? Differential Diagnosis and Pitfalls

- Psoriasis
- Granuloma annulare—no scale
- Cutaneous candidiasis—often beefy red with satellite lesions
- Allergic contact dermatitis
- Irritant contact dermatitis
- Erythrasma—tan/brown with slight scaling and no active border
- Familial benign pemphigus (Hailey-Hailey disease)
- Folliculitis
- Intertrigo
- Lichen simplex chronicus
- Bowen disease
- Extramammary Paget disease
- Glucagonoma syndrome

✓ Best Tests

Scrape the scaly, active border with a scalpel blade or edge of a glass slide. Collect scale on a slide and coverslip. Direct a drop of 10% KOH (potassium hydroxide) to the edge of the coverslip, or put a drop of the KOH on the scales before covering with the coverslip. Wait for about 5 min, then examine with the microscope. Observe for branching or curving fungal hyphae, which cross the keratin cell borders.

▲▲ Management Pearls

- Treat all active areas of infection simultaneously to prevent reinfection of the groin from other body sites.

Treat clinically affected areas and a 2 cm margin of healthy-appearing skin, and continue to treat for 1 week after clinical resolution.
- Also advise drying the inguinal folds completely after bathing. Explain to the patient that permanent cure is rare, but proper treatment results in excellent control that will, however, require periodic re-treatment.

Therapy

Limited, localized disease should be treated topically. Allylamines (e.g., terbinafine, naftifine) and imidazoles (e.g., clotrimazole) are the mainstays of therapy. Allylamines may require shorter courses, but imidazoles are less expensive.

Use topical antifungals for 1 to 6 weeks, based on clinical response:

- Terbinafine 1% cream or spray—apply once to twice daily
- Clotrimazole 1% cream—apply twice daily
- Econazole 1% cream—apply once to twice daily
- Oxiconazole 1% cream—apply twice daily
- Ciclopirox 0.77% cream, gel, or lotion—apply twice daily
- Ketoconazole 2% cream—apply once to twice daily
- Miconazole 2% cream—apply twice daily
- Naftifine 1% cream—apply once to twice daily
- Butenafine 1% cream—apply once to twice daily

Topical corticosteroids, by themselves or in combination with antifungals, are generally not indicated and are absolutely contraindicated in immunosuppressed patients.

(Continued)

Use of corticosteroid–antifungal combinations in cases of diagnostic uncertainty may lead to persistent fungal infections and is not recommended.

Extensive disease, particularly when other body parts are involved, may require weeks of oral antifungal agents:

- Terbinafine 250 mg once a day for 2 to 4 weeks
- Itraconazole 100 to 200 mg twice a day for 1 week
- Fluconazole 150 to 300 mg once a week for 2 to 4 weeks
- Griseofulvin ultramicrosize 5 mg/kg/day for 4 to 8 weeks (generally reserved for severe cases)

Systemic antifungals are contraindicated in patients with liver disease; monitoring of liver enzymes is generally recommended.

Immunocompromised Patient Considerations

Localized disease may still be treated topically in immunocompromised patients.

Extensive disease may require longer courses of systemic antifungals than are used in immunocompetent patients:

- Terbinafine 250 mg per day for 2 to 6 weeks, depending on response

- Itraconazole 200 mg twice daily for 2 to 6 weeks, depending on response
- Griseofulvin ultra-microsize 5 mg/kg/day for 4 to 8 weeks

Avoid topical corticosteroids in immunocompromised patients.

Suggested Readings

Drake LA, Dinehart SM, Farmer ER, et al. Guidelines of care for superficial mycotic infections of the skin: Tinea corporis, tinea cruris, tinea faciei, tinea manuum, and tinea pedis. Guidelines/Outcomes Committee. American Academy of Dermatology. *J Am Acad Dermatol.* 1996 Feb;34 (2 Pt 1):282–286.

Gupta AK, Chaudhry M, Elewski B. Tinea corporis, tinea cruris, tinea nigra, and piedra. *Dermatol Clin.* 2003 Jul;21(3):395–400, v.

Gupta AK, Cooper EA. Update in antifungal therapy of dermatophytosis. *Mycopathologia.* 2008 Nov-Dec;166(5–6):353–367.

Kyle AA, Dahl MV. Topical therapy for fungal infections. *Am J Clin Dermatol.* 2004;5(6):443–451.

Lebwohl M, Elewski B, Eisen D, et al. Efficacy and safety of terbinafine 1% solution in the treatment of interdigital tinea pedis and tinea corporis or tinea cruris. *Cutis.* 2001 Mar;67(3):261–266.

van Heerden JS, Vismer HF. Tinea corporis/cruris: New treatment options. *Dermatology.* 1997;194(Suppl. 1):14–18.

Verma S, Heffernan MP. Superficial fungal infection: Dermatophytosis, Onychomycosis, Tinea Nigra, Piedra. In: Fitzpatrick TB, Wolff K, eds. *Fitzpatrick's Dermatology in General Medicine.* 7th Ed. New York, NY: McGraw-Hill; 2008:1815.

Candidiasis (Thrush)

◾◾ Diagnosis Synopsis

Oral candidiasis, also known as moniliasis or thrush, is a common yeast infection of the oral mucosal membranes, typically caused by the overgrowth of *Candida albicans*. *C. albicans* also frequently affects immunocompromised individuals such as those receiving immunosuppressive agents (e.g., systemic or inhaled corticosteroids and chemotherapy). *Candida* is also seen in patients with diabetes mellitus and in HIV and AIDS patients.

Frequent or chronic antibiotic use will predispose normal individuals as well as immunosuppressed patients to oral candidiasis. Hyposalivation states leading to dry mouth (post–head and neck radiation and anticholinergic medications) and persons wearing dentures that do not adequately support the oral musculature or with normal age-related facial sagging causing drooping of the corners of the mouth and pooling of saliva are also susceptible.

Immunocompromised Patient Considerations

Species of *Candida* that are occasional causes of disease, particularly in AIDS patients and patients with a history of head and neck radiation, are *C. glabrata* (formerly known as *Torulopsis glabrata*), *C. tropicalis*, *C. krusei*, *C. dubliniensis*, and others.

Oral *Candida* infection may present as pseudomembranous candidiasis (thrush), erythematous candidiasis (chronic atrophic candidiasis or denture sore mouth), plaque-like candidiasis (*Candida* leukoplakia), angular cheilitis (perlèche), and, rarely, chronic nodular candidiasis (giving the tongue a cobbled appearance). Chronic mucocutaneous candidiasis is associated with persistent infection of the mouth, skin, and nails.

Symptoms include roughness, soreness, burning, and pain, which may limit eating. Palatal disease is often asymptomatic.

Patients with defective T-cell function are susceptible to mucosal *Candida* infection. Oral *Candida* carriage rates are higher in HIV-infected individuals, intravenous drug abusers, and denture wearers. *C. albicans* frequently affects immunocompromised individuals such as those receiving immunosuppressive agents (e.g., systemic corticosteroids, azathioprine, cyclosporine A, or tacrolimus). *Candida* is also seen in patients with leukemia or other malignancies who may be undergoing chemotherapy, head and neck radiotherapy, and in HIV and AIDS patients. It is common during infancy when the immune system and immune responses are developing. Dentures, xerostomia, diabetes, and nutritional deficiencies are other risk factors.

◉ Look For

There are three main clinical forms that exist:

- Pseudomembranous (thrush) is the most common—curdy, white papules and plaques are seen that wipe off with some difficulty, leaving a raw, bleeding surface. Any mucosal surface may be involved (Figs. 4-792 and 4-793).
- Atrophic/erythematous form—This occurs more commonly than thrush in the population of HIV-infected individuals and appears red, atrophic (Fig. 4-794), and eroded. It also often occurs underneath dentures (also called denture sore mouth) and on the dorsum of the tongue. When it occurs at the corners of the mouth, it is called angular cheilitis (perlèche).
- Hyperplastic form (less common)—White papules and plaques are present that do not wipe off, are often indistinguishable from leukoplakia, and are often associated with mucocutaneous disease.

Median rhomboid glossitis is a form of chronic oral candidiasis that presents as an ovoid or rhomboidal area in the midline of the tongue just anterior to the circumvallate papillae.

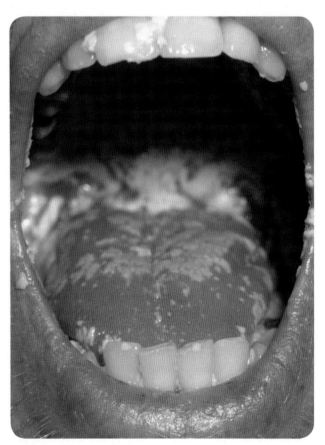

Figure 4-792 Extensive white plaques of *Candida* on the tongue and soft palate.

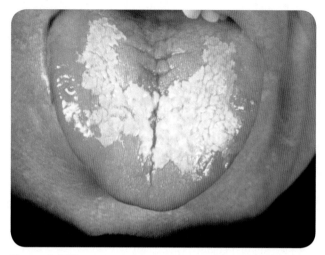

Figure 4-793 Thick, white plaques of *Candida* on the tongue.

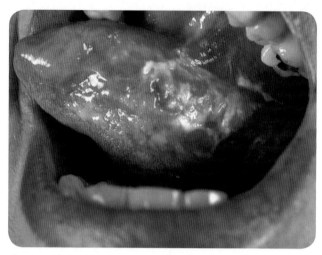

Figure 4-794 Thick, white plaques on the tongue with regions of atrophy.

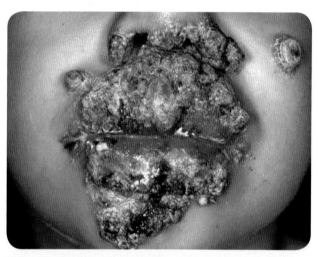

Figure 4-795 Thick, granuloma-like lesions of *Candida* are associated with genetic or acquired immunodeficiencies.

Immunocompromised Patient Considerations

White plaques of the tongue and/or buccal mucosa sometimes spreading to the commissure of the lips. Whereas the lesions are gray-white in color, their bases are red and moist. Smooth, red, glazed oral plaques. Fissure and erythema at mouth corners. (Fig. 4-795)

●● Diagnostic Pearls

- Dentures and malocclusion can predispose to candidiasis. Candidiasis beneath dentures can present as redness and soreness of the palate with few organisms on KOH prep.

?? Differential Diagnosis and Pitfalls

- Oral hairy leukoplakia—and HIV-associated disease—often has an associated secondary candidal infection and is most common on the lateral borders of the tongue, often (but not always) in a bilateral and symmetric distribution.
- Chronic bite injury—usually painless with a gelatinous, shaggy consistency
- Leukoplakia
- Erythroplakia
- Hypersensitivity reaction to denture base material
- Lichen planus—usually reticulated and erythematous rather than plaque-like
- Geographic tongue
- Diphtheria—the membrane is often associated with hemorrhagic crusts around the mouth and nares
- Hairy tongue

Immunocompromised Patient Differential Diagnosis

- Oral hairy leukoplakia
- Leukoplakia
- Squamous cell carcinoma
- Lichen planus
- Aphthous ulcers
- Geographic tongue
- White sponge nevus
- Diphtheria

✓ Best Tests

- Scrape white plaques with a tongue blade, apply to glass slide, and stain with KOH. Look for budding yeast forms and nonseptate hyphae (pseudohyphae).
- Cultures are not recommended because 20% of the population is a carrier. However, in immunocompromised patients, culture for speciation is important because some species (e.g., *C. tropicalis*) may be resistant to standard therapy.

▲▲▲ Management Pearls

- One dose of oral fluconazole (Diflucan) 200 mg may be curative, especially in those patients in whom antibiotic usage has allowed *Candida* overgrowth. Regular use (e.g., once weekly) may be necessary for those with predisposing conditions.
- If using nystatin (see below), make sure that the patient removes any dentures before using the rinse to make sure that the nystatin contacts the infected mucosa under the denture.
- Also, any denture needs to be treated to kill yeast that it may be harboring. If possible, discontinue the antibiotic and/or immunosuppressive agent.
- Voriconazole, both peroral and parenteral formulations, and parenteral caspofungin are new agents effective against resistant *Candida* species.

Therapy

Nystatin rinse (1:100,000 IU/mL), swish and spit out 5 mL three to four times daily. Be careful about using this in patients with dry mouths (especially patients who have received head and neck radiation) because nystatin contains sucrose and can aggravate a tendency to develop caries in these patients.

Clotrimazole troches (Mycelex troches)—10 mg troche five times daily for 2 weeks. This does not work well if the mouth is dry since saliva is necessary for the troches to dissolve.

One dose of oral fluconazole (Diflucan) 200 mg may be curative, especially in those patients in whom antibiotic usage has allowed *Candida* overgrowth. Regular use (e.g., once weekly) may be necessary for those with predisposing conditions.

Nystatin and triamcinolone (Mycolog) cream or topical ketoconazole ointment for corners of mouth, applied three times daily.

Immunocompromised Patient Considerations

Mouth and dental hygiene.

Topical therapy (nystatin and clotrimazole troches) may be ineffective for the immunocompromised and difficult for patients with xerostomia and pain. Clotrimazole 10 mg troche five times daily for 2 weeks.

Systemic therapy with fluconazole or itraconazole (100 to 200 mg daily) may be necessary.

Therapy is given until there is symptomatic recovery. Therapy for recurrence may be necessary and is preferred to continuous therapy because of the risk of resistance developing.

Suggested Readings

Appleton SS. Candidiasis: Pathogenesis, clinical characteristics, and treatment. *J Calif Dent Assoc*. 2000 Dec;28(12):942–948.

Farah CS, Ashman RB, Challacombe SJ. Oral candidosis. *Clin Dermatol*. 2000 Sep–Oct;18(5):553–562.

Liu X, Hua H. Oral manifestation of chronic mucocutaneous candidiasis: Seven case reports. *J Oral Pathol Med*. 2007 Oct;36(9):528–532.

Pappas PG, Rex JH, Sobel JD, et al.; Infectious Diseases Society of America. Guidelines for treatment of candidiasis. *Clin Infect Dis*. 2004 Jan;38(2):161–189.

Patton LL, van der Horst C. Oral infections and other manifestations of HIV disease. *Infect Dis Clin North Am*. 1999 Dec;13(4):879–900.

Pienaar ED, Young T, Holmes H. Interventions for the prevention and management of oropharyngeal candidiasis associated with HIV infection in adults and children. *Cochrane Database Syst Rev*. 2006;3:CD003940.

Vazquez JA, Skiest DJ, Tissot-Dupont H, et al. Safety and efficacy of posaconazole in the long-term treatment of azole-refractory oropharyngeal and esophageal candidiasis in patients with HIV infection. *HIV Clin Trials*. 2007 Mar–Apr;8(2):86–97.

Diagnosis Synopsis

Aphthous ulcers, or aphthae (canker sores), are the most common cause of recurring ulcers of the mucous membranes. They affect approximately 25% of the general population (estimates range from 20% up to 50%), and their precise cause is unknown. They consist of three morphologic types: minor aphthae, major aphthae, and herpetiform aphthae. The mouth is the most common site.

Minor aphthae (80% of cases) are single or multiple lesions, 1.0 cm or less in diameter, and mildly painful; they heal within 1 to 2 weeks. Major aphthae (Sutton disease, approximately 10% of cases) are deep ulcers that are 1 to 3 cm in diameter. These lesions are extremely painful, last from 2 to 6 weeks, and generally heal with scarring. Herpetiform aphthae (10% of cases) are characterized by multiple ulcerations, 1 to 3 mm in diameter, and have a clinical course similar to minor aphthous ulcers.

Oral ulcers morphologically indistinguishable from aphthae that arise in the context of another disease process, such as Behçet disease, are referred to as aphthous-like ulcers.

Most patients with aphthous ulcers or aphthous-like ulcers suffer from a recurring/relapsing process termed recurrent aphthous stomatitis (RAS). There are a few well-recognized patterns for recurring oral ulcerations. Simple aphthosis is primarily marked by minor aphthae that recur intermittently with disease-free intervals of weeks to months. Patients are generally young and healthy, with lesions limited to the mouth and no underlying systemic disease. Complex aphthosis is marked by the near-constant presence of three or more aphthae, major aphthae, and frequently an underlying disease such as HIV, gluten-sensitive enteropathy, inflammatory bowel disease, or others. Finally, oral ulceration is characteristic of Behçet disease, but by definition, is accompanied by other findings such as genital ulcers, uveitis, and other skin and systemic inflammatory processes.

Most cases of simple aphthosis begin in childhood or adolescence. Patients frequently report a family history of oral ulceration. In addition to presumed genetic risk, epidemiologic studies (and patient reports) support an association between new lesions and oral trauma, emotional stress, and smoking cessation. Pregnancy and hormonal changes in menses appear to increase risk. Some studies suggest that those who were breast-fed as infants may be at decreased risk.

The cause of aphthous ulceration is generally unknown, but studies point to a defect in the regulation of cellular immunity that results in an increased T-cell reactivity to either mucous membrane keratinocytes or microorganisms on the mucosal surface. Ulcers show a dysregulated Th1-type immune response (including increased levels of TNF-α), and patients prone to aphthae demonstrate quantitative and functional deficits in regulatory T-cells. There are HLA haplotype associations with RAS that may reflect linkage to an as yet uncharacterized gene on the short arm of chromosome 6.

No single organism, including herpes simplex virus (HSV), has emerged as a distinctive cause of RAS, though individual aphthous-like ulcers may, on occasion, have HSV as a cause.

Immunocompromised Patient Considerations

Individuals infected with HIV are commonly affected by severe RAS.

Look For

Painful crater-like ulcers that localize inside the mouth on the nonkeratinized mucosa of the lips, buccal mucosa, or tongue (Figs. 4-796–4-799). These round to ovoid ulcers have a white, gray, or yellow base with an erythematous halo.

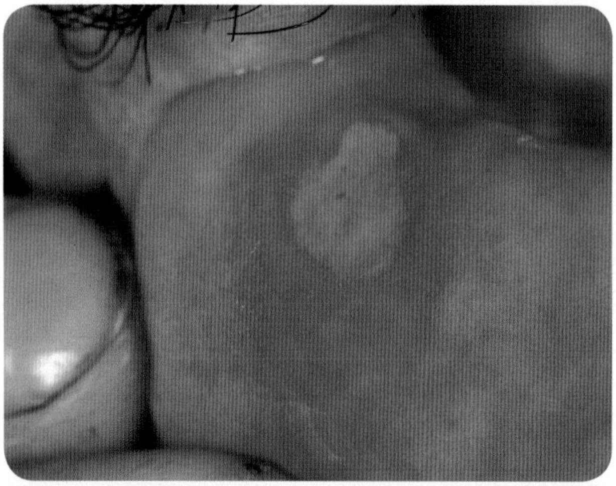

Figure 4-796 A gray crust with a large rim of erythema is characteristic of an aphthous ulcer.

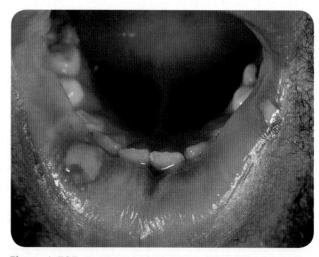

Figure 4-797 The border of an aphthous ulcer may be irregular.

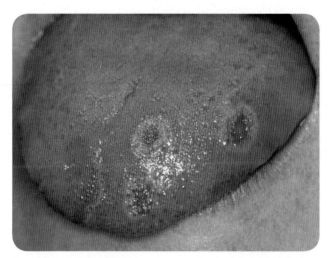

Figure 4-798 Small aphthae on the tongue with a rim of hyperkeratosis.

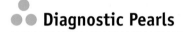

Diagnostic Pearls

- Cases of simple aphthosis (i.e., recurring minor aphthae in otherwise well individuals with onset during childhood or adolescence) require no additional diagnostic evaluation.
- Complex aphthosis, severe cases, or cases with onset later in life should prompt evaluation for an underlying cause. Aphthous-like ulcers have been associated with iron; zinc; folate; and vitamin B_1, B_2, B_6, and B_{12} deficiencies. They are also seen in Behçet disease, systemic lupus erythematosus, AIDS, inflammatory bowel disease, and other systemic illnesses.
- Lesions recurring at the same anatomic site may suggest HSV infection.

?? Differential Diagnosis and Pitfalls

Diseases with Oral Ulcerations Clinically Distinguishable from Aphthae

- Hand-foot-and-mouth disease usually has skin lesions.
- Herpangina is characteristically located on the soft palate and adjacent mucosae.
- Chemotherapy-induced lesions
- Erosive lichen planus
- Pemphigus
- Pemphigoid
- Dermatitis herpetiformis
- Chronic ulcerative stomatitis
- Herpes zoster
- Varicella
- Herpes simplex virus, including primary herpes gingivostomatitis
- Chemical burn (e.g., from holding aspirin near the mucosae)
- Oral candidiasis—typically painless
- Squamous cell carcinoma

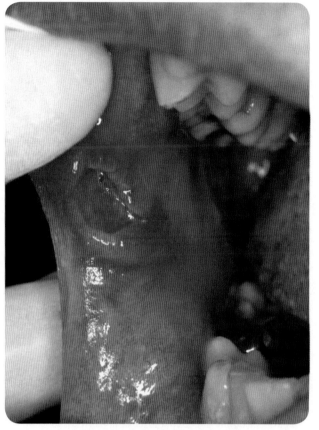

Figure 4-799 Deep aphthous ulcer in an HIV-infected individual.

Systemic Diseases with Aphthous-like Ulcerations

- Behçet disease
- Inflammatory bowel disease
- HIV
- Celiac disease—gluten-sensitive enteropathy
- Systemic lupus erythematosus
- Hematinic deficiencies—iron; zinc; folate; and vitamins B_1, B_2, B_6, and B_{12}
- Cyclic neutropenia
- Sweet syndrome
- FAPA syndrome (fever, aphthae, pharyngitis, and cervical adenitis)
- MAGIC syndrome (mouth and genital ulcers with inflamed cartilage)

✓ Best Tests

This is usually a clinical diagnosis. However, a biopsy can confirm the diagnosis and rule out other causes of oral ulcers. Oral ulcerations lasting longer than 3 weeks should be biopsied to exclude malignancy.

Consider the following tests:

- CBC
- Vitamin B_{12}, B_6, B_2, and B_1 levels, serum folate, zinc, iron, and ferritin
- Tzanck smear, viral culture, direct fluorescent antibody testing, or PCR for HSV

▲▲ Management Pearls

- Most patients with simple aphthosis can be successfully treated with topical agents. The goals are symptomatic relief and accelerated ulcer healing. Systemic treatments should be reserved for severe cases.
- Counsel the patient regarding trigger avoidance. Inciting factors include emotional stress, oral trauma from sharp or hard foods, and menstruation. Acidic foods and beverages increase ulcer pain.
- Limited data support the use of toothpastes free of the detergent sodium lauryl sulfate to decrease the frequency of attacks of RAS. Chlorhexidine-containing mouthwashes may also decrease frequency of attacks.

Therapy

Patients with aphthous-like ulcers benefit from the treatment of any underlying disease in addition to treatments targeted at simple aphthosis. Correct any underlying vitamin or mineral deficiencies. Advise all patients on trigger avoidance.

Patient-Directed Treatments to Palliate Symptoms from Aphthae

- Topical local anesthetics—lidocaine, benzocaine, or dyclonine (some over the counter) available in a variety of preparations designed for oral use
- Anesthetic mouthwashes combining aluminum and magnesium hydroxide, lidocaine, and diphenhydramine
- Sucralfate
- Oral nonsteroidal analgesics
- Opioid analgesics in severe cases

Patient-Directed Topical Treatments to Accelerate Healing of Aphthae (Best Used at Earliest Onset of a New Ulceration)

- Topical corticosteroids (e.g., triamcinolone, halobetasol, and clobetasol) available in gels or oral preparations such as carboxymethylcellulose base—applied two to four times daily
- Diclofenac in hyaluronic acid—single treatment
- Amlexanox 5% oral paste four times daily for 5 days
- Oral suspensions of tetracyclines, used for anti-inflammatory effect. Data support the use of tetracycline, doxycycline, and minocycline though topical

forms are not widely available. A 250 mg capsule of tetracycline may be dissolved in a tablespoon of water and swished around the mouth for 5 min three to four times a day

- Hyaluronic acid 0.2% twice daily for 2 weeks
- 5-Aminosalicylic acid 5% cream three times a day

Clinician-Directed Treatment for Individual Stubborn or Severe Aphthae

- Chemical cautery with silver nitrate 1% to 2%
- Chemical cautery with 50% sulfonated phenolics in 30% sulfuric acid (also available in applicators intended for patient-directed use)
- Intralesional injection with triamcinolone acetonide 5 to 10 mg/mL

Systemic Treatments for Severe Cases or Patients Prone to Severe Recurrences

- Prednisone 10 to 20 mg per day for 5 to 7 days or other oral corticosteroids
- Colchicine 0.6 mg two to three times daily
- Pentoxifylline 400 mg three times daily
- Doxycycline 20 mg two times daily
- Methotrexate 7.5 to 20 mg weekly
- Dapsone 100 mg daily
- Thalidomide 50 to 300 mg per day
- Azathioprine 50 to 150 mg per day
- Cyclosporine A 3 to 6 mg/kg daily
- Biologic anti-TNF-α agents (e.g., etanercept, infliximab, and adalimumab) have demonstrated efficacy in case reports
- Other systemic therapies include levamisole, alkylating agents, and antimetabolites

Combination therapy should be considered when a single agent does not suffice.

Suggested Readings

Altenburg A, Zouboulis CC. Current concepts in the treatment of recurrent aphthous stomatitis. *Skin Therapy Lett.* 2008 Sep;13(7):1–4.

Greer RO, Lindenmuth JE, Juarez T, et al. A double-blind study of topically applied 5% amlexanox in the treatment of aphthous ulcers. *J Oral Maxillofac Surg.* 1993 Mar;51(3):243–248; discussion 248–249.

Letsinger JA, McCarty MA, Jorizzo JL. Complex aphthosis: A large case series with evaluation algorithm and therapeutic ladder from topicals to thalidomide. *J Am Acad Dermatol.* 2005 Mar;52(3 Pt 1):500–508.

MacPhail L. Topical and systemic therapy for recurrent aphthous stomatitis. *Semin Cutan Med Surg.* 1997 Dec;16(4):301–307.

Sciubba JJ. Oral mucosal diseases in the office setting—part I: Aphthous stomatitis and herpes simplex infections. *Gen Dent.* 2007 Jul–Aug; 55(4):347–354; quiz 355–356, 376.

Scully C. Clinical practice. Aphthous ulceration. *N Engl J Med.* 2006 Jul;355(2):165–172.

Woo SB, Sonis ST. Recurrent aphthous ulcers: a review of diagnosis and treatment. *J Am Dent Assoc.* 1996 Aug;127(8):1202–1213.

CHAPTER 5

Dermatologic Therapies

Dermatologic care makes extensive use of topical agents, and this chapter emphasizes important practical points for the safe and optimal use of these topical medications. Details of drug use for specific diseases are covered when specific diseases are considered.

Percutaneous Absorption of Topical Medications

The total systemic absorption of topical medicines is related to the concentrations of the medication, the vehicle in which the medication is compounded, intactness of the epidermis, the maturity of the epidermis, and the percentage of the body to which the medication is applied.

General Considerations

Body Surface Area and Topical Medications

Percentage of body surface area (BSA) is useful in determining the extent of dermatologic disease and in estimating the amount of topical medication to be prescribed. If the BSA of a patient is known, one can utilize percentages found in the Lund-Browder chart to calculate the amount of topical medication required for a patient to treat his or her dermatosis (Table 5-1).

Vehicle Recommendations

Vehicles, or bases, are major determinants of medication stability, tolerability, absorption, efficacy, ease of application, and patient acceptance. The fundamental ingredients of vehicles are liquids, powders, and lipids. For most dermatologic conditions, vehicles with higher lipid content are preferred (i.e., ointments and oils) due to their increased moisturizing properties, decreased burning on application, and ability to increase percutaneous absorption of most medications. For locations of the body where the skin is thin or naturally occluded (intertriginous areas) or for dermatoses that are weeping or oozing, vehicles with higher liquid content should

be considered (i.e., creams, lotions, gels, and solutions). These enhance spreadability and are better tolerated in moist areas of the body and for "wet" dermatoses. Vehicles with powder added (i.e., pastes and shake lotions) are also useful in intertriginous areas, where they can be used to decrease friction and absorb excess moisture.

Special Therapeutic Agents

Topical Corticosteroids

Topical corticosteroids are antiinflammatory and antiproliferative agents that are used extensively in dermatology. Multiple assays have been developed to rank the clinical efficacy of topical steroids, and potency ratings may vary slightly depending on the reference utilized. The Stoughton vasoconstriction assay, in which steroids are classed based on their vasoconstrictive activities, is the most commonly used rating system for the potency of steroids. For most topical corticosteroids, clinical efficacy is well correlated with their position on this ladder (Table 5-2). This is a numerical scale, not a linear ladder, and patients are often confused when they look at the concentration of a steroid

TABLE 5-1 Lund-Browder Chart and Topical Coverage Requirements

Area	Percentage of BSA	Grams of Topical Ointment Required for 1-month Supply for Each Body Part Using Twice Daily Dosing
Whole body	100	2250
Head (back or front)	3.5	85
Upper leg	9.5	215
Lower leg	7	150
Trunk (back or front)	13	300
Upper arm	4	90
Lower arm	3	65

TABLE 5-2 Steroid Potency Ladder: From Most Potent (Class 1) to Least Potent (Class 7)

Ointments and Creams

Class 1

Clobetasol propionate 0.05% ointment and cream

Halobetasol propionate 0.05% ointment and cream

Class 2

Betamethasone dipropionate 0.05% ointment and cream

Amcinonide 0.1% ointment

Mometasone furoate 0.1% ointment

Fluocinonide 0.05% ointment and cream

Diflorasone diacetate 0.05% ointment and cream

Desoximetasone 0.25% ointment and cream

Halcinonide 0.1% cream

Class 3

Triamcinolone acetonide 0.1% ointment

Triamcinolone acetonide 0.5% cream

Betamethasone valerate 0.1% ointment

Fluticasone propionate 0.005% ointment

Halcinonide 0.1% ointment

Amcinonide 0.1% cream

Desoximetasone 0.05% cream

Class 4

Flurandrenolide 0.05% ointment

Fluocinolone acetonide 0.025% ointment

Hydrocortisone valerate 0.2% ointment

Triamcinolone acetonide 0.1% cream

Mometasone furoate 0.1% cream

Class 5

Flurandrenolide 0.025% ointment

Prednicarbate 0.1% ointment and cream

Hydrocortisone butyrate 0.1% ointment and cream

Betamethasone valerate 0.1% cream

Clocortolone pivalate 0.1% cream

Flurandrenolide 0.05% cream

Fluocinolone acetonide 0.025% cream

Hydrocortisone probutate 0.1% cream

Fluocinolone acetonide 0.01% cream

Hydrocortisone valerate 0.2% cream

Fluocinolone acetonide 0.01% oil

Class 6

Alclometasone dipropionate 0.05% ointment and cream

Desonide 0.05% ointment and cream

Triamcinolone acetonide 0.025% cream

Flurandrenolide 0.025% cream

Class 7

Hydrocortisone 1% and 2.5% ointment and cream

and try to correlate that with its potency. Stronger steroids have lower class numbers. It is also important to remember that corticosteroids of the same strength will be of higher potency in lipophilic vehicles (ointments) than in aqueous (lotion) vehicles. Understanding this relationship is imperative to choosing the correct topical corticosteroid in the most appropriate vehicle. Attention to these factors will optimize treatment while avoiding undesired corticosteroid side effects.

Potential Adverse Effects of Topical Steroids

The risk for adverse effects from topical corticosteroids is increased in areas of the body where skin is thinnest (eyelids, face, or intertriginous areas where skin touches skin). Although rare in adults, the suppression of the hypothalamic-pituitary-adrenal axis may result within a week of exposure to small amounts of superpotent topical steroids (class 1) or extensive and prolonged exposure to medium-potency topical steroids (classes 3 to 4). Serious adverse effects, however, have been reported only after gross misuse over years of topical corticosteroid application.[1-3] Local atrophy can occur with repeated exposure of normal skin to superpotent topical corticosteroids.

Potential Systemic Adverse Effects

- Suppression of the hypothalamic-pituitary-adrenal axis
- Iatrogenic Cushing syndrome

Potential Local Adverse Effects

- Epidermal atrophy
- Striae
- Purpura
- Hypopigmentation
- Glaucoma (from absorption around the eyes)
- Cataracts (from absorption around the eyes)
- Hypertrichosis
- Folliculitis or steroid-induced acne
- Perioral dermatitis
- Delayed wound healing

Guidelines and Tips for the Use of Topical Steroids

- Familiarize yourself with a small group of generic topical corticosteroid ointments to use as a practical therapeutic ladder (Table 5-3).[4,5] Build upon this ladder as you gain experience with topical corticosteroids. In the United States, 1% hydrocortisone is available without a prescription.
- Utilize the lowest-strength corticosteroid that will clear dermatitis in a short amount of time (i.e., <7 days).
- If long-term chronic therapy is required (e.g., for atopic dermatitis), intermittent therapy is recommended over continuous therapy. An ideal topical corticosteroid will clear the patient's dermatitis within 3 days and maintain clearance for a week before more topical corticosteroid is required.
- Use only very mild topical corticosteroids on eyelids or intertriginous areas.

TABLE 5-3 Suggested Therapeutic Ladder

Potency (Example)	Dermatosis	Skin Thickness	Location	Length of Continuous Use
Superpotent (Clobetasol propionate 0.05% ointment)	Resistant and chronic	Very thick or lichenified	Avoid face and skin folds Caution on torso	Monitor closely if >2–3 weeks
High (Fluocinonide 0.05% ointment)	Severe and chronic	Very thick or lichenified	Peripheral extremities Avoid face and skin folds Caution on torso	Monitor closely
Intermediate (Triamcinolone Acetonide 0.1% ointment)	Moderate acute or chronic	Moderately thick Mildly lichenified	Torso and extremities Caution on face and skin folds	Monitor closely if >2–3 weeks on face or skin folds or >3 months on body
Low (Desonide 0.05% ointment)	Mild and acute	Minimal thickness No lichenification	Face and skin folds	Monitor regularly if >4 weeks on face or skin folds
Very low (Hydrocortisone 2.5% ointment)	Very mild and acute	No thickening No lichenification	Face, skin folds, occluded areas	Monitor regularly if >4 weeks on face

- Recognize that ointments are usually stronger than other formulations when changing vehicles (e.g., changing from an ointment to a solution to treat a dermatosis of the scalp).

Systemic Corticosteroids

The use of systemic corticosteroids is limited to specific severe disorders in dermatology, including lupus erythematosus, autoimmune disease, bullous dermatoses, acute allergic reactions, and severe drug reactions. Systemic steroids are very rarely indicated for psoriasis or atopic dermatitis. The most commonly used steroids are prednisone and prednisolone, typically at doses between 0.5 and 2 mg/kg/day (Table 5-4). While on long-term therapy (longer than 2 to 4 weeks), patients should be closely monitored for adverse effects (see below); have their blood pressure followed; and be started on vitamin D, calcium, and a bisphosphonate to prevent osteoporosis. Peptic ulcer prophylaxis can be achieved with proton pump inhibitors.

Potential Adverse Effects of Systemic Steroids

- Suppression of the hypothalamic-pituitary-adrenal axis
- Adrenal crisis

TABLE 5-4 Systemic Corticosteroid Equivalent Dosing (mg)

Cortisone	25
Hydrocortisone	20
Prednisone	5
Prednisolone	5
Methylprednisolone	4
Triamcinolone	4
Dexamethasone	0.75
Betamethasone	0.75

- Hyperglycemia
- Hypertension
- Congestive heart failure
- Hyperlipidemia
- Cushingoid changes
- Osteoporosis
- Osteonecrosis
- Peptic ulcer disease
- Bowel perforation
- Cataracts
- Agitation
- Immunosuppression
- Myopathy
- Delayed wound healing
- Pseudotumor cerebri
- Perioral dermatitis
- Steroid acne
- Striae

Antiparasitic Agents

Most cases of lice and scabies are treatable with topical agents and sometimes systemic agents. These agents and their usage are listed in Table 5-5.

Topical Anesthetics

Topical anesthetics are useful for minor procedures on intact skin (needle or laser procedures). More invasive procedures, such as excisions, require the addition of local anesthetics or general anesthesia. Contraindications to topical anesthetics include allergy to amide anesthetics, nonintact skin, and for EMLA, recent sulfonamide antibiotic use and methemoglobinemia. Dosing and proper application of topical anesthetics are described in Table 5-6.[6–8]

Local Anesthetics

Local anesthetics are required for invasive dermatologic procedures (e.g., biopsies and excisions).[9] Onset-of-action information for local anesthetics can be found in Table 5-7.

TABLE 5-5 Common Antiparasitic Agents and Their Uses

Name	Available Formulations	Use
Pyrethrins with piperonyl butoxide	0.3% shampoo or lotion 0.18% lotion	Pediculosis
Permethrin	1% and 5% cream	Pediculosis and scabies
Ivermectin (200 μg/kg)	3 or 6 mg tablets	Pediculosis and scabies
Lindane	1% shampoo or lotion	Pediculosis and scabies
Crotamiton	10% cream or lotion	Scabies
Malathion	0.5% lotion	Pediculosis
Benzyl benzoate	20%–25% solution	Scabies
Thiabendazole (1.5 g p.o. bid × 2 days)	500 mg tablets	Cutaneous larva migrans
Precipitated sulfur	6% ointment	Scabies

TABLE 5-6 Onset of Action for Topical Anesthetics

Brand	Active Ingredients	Onset of Action (min)
EMLA	2.5% lidocaine and 2.5% prilocaine	60–120
LMX-4	4% lidocaine	30–60
LMX-5	5% lidocaine	30–60
Topicaine	4% lidocaine	30–60

TABLE 5-7 Onset of Action for Local Anesthetics

Name	Onset of Action (min)	Duration (min)
Lidocaine	<1	30–120
Lidocaine with epinephrine	<1	60–400
Bupivacaine	2–10	120–240
Bupivacaine with epinephrine	2–10	240–480
Mepivacaine	3–20	30–120

Topical Antifungal Agents

Many topical antifungal agents are available for the treatment of superficial dermatophyte and yeast infections (Table 5-8). They are usually applied twice daily, but more frequent application may be required if agents are removed by bathing or perspiration. Several agents, such as clotrimazole, miconazole, and terbinafine, are available as over-the-counter medications and are good first-line agents. Undecylenic acid and tolnaftate are usually less effective than prescription medications. The use of combination products containing corticosteroids is not recommended.

Acne Medications

The basic principle in treating acne is to utilize the simplest regimen possible that adequately controls the disease. Once a treatment regimen is begun, medications should be titrated regularly to optimize clinical response and minimize irritation, but allowed at least 6 to 8 weeks before alterations are made for lack of efficacy.

As retinoids affect all acne lesions, they should be included as first-line agents in every acne regimen. Topical retinoids are ranked by the efficacy of their antiacne action in increasing strength from azelaic acid as the weakest retinoid to adapalene, to tretinoin, and to tazarotene as the strongest agent in the retinoid class (Table 5-9). Irritancy parallels efficacy, such that tazarotene—the strongest retinoid—is

also the most irritating. Many physicians start with a topical tretinoin product (e.g., tretinoin 0.05% cream) and titrate up or down the retinoid ladder based on clinical response and level of irritation.

Other medications may be used in addition to topical retinoids to reduce specific acne lesions. Topical antibiotics are most useful in decreasing inflammatory (erythematous or pustular) acne lesions. Oral antibiotics are most useful in decreasing deep acne nodules. Hormonal therapies are especially useful in females who have acne flares around their periods. Combination products are used to simplify a patient's acne regimen.

Isotretinoin is used when the above regimens fail. Treatment usually lasts approximately 5 to 6 months, after which patients are either "cured" of their acne or have residual acne that is much more sensitive to standard therapies. The use of isotretinoin is highly regulated and requires close monitoring. Proper training in the regulatory system and treatment guidelines is important for prescribers.

Over-the-Counter Medications

Sunscreens

The American Academy of Dermatology recommends use of broad-spectrum sunscreens that are water resistant, SPF 15 and above.

TABLE 5-8 Topical Antifungal Agents

Name	Spectrum	Formulation
Undecylenic acid	Dermatophytes, *Candida*	Cream, foam, spray, powder, and ointment
Tolnaftate	Dermatophytes	Cream, gel, spray, and powder
Ciclopirox	Dermatophytes, yeast	Cream, gel, lotion, solution, and nail lacquer
Clotrimazole	Dermatophytes, yeast	Cream, lotion, and spray
Miconazole nitrate	Dermatophytes, yeast	Cream
Econazole nitrate	Dermatophytes, yeast	Cream
Sulconazole	Dermatophytes, yeast	Cream, solution
Ketoconazole	Dermatophytes, *Candida*, *Pityrosporum*	Shampoo and cream
Oxiconazole	Dermatophytes, yeast, *Pityrosporum*	Cream and lotion
Naftifine	Dermatophytes, *Candida*, *Pityrosporum*	Cream and gel
Terbinafine	Dermatophytes, *Pityrosporum*	Cream, solution, and spray
Butenafine	Dermatophytes, *Candida*, *Pityrosporum*	Cream
Nystatin	*Candida*	Cream, ointment, and powder

TABLE 5-9 Dosage of Acne Medications

Class	Name	Dosage/Application
Topical Retinoids—prevent formation of precursor lesions, and decrease comedones and inflammatory lesions		
	Tazarotene	0.05%–0.1% gel or cream qhs
	Tretinoin	0.025%–0.1% cream, gel, or solution qhs
	Adapalene	0.3%–0.1% cream, gel, solution, or swab qhs
	Azelaic acid	15%–20% cream or gel qhs
Topical Antibiotics—decrease inflammatory lesions		
	Clindamycin phosphate	1% solution, lotion, pad, or gel qd to bid
	Erythromycin	2% ointment, solution, or pad bid
	Benzoyl peroxide	2.5%–10% cream, gel, lotion, liquid, pad, soap, or solution qd to bid
	Sulfur	1%–10% lotion, ointment, cream, soap qd to tid
	Sodium sulfacetamide	10% lotion, pad, cream, or soap bid
Combination Products—combined effects of 2 topical therapies in 1 formulation		
	Benzoyl peroxide/erythromycin	3%/5% cream bid
	Benzoyl peroxide/clindamycin	1%/5% cream qd
	Clindamycin/tretinoin	1.2%/0.025% gel qhs
Systemic Antibiotics—decrease superficial and deep inflammatory lesions		
	Tetracycline	500 mg bid
	Doxycycline	100 mg bid
	Minocycline	100 mg bid
Systemic Retinoids—decrease comedones and superficial and deep inflammatory lesions		
	Isotretinoin	Up to 2 mg/kg daily or divided bid
Hormonal Therapies—decrease comedones and superficial and deep inflammatory lesions in women		
	Spironolactone	50–100 mg bid
	Oral contraceptives	Various

TABLE 5-10 Commonly Used Oral Antibiotics

Name	Formulations	Dose	Max Dose
Amoxicillin	Drops: 50 mg/mL Suspension: 125, 200, 250, or 400 mg/5 mL Caps: 250, 500 mg Tabs: 500, 875 mg Chewable tabs: 125, 200, 250, 400 mg Tabs for oral suspension: 200, 400, 600 mg	250–500 mg/dose tid	2–3 g/24 h
Amoxicillin-clavulanic acid	Tabs: 250, 500, 875 mg amoxicillin Extended release tabs: 1 g amoxicillin Chewable tabs: 125, 200, 250, 400 mg amoxicillin Suspension 125, 200, 250, 400 mg amoxicillin/5 mL	250–500 mg/dose tid	2–3 g/24 h
Ampicillin	Suspension: 125, 250 mg/5 mL Caps: 250, 500 mg	250–500 mg q6 hour	2–3 g/24 h
Azithromycin	Tabs: 250, 500, 600 mg Suspension: 100, 200 mg/5 mL	500 mg on day 1 followed by 250 mg × 4 days	Multiple day regimens: 500 mg/24 h 1-day regimen: 1,500 mg/24 h
Cefaclor	Caps: 250, 500 mg Suspension: 125, 187, 250, 375 mg/5 mL	250–500 mg/dose q8 h	4 g/24 h
Cephalexin	Tabs: 250, 500 mg Caps: 250, 500 mg Suspension: 125, 250 mg/5 mL	1–4 g/24 h divided bid to qid	4 g/24 h
Clarithromycin	Film tablets: 250, 500 mg Extended-release tabs: 500 mg Granules for suspension: 125, 250 mg/5 mL	250–500 mg/dose bid	1 g/24 h
Ciprofloxacin	Tabs: 100, 250, 500, 750 mg Extended-release tabs: 500, 1000 mg Suspension: 250, 500 mg/5 mL	250–750 mg/dose bid	2 g/24 h
Clindamycin	Caps: 75, 150, 300 mg Oral solution: 75 mg/5 mL	150–450 mg/dose q6–8 h	1.8 g/24 h
Dicloxacillin sodium	Caps: 250, 500 mg	125–500 mg/dose q6 h	4 g/24 h
Doxycycline	Caps: 20, 50, 75, 100 Tabs: 20, 50, 100 Syrup: 50 mg/5 mL Suspension: 25 mg/5 mL	100–200 mg/24 h divided qd to bid	200 mg/24 h
Erythromycin	Estolate: Suspension: 125, 250 mg/5 mL Ethyl succinate: Suspension: 200, 400 mg/5 mL Oral drops: 100 mg/2.5 mL Chewable tabs: 200 mg Tabs: 400 mg Base: Tabs: 250, 333, 500 mg	1–4 g/24 h divided q6 h	4 g/24 h
Minocycline	Tabs: 50, 75, 100 mg Caps: 50, 75, 100 mg Caps (pellet filled): 50, 100 mg Oral suspension: 50 mg/5 mL	50–100 mg/dose qd to tid	200 mg/24 h
Nafcillin	Caps: 250 mg	250–1000 mg q4–6 h	12 g/24 h
Oxacillin	Oral solution: 250 mg/5 mL	500–1000 mg/dose q4–6 h	12 g/24 h
Penicillin V potassium	Tabs: 250, 500 mg Oral solution: 125, 250 mg/5 mL	250–500 mg/dose divided q6–8 h	3 g/24 h
Tetracycline	Caps: 250, 500 mg Suspension: 125 mg/5 mL	1–2 g/24 h divided q6–12 h	3 g/24 h
Trimethoprim-sulfamethoxazole	Tabs (regular strength): 80 mg TMP/400 mg SMX Tabs (double strength): 160 mg TMP/800 mg SMX Suspension: 40 mg TMP/200 mg SMX/5 mL	160 mg TMP/dose bid	320 mg TMP/24 h

TABLE 5-11 H1-Antihistamines

Name	Antihistamine Effect	Anticholinergic Effect	Sedative Effect
Chlorpheniramine	Moderate	Moderate	Mild
Cyproheptadine	Moderate	Moderate	Mild
Diphenhydramine	Mild	Strong	Strong
Hydroxyzine	Strong	Moderate	Strong
Loratadine	Strong	Weak	Rare
Fexofenadine	Strong	Weak	Rare
Cetirizine	Strong	Weak	Occasional
Promethazine	Very strong	Strong	Strong

Sunscreen Labeling

- SPF (sun protection factor)—time to produce erythema (redness) on protected skin divided by time to produce erythema on unprotected skin
- Broad-spectrum protection—protection over UVA and UVB spectra
- Water resistant—maintains SPF after 40 min of water immersion
- Very water resistant/waterproof—maintains SPF after 80 min of water immersion

Insect Repellants

Products containing DEET (N, N-Diethyl-meta-toluamide) or picaridin are formulated for use directly on the skin.[10] Repellants containing permethrin are formulated for use on clothing. DEET is sold over the counter in concentrations ranging up to 100% DEET. The higher the concentration, the longer the protection will last. The CDC recommends 30% to 50% DEET formulations to repel most insects.

Systemic Medications

Commonly Used Oral Antibiotics

Some of the antibiotics commonly used for cutaneous infections are outlined in Table 5-10. The choice for specific antibiotics is discussed in the section for each disease.

TABLE 5-12 Dosing of Commonly Used H1-Antihistamines

First-Generation H1-Antihistamines	
Diphenhydramine	25–50 mg every 4–6 h; maximum 300 mg/day
Hydroxyzine	2 mg/kg/24 h divided q6–8 h
Second-Generation H1-Antihistamines	
Cetirizine	10 mg daily
Levocetirizine	5 mg daily
Loratadine	10 mg daily
Desloratadine	5 mg daily
Fexofenadine	60 mg bid or 180 mg daily

H1-Antihistamines[11]

Antihistamines can be very useful for pruritus. Specific dosing is important to prevent adverse effects (Tables 5-11 and 5-12).

Immunomodulators

Systemic immunomodulators are important agents for patients with significant cutaneous and systemic disorders and should be used by those with experience with these agents and their side effects (Table 5-13).

TABLE 5-13 Dosage of Commonly Used Immunomodulators

Name	Dermatologic Indications	Dosage Range
Methotrexate	Psoriasis Morphea Immunobullous disease	5–25 mg weekly
Azathioprine	Atopic dermatitis Immunobullous disease Lupus erythematosus	3–5 mg/kg/day[a]
Mycophenolate mofetil	Atopic dermatitis Psoriasis Immunobullous disease	2–3 g/day divided bid
Cyclosporine	Psoriasis Atopic dermatitis	2.5–5 mg/kg/day
Etanercept	Psoriasis	0.8 mg/kg 2×/week 50 mg SQ BIW, then QW
Hydroxy-chloroquine	Lupus erythematosus Polymorphous light eruption	200–400 mg qd
Dapsone	Immunobullous disease Pyoderma gangrenosum Pustular psoriasis	50–100 mg qd

[a]Initial dosing based on blood testing for TPMT level.

TABLE 5-14 **Commonly Used Systemic Retinoids**		
Name	**Indication**	**Dose**
Acitretin	Psoriasis	0.5 mg/kg/day
Isotretinoin	Acne	0.5–2 mg/kg/day

Systemic Retinoids

Both systemic retinoids have the potential for causing birth defects in females of child-bearing potential, and established guidelines for their use *must* be followed (Table 5-14).

References

1. Katz HI, Prawer SE, Mooney JJ, et al. Preatrophy: Covert sign of thinned skin. *J Am Acad Dermatol* 1989;20(5 Pt 1):731–735.

2. Gilbertson EO, Spellman MC, Piacquadio DJ, et al. Super potent topical corticosteroid use associated with adrenal suppression: clinical considerations. *J Am Acad Dermatol* 1998;38(2 Pt 2):318–321.

3. Warner MR, Camisa C. Topical corticosteroids. In: Wolverton SE, ed. *Comprehensive Dermatologic Drug Therapy.* 2nd Ed. Philadelphia, PA: Saunders Elsevier; 2007:595–624.

4. Drake LA, Dinehart SM, Farmer ER, et al. Guidelines of care for the use of topical glucocorticosteroids. *J Am Acad Dermatol.* 1996;35(4):615–619.

5. Micromedex® Healthcare Series. Englewood, Co: Micromedex, Inc; 1990s. http://www.micromedex.com/.

6. Soriano TT, Lask GP, Dinehart SM. Anesthesia and analgesia. In: Robinson JK, Hanke WC, Sengelmann R, Siegel D, eds. *Surgery of the Skin: Procedural Dermatology.* Philadelphia, PA: Elsevier Mosby; 2005:39–58.

7. *Physicians' Desk Reference: PDR 2009.* 63rd Ed. Montvale, NJ: Thomson PDR; 2008.

8. DRUGDEX. Englewood, Co: Micromedex, Inc; 1990s. http://www.micromedex.com/products/drugdex/.

9. Lubenow TR, Ivankovich AD, Barkin RL. Management of acute postoperative pain. In: Barash PG, Cullen BF, Stoelting RK, eds. *Clinical Anesthesia.* 5th Ed. Philadelphia, PA: Lippincott Williams & Wilkins; 2006: 1405–1440.

10. Katz TM, Miller JH, Herbert AA. Insect repellents: Historical perspectives and new developments. *J Am Acad Dermatol* 2008;58: 865–871.

11. AJ, Severson DL, eds. *Pocket Guide to Medications Used in Dermatology.* Philadelphia, PA: Lippincott Williams & Wilkins; 2003.

Index

Page numbers in *italics* denote figures; those followed by a "t" denote tables.